Advances in Experimental Medicine and Biology

Volume 816

For further volumes:
http://www.springer.com/series/5584

Bharat B. Aggarwal · Bokyung Sung
Subash Chandra Gupta
Editors

Inflammation and Cancer

Springer

Editors
Bharat B. Aggarwal
Bokyung Sung
Subash Chandra Gupta
Department of Experimental Therapeutics
The University of Texas M.D. Anderson
Cancer Center
Houston, TX
USA

ISSN 0065-2598 ISSN 2214-8019 (electronic)
ISBN 978-3-0348-0836-1 ISBN 978-3-0348-0837-8 (eBook)
DOI 10.1007/978-3-0348-0837-8
Springer Basel Heidelberg New York Dordrecht London

Library of Congress Control Number: 2014937690

Printed on acid-free paper

Springer is part of Springer Science+Business Media (www.springer.com)

Preface

It was Aulus Cornelius Celsus, a physician in first-century Rome, who first defined *inflammation* as *calor* (heat), *dolor* (pain), *rubor* (redness), and *tumor* (swelling). However, it was Rudolf Virchow who in the mid-1800s linked inflammation with atherosclerosis, rheumatoid arthritis, multiple sclerosis, asthma, Alzheimer's disease, cancer, and other chronic diseases. The suffix "*-itis*" was introduced to indicate inflammation in words such as *bronchitis* (inflammation of the bronchus) and *colitis* (inflammation of the colon). Extensive research has revealed that inflammation precedes most cancers; for example, cancers of the liver, lung, colon, cervix, pancreas, stomach, and prostate are preceded by hepatitis, bronchitis, colitis, cervicitis, pancreatitis, gastritis, and prostatitis, respectively.

Within the past three decades, researchers have determined the molecular basis of most kinds of inflammation. Furthermore, various cell-signaling pathways that lead to inflammation have also been relatively well defined, leading to the development of various therapeutics that can modulate these pathways and thus alter the course of disease.

The current monograph deals with the role of inflammation in cancer, and some of the leaders in the field have contributed to this volume. We would like to thank these experts for their contributions and the publisher for giving us the opportunity to edit this volume.

Bharat B. Aggarwal
Bokyung Sung
Subash Chandra Gupta

Preface

Contents

Contributors

António Araújo Chief of the Medical Oncology Service of Centro Hospitalar do Porto, Porto, Portugal; Chief of the Medical Oncology Service of Centro Hospitalar de Entre Douro e Vouga, Santa Maria da Feira, Portugal; Instituto de Ciências Biomédicas de Abel Salazar, Porto, Portugal

Anupam Bishayee Department of Pharmaceutical Sciences, School of Pharmacy, American University of Health Sciences, Signal Hill, CA, USA

Marcelo Bonomi Head and Neck Oncology Program, Wake Forest School of Medicine, Winston-Salem, NC, USA

Ronald Bukowski Cleveland Clinic Lerner College of Medicine, Case Western Reserve University, Cleveland, OH, USA

Antonino Carbone Department of Pathology, Centro di Riferimento Oncologico Aviano, Istituto Nazionale Tumori, IRCCS, Aviano, Italy

Carmelo Carlo-Stella Department of Oncology and Hematology, Humanitas Cancer Center, Humanitas Clinical and Research Center, Rozzano, Milan, Italy

Ana Coelho Instituto Português de Oncologia do Porto Francisco Gentil, EPE, Grupo de Oncologia Molecular—CI, Porto, Portugal; Faculty of Medicine of University of Porto, Porto, Portugal; LPCC Research Department-Portuguese League Against Cancer (NRNorte), Porto, Portugal

Charles Conrad Department of Neuro-Oncology, The University of Texas MD Anderson Cancer Center, Houston, TX, USA

Angelo M. De Marzo Department of Pathology, The Johns Hopkins University School of Medicine, Baltimore, MD, USA

Antonio Roma de Vivar Chevez Cleveland Clinic Lerner College of Medicine, Case Western Reserve University, Cleveland, OH, USA

S. Deivendran Cancer Research Program, Rajiv Gandhi Centre for Biotechnology, Thiruvananthapuram, India

Mert Erkan Department of Surgery, Klinikum rechts der Isar, Technische Universität München, Munich, Germany

James Finke Cleveland Clinic Lerner College of Medicine, Case Western Reserve University, Cleveland, OH, USA

Tamer M. Fouad Department of Breast Medical Oncology, Morgan Welch Inflammatory Breast Cancer Research Program and Clinic, The University of Texas MD Anderson Cancer Center, Houston, TX, USA; Department of Medical Oncology, The National Cancer Institute, Cairo University, Cairo, Egypt

Ciara Freeman Department of Haematology, Barts and the Royal London NHS Trust, London, UK

Helmut Friess Department of Surgery, Klinikum rechts der Isar, Technische Universität München, Munich, Germany

Georgios Gakis Department of Urology, University Hospital Tübingen, Eberhard-Karls University, Tübingen, Germany

Khushboo Gandhi Maru Lab, Advanced Centre for Treatment, Research and Education in Cancer (ACTREC), Tata Memorial Centre (TMC), Kharghar, Navi Mumbai, India

Francis J Giles Northwestern Medicine Developmental Therapeutics Institute, Robert H. Lurie Comprehensive Cancer Center of Northwestern University, Chicago, USA

Annunziata Gloghini Department of Diagnostic Pathology and Laboratory Medicine, Fondazione IRCCS Istituto Nazionale dei Tumori, Milan, Italy

Mónica Gomes Instituto Português de Oncologia do Porto Francisco Gentil, EPE, Grupo de Oncologia Molecular—CI, Porto, Portugal; ICBAS, Abel Salazar Institute for the Biomedical Sciences, University of Porto, Porto, Portugal; LPCC Research Department-Portuguese League Against Cancer (NRNorte), Porto, Portugal

Simone Hausmann Department of Surgery, Klinikum rechts der Isar, Technische Universität München, Munich, Germany

Heidi A. Hempel Department of Pathology, The Johns Hopkins University School of Medicine, Baltimore, MD, USA

Naveena B. Janakiram Center for Cancer Prevention and Drug Development, Department of Medicine, Hematology Oncology Section, PCS Cancer Center, University of Oklahoma Health Sciences Center, Oklahoma City, OK, USA

Kenneth M. Johnson Department of Pharmacology and Toxicology, The University of Texas Medical Branch (UTMB), Galveston, TX, USA

Takahiro Kogawa Department of Breast Medical Oncology, Morgan Welch Inflammatory Breast Cancer Research Program and Clinic, The University of Texas MD Anderson Cancer Center, Houston, TX, USA

Bo Kong Department of Surgery, Klinikum rechts der Isar, Technische Universität München, Munich, Germany

Janusz Krawczyk Department of Haematology, Galway University Hospital, Galway, Ireland

Gaurav Kumar Maru Lab, Advanced Centre for Treatment, Research and Education in Cancer (ACTREC), Tata Memorial Centre (TMC), Kharghar, Navi Mumbai, India

Girish B. Maru Maru Lab, Advanced Centre for Treatment, Research and Education in Cancer (ACTREC), Tata Memorial Centre (TMC), Kharghar, Navi Mumbai, India

K. Hezlin Marzook Cancer Research Program, Rajiv Gandhi Centre for Biotechnology, Thiruvananthapuram, India

Rui Medeiros Instituto Português de Oncologia do Porto Francisco Gentil, EPE, Grupo de Oncologia Molecular—CI, Porto, Portugal; ICBAS, Abel Salazar Institute for the Biomedical Sciences, University of Porto, Porto, Portugal; LPCC Research Department-Portuguese League Against Cancer (NRNorte), Porto, Portugal; CEBIMED, Health Sciences Faculty, Fernando Pessoa, University of Porto, Porto, Portugal

Christoph Michalski Department of Surgery, Klinikum rechts der Isar, Technische Universität München, Munich, Germany

Michael O'Dwyer Biosciences, National University of Ireland Galway, Galway, Ireland

Murat Bulut Özkan Department of General Surgery, Ankara Numune Research and Training Hospital, Ankara, Turkey

Alexis Patsias Head and Neck Oncology Program, Mount Sinai School of Medicine, New York, USA

Joel T. Patterson Department of Surgery, Division of Neurosurgery, UTMB, Galveston, TX, USA

Marshall Posner Head and Neck Oncology Program, Mount Sinai School of Medicine, New York, USA

M. Radhakrishna Pillai Cancer Research Program, Rajiv Gandhi Centre for Biotechnology, Thiruvananthapuram, India

Jürgen Radons Department of Radiotherapy and Radiation Oncology, Klinikum rechts der Isar, Technische Universität München, Munich, Germany

Asha Ramchandani Maru Lab, Advanced Centre for Treatment, Research and Education in Cancer (ACTREC), Tata Memorial Centre (TMC), Kharghar, Navi Mumbai, India

Chinthalapally V. Rao Center for Cancer Prevention and Drug Development, Department of Medicine, Hematology Oncology Section, PCS Cancer Center, University of Oklahoma Health Sciences Center, Oklahoma City, OK, USA

James M. Reuben Department of Hematopathology, Morgan Welch Inflammatory Breast Cancer Research Program and Clinic, The University of Texas MD Anderson Cancer Center, Houston, TX, USA

Domenico Ribatti Department of Basic Medical Sciences, Neurosciences and Sensory Organs, Section of Human Anatomy and Histology, University of Bari Medical School, Bari, Italy; National Cancer Institute, Bari, Italy

Armando Santoro Department of Oncology and Hematology, Humanitas Cancer Center, Humanitas Clinical and Research Center, Rozzano, Milan, Italy

Kazım Şenol Department of General Surgery, Ankara Numune Research and Training Hospital, Ankara, Turkey

Karen S. Sfanos Department of Pathology, The Johns Hopkins University School of Medicine, Baltimore, MD, USA

Andrew Sikora Head and Neck Oncology Program, Mount Sinai School of Medicine, New York, USA

James L. Sowers Department of Pharmacology and Toxicology, The University of Texas Medical Branch (UTMB), Galveston, TX, USA; Combined Degree Program, UTMB, Galveston, TX, USA

Lawrence C. Sowers Department of Pharmacology and Toxicology, The University of Texas Medical Branch (UTMB), Galveston, TX, USA; Department of Internal Medicine, Division of Oncology, UTMB, Galveston, TX, USA

Ronan Swords Sylvester Comprehensive Cancer Center, University of Miami, Miami, USA

Ana Luísa Teixeira Instituto Português de Oncologia do Porto Francisco Gentil, EPE, Grupo de Oncologia Molecular—CI, Porto, Portugal; ICBAS, Abel Salazar Institute for the Biomedical Sciences, University of Porto, Porto, Portugal; LPCC Research Department-Portuguese League Against Cancer (NRNorte), Porto, Portugal

Mesut Tez Department of General Surgery, Ankara Numune Research and Training Hospital, Ankara, Turkey

Claudio Tripodo Tumor Immunology Unit, Human Pathology Section, Department of Health Sciences, University of Palermo, Palermo, Italy

Naoto T. Ueno Department of Breast Medical Oncology, Morgan Welch Inflammatory Breast Cancer Research Program and Clinic, The University of Texas MD Anderson Cancer Center, Houston, TX, USA

Angelo Vacca Department of Biomedical Sciences and Human Oncology (DIMO), Section of Internal Medicine and Clinical Oncology, University of Bari Medical School, Bari, Italy

Selahattin Vural Department of General Surgery, Ankara Numune Research and Training Hospital, Ankara, Turkey

Chapter 1
The Role of Inflammation in Lung Cancer

Mónica Gomes, Ana Luísa Teixeira, Ana Coelho, António Araújo and Rui Medeiros

Abstract Lung cancer remains a serious public health problem and is the first cause of cancer death worldwide, and the overall 5-year survival rate for all stages is 14–17 % for Non-small-cell lung cancer and 6 % for small-cell lung cancer. Clinical and epidemiologic studies have suggested a strong association among chronic infection, inflammation, and cancer. Immune system plays a critical role in maintaining tissue homeostasis, cell turnover, tissue remodeling, and preventing

M. Gomes (✉) · A. L. Teixeira · A. Coelho · R. Medeiros
Instituto Português de Oncologia do Porto Francisco Gentil, EPE, Grupo de Oncologia Molecular—CI, Edifício Laboratórios, 4° piso Rua Dr. António Bernardino de Almeida, Porto 4200-072, Portugal
e-mail: monicagomes26@gmail.com

M. Gomes · A. L. Teixeira · R. Medeiros
ICBAS, Abel Salazar Institute for the Biomedical Sciences, University of Porto, Porto, Portugal

A. Coelho
Faculty of Medicine of University of Porto, Porto, Portugal

M. Gomes · A. L. Teixeira · A. Coelho · R. Medeiros
LPCC Research Department-Portuguese League Against Cancer (NRNorte), Porto, Portugal

R. Medeiros
CEBIMED, Health Sciences Faculty, Fernando Pessoa, University of Porto, Porto, Portugal

A. Araújo
Chief of the Medical Oncology Service of Centro Hospitalar do Porto, Porto, Portugal

A. Araújo
Chief of the Medical Oncology Service of Centro Hospitalar de Entre Douro e Vouga, Santa Maria da Feira, Portugal

A. Araújo
Instituto de Ciências Biomédicas de Abel Salazar, Porto, Portugal

B. B. Aggarwal et al. (eds.), *Inflammation and Cancer*, Advances in Experimental Medicine and Biology 816, DOI: 10.1007/978-3-0348-0837-8_1, © Springer Basel 2014

infection and cell transformation. The inflammatory component in the development of the neoplasm includes a diverse leukocyte population; these components are considered inflammatory tumor key factors promoting tumor progression due to its ability to release a variety of cytokines, chemokines, and cytotoxic mediators such as reactive oxygen species (ROS), metalloproteinases, interleukins, and interferons. Cancer-related inflammation affects many aspects of malignancy, including the proliferation and survival of malignant cells, angiogenesis, tumor metastasis, and tumor response to chemotherapeutic drugs and hormones. Moreover, epidemiologic studies and meta-analysis have shown that prolonged use of non-steroid anti-inflammatory (NSAID) drugs reduces the risk of several solid tumor including lung cancer. Strong lines of evidence suggest that the chemopreventive properties of chronic NSAID administration are based on their COX-inhibitory activity. However, the prevention is a much better and more economical way to fight against cancer than treating an already advanced and often incurable disease.

1.1 Introduction: Incidence, Survival, Major Gene Products and Current Therapies for Lung Cancer

In 2008, about 12.7 million cancer cases and 7.6 million cancer deaths are estimated to have occurred in this year in worldwide, with 56 % of cases and 64 % of the deaths in the economically developing world (Jemal et al. 2011). Lung cancer was found to be the most commonly diagnosed cancer as well as the primary cause of cancer-related mortality for males worldwide and the second leading cause of cancer-related deaths for women (Jemal et al. 2011; Siegel et al. 2012). For the year 2012, it is estimated that lung cancer will account for 26 % of all female cancer deaths and 29 % of all male cancer deaths (Siegel et al. 2012). Breast cancer in females and lung cancer in males are the most frequently diagnosed cancers and the leading cause of cancer death for each sex in both economically developed and developing countries, except lung cancer is preceded by prostate cancer as the most frequent cancer among males in economically developed countries (Jemal et al. 2011).

Lung cancer was the most commonly diagnosed cancer as well as the leading cause of cancer death in males in 2008, globally. Among females, it was the fourth most commonly diagnosed cancer and the second leading cause of cancer death (Jemal et al. 2011; Ferlay et al. 2010). Lung cancer accounts for 13 % (1.6 million) of the total cases and 18 % (1.4 million) of the deaths in 2008 (Ferlay et al. 2010; Jemal et al. 2011).

The observed variations in lung cancer rates and trends across countries or between males and females within each country largely reflect differences in the stage and degree of the tobacco epidemic (Jemal et al. 2011).

Lung cancer can be divided into two major groups: small-cell lung cancer (SCLC) and non-small-cell cancer (NSCLC) (Hoffman et al. 2000; Molina et al. 2008), NSCLC accounts for approximately 85 % of all cases of lung cancer

(Molina et al. 2008; Araujo et al. 2007). These lung cancer cells can again be categorized based on their histological characteristics as squamous cell carcinoma, large cell carcinoma, and adenocarcinoma (Tang et al. 2013). NSCLC spreads slower than SCLC, so many patients who are diagnosed at an earlier stage are potentially curable, though NSCLC may often relapse at other metastatic site. Furthermore, NSCLC is generally less responsive to chemotherapy than SCLC, so that even with surgical resection at early diagnosis, approximately 50 % of NSCLC patients face recurring cancers (Tang et al. 2013).The 1-year survival rate for lung cancer was 43 % in 2003–2006. However, despite extensive preclinical and clinical research, the overall 5-year survival rate for all stages is still as low as 14–17 % for NSCLC (Araujo et al. 2007; Peebles et al. 2007) and even lower in SCLC (6 %) (Wu et al. 2012).

In recent years, knowledge concerning the molecular mechanisms underlying cellular transformation and development of cancer has been greatly expanded (Araujo et al. 2007). Alteration of the major cell signaling and regulatory pathways either by overexpression or gene sequence variation is a frequent event in lung cancer. These changes include alterations in receptor tyrosine kinases (TKs), such as epidermal growth factor receptor (EGFR), and alterations in angiogenesis pathways, apoptosis, proteasome regulation, and cell cycle control, among others (Molina et al. 2008).

The EGFR is a tyrosine kinase that contributes to the regulation of cellular homeostasis. It is a 170-KDa membrane protein that stimulates downstream cell proliferation, survival, and tumorigenesis (Wheeler et al. 2010; Cohen 1965). EGFR has been implicated in the growth of several human epithelial malignancies, including lung cancer. It is overexpressed in several cancers, including approximately 40–80 % of NSCLC, which made EGFR a popular target for new drug treatment exploration (Tang et al. 2013).

The ALK tyrosine kinase receptor has gained much attention recently as a newly emerging relevant biomarker and therapeutic target in NSCLC (Wu et al. 2012). The activation of ALK is primarily through the formation of fusion genes. EML4-ALK translocation is the most common ALK gene rearrangement. This rearrangement in NSCLC patients is mainly found in younger non-smoking patients with adenocarcinoma (Wu et al. 2012; Kwak et al. 2010). EML4-ALK rearrangements are mutually exclusive with EGFR or KRAS mutations (Wu et al. 2012; Li et al. 2013). It has been reported that approximately 2–11 % of tumors carrying positive EML4-ALK (Li et al. 2013).

KRAS mutations are a negative predictor of response to EGFR TKs, mainly accounting for primary resistence (Linardou et al. 2008; de Mello et al. 2011). Most KRAS mutations in lung adenocarcinoma are associated with smoking. KRAS positive mutations are limited to NSCLC and are mutually exclusive to mutations in EGFR and ALK (Linardou et al. 2008; Wu et al. 2012).

Lung cancer is a very aggressive cancer and its treatment still remains a challenge for health professionals. Conventional treatments are based on surgery, radiation therapy, and chemotherapy. The selection of therapeutic regimen is based on the cancer type (small-cell or non-small-cell), stage of disease, patient's functional ability, and genetic characterization (Wu et al. 2012; Tang et al. 2013; Hoffman et al. 2000).

The majority of stage I through stage IIIA lung cancer patients generally choose surgery as their primary option. Another popular option is preoperative chemotherapy, which has been shown to improve survival rate in patients with NSCLC. Patients who require complete resection and no preoperative chemotherapy usually invest in adjuvant chemotherapy. For patients with unresectable NSCLC, RT and chemotherapy are excellent options for treatment (Tang et al. 2013). Further, certain agents have been combined with the chemotherapy to enhance its effects. The anti-vascular endothelial growth factor agent, bevacizumab, for example, when combined with chemotherapy, has resulted in increased survival rate when compared to chemotherapy treatment alone (Tang et al. 2013).

For first-line chemotherapy, a platinum-based two-drug combination is suggested for patients (Azzoli et al. 2009; Molina et al. 2008). Studies show that the cisplatin, when used in combination chemotherapy, is associated with improved response rates, no change in survival rate, and increased toxicity when compared with the carboplatin (Tang et al. 2013). Also, another drug bevacizumab has demonstrated great potential when used in combination with carboplatin or paclitaxel in NSCLC patients (Tang et al. 2013; Molina et al. 2008).

The second-line chemotherapy treatment options, after primary treatment fails to yield effective results, do differ from the first-line drugs. Approximately 30 % of NSCLC patients who undergo first-line cancer treatment are candidates for second- or third-line therapeutics. The first agent that was approved for second-line therapeutics was docetaxel (Fossella et al. 2000). Other drugs that were also soon approved include pemetrexed, erlotinib, and gefitinib (Tang et al. 2013). Undergoing research is currently evaluating other possible strategies for second-line therapeutics.

1.2 Inflammatory Signaling Pathways Associated with Lung Cancer

Cancer is a hyperproliferative disorder that involves morphological cellular transformation, dysregulation of apoptosis, uncontrolled cellular proliferation, invasion, angiogenesis, and metastasis (Lin and Karin 2007; Hanahan and Weinberg 2011).

Clinical and epidemiologic studies have suggested strong association between chronic infection, inflammation, and cancer (Coussens and Werb 2002; Lin and Karin 2007; Ribeiro et al. 2007). Up to 20 % of cancers are linked to chronic infections, 30 % can be attributed to tobacco smoking and inhaled pollutants (such as silica and asbestos), and 35 % to dietary factors (20 % of cancer burden is linked to obesity) (Aggarwal et al. 2009).

Approximately 150 ago, Virchow postulated that inflammation is a predisposing factor of tumorigenesis (Lu et al. 2006; Balkwill and Mantovani 2001; Schottenfeld and Beebe-Dimmer 2006). This hypothesis was based on his observation that

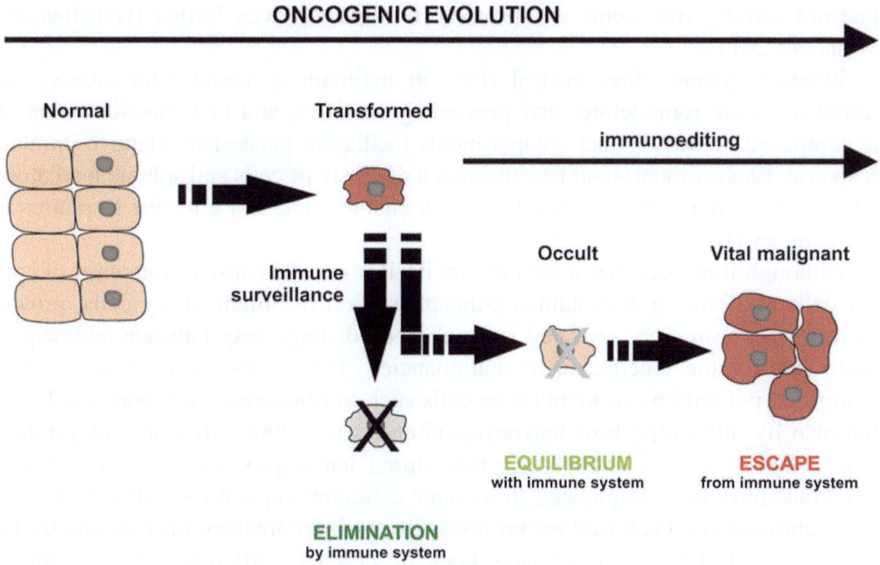

Fig. 1.1 Oncogenic evolution (adapted from Bremnes et al. 2011)

cancerous tissue often arose at sites of chronic inflammation and that inflammation cells were present in the resect tumors (Bremnes et al. 2011; Mantovani et al. 2008; Balkwill and Mantovani 2001). In contrast, Burnet proposed, in 1970, the concept of immunological surveillance: the immune system spontaneously identifies and eliminates cancer cells, thus protecting against tumor development (Bremnes et al. 2011; Van Ginderachter et al. 2006) (Fig. 1.1).

During the last decades, and according to Virchow hypothesis, epidemiological studies have shown that individuals prone to chronic inflammatory diseases have an increased risk of cancer development and that the underlying infections and inflammatory responses have been linked to 15–20 % of all cancer deaths worldwide (Bremnes et al. 2011).

The ultimate recognition of inflammation as a major player in cancer development was reinforced with the 2011 update article on cancer hallmarks by Hanahan and Weinberg, where it was classified as an enabling characteristic of tumors (Mantovani et al. 2008; Hanahan and Weinberg 2011).

These evidence gathered over the last years showed that inflammation contributes to the appearance of multiple cancer hallmark capabilities by supplying important molecules to the tumor microenvironment. Those molecules include growth factors that sustain the proliferative signaling, survival factors that limit apoptosis, pro-angiogenic factors, extracellular matrix-modifying enzymes that favor angiogenesis, invasion, and metastasis (Ben-Baruch 2006). Furthermore, inflammation manifestations are observed at the earliest stages of tumor progression and are capable of nurturing insipient neoplasias into developed cancers. In addition, inflammatory cells can release a number of chemicals, such as ROS, that are actively mutagenic and promote malignancy even further (Hanahan and Weinberg 2011).

Immune system plays critical roles in maintaining tissue homeostasis, cell turnover, tissue remodeling, and preventing infection and cell transformation. It is composed of two distinct compartments mediating innate and adaptive immune response. Each compartment has, through a diversity of cells and soluble mediators, advanced communication networks, which enable rapid and effective responses to tissue injury (Bremnes et al. 2011).

Although it is clear that inflammation itself is not the cause of the onset of cancer cell proliferation, a sustained atmosphere rich in inflammatory cells, growth factors, and promoters activated stromal DNA damage may enhance and/or promote risk for the emergence of malignancies. This tumor microenvironment is composed not only by resident tissue cells such as fibroblasts and endothelial cells but also by infiltrating host leukocytes (Ben-Baruch 2006). Tumor cells produce several cytokines and chemokines that attract leukocytes. Several inflammatory cytokines have been implicated to mediate different steps in the pathway leading to carcinogenesis. Increased serum levels of pro-inflammatory interleukins IL-1β, IL-6, IL-8, IL-12, and IL-18 have been observed in different types of cancer, including lung cancer (Tsai et al. 1999; Srivani and Nagarajan 2003; Michalaki et al. 2004; Ye et al. 2007; Azevedo et al. 2011).

On the other hand, the pleiotropic anti-inflammatory interleukins, IL-4 and IL-10, stimulate the growth of many tumors, such as ovarian, prostate, and lung although they have an inhibitory effect on growth or invasion of other types of cancer (Toi et al. 1992; Takeshi et al. 2005; Lan et al. 2006; Gomes et al. 2012) (Fig. 1.2).

The inflammatory component in the development of the neoplasm includes a diverse leukocyte population, which stand macrophages (abundant in many types of tumors), lymphocytes, natural killer (NK) cells, neutrophils, and dendritic cells.

These components are considered inflammatory tumor key factors in promoting tumor progression due to its ability to release a variety of cytokines, chemokines, cytotoxic mediators such as reactive oxygen species, metalloproteinases (MMPs) and agents perforator membrane, and soluble mediators of cell death, such as TNF-α (Tumor Necrosis Factor-α), interleukins (IL), and interferons (IFNs) (Coussens and Werb 2002).

Many of the mediators released during chronic inflammation promote unregulated cell proliferation and invasion, induce angiogenesis, and increase mutagenesis. Due to these characteristics, the transformation and initiation of a malignant phenotype may occur and tumor progression may be promoted. In addition, many of the factors released by inflammatory cells may lead directly or indirectly to a marked suppression of the immune response, which otherwise could have an important role in tumor eradication (Ben-Baruch 2006).

The lung cancer tumor microenvironment is composed of extracellular matrix, tumor cells, fibroblasts, inflammatory cells, vascular and lymphatic endothelial cells, growth factors, cytokine, chemokines, hormones, proteases, among others. Fibroblasts exist normally in the connective tissue and produce extracellular

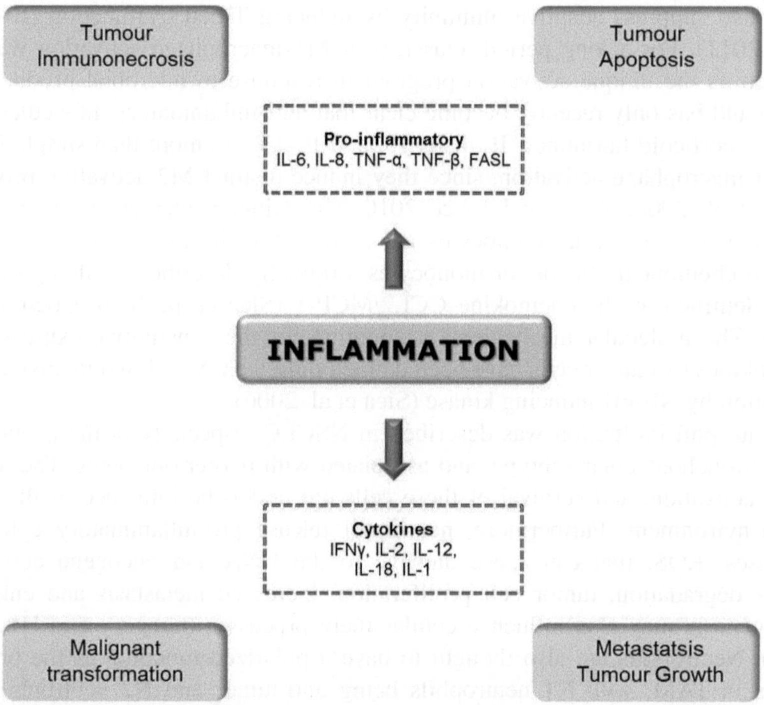

Fig. 1.2 The tumor microenvironment associated with inflammation and its consequence in cancer processes (adapted from Serefoglou et al. 2008)

matrix and collagen. They are essential in wound repairing but when exposed to cigarette smoke, they secrete pro-inflammatory mediators such as prostaglandin-E2 (PGE_2), IL-8, IL-6, and MCP-1, leading to a prolonged inflammatory response (Martey et al. 2004). Macrophages are recruited by granulocyte colony-stimulating factor (G-CSF), GM-CSF, macrophage-stimulating protein (MSP), vascular endothelial growth factor (VEGF), transforming growth factor-β (TGF-β), and macrophage migration inhibitory factor (MIF).

It is known that macrophages can be activated in response to microbiological agents and in particular cytokines interferon-γ (IFN-γ) (classical macrophage activation). However, it was recently discovered that anti-inflammatory molecules, such as glucocorticoid hormones and cytokines IL-4, IL-13, and IL-10, induce a different program activation of macrophages (alternative macrophage activation) (Sica et al. 2006; Mantovani et al. 2002, 2004). Tumor-associated macrophages (TAM) that interact with tumor cells to produce cytokines and growth factors that influence tumor development have two different phenotypes: M1 and M2 (O'Callaghan et al. 2010). The M1 macrophages have been associated with better prognosis in NSCLC, are efficient immune cells and are associated with an antitumor behavior (Bremnes et al. 2011). Nonetheless, the most prevalent phenotype is the M2, which promotes tumor growth, angiogenesis, invasion, and metastasis.

They also suppress adaptive immunity by inducing T cell dysfunction (Bremnes et al. 2011). For a long period, classical or M1 macrophage activation was recognized as the unique activation program in response to microbial products and IFN-γ and has only recently become clear that anti-inflammatory molecules, such as glucocorticoid hormones, IL-4, IL-13, and IL-10, are more than simple inhibitors of macrophage activation, since they induce distinct M2 activation programs (Sica et al. 2006; Wang and Joyce 2010; Van Ginderachter et al. 2006). TAM derived from circulating monocytes are recruited at the tumor site by a tumor-derived chemotactic factor for monocytes, originally described by this group and later identified as the chemokine CCL2/MCP-1 (Sica et al. 2006; Coelho et al. 2006). The molecular mechanisms accounting for the constitutive expression of chemokines by cancer cells have been defined only for CXCL1 and involve NF-κB activation by NF-κB-inducing kinase (Sica et al. 2006).

Neutrophil infiltration was described in NSCLC, especially in the adenocarcinoma bronchoalveolar subtype, and associated with poorer outcomes. The recruitment, activation, and survival of these cells are under the influence of the tumor microenvironment. Furthermore, neutrophil release pro-inflammatory cytokines, proteases, ROS, that can cause damage to the DNA and oncogene activation, matrix degradation, tumor cell proliferation, increased metastasis and enhanced angiogenesis may also influence celular there processes (Gregory and Houghton 2011). Neutrophils are also thought to have a polarized function, as the one that occurs in TAM, with N1 neutrophils being anti-tumor and N2 neutrophils pro-tumor (88). CD8+ T cells are proposed to have a protective role against tumors, by modifying the tumor stromal and epithelium and therefore reducing disease progression and metastasis, but sometimes fail to mount a robust anti-tumor response due to suppressive factors that affect their survival (Bremnes et al. 2011; Gregory and Houghton 2011). Nevertheless, CD8+ T cells in the stromal correlated with disease-specific survival (DSS) in NSCLC (Bremnes et al. 2011). Stromal levels of helper CD4+ T cells correlated significantly with DSS and were a favorable independent prognostic factor in NSCLC patients (Bremnes et al. 2011). The localization of CD8+ and CD4+ T cells is associated with an improved survival (Suzuki et al. 2011). Regulatory T cells suppress host immune responses and are thought to promote tumor growth. Their levels correlated positively with cyclooxygenase-2 (COX-2) expression levels in NSCLC tumors and were associated with increased recurrence (Suzuki et al. 2011). Increased numbers of epithelial and stromal B lymphocytes correlated with DSS in NSCLC. This good prognosis is thought be related to limited tumor dissemination and to the antibody-mediated action of NK cells (Bremnes et al. 2011). Increasing numbers of stromal NK cells were associated with DSS and considered a favorable prognostic factor (Bremnes et al. 2011). An effective anti-tumor response depends on the action of dendritic cells given their important role as antigen-presenting cells (Bremnes et al. 2011). Increasing numbers of these cells were associated with DSS, and the density of mature dendritic cells was a better predictor of NSCLC clinical outcome (Bremnes et al. 2011). Mast cell density was also significantly associated with angiogenesis, microvessel density, and poor prognosis of NSCLC patients (Bremnes et al. 2011).

1.3 Role of Inflammatory Molecules in the Development of Lung Cancer: Evidence from in Vitro Studies

Chronic inflammation has been postulated to play a central role in orchestrating these processes in concert with irreversible mutational events and may provide reversible targets for lung cancer prevention and treatment. Cancer-related inflammation affects many aspects of malignancy, including the proliferation and survival of malignant cells, angiogenesis, tumor metastasis, and tumor response to chemotherapeutic drugs and hormones (Mantovani et al. 2008). When tissue homeostasis is persistently perturbed as in chronic inflammation, interactions between innate and adaptive immune cells as well as composition of cells and mediators will change. The inability to properly regulate the innate and adaptive immune system can result in excessive tissue remodeling, loss of tissue architecture due to destruction, protein alterations and genotoxic DNA damage due to oxidative stress and subsequently increased cancer risk (de Visser et al. 2006).

1.3.1 Role of Inflammatory Molecules in the Transformation of Lung Cancer Cells

There are some events that are required to drive from initiated cells to malignant tumors (Hanahan and Weinberg 2011). The infiltration of immune cells to tumors may repress tumor growth (Dunn et al. 2002). However, the increasing concern hypothesis is that inflammatory cells act as tumor promoters in inflammation-associated cancers (Smyth et al. 2004). Accumulated mutations in epithelial cells lead to dysregulation of their growth and migration. These dysregulated may also produce cytokines and chemokines to attract immune cells to facilitate cancer development (Lin and Pollard 2004; Coelho et al. 2006).

Several studies on tumor–host interaction have highlighted the importance of inflammatory response in the early steps of carcinogenesis as well as in established progressive tumors and are beginning now to identify the contribution of polarized inflammatory responses in cancer progression (Sica et al. 2006; Wang and Joyce 2010).

TNF is a transforming agent for carcinogen-treated fibroblast. Two weeks of exposure to the cytokine in vitro is sufficient to render cells capable of tumor formation in nude mice (Komori et al. 1993). The molecular basis may involve induction of reactive oxygen. Reactive oxygen in the form of NO is often generated by inflammatory cytokine induction of NO synthase. NO is an important regulatory molecule in both inflammation and cancer development (Lu et al. 2006). NO can directly oxidize DNA, resulting in mutagenic changes, and may damage some DNA repair proteins (Jaiswal et al. 2000). In study of Yan and co-workers, they revealed that TNF-α is potent mutagen that causes DNA damage through the induction of ROS (Yan et al. 2006; Aggarwal et al. 2006). This study brings up two new concepts, a mechanism through which a cytokine can induce genetic instability and the involvement of the TNF-α-mediated DNA damage pathway in inflammation-associated carcinogenesis (Yan et al. 2006). DNA damage can be induced by conventional mutagens, such as radiation and chemicals, or endogenous from errors in DNA replication or ROS produced cell metabolism. Yan and co-workers found that endogenous cytokine TNF-α is potent mutagen by virtue of its ability to induce ROS (Yan et al. 2006). Therefore, TNF-α drives tumor development by promoting the accumulation of mutations and survival of precancerous or transformed cells (Yan et al. 2006).

1.3.2 Role of Inflammatory Molecules in the Survival of Lung Cancer Cells

A large number of studies suggest that TNF and chemokines are candidate linking molecules between inflammation and cancer (Lu et al. 2006). The TNF, which is produced mainly by activated macrophages but also by tumor cells, binds to membrane-bound homotrimeric receptors (Lu et al. 2006).

It is well established the critical role of TNF-α in chronic inflammatory diseases, and its tumor-promoting effects have been demonstrated (Lin and Karin 2007). The production of TNF-α by tumor cells or inflammatory cells in the tumor microenvironment can promote tumor cell survival through the induction of genes encoding NF-κB-dependent anti-apoptotic molecules (Lin and Karin 2007; Luo et al. 2004). Furthermore, TNF-α promotes cell survival and thereby reduces asbestos-induced cytotoxicity, increasing the pool of asbestos-damaged mesothelial cells that are susceptible to malignant transformation (Yang et al. 2006; Lin and Karin 2007). Other actions of TNF-α that might enhance tumor progression, as opposed to tumor initiation, include promotion of angiogenesis and metastasis, as well as impairment of immune surveillance by strongly suppressing many T cell responses and the cytotoxic activity of activated macrophages (Elgert et al. 1998; Lin and Karin 2007).

Transforming growth factor-β (TGFβ), an immunosuppressive cytokine (Flavell et al. 2010), with a pleiotropic role in tumor biology, is a cytokine frequently overexpressed in many cancers, including NSCLC (Bruno et al. 2013; Teixeira et al. 2011; Siegel and Massague 2003). TGFβ belong to widely expressed family of cytokines with pleiotropic effects on a variety of cellular functions such as cell growth, proliferation, differentiation, and apoptosis (Luo et al. 2010).

TGFβ also has a role in the tumor microenvironment immune cell polarization, including macrophages, neutrophils, and NK cells associated with tumor immune evasion (Flavell et al. 2010; Siegel and Massague 2003). High expression of TGFβ is characteristic of NSCLC and predictive of poor survival (Teixeira et al. 2011).

Interleukin-10 (IL-10) is a multifunctional cytokine with both immunosuppressive and anti-angiogenic functions and consequently has both tumor-promoting and tumor-inhibiting properties (Shih et al. 2005). Raised levels of serum and peri-tumoral IL-10 production have been reported in many malignant (Dummer et al. 1995), including lung cancer (Shih et al. 2005), which have been interpreted in support of a role for IL-10 in tumor escape from the immune response. Furthermore, increased production of immunosuppressive IL-10 by NSCLC and increased serum concentrations of IL-10 in NSCLC patients have both been shown recently to correlate with reduced survival (Shih et al. 2005). Serum levels of IL-10 were found to be elevated in NSCLC patients when compared to healthy controls; moreover, IL-10 serum levels were demonstrated to be higher in patients with metastatic disease as opposed to the values recorded in patients with undisseminated cancer (De Vita et al. 2000). IL-10 promotes tumor malignancy by promoting T cell apoptosis and tumor cell survival (Wang et al. 2012). In lung carcinomas, IL-10 production can inhibit tumor cell susceptibility to cytotoxic T-lymphocyte-mediated killing (Asselin-Paturel et al. 2001). IL-10 transgenic cytotoxic mice injected with Lewis lung carcinoma cells developed larger tumors than control mice, suggesting that the production of IL-10 prevents the development of an effective immune response against the tumor cells (Montuenga and Pio 2007).

1.3.3 Role of Inflammatory Molecules in the Proliferation of Lung Cancer Cells

NK-κB is a positive mediator of cell growth and proliferation. NF-κB increases the expression of several factors involved cell cycle progression such as cyclins D and E (Chen et al. 2011). Upregulation of cyclin D1 expression by NF-κB is associated with enhanced transition from G1 to S phase (Chen et al. 2011; Nogueira et al. 2013). Furthermore, NF-κB negatively regulates expression of growth arrest and DNA damage-inducible protein 45 (GADD45), a cell cycle checkpoint protein that keeps cell at the G2/M phase transition (Chen et al. 2011). Additionally, the mutual interplay between NF-κB and proinflammatory cytokines such as TNF-α and IL-1β is also involved in stimulating cancer cell proliferation, particularly during chronic inflammation (Karin 2008). The contributions of NF-κB to lung cancer development are complex, underlying mechanism of which have not been fully understood (Chen et al. 2011). There is considerable evidence that NF-κB is constitutively activated in a variety of solid tumors, including prostate, breast, cervical, pancreatic, and lung cancer (Chen et al. 2011; Karin 2008). Although lung tumors are histologically heterogenic, tumor samples obtained from lung cancer patients showed high levels of NF-κB activation in both SCLC and NSCLC and are significantly associated with disease advancement in TNM stages and poor prognosis in lung cancer patients (Chen et al. 2011). Inhibiting NF-κB with different approaches such as siRNA, IKK inhibitors, and IkappaB super suppressor inhibited lung cancer cell's survival and proliferation (Chen et al. 2011; Karin 2008).

IL-6 is a potent pleiotropic inflammatory cytokine that is considered a key growth-promoting and anti-apoptotic factor, and this interleukin was responsible of biological activities in immune regulation, hematopoiesis, inflammation, and oncogenesis which is produced by various types of human normal and transformed tumor cells and transformed tumor cells (Ishihara and Hirano 2002; Lin and Karin 2007; Chang et al. 2005). IL-6 is of particular interest because they are expressed in malignant epithelial cells, and their expression is associated with a poor prognosis in lung cancer patients (Pine et al. 2011). Consistent with this prominent role in cell proliferation, IL-6 has been detected in primary squamous cell carcinomas, adenocarcinomas, as well as in tumor cell lines (Chang et al. 2005; Azevedo et al. 2011).

Increased serum levels of IL-6 was found in 39 % of lung cancer patients, whereas IL-6 was not detected in the serum of healthy people as well as patients with benign lung diseases (Chang et al. 2005; Yanagawa et al. 1995). Bihl and coworkers have demonstrated that IL-6 may be required in the control of cell proliferation in a subset of NSCLC cell lines, and there are two subgroups of NSCLC IL-6 dependent and independent (Bihl et al. 1998). Paradoxically, anti-tumor effects of IL-6 have been demonstrated in vitro and in vivo patients with NSCLC and breast cancer (Chang et al. 2005).

1.3.4 Role of Inflammatory Molecules in the Invasion, Metastasis, and Angiogenesis of Lung Cancer Cells

The tumor vasculature is derived from sprouting of local blood vessels (angiogenesis) and circulating vasculogenic progenitor cells derived from the bone marrow (vasculogenesis). The new vessels are often irregular and leaky due to lack of the pericyte cover, with the result that tumor cells can penetrate them more easily. As compared to blood capillaries, lymphatic endothelial cells have even less developed junctions with frequently large interendothelial gaps and impaired basement membranes (Kessenbrock et al. 2010). The invasive margin is a critical area for stimulation of angiogenesis and lymphangionesis in tumors, which contributes to tumor invasion and metastasis (Padera et al. 2002).

The major MMPs involved in tumor angiogenesis are MMP-2, MMP-9, and MMP-14, and to a lesser extent MMP-1 and MMP-7 (Kessenbrock et al. 2010; Rao et al. 2005).

MMPs are a family of proteolytic enzymes that are capable of degrading various components of the extracellular matrix (Liu et al. 2012). They are involved in all stages of cancer progression, not only in the process of tumor invasion and metastasis (Hu et al. 2005) but also in as proliferation, adhesion, migration, differentiation, angiogenesis, senescence, autophagy, apoptosis, and evasion of the immune system (Gonzalez-Arriaga et al. 2012; Deryugina and Quigley 2006). The expression of these MMPs by tumor cells may help to increase the invasive potential of tumor cells by allowing the remodeling of the extracellular matrix

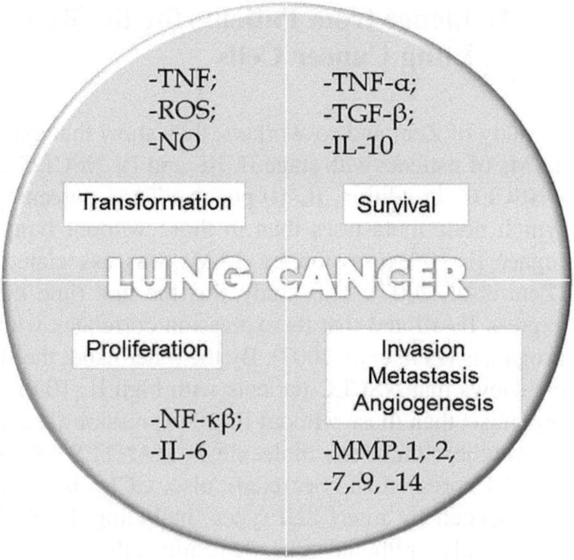

Fig. 1.3 Overview of the role of inflammatory molecules in development of lung cancer

(Hu et al. 2005; Gomes et al. 2011). The proteolytic activity is also required for a cancer cell to invade a nearby blood vessel (intravasation) and then extravasate at a distant location and invade the distant tissue in order to seed a new metastatic site (Roy et al. 2009). Increased expression of MMP-2 and MMP-9 was shown to correlate with an invasive phenotype of cancer cells (Vihinen and Kahari 2002). Several recent reports confirmed lung neoplastic cells produce both and their inhibitors (Brown et al. 1993).

MMPs have also been implicated in the epithelial to mesenchymal transition (EMT), a hallmark of cancer progression to metastasis (Thiery 2002; Roy et al. 2009; Rao et al. 2005). During EMT, tumor cells acquire migratory characteristics and more readily invade into surrounding tissues and metastasize to secondary sites (Roy et al. 2009; Rao et al. 2005).

Several studies have reported that plasma and/or serum levels of MMP-9 and TIMP-1 are elevated in patient with stage III or IV lung cancer, when compared with those in patients with nonmalignant lung diseases (Jumper et al. 2004; Koc et al. 2006). Retrospective studies of NSCLC tissue found that MMP-7 expression was higher in squamous cell carcinomas than in adenocarcinomas and correlated with significantly lower overall in patients (Liu et al. 2007). In the normal lung, MMP-9 is not produced by resident cells, but under various forms of stimulation, bronchial epithelial cells, alveolar type II cells, fibroblasts, smooth muscle cells, and endothelial cells produce MMP-9 (Atkinson and Senior 2003). Leukocytes in the lung can also be a source of MMP-9. Macrophages, eosinophils, mast cells, lymphocytes, NK cells, and dendritic cells all can produce MMP-9 (Atkinson and Senior 2003). Lung cancer cells, both primary and metastatic, can express MMP-9 constitutively, which may correlate with metastatic potential (Atkinson and Senior 2003; Zucker et al. 1992; Baruch et al. 2001) (Fig. 1.3).

1.4 Evidence from Patients for the Role of Inflammation in Lung Cancer Cells

In study of Zeni and co-workers, they show that expression of IL-10 is increased in TAMs of patients with stage II, III, and IV NSCLC compared with those with stage I NSCLC. In adition, IL-10 positive TAM percentage was higher in patients with lymph node metastases than in those without lymph node metastases. Moreover, higher IL-10 expression by TAMs was associated with shorter overall survival (Zeni et al. 2007). This study was the first time they showed, in NSCLC, TAMs express IL-10 and that its expression correlates with both disease progression and prognosis (Zeni et al. 2007). By the other hand, the study of Hatanaka and co-workers shows that NSCLC patients with high IL-10-expressing tumors showed poorer prognosis than those without IL-10 expression (Hatanaka et al. 2000).

Another important molecule is RANTES (Regulated on Activation, Normal T cell Expressed and Secreted); also, CCL5 is a known chemotactic cytokine that is produced by many cell types, including T-lymphocytes, monocytes, platelets, eosinophils, epithelial cells, dendritic cells, and mast cells (Umekawa et al. 2013). RANTES has been used as a prognostic indicator in both breast and cervical cancers, and high levels of RANTES in these malignancies correlate with poor outcome (Borczuk et al. 2008; Niwa et al. 2001).

Umekawa and co-workers showed that, in NSCLC patients, high level of plasma RANTES at diagnosis was associated with the severity of general fatigue. Low level of plasma RANTES at diagnosis was significantly associated with long-term survival. Thus, patients with high systemic inflammation, as represented by RANTES, may experience severe general fatigue and shorter survival time (Umekawa et al. 2013). In another study, Moran and co-workers found a correlation between increased RANTES expression and tumor lymphocytic response in lung cancer patients (Moran et al. 2002).

De Vita, in 1998, has evaluated serum levels of IL-6 in a group of advanced NSCLC patients and found that patients who respond to cisplatin-based chemotherapy have lower serum IL-6 levels when compared with unresponsive patients. Their data suggest that NSCLC patients with high levels of IL-6 have a worse clinical outcome and may manifest resistance to cisplatin chemotherapy (De Vita et al. 1998). However, in study of Chang and co-workers, they failed to demonstrate that exogenous or endogenous IL-6 could influence cisplatin or etoposide sensitivity of the tested NSCLC cells at cellular level (Chang et al. 2005).

1.5 Inhibitors of Inflammation for the Prevention and Treatment of Lung Cancer

Epidemiologic studies and meta-analysis have shown that prolonged use of NSAIDs reduces the risk of several solid tumor including lung cancer, and recent meta-analysis suggests that low-dose aspirin could reduce the relative risk of cancer mortality (Zhan et al. 2013; Vaish and Sanyal 2011; Setia and Sanyal 2012). Both clinical and experimental studies support the anti-neoplastic effects of NSAIDs mediated by regulation of COX-2 levels and induction of apoptosis (Haynes et al. 2003). A daily intake of NSAIDs for 1 or 2 years is reported to reduce 60–68 % of relative risk of lung cancer (Harris et al. 2007). The best known target of NSAIDs, including aspirin, is the enzyme COX-2, a key enzyme involved in the production of prostaglandins and other eicosanoids from arachidonic acid (Menter et al. 2010; Pereira et al. 2010). Due primarily to the action of COXs on the free arachidonic acid (AA) liberated from membrane phospholipids, overproduction of PGE_2 which is predominantly generated by upregulation of COX-2 is associated with a variety of carcinogenic mechanisms (Mao et al. 2005, 2011).

The association between COX-2 overexpression and survival in lung cancer patients has been studied for over a decade (Dalwadi et al. 2005). COX-2 expression has also been shown to be a poor prognostic indicator in non-small-cell lung cancer (Khuri et al. 2001; Li et al. 2011). Inhibition of COX-2 and thus of PGE_2 synthesis suppresses lung tumorigenesis in animal models (Mao et al. 2011). According to these evidences, COX-2 is one of the targets under investigation for lung cancer therapy and chemoprevention (Dubinett et al. 2003; Lee et al. 2007). Some reports indicate that the regular use of aspirin and other is associated with reduced risks of developing lung cancer in animal models and in smokers (Smith et al. 2006; Brody and Spira 2006; Peebles et al. 2007). Later epidemiologic studies have confirmed the chemopreventive effect of NSAIDs in colorectal cancer (Gupta and Dubois 2001). More recently, it has become clear that effects of aspirin may not be restricted to gastrointestinal tract cancers, but may also be relevant in the prevention of breast cancer and lung cancer (Ballaz and Mulshine 2003). In animal model of lung cancer, anti-inflammatory treatment resulted in a significance (34–52 %) reduction of tumor multiplicity (i.e., in number of tumors per animal), although treatment with anti-inflammatory drugs did not completely inhibit tumor growth (Rioux and Castonguay 1998; Duperron and Castonguay 1997; Ballaz and Mulshine 2003).

Strong lines of evidence suggest that the chemopreventive properties of chronic NSAID administration are based on their COX-inhibitory activity. Overexpression of COX-2 is associated with poorer prognosis in some cancers, including NSCLC (Brabender et al. 2002; Ballaz and Mulshine 2003).

However, increasing evidences showing that NF-κB plays a critical role in lung cancer development suggest NF-κB as a target for lung cancer chemoprevention (Chen et al. 2011). Interestingly, some agents that have lung cancer preventive potential, including NSAIDs and dietary compounds, possess inhibitory activity on NF-κB (Cuzick et al. 2009). Oral administration of pomegranate fruit extract, which inhibits NF-κB, significantly reduced multiplicity of lung tumor induced by benzo(a)pyrene and N-nitroso-tris-chloroethylurea (Khan et al. 2007a, b). Chemoprevention involves prolonged use of preventive agents. The long-time use of the NF-κB inhibitors or anti-inflammatory drugs is likely to result in un-tolerable side effects (Karin 2006). Thus, dedicated single NF-κB inhibitors are unlikely to be used as chemoprevention agents (Cuzick et al. 2009). It has been proposed that logically constructed mixtures of agents or combination treatments are better choice for lung cancer chemoprevention (Chen et al. 2011). This strategy would improve the efficacy of cancer prevention while eliminate the possible side effects.

1.6 Conclusions and Future Directions

Inflammation can affect all hallmarks of tumor development and prognosis as well as the response to therapy. During the inflammation progress, various types of leukocytes, lymphocytes, and other inflammatory cells are activated and attracted to the inflamed site by a signaling network involving a great number of growth factors, cytokines, and chemokines (Lu et al. 2006).

In the NSCLC microenvironment, there is a complex interaction between immune cells and tumor cells as well as other stromal cell types and tissue components. The distribution of these cells and the expression of different inflammatory molecules throughout the tumor microenvironment are, to various extents, related to tumor progression and survival.

We believe that further studies are needed and further research in order to find new predictive and prognosis biomarkers in NSCLC. Also needed are new measures to reduce the risk of cancer. Thereby, prevention is a much better and more economical way to fight cancer than treating an already advanced and often incurable disease.

References

Aggarwal BB, Shishodia S, Sandur SK, Pandey MK, Sethi G (2006) Inflammation and cancer: how hot is the link? Biochem Pharmacol 72(11):1605–1621. doi:10.1016/j.bcp.2006.06.029

Aggarwal BB, Vijayalekshmi RV, Sung B (2009) Targeting inflammatory pathways for prevention and therapy of cancer: short-term friend, long-term foe. Clin Cancer Res 15(2):425–430. doi:10.1158/1078-0432.CCR-08-0149

Araujo A, Ribeiro R, Azevedo I, Coelho A, Soares M, Sousa B, Pinto D, Lopes C, Medeiros R, Scagliotti GV (2007) Genetic polymorphisms of the epidermal growth factor and related receptor in non-small cell lung cancer—A review of the literature. Oncologist 12(2):201–210. doi:10.1634/theoncologist.12-2-201

Asselin-Paturel C, Megherat S, Vergnon I, Echchakir H, Dorothee G, Blesson S, Gay F, Mami-Chouaib F, Chouaib S (2001) Differential effect of high doses versus low doses of interleukin-12 on the adoptive transfer of human specific cytotoxic T lymphocyte in autologous lung tumors engrafted into severe combined immunodeficiency disease-nonobese diabetic mice: relation with interleukin-10 induction. Cancer 91(1):113–122

Atkinson JJ, Senior RM (2003) Matrix metalloproteinase-9 in lung remodeling. Am J Respir Cell Mol Biol 28(1):12–24. doi:10.1165/rcmb.2002-0166TR

Azevedo A, Cunha V, Teixeira AL, Medeiros R (2011) IL-6/IL-6R as a potential key signaling pathway in prostate cancer development. World J Clin Oncol 2(12):384–396. doi:10.5306/wjco.v2.i12.384

Azzoli CG, Baker S Jr, Temin S, Pao W, Aliff T, Brahmer J, Johnson DH, Laskin JL, Masters G, Milton D, Nordquist L, Pfister DG, Piantadosi S, Schiller JH, Smith R, Smith TJ, Strawn

JR, Trent D, Giaccone G (2009) American Society of Clinical Oncology Clinical Practice Guideline update on chemotherapy for stage IV non-small-cell lung cancer. J Clin Oncol 27(36):6251–6266. doi:10.1200/JCO.2009.23.5622

Balkwill F, Mantovani A (2001) Inflammation and cancer: back to Virchow? Lancet 357(9255):539–545. doi:10.1016/S0140-6736(00)04046-0

Ballaz S, Mulshine JL (2003) The potential contributions of chronic inflammation to lung carcinogenesis. Clin Lung Cancer 5(1):46–62. doi:10.3816/CLC.2003.n.021

Baruch RR, Melinscak H, Lo J, Liu Y, Yeung O, Hurta RA (2001) Altered matrix metalloproteinase expression associated with oncogene-mediated cellular transformation and metastasis formation. Cell Biol Int 25(5):411–420. doi:10.1006/cbir.2000.0647

Ben-Baruch A (2006) Inflammation-associated immune suppression in cancer: the roles played by cytokines, chemokines and additional mediators. Semin Cancer Biol 16(1):38–52. doi:10.1016/j.semcancer.2005.07.006

Bihl M, Tamm M, Nauck M, Wieland H, Perruchoud AP, Roth M (1998) Proliferation of human non-small-cell lung cancer cell lines: role of interleukin-6. Am J Respir Cell Mol Biol 19(4):606–612. doi:10.1165/ajrcmb.19.4.3247

Borczuk AC, Papanikolaou N, Toonkel RL, Sole M, Gorenstein LA, Ginsburg ME, Sonett JR, Friedman RA, Powell CA (2008) Lung adenocarcinoma invasion in TGFbetaRII-deficient cells is mediated by CCL5/RANTES. Oncogene 27(4):557–564. doi:10.1038/sj.onc.1210662

Brabender J, Park J, Metzger R, Schneider PM, Lord RV, Holscher AH, Danenberg KD, Danenberg PV (2002) Prognostic significance of cyclooxygenase 2 mRNA expression in non-small cell lung cancer. Ann Surg 235(3):440–443

Bremnes RM, Al-Shibli K, Donnem T, Sirera R, Al-Saad S, Andersen S, Stenvold H, Camps C, Busund LT (2011) The role of tumor-infiltrating immune cells and chronic inflammation at the tumor site on cancer development, progression, and prognosis: emphasis on non-small cell lung cancer. J Thoracic Oncol: Official Pub Int Assoc Study Lung Cancer 6(4):824–833. doi:10.1097/JTO.0b013e3182037b76

Brody JS, Spira A (2006) State of the art. Chronic obstructive pulmonary disease, inflammation, and lung cancer. Proc Am Thorc Soc 3(6):535–537. doi:10.1513/pats.200603-089MS

Brown PD, Bloxidge RE, Stuart NS, Gatter KC, Carmichael J (1993) Association between expression of activated 72-kilodalton gelatinase and tumor spread in non-small-cell lung carcinoma. J Natl Cancer Inst 85(7):574–578

Bruno A, Focaccetti C, Pagani A, Imperatori AS, Spagnoletti M, Rotolo N, Cantelmo AR, Franzi F, Capella C, Ferlazzo G, Mortara L, Albini A, Noonan DM (2013) The proangiogenic phenotype of natural killer cells in patients with non-small cell lung cancer. Neoplasia 15(2):133–142

Chang KT, Huang CY, Tsai CM, Chiu CH, Lok YY (2005) Role of IL-6 in neuroendocrine differentiation and chemosensitivity of non-small cell lung cancer. Am J Physiol Lung Cell Mol Physiol 289(3):L438–L445. doi:10.1152/ajplung.00033.2005

Chen W, Li Z, Bai L, Lin Y (2011) NF-kappaB in lung cancer, a carcinogenesis mediator and a prevention and therapy target. Front Biosci: J Virtual Libr 16:1172–1185

Coelho A, Calcada C, Catarino R, Pinto D, Fonseca G, Medeiros R (2006) CXCL12-3' A polymorphism and lung cancer metastases protection: new perspectives in immunotherapy? Cancer Immunol Immunother 55(6):639–643. doi:10.1007/s00262-005-0062-1

Cohen S (1965) The stimulation of epidermal proliferation by a specific protein (EGF). Dev Biol 12(3):394–407

Coussens LM, Werb Z (2002) Inflammation and cancer. Nature 420(6917):860–867. doi:10.1038/nature01322

Cuzick J, Otto F, Baron JA, Brown PH, Burn J, Greenwald P, Jankowski J, La Vecchia C, Meyskens F, Senn HJ, Thun M (2009) Aspirin and non-steroidal anti-inflammatory drugs for cancer prevention: an international consensus statement. Lancet Oncol 10(5):501–507. doi:10.1016/S1470-2045(09)70035-X

Dalwadi H, Krysan K, Heuze-Vourc'h N, Dohadwala M, Elashoff D, Sharma S, Cacalano N, Lichtenstein A, Dubinett S (2005) Cyclooxygenase-2-dependent activation of signal transducer and activator of transcription 3 by interleukin-6 in non-small cell lung cancer. Clin Cancer Res 11(21):7674–7682. doi:10.1158/1078-0432.CCR-05-1205

de Mello RA, Marques DS, Medeiros R, Araujo AM (2011) Epidermal growth factor receptor and K-Ras in non-small cell lung cancer-molecular pathways involved and targeted therapies. World J Clin Oncol 2(11):367–376. doi:10.5306/wjco.v2.i11.367

de Visser KE, Eichten A, Coussens LM (2006) Paradoxical roles of the immune system during cancer development. Nat Rev Cancer 6(1):24–37. doi:10.1038/nrc1782

De Vita F, Orditura M, Auriemma A, Infusino S, Roscigno A, Catalano G (1998) Serum levels of interleukin-6 as a prognostic factor in advanced non-small cell lung cancer. Oncol Rep 5(3):649–652

De Vita F, Orditura M, Galizia G, Romano C, Roscigno A, Lieto E, Catalano G (2000) Serum interleukin-10 levels as a prognostic factor in advanced non-small cell lung cancer patients. Chest 117(2):365–373

Deryugina EI, Quigley JP (2006) Matrix metalloproteinases and tumor metastasis. Cancer Metastasis Rev 25(1):9–34. doi:10.1007/s10555-006-7886-9

Dubinett SM, Sharma S, Huang M, Dohadwala M, Pold M, Mao JT (2003) Cyclooxygenase-2 in lung cancer. Prog Exp Tumor Res 37:138–162

Dummer W, Becker JC, Schwaaf A, Leverkus M, Moll T, Brocker EB (1995) Elevated serum levels of interleukin-10 in patients with metastatic malignant melanoma. Melanoma Res 5(1):67–68

Dunn GP, Bruce AT, Ikeda H, Old LJ, Schreiber RD (2002) Cancer immunoediting: from immunosurveillance to tumor escape. Nat Immunol 3(11):991–998. doi:10.1038/ni1102-991

Duperron C, Castonguay A (1997) Chemopreventive efficacies of aspirin and sulindac against lung tumorigenesis in A/J mice. Carcinogenesis 18(5):1001–1006

Elgert KD, Alleva DG, Mullins DW (1998) Tumor-induced immune dysfunction: the macrophage connection. J Leukoc Biol 64(3):275–290

Ferlay J, Parkin DM, Steliarova-Foucher E (2010) Estimates of cancer incidence and mortality in Europe in 2008. Eur J Cancer 46(4):765–781. doi:10.1016/j.ejca.2009.12.014

Flavell RA, Sanjabi S, Wrzesinski SH, Licona-Limon P (2010) The polarization of immune cells in the tumour environment by TGFbeta. Nat Rev Immunol 10(8):554–567. doi:10.1038/nri2808

Fossella FV, DeVore R, Kerr RN, Crawford J, Natale RR, Dunphy F, Kalman L, Miller V, Lee JS, Moore M, Gandara D, Karp D, Vokes E, Kris M, Kim Y, Gamza F, Hammershaimb L (2000) Randomized phase III trial of docetaxel versus vinorelbine or ifosfamide in patients with advanced non-small-cell lung cancer previously treated with platinum-containing chemotherapy regimens. The TAX 320 Non-Small Cell Lung Cancer Study Group. J Clin Oncol 18(12):2354–2362

Gomes M, Coelho A, Araújo A, Catarino R, Medeiros R (2011) 1137 POSTER Is MMP-9 Q279R a possible marker of prognostic in non small cell lung cancer? Eur J Cancer (Oxford 1990) 47:S134–S135

Gomes M, Coelho A, Araujo A, Teixeira AL, Catarino R, Medeiros R (2012) Influence of functional genetic polymorphism (−590C/T) in non-small cell lung cancer (NSCLC) development: the paradoxal role of IL-4. Gene 504(1):111–115. doi:10.1016/j.gene.2012.05.008

Gonzalez-Arriaga P, Pascual T, Garcia-Alvarez A, Fernandez-Somoano A, Lopez-Cima MF, Tardon A (2012) Genetic polymorphisms in MMP 2, 9 and 3 genes modify lung cancer risk and survival. BMC Cancer 12:121. doi:10.1186/1471-2407-12-121

Gregory AD, Houghton AM (2011) Tumor-associated neutrophils: new targets for cancer therapy. Cancer Res 71(7):2411–2416. doi:10.1158/0008-5472.CAN-10-2583

Gupta RA, Dubois RN (2001) Colorectal cancer prevention and treatment by inhibition of cyclooxygenase-2. Nat Rev Cancer 1(1):11–21. doi:10.1038/35094017

Hanahan D, Weinberg RA (2011) Hallmarks of cancer: the next generation. Cell 144(5):646–674. doi:10.1016/j.cell.2011.02.013

Harris RE, Beebe-Donk J, Alshafie GA (2007) Reduced risk of human lung cancer by selective cyclooxygenase 2 (COX-2) blockade: results of a case control study. Int J Biol Sci 3(5):328–334

Hatanaka H, Abe Y, Kamiya T, Morino F, Nagata J, Tokunaga T, Oshika Y, Suemizu H, Kijima H, Tsuchida T, Yamazaki H, Inoue H, Nakamura M, Ueyama Y (2000) Clinical implications of interleukin (IL)-10 induced by non-small-cell lung cancer. Ann Oncol 11(7):815–819

Haynes A, Shaik MS, Chatterjee A, Singh M (2003) Evaluation of an aerosolized selective COX-2 inhibitor as a potentiator of doxorubicin in a non-small-cell lung cancer cell line. Pharm Res 20(9):1485–1495

Hoffman PC, Mauer AM, Vokes EE (2000) Lung cancer. Lancet 355(9202):479–485. doi:10.1016/S0140-6736(00)82038-3

Hu Z, Huo X, Lu D, Qian J, Zhou J, Chen Y, Xu L, Ma H, Zhu J, Wei Q, Shen H (2005) Functional polymorphisms of matrix metalloproteinase-9 are associated with risk of occurrence and metastasis of lung cancer. Clin Cancer Res 11(15):5433–5439. doi:10.1158/1078-0432.CCR-05-0311

Ishihara K, Hirano T (2002) IL-6 in autoimmune disease and chronic inflammatory proliferative disease. Cytokine Growth Factor Rev 13(4-5):357–368

Jaiswal M, LaRusso NF, Burgart LJ, Gores GJ (2000) Inflammatory cytokines induce DNA damage and inhibit DNA repair in cholangiocarcinoma cells by a nitric oxide-dependent mechanism. Cancer Res 60(1):184–190

Jemal A, Bray F, Center MM, Ferlay J, Ward E, Forman D (2011) Global cancer statistics. CA Cancer J Clin 61(2):69–90. doi:10.3322/caac.20107

Jumper C, Cobos E, Lox C (2004) Determination of the serum matrix metalloproteinase-9 (MMP-9) and tissue inhibitor of matrix metalloproteinase-1 (TIMP-1) in patients with either advanced small-cell lung cancer or non-small-cell lung cancer prior to treatment. Respir Med 98(2):173–177

Karin M (2006) Nuclear factor-kappaB in cancer development and progression. Nature 441(7092):431–436. doi:10.1038/nature04870

Karin M (2008) The IkappaB kinase—a bridge between inflammation and cancer. Cell Res 18(3):334–342. doi:10.1038/cr.2008.30

Kessenbrock K, Plaks V, Werb Z (2010) Matrix metalloproteinases: regulators of the tumor microenvironment. Cell 141(1):52–67. doi:10.1016/j.cell.2010.03.015

Khan N, Afaq F, Kweon MH, Kim K, Mukhtar H (2007a) Oral consumption of pomegranate fruit extract inhibits growth and progression of primary lung tumors in mice. Cancer Res 67(7):3475–3482. doi:10.1158/0008-5472.CAN-06-3941

Khan N, Hadi N, Afaq F, Syed DN, Kweon MH, Mukhtar H (2007b) Pomegranate fruit extract inhibits prosurvival pathways in human A549 lung carcinoma cells and tumor growth in athymic nude mice. Carcinogenesis 28(1):163–173. doi:10.1093/carcin/bgl145

Khuri FR, Wu H, Lee JJ, Kemp BL, Lotan R, Lippman SM, Feng L, Hong WK, Xu XC (2001) Cyclooxygenase-2 overexpression is a marker of poor prognosis in stage I non-small cell lung cancer. Clin Cancer Res 7(4):861–867

Koc M, Ediger D, Budak F, Karadag M, Oral HB, Uzaslan E, Ege E, Gozu RO (2006) Matrix metalloproteinase-9 (MMP-9) elevated in serum but not in bronchial lavage fluid in patients with lung cancer. Tumori 92(2):149–154

Komori A, Yatsunami J, Suganuma M, Okabe S, Abe S, Sakai A, Sasaki K, Fujiki H (1993) Tumor necrosis factor acts as a tumor promoter in BALB/3T3 cell transformation. Cancer Res 53(9):1982–1985

Kwak EL, Bang YJ, Camidge DR, Shaw AT, Solomon B, Maki RG, Ou SH, Dezube BJ, Janne PA, Costa DB, Varella-Garcia M, Kim WH, Lynch TJ, Fidias P, Stubbs H, Engelman JA, Sequist LV, Tan W, Gandhi L, Mino-Kenudson M, Wei GC, Shreeve SM, Ratain MJ, Settleman J, Christensen JG, Haber DA, Wilner K, Salgia R, Shapiro GI, Clark JW, Iafrate AJ (2010) Anaplastic lymphoma kinase inhibition in non-small-cell lung cancer. N Engl J Med 363(18):1693–1703. doi:10.1056/NEJMoa1006448

Lan Q, Zheng T, Rothman N, Zhang Y, Wang SS, Shen M, Berndt SI, Zahm SH, Holford TR, Leaderer B, Yeager M, Welch R, Boyle P, Zhang B, Zou K, Zhu Y, Chanock S (2006) Cytokine polymorphisms in the Th1/Th2 pathway and susceptibility to non-Hodgkin lymphoma. Blood 107(10):4101–4108. doi:10.1182/blood-2005-10-4160

Lee JM, Mao JT, Krysan K, Dubinett SM (2007) Significance of cyclooxygenase-2 in prognosis, targeted therapy and chemoprevention of NSCLC. Future Oncol 3(2):149–153. doi:10.2217/14796694.3.2.149

Li F, Liu Y, Chen H, Liao D, Shen Y, Xu F, Wang J (2011) EGFR and COX-2 protein expression in non-small cell lung cancer and the correlation with clinical features. J Exp Clin Cancer Res 30:27. doi:10.1186/1756-9966-30-27

Li Y, Yang T, Wei S, Wang J, Wang M, Wang Y, Zhou Q, Liu H, Chen J (2013) Clinical significance of EML4-ALK fusion gene and association with EGFR and KRAS gene mutations in 208 Chinese patients with non-small cell lung cancer. PLoS One 8(1):e52093. doi:10.1371/journal.pone.0052093

Lin EY, Pollard JW (2004) Role of infiltrated leucocytes in tumour growth and spread. Br J Cancer 90(11):2053–2058. doi:10.1038/sj.bjc.6601705

Lin WW, Karin M (2007) A cytokine-mediated link between innate immunity, inflammation, and cancer. J Clin Invest 117(5):1175–1183. doi:10.1172/JCI31537

Linardou H, Dahabreh IJ, Kanaloupiti D, Siannis F, Bafaloukos D, Kosmidis P, Papadimitriou CA, Murray S (2008) Assessment of somatic k-RAS mutations as a mechanism associated with resistance to EGFR-targeted agents: a systematic review and meta-analysis of studies in advanced non-small-cell lung cancer and metastatic colorectal cancer. Lancet Oncol 9(10):962–972. doi:10.1016/S1470-2045(08)70206-7

Liu D, Guo H, Li Y, Xu X, Yang K, Bai Y (2012) Association between polymorphisms in the promoter regions of matrix metalloproteinases (MMPs) and risk of cancer metastasis: a meta-analysis. PLoS One 7(2):e31251. doi:10.1371/journal.pone.0031251

Liu D, Nakano J, Ishikawa S, Yokomise H, Ueno M, Kadota K, Urushihara M, Huang CL (2007) Overexpression of matrix metalloproteinase-7 (MMP-7) correlates with tumor proliferation, and a poor prognosis in non-small cell lung cancer. Lung Cancer 58(3):384–391. doi:10.1016/j.lungcan.2007.07.005

Lu H, Ouyang W, Huang C (2006) Inflammation, a key event in cancer development. Molecular cancer research : MCR 4(4):221–233. doi:10.1158/1541-7786.MCR-05-0261

Luo JL, Maeda S, Hsu LC, Yagita H, Karin M (2004) Inhibition of NF-kappaB in cancer cells converts inflammation- induced tumor growth mediated by TNFalpha to TRAIL-mediated tumor regression. Cancer Cell 6(3):297–305. doi:10.1016/j.ccr.2004.08.012

Luo X, Ding Q, Wang M, Li Z, Mao K, Sun B, Pan Y, Wang Z, Zang YQ, Chen Y (2010) In vivo disruption of TGF-beta signaling by Smad7 in airway epithelium alleviates allergic asthma but aggravates lung carcinogenesis in mouse. PLoS One 5(4):e10149. doi:10.1371/journal.pone.0010149

Mantovani A, Allavena P, Sica A, Balkwill F (2008) Cancer-related inflammation. Nature 454(7203):436–444. doi:10.1038/nature07205

Mantovani A, Sica A, Sozzani S, Allavena P, Vecchi A, Locati M (2004) The chemokine system in diverse forms of macrophage activation and polarization. Trends Immunol 25(12):677–686. doi:10.1016/j.it.2004.09.015

Mantovani A, Sozzani S, Locati M, Allavena P, Sica A (2002) Macrophage polarization: tumor-associated macrophages as a paradigm for polarized M2 mononuclear phagocytes. Trends Immunol 23(11):549–555

Mao JT, Cui X, Reckamp K, Liu M, Krysan K, Dalwadi H, Sharma S, Hazra S, Strieter R, Gardner B, Dubinett SM (2005) Chemoprevention strategies with cyclooxygenase-2 inhibitors for lung cancer. Clin Lung Cancer 7(1):30–39. doi:10.3816/CLC.2005.n.019

Mao JT, Roth MD, Fishbein MC, Aberle DR, Zhang ZF, Rao JY, Tashkin DP, Goodglick L, Holmes EC, Cameron RB, Dubinett SM, Elashoff R, Szabo E, Elashoff D (2011) Lung cancer chemoprevention with celecoxib in former smokers. Cancer Prev Res (Phila) 4(7):984–993. doi:10.1158/1940-6207.CAPR-11-0078

Martey CA, Pollock SJ, Turner CK, O'Reilly KM, Baglole CJ, Phipps RP, Sime PJ (2004) Cigarette smoke induces cyclooxygenase-2 and microsomal prostaglandin E2 synthase in human lung fibroblasts: implications for lung inflammation and cancer. Am J Physiol Lung Cell Mol Physiol 287(5):L981–L991. doi:10.1152/ajplung.00239.2003

Menter DG, Schilsky RL, DuBois RN (2010) Cyclooxygenase-2 and cancer treatment: understanding the risk should be worth the reward. Clin Cancer Res 16(5):1384–1390. doi:10.1158/1078-0432.CCR-09-0788

Michalaki V, Syrigos K, Charles P, Waxman J (2004) Serum levels of IL-6 and TNF-alpha correlate with clinicopathological features and patient survival in patients with prostate cancer. Br J Cancer 90(12):2312–2316. doi:10.1038/sj.bjc.6601814

Molina JR, Yang P, Cassivi SD, Schild SE, Adjei AA (2008) Non-small cell lung cancer: epidemiology, risk factors, treatment, and survivorship. Mayo Clin Proc Mayo Clin 83(5):584–594. doi:10.4065/83.5.584

Montuenga LM, Pio R (2007) Tumour-associated macrophages in nonsmall cell lung cancer: the role of interleukin-10. Eur Respir J 30(4):608–610. doi:10.1183/09031936.00091707

Moran CJ, Arenberg DA, Huang CC, Giordano TJ, Thomas DG, Misek DE, Chen G, Iannettoni MD, Orringer MB, Hanash S, Beer DG (2002) RANTES expression is a predictor of survival in stage I lung adenocarcinoma. Clin Cancer Res 8(12):3803–3812

Niwa Y, Akamatsu H, Niwa H, Sumi H, Ozaki Y, Abe A (2001) Correlation of tissue and plasma RANTES levels with disease course in patients with breast or cervical cancer. Clin Cancer Res 7(2):285–289

Nogueira A, Assis J, Catarino R, Medeiros R (2013) DNA repair and cytotoxic drugs: the potential role of RAD51 in clinical outcome of non-small-cell lung cancer patients. Pharmacogenomics 14(6):689–700. doi:10.2217/pgs.13.48

O'Callaghan DS, O'Donnell D, O'Connell F, O'Byrne KJ (2010) The role of inflammation in the pathogenesis of non-small cell lung cancer. J Thoracic Oncol: Off Pub Int Assoc Study Lung Cancer 5(12):2024–2036

Padera TP, Kadambi A, di Tomaso E, Carreira CM, Brown EB, Boucher Y, Choi NC, Mathisen D, Wain J, Mark EJ, Munn LL, Jain RK (2002) Lymphatic metastasis in the absence of functional intratumor lymphatics. Science 296(5574):1883–1886. doi:10.1126/science.1071420

Peebles KA, Lee JM, Mao JT, Hazra S, Reckamp KL, Krysan K, Dohadwala M, Heinrich EL, Walser TC, Cui X, Baratelli FE, Garon E, Sharma S, Dubinett SM (2007) Inflammation and lung carcinogenesis: applying findings in prevention and treatment. Expert Rev Anticancer Ther 7(10):1405–1421. doi:10.1586/14737140.7.10.1405

Pereira C, Pimentel-Nunes P, Brandao C, Moreira-Dias L, Medeiros R, Dinis-Ribeiro M (2010) COX-2 polymorphisms and colorectal cancer risk: a strategy for chemoprevention. Eur J Gastroenterol Hepatol 22(5):607–613. doi:10.1097/MEG.0b013e3283352cbb

Pine SR, Mechanic LE, Enewold L, Chaturvedi AK, Katki HA, Zheng YL, Bowman ED, Engels EA, Caporaso NE, Harris CC (2011) Increased levels of circulating interleukin 6, interleukin 8, C-reactive protein, and risk of lung cancer. J Nat Cancer Inst 103(14):1112–1122. doi:10.1093/jnci/djr216

Rao JS, Gondi C, Chetty C, Chittivelu S, Joseph PA, Lakka SS (2005) Inhibition of invasion, angiogenesis, tumor growth, and metastasis by adenovirus-mediated transfer of antisense uPAR and MMP-9 in non-small cell lung cancer cells. Mol Cancer Ther 4(9):1399–1408. doi:10.1158/1535-7163.MCT-05-0082

Ribeiro R, Araujo A, Lopes C, Medeiros R (2007) Immunoinflammatory mechanisms in lung cancer development: is leptin a mediator? J Thoracic Oncol: Off Pub Int Assoc Study Lung Cancer 2(2):105–108

Rioux N, Castonguay A (1998) Prevention of NNK-induced lung tumorigenesis in A/J mice by acetylsalicylic acid and NS-398. Cancer Res 58(23):5354–5360

Roy R, Yang J, Moses MA (2009) Matrix metalloproteinases as novel biomarkers and potential therapeutic targets in human cancer. J Clin Oncol 27(31):5287–5297. doi:10.1200/JCO.2009.23.5556

Schottenfeld D, Beebe-Dimmer J (2006) Chronic inflammation: a common and important factor in the pathogenesis of neoplasia. CA Cancer J Clin 56(2):69–83

Serefoglou Z, Yapijakis C, Nkenke E, Vairaktaris E (2008) Genetic association of cytokine DNA polymorphisms with head and neck cancer. Oral Oncol 44(12):1093–1099. doi:10.1016/j.oraloncology.2008.02.012

Setia S, Sanyal SN (2012) Upregulation of intrinsic apoptotic pathway in NSAIDs mediated chemoprevention of experimental lung carcinogenesis. Pharmacol Rep: PR 64(3):615–624

Shih CM, Lee YL, Chiou HL, Hsu WF, Chen WE, Chou MC, Lin LY (2005) The involvement of genetic polymorphism of IL-10 promoter in non-small cell lung cancer. Lung Cancer 50(3):291–297. doi:10.1016/j.lungcan.2005.07.007

Sica A, Schioppa T, Mantovani A, Allavena P (2006) Tumour-associated macrophages are a distinct M2 polarised population promoting tumour progression: potential targets of anti-cancer therapy. Eur J Cancer 42(6):717–727. doi:10.1016/j.ejca.2006.01.003

Siegel PM, Massague J (2003) Cytostatic and apoptotic actions of TGF-beta in homeostasis and cancer. Nat Rev Cancer 3(11):807–821. doi:10.1038/nrc1208

Siegel R, Naishadham D, Jemal A (2012) Cancer statistics, 2012. CA Cancer J Clin 62(1):10–29. doi:10.3322/caac.20138

Smith CJ, Perfetti TA, King JA (2006) Perspectives on pulmonary inflammation and lung cancer risk in cigarette smokers. Inhalation Toxicol 18(9):667–677. doi:10.1080/08958370600742821

Smyth MJ, Cretney E, Kershaw MH, Hayakawa Y (2004) Cytokines in cancer immunity and immunotherapy. Immunol Rev 202:275–293. doi:10.1111/j.0105-2896.2004.00199.x

Srivani R, Nagarajan B (2003) A prognostic insight on in vivo expression of interleukin-6 in uterine cervical cancer. Int J Gynecol Cancer: Off J Int Gynecol Cancer Soc 13(3):331–339

Suzuki K, Kachala SS, Kadota K, Shen R, Mo Q, Beer DG, Rusch VW, Travis WD, Adusumilli PS (2011) Prognostic immune markers in non-small cell lung cancer. Clin Cancer Res 17(16):5247–5256. doi:10.1158/1078-0432.CCR-10-2805

Takeshi U, Sadar MD, Suzuki H, Akakura K, Sakamoto S, Shimbo M, Suyama T, Imamoto T, Komiya A, Yukio N, Ichikawa T (2005) Interleukin-4 in patients with prostate cancer. Anticancer Res 25(6C):4595–4598

Tang J, Salama R, Gadgeel SM, Sarkar FH, Ahmad A (2013) Erlotinib resistance in lung cancer: current progress and future perspectives. Front Pharmacol 4:15. doi:10.3389/fphar.2013.00015

Teixeira AL, Araujo A, Coelho A, Ribeiro R, Gomes M, Pereira C, Medeiros R (2011) Influence of TGFB1+869T>C functional polymorphism in non-small cell lung cancer (NSCLC) risk. J Cancer Res Clin Oncol 137(3):435–439. doi:10.1007/s00432-010-0896-6

Thiery JP (2002) Epithelial-mesenchymal transitions in tumour progression. Nat Rev Cancer 2(6):442–454. doi:10.1038/nrc822

Toi M, Bicknell R, Harris AL (1992) Inhibition of colon and breast carcinoma cell growth by interleukin-4. Cancer Res 52(2):275–279

Tsai CC, Chen CC, Lin CC, Chen CH, Lin TS, Shieh TY (1999) Interleukin-1 beta in oral submucous fibrosis, verrucous hyperplasia and squamous cell carcinoma tissues. Kaohsiung J Med Sci 15(9):513–519

Umekawa K, Kimura T, Kudoh S, Suzumura T, Oka T, Nagata M, Mitsuoka S, Matsuura K, Nakai T, Yoshimura N, Kira Y, Hirata K (2013) Plasma RANTES, IL-10, and IL-8 levels in non–small-cell lung cancer patients treated with EGFR-TKIs. BMC Res Notes 6(1):139. doi:10.1186/1756-0500-6-139

Vaish V, Sanyal SN (2011) Chemopreventive effects of NSAIDs on cytokines and transcription factors during the early stages of colorectal cancer. Pharmacol Rep: PR 63(5):1210–1221

Van Ginderachter JA, Movahedi K, Hassanzadeh Ghassabeh G, Meerschaut S, Beschin A, Raes G, De Baetselier P (2006) Classical and alternative activation of mononuclear phagocytes: picking the best of both worlds for tumor promotion. Immunobiology 211(6–8):487–501. doi:10.1016/j.imbio.2006.06.002

Vihinen P, Kahari VM (2002) Matrix metalloproteinases in cancer: prognostic markers and therapeutic targets. Int J Cancer 99(2):157–166. doi:10.1002/ijc.10329

Wang HW, Joyce JA (2010) Alternative activation of tumor-associated macrophages by IL-4: priming for protumoral functions. Cell Cycle 9(24):4824–4835

Wang YC, Sung WW, Wu TC, Wang L, Chien WP, Cheng YW, Chen CY, Shieh SH, Lee H (2012) Interleukin-10 haplotype may predict survival and relapse in resected non-small cell lung cancer. PLoS One 7(7):e39525. doi:10.1371/journal.pone.0039525

Wheeler DL, Dunn EF, Harari PM (2010) Understanding resistance to EGFR inhibitors-impact on future treatment strategies. Nat Rev Clin Oncol 7(9):493–507. doi:10.1038/nrclinonc.2010.97

Wu K, House L, Liu W, Cho WC (2012) Personalized targeted therapy for lung cancer. Int J Mol Sci 13(9):11471–11496. doi:10.3390/ijms130911471

Yan B, Wang H, Rabbani ZN, Zhao Y, Li W, Yuan Y, Li F, Dewhirst MW, Li CY (2006) Tumor necrosis factor-alpha is a potent endogenous mutagen that promotes cellular transformation. Cancer Res 66(24):11565–11570. doi:10.1158/0008-5472.CAN-06-2540

Yanagawa H, Sone S, Takahashi Y, Haku T, Yano S, Shinohara T, Ogura T (1995) Serum levels of interleukin 6 in patients with lung cancer. Br J Cancer 71(5):1095–1098

Yang H, Bocchetta M, Kroczynska B, Elmishad AG, Chen Y, Liu Z, Bubici C, Mossman BT, Pass HI, Testa JR, Franzoso G, Carbone M (2006) TNF-alpha inhibits asbestos-induced cytotoxicity via a NF-kappaB-dependent pathway, a possible mechanism for asbestos-induced oncogenesis. Proc Natl Acad Sci USA 103(27):10397–10402. doi:10.1073/pnas.0604008103

Ye ZB, Ma T, Li H, Jin XL, Xu HM (2007) Expression and significance of intratumoral interleukin-12 and interleukin-18 in human gastric carcinoma. World J Gastroenterol 13(11):1747–1751

Zeni E, Mazzetti L, Miotto D, Lo Cascio N, Maestrelli P, Querzoli P, Pedriali M, De Rosa E, Fabbri LM, Mapp CE, Boschetto P (2007) Macrophage expression of interleukin-10 is a prognostic factor in nonsmall cell lung cancer. Eur Respir J 30(4):627–632. doi:10.1183/09031936.00129306

Zhan P, Qian Q, Yu LK (2013) Prognostic value of COX-2 expression in patients with non-small cell lung cancer: a systematic review and meta-analysis. J Thoracic Dis 5(1):40–47. doi:10.3978/j.issn.2072-1439.2013.01.02

Zucker S, Lysik RM, Malik M, Bauer BA, Caamano J, Klein-Szanto AJ (1992) Secretion of gelatinases and tissue inhibitors of metalloproteinases by human lung cancer cell lines and revertant cell lines: not an invariant correlation with metastasis. Int J Cancer 52(3):366–371

Chapter 2
The Role of Inflammation in Colon Cancer

Naveena B. Janakiram and Chinthalapally V. Rao

Abstract Colorectal cancer (CRC) is the one of the leading causes of cancer-related deaths in the world. CRC is responsible for more than 600,000 deaths annually and incidence rates are increasing in most of the developing countries. Epidemiological and laboratory investigations suggest that environmental factors such as western style dietary habits, tobacco-smoking, and lack of physical activities are considered as risks for CRC. Molecular pathobiology of CRC implicates pro-inflammatory conditions to promote the tumor malignant progression, invasion, and metastasis. It is well known that patients with inflammatory bowel disease are at higher risk of CRC. Many evidences exist reiterating the link between Inflammation and CRC. Inflammation involves interaction between various immune cells, inflammatory cells, chemokines, cytokines, and pro-inflammatory mediators, such as cyclooxygenase (COX) and lipoxygenase (LOX) pathways, which may lead to signaling towards, tumor cell proliferation, growth, and invasion. Thus, this review will focus on mechanisms by which pro-inflammatory mediators and reactive oxygen/nitrogen species play a role in promoting CRC. Based on these mechanisms, various preventive strategies, involving anti-inflammatory agents, such as COX inhibitors, COX-LOX inhibitors, iNOS inhibitors, natural supplements/agents, and synthetic agents, that blocks the inflammatory pathways and suppress CRC are discussed in this review.

N. B. Janakiram (✉) · C. V. Rao (✉)
Center for Cancer Prevention and Drug Development, Department of Medicine, Hematology Oncology Section, PCS Cancer Center, University of Oklahoma Health Sciences Center, Oklahoma City, OK 73104, USA
e-mail: naveena-janakirram@ouhsc.edu

C. V. Rao
e-mail: cv-rao@ouhsc.edu

B. B. Aggarwal et al. (eds.), *Inflammation and Cancer*, Advances in Experimental Medicine and Biology 816, DOI: 10.1007/978-3-0348-0837-8_2, © Springer Basel 2014

Abbreviations

CRC	Colorectal cancer
CAC	Colitis-associated cancer
IBD	Inflammatory bowel disease
NSAIDs	Non-steroidal anti-inflammatory drugs
NK	Natural killer cells
DC	Dendritic cells
ACF	Aberrant crypt foci
T reg	T regulatory cells
5-ASA	5-aminosalicylic acid
MCP-1	Monocytes chemo attractant protein 1
PGE_2	Prostaglandin E_2
IL-8	Interleukin-8
IL-6	Interleukin-6
IL-10	Interleukin 10
TNF-α	Tumor necrosis factor- α
COX-2	Cyclooxygenase-2
PGI_2	Prostaglandin I_2
PGD_2	Prostaglandin D_2
LT	Leukotriene
HPETE	Hydroperoxyeicosatetraenoic acid
EETs	Epoxy-eicosatrienoic acids
EPA	Eicosapentaenoic acid
DHA	Decosahexaenoic acid
PUFAs	Polyunsaturated fatty acids (PUFAs)
LX	Lipoxins
RVs	Resolvins
AOM	Azoxymethane
NO	Nitric oxide
NF-κB	Nuclear factor–κB
MMP	Matrix metalloproteinase
PI3K	Phosphatidylinositol 3-kinase
mPGES	Microsomal prostaglandin E synthase
VEGF	Vascular endothelial growth factor
FLAP	Five lox activating protein
DP1	PGD_2 receptor
ROS	Reactive oxygen species
RNS	Reactive nitrogen species
NO	Nitric oxide
iNOS	Inducible nitric oxide synthase
nNOS	Neuronal nitric oxide synthase
eNOS	Endothelial nitric oxide synthase
APC	Adenomatous polyposis coli
LPS	Lipopolysaccharide

IL-1β	Interleukin-1β
AA	Arachidonic acid
NO-NSAID	NO-releasing NSAID
IL-4	Interleukin 4
COXibs	COX-2-specific inhibitors
FAP	Familial adenomatous polyposis
L-NAME	*L*-nitro arginine methyl ester
Se-PBIT	Selenium [*S,S'*-1,4-phenylene*bis*(1,2-ethanediyl) *bis*-isothiourea]
GI	Gastrointestinal
MIP	Macrophage inflammatory protein
MCP	Monocytes chemo attractant protein
ABC	ATP-binding cassette
DMH	Dimethyl hydrazine
MDFs	Mucin depleted foci
DSS	Dextran sulfate sodium
EPA-FFA	Eicosapentaenoic acid-free fatty acid
ONA	Oleanolic acid
OT	18α-olean-12-ene-3β-23,28-triol
18*R*-*Rv*E1	5,12,18*R*-trihydroxy-EPA
LXA_4	lipoxins A_4
ABC	ATP-binding cassette

2.1 Colorectal Cancer: A Major Health Problem

Colorectal cancer (CRC) is one of the leading causes of cancer-related deaths in the United States (US). Early diagnosis, though, often can lead to a complete cure. Each year, worldwide more than 1.2 million cases are diagnosed with about 600,000 deaths. CRC is the third most common cancer diagnosed in both men and women in the US and the fourth most common cause of cancer mortality worldwide (Tenesa and Dunlop 2009). It is the second most common cause of cancer deaths in the US. Overall, the lifetime risk of developing CRC is ~6 %. As per American Cancer Society statistics, it is expected to cause about 50,830 deaths during 2013 (ACS). Most of the CRC cases are sporadic and about 25 % are linked to genetic disorders. The majority of CRC cases are linked to environmental factors, including diet, exercise, weight, food borne mutagens, intestinal commensals, and chronic intestinal inflammation, which precedes tumor development.

2.2 Inflammatory Bowel Disease as Risk Factor for Colorectal Cancer

Inflammatory bowel disease (IBD) may lead to colitis-associated cancer (CAC), which is a usually difficult-to-treat cancer having high mortality (Feagins et al. 2009). It is reported that more than 20 % of IBD patients develop cancer and 50 % of these will die of colon cancer (Lakatos and Lakotos 2008). These patients are reported to have increased inflammatory infiltration and increased expression of inflammatory genes (Atreya and Neurath 2008; Atreya et al. 2008; Waldner and Neurath 2008; Clevers 2004). A higher risk for colon cancer is observed in IBD patients who have a family history of CRC (Askling et al. 2001). This increased risk suggests an overlap of signaling pathways and mechanisms that drive cancer development in CAC and CRC. Anti-inflammatory therapy has been reported to reduce the risk or prevent CRC and colitis-related CRC in several observational studies. Non-steroidal anti-inflammatory drugs (NSAIDs) have been reported to reduce colorectal neoplasia by 40–50 % (Thun et al. 1991; Smalley and Dubois 1997) and also have been reported to reduce CRC mortality odds by 49 % in a population of US military veterans with IBD (Bansal and Sonnenberg 1996). A recent meta-analysis of 9 observational studies reported that use of 5-aminosalicylic acid (5-ASA), mesalamine reduced the odds of colitis-related CRC by 49 % (Velayos et al. 2006). It is noteworthy that anti-inflammatory drugs such as 5-aminosalicylate-based compounds have remained in the mainstream for the treatment of IBD patients for >50 years. The findings in the human studies confirm observations in animal models, which show that NSAIDs reduce the occurrence of intestinal neoplasia. More than 90 % of 110 preclinical animal studies examining the effects of NSAIDs on tumorigenesis reported an anti-neoplastic effect (Hawk and Levin 2005). The large volume of compelling data on the use of anti-inflammatory agents/NSAIDs to reduce the risk of CRC suggests a potential role of inflammation in CRC.

2.3 Inflammation in CRC

Inflammation is driven by the accumulation of various immune and inflammatory cells and soluble inflammatory mediators, such as cytokines, chemokines, growth factors, lipid molecules, reactive oxygen, and nitrogen species. The interaction between these immune and inflammatory cells and cytokines leads to generation of autocrine and paracrine signals that foster tumor cell progression, growth, and metastases. A clear link exits between inflammation and CRC. Even CRC that is linked to genetic mutations shows a contribution from inflammation to tumor development, as shown by the decreased CRC mortality with regular use of NSAIDs. These data strongly support a pro-tumorigenic role of inflammation in colon cancer. Various factors can influence the initiation of inflammation and establishment of CRC.

2.4 Role of Immune and Inflammatory Cells in CRC

Pathological analysis of CRC shows infiltration with various types of cells that function in innate immunity, such as neutrophils, mast cells, natural killer (NK) cells, dendritic cells (DC), and tumor-associated macrophages (Atreya and Neurath 2008).

These cells help in anti-tumor immune responses by suppressing tumor growth and angiogenesis. They also help to recruit and interact with other cells involved in adaptive immune responses. Collectively, these responses lead to a balancing of immune surveillance with tumor-promoting inflammatory functions. Immune surveillance helps in early detection of aberrant crypt foci (ACF) and elimination of aberrant cells, which may progress into adenomas and adenocarcinomas in CRC. However, when a chronic inflammation persists, it creates an environment that outcompetes immune surveillance mechanisms and creates a microenvironment that favors inhibition of anti-tumor immune responses and leads to formation of tolerogenic DCs and infiltration of T regulatory cells (T reg), which help in establishment of tumor cell growth. T reg infiltration is associated with bad prognosis (Erdman et al. 2005; Dunn et al. 2004). Thus, it is necessary to design drugs and standardize doses that will inhibit only tumor-promoting immune responses and will spare tumor-inhibiting responses.

2.5 Resolution of Inflammation and Pro-Inflammatory Mediators in CRC

Macrophages accumulate at the site of inflammation or injury and are activated by the cytokines interleukin-10 (IL-10), tumor necrosis factor-α (TNF-α), and monocytes chemoattractant protein (MCP-1). Neutrophils follow for resolution of inflammation. Eventually, fibroblasts play a role in tissue repair by secreting pro-inflammatory cytokines such as interleukin-6 (IL-6), interleukin-8 (IL-8), and prostaglandin E_2 (PGE_2), which will help in the neutrophil response. Epithelial cells and stromal cells together help in repairing/healing the wound. Resolution of inflammation by recruitment of neutrophils can lead to complete remission of inflammation and stop the aberrant proliferation, which can extend into tumor growth. However, if this active process of resolution of inflammation is impaired, the on-going tissue repair eventually may lead to chronic inflammation, which predisposes to cancer. Cyclooxygenase (COX) and lipoxygenase (LOX) pathways and persisting inflammatory cells are involved in generating pro-inflammatory lipid mediators and gene responses, creating a favorable microenvironment that eventually can lead to tumor cell growth, proliferation, and metastases.

2.6 Role of Inflammatory Bioactive Arachidonic Acid Lipid Metabolites in CRC

Arachidonic acid (AA) is an omega-6 polyunsaturated fatty acid (PUFA) present in the phospholipids of cell membranes. It acts as a precursor for production of various eicosanoids usually generated by three enzymes: COX, LOX, and cytochrome p450. The metabolites formed by action of COX and LOX are prostaglandin I_2

(PGI_2), prostaglandin D_2 (PGD_2), PGE_2 and thromboxane A_4 and Leukotrienes (LT)-A_4, C_4, D_4 and B_4, respectively. The LOX metabolites involve hydroperoxyeicosatetraenoic acids (HPETE) such as 5-HPETE, 12-HPETE, and 15-HPETE. The metabolites of P450 are epoxy-eicosatrienoic acids (EETs) resulting in four regioisomeric EETs (5,6-EET, 8,9-EET, 11,12-EET, and 14,15-EET). The other metabolites that play a role during inflammatory processes are omega-3FAs [eicosapentaenoic acid (EPA) and decosahexaenoic acid (DHA)] derived from PUFAs. The other important bioactive molecules derived from these intermediates are lipoxins (LX) and resolvins (RVs). Unlike some of the COX and LOX metabolites, these bioactive molecules display potent anti-inflammatory, immunoregulatory, pro-resolving and anti-tumorigenic properties.

2.6.1 Role of Inflammatory Lipid Molecules Derived from the COX-2 Pathway in CRC

COX-2 is the inducible COX gene that mediates prostaglandin synthesis and pro-inflammatory functions. The expression of COX-2 is elevated in 50 % of adenomas and in 85 % of adenocarcinomas. In human intestinal tumors, COX-2 is expressed in epithelial and stromal cells; it usually is induced by interleukin 1β (IL-1β) and TNF-α. Over-expression of COX-2 increased azoxymethane (AOM)-induced tumor formation (Al-Salihi et al. 2009); and COX-2 deficiency significantly diminished tumorigenesis in mouse models of colon cancer (Chulada et al. 2000a, b; Oshima et al. 1996a, b), confirming a role for COX-2 in tumorigenesis. The pro-inflammatory and pro-tumorigenic effects of COX-2 are mediated by its major end product, PGE_2, which stimulates tumor cell proliferation/growth, angiogenesis, and survival and inhibits apoptosis in CRC (Wang and Dubois 2006; Castellone et al. 2006). PGE_2 activates a number of oncogenic signaling pathways, including β-catenin/transcription factors (TCF), Ras, and the phosphatidylinositol 3-kinase (PI3K) pathways. The generation of microsomal prostaglandin E synthase (mPGES-1)-deficient mice has revealed a dominant role of this enzyme in PGE_2 generation relevant to promotion of inflammation (Trebino et al. 2003). The mPGES-1-derived-PGE_2 exhibits similar inflammatory responses during tumor growth. mPGES-1 deficiency was linked to reduced vascular endothelial growth factor (VEGF). Together, these findings show that deletion or inhibition of mPGES-1 markedly reduces inflammatory responses in mouse models and eventually may lead to inhibition of tumor cell proliferation.

PGD_2, another important metabolite of COX-2, appears to be a negative regulator of tumorigenesis; it has been demonstrated to possess anti-tumor properties (Murata et al. 2008). It is produced locally by inflammatory cells at sites of inflammation; and its receptor (DP1) also is expressed highly in tumor endothelial cells. The DP1 receptor is expressed on DCs that play a key role in initiating an adaptive immune response to foreign antigens (Hammad et al. 2003). These studies suggest that different COX-2-derived prostaglandins have opposing effects on inflammation and tumor cell proliferation and that selective modulation of these prostaglandins may prevent tumor growth in CRC.

2.6.2 *Role of Lipid Molecules Derived from the LOX Pathway in Inflammation and CRC*

Among the LOX pathways, 5-LOX and 12-LOX pathways are closely related to inflammation and carcinogenesis; however, metabolites from another LOX pathway, 15-LOX are linked positively and shown to inhibit inflammation and carcinogenesis. A number of reports suggest the involvement of 5-LOX in early stages of CRC (Qiao et al. 1995; Bortuzzo et al. 1996; Avis et al. 2001; Ding et al. 2003; Tong et al. 2005). Hong et al. (1999) reported high expression of 5-LOX and 5-LOX-activating protein in cancer cell lines. High expression of 5-LOX and its receptors was observed in CRC patients showing poor prognosis (Ohd et al. 2003). Accumulation of 5-HETE and LT upon activation of 5-LOX resulted in cancer cell proliferation (Ding et al. 1999). COX and LOX pathways are both linked in such a way that disturbance in one pathway may lead to over-expression of the other pathway; thus, balanced inhibition of these two pathways is favorable for inhibiting CRC (Byrum et al. 1997; Griffiths et al. 1997; Goulet et al. 1994). Many studies have suggested that removal of 5-LOX and 5-LOX-activating protein (FLAP) results in increased expression of COX metabolites (Byrum et al. 1997; Goulet et al. 1994). These studies provide evidence for an important role of 5-LOX in CRC and suggest the potential for chemoprevention and treatment for CRC. Thus, targeting both COX-2 and 5-LOX pathways together and increasing production of LX and RVs is a better approach for prevention/treatment of CRC.

2.6.3 *Role of Reactive Oxygen and Nitrogen Species in Inflammation and CRC*

Inflammation also is associated with generation of reactive oxygen species (ROS) and reactive nitrogen species (RNS). Free radicals are known to be involved in carcinogenesis (Goldstein and Witz 1990; Cerutti 1985). Inflammatory phagocytic cells make ROS. $O_2^{\cdot -}$ is the initial ROS and undergoes sequential metabolic changes that generate other species (i.e., OH, OCl^-, and H_2O_2). Usually, these reactive species lead to mutations in DNA that may be mutagenic and involved in the etiology of cancer (Babbs 1990). A significant increased expression in ROS was reported by Haklar et al. (2001) in patient colon tumors.

The literature in this area generally is consistent with the view that the enhanced production of ROS and bioavailability of nitric oxide (NO) that accompany an inflammatory response play pivotal roles in mediating formation of microvessels during tumor growth. Activated inflammatory cells produce ROS and reactive nitrogen intermediates that can induce DNA damage and mutation in adjacent epithelial cells. These changes can stimulate ROS production within the epithelial cells may cause epigenetic silencing of tumor suppressor genes (Meira et al. 2008; Westbrook et al. 2009). The discovery of NO as a product of immune system cells has implicated this chemical in the mechanism of carcinogenesis (Tamir and Tannenbaus 1996). Produced NO can interact with $O_2^{\cdot -}$ resulting in the propagation of the highly reactive species peroxynitrite (Oshima and Bartsch 1994). Peroxynitrite, which is formed from the reaction between $O_2^{\cdot -}$ and NO, reacts with all classes of biomolecules and thereby is thought to be involved in many pathologic phenomena (Bartosz 1996). NO and peroxynitrite concentrations were reported to be increased in cancerous samples (Haklar et al. 2001). NO is produced by three isoforms of nitric oxide synthase (NOS) [neuronal nitric oxide synthase (nNOS), endothelial nitric oxide synthase (eNOS), and inducible NOS (iNOS)]. nNOS and eNOS are constitutive NOS isoforms, whereas iNOS is induced upon exposure to inflammatory stimulation. iNOS is expressed in many cells: extravascular resident leukocytes (macrophages), intravascular and/or infiltrating leukocytes (neutrophils and monocytes), endothelium, and parenchymal cells, including intestinal epithelium. Its production is stimulated by lipopolysaccharide (LPS), TNF-α, or interleukin-1β (IL-1β). The role of NO in colon cancer is controversial. Increased production of NO for a limited time is considered to produce positive results in inhibiting CRC, whereas chronic and continuous production of NO produced by iNOS is implicated in neoplastic transformation, a very crucial step during carcinogenesis. Studies with iNOS knockout mice suggested a positive role for iNOS in inducing polyps in adenomatous polyposis coli (APC) min/+ mice (Hofseth et al. 2003; Crowell et al. 2003; Ahn and Ohshima 2001; Nam et al. 2004). High expression of iNOS in CRC xenografts suggested an inhibitory role for iNOS in tumor growth (Xu et al. 2002). In various preclinical studies in animal models, we noted that iNOS inhibitors show promise for inhibiting CRC (Rao et al. 1999, 2002). In summary, both increased expression and decreased expression of NO is observed to have beneficial effects on CRC. Carefully designed, detailed studies to understand the role of NO during inflammation are necessary in order to understand how to modulate its effects in CRC. Interactions between NO and COX-2 are well documented, and combinations of iNOS inhibitors and COX-2 inhibitors have provided inhibition of invasive adenocarcinomas in animal models of colon cancer (Janakiram and Rao 2012).

2.7 Anti-inflammatory Agents in Prevention of CRC

Since it is evident that inflammation is a significant contributor to CRC, anti-inflammatory agents, both from synthetic and natural origin, have gained importance for use in prevention and treatment of CRC. As mentioned previously, NSAIDs are the main anti-inflammatory agents shown to possess anti-tumorigenic properties. They function by inhibiting AA-related pathways and by enhancing immune responses against tumor development. iNOS inhibitors also have gained importance as anti-inflammatory agents in CRC and in other cancers. CRC is associated with lower consumption of fruits and vegetables and greater consumptions of fatty foods implicated in causing CRC, thus natural constituents in these and other foods may contribute to reduce cancer risk or prevention. Here, we discuss various synthetic and natural bioactive compounds that can activate or deactivate signaling cascades implicated during tumor development and that may exhibit chemopreventive properties.

2.7.1 Synthetic Anti-Inflammatory Agents for Prevention of CRC

Preclinical and clinical evidences suggest the presence of high levels of prostaglandins, such as PGE_2 as mentioned earlier, which affect tumor cell proliferation by suppressing immune responses (Marnett 1992; Smith 1992). Hence, it is reasonable to use NSAIDs that can suppress the synthesis of these prostaglandins by inhibiting COX enzymes may in turn suppress tumor development and growth in colon.

Epidemiological studies, intervention trials, and animal studies have provided compelling data for inhibition of colorectal carcinogenesis by aspirin and other NSAIDs (Giovannuci 1999; Brown and Dubois 2005). The first epidemiological report suggested use of aspirin to decrease risk for CRC (Kune et al. 1988). Most of the subsequent case–control studies and prospective studies supported these results (Thun et al. 1991; Freedman et al. 1998; La Vecchia et al. 1977; Muscat et al. 1994; Peleg et al. 1994; Suh et al. 1993; Giovannucci et al. 1994; Schreinemachers and Everson 1994; Chan et al. 2005). The relative risks were very consistent in reducing the risk to 50 % in aspirin users compared with non-aspirin users. Studies on precursors of CRC such as adenomatous polyps have shown similarly decreased risks (Suh et al. 1993; Greenberg et al. 1993; Logan et al. 1993; Martinez et al. 1995). Whereas, the risk reduction of CRC is linked to the dose intake and also the duration of aspirin use which is explored in a subset of studies. Across-study comparisons indicate a dose—response relationship between aspirin and CRC or other cancer types (Harris et al. 2005). A greatest risk reduction was seen among women who took more than two aspirin tablets daily reported by the Nurses' Health Study support a strong dose—response relationship with colon cancer (Chan et al. 2005). Ten years of consistent aspirin use seems to be having reduced risks of CRC which is evidenced and seems consistent (Chan et al. 2005). Further, the role of NSAIDs/aspirin use is substantially strengthened in secondary prevention for reduction of metachronous lesions among patients with primary colorectal adenomas or CRC by two randomized controlled trials. In this trial, aspirin had a modest effect on patients with previous adenomas in reducing the risk of developing new adenomas or cancer that differed by dose. In this study, a lower dose (81 mg/day) showed better response of 19 % reduced risk of adenomas than a higher dose (325 mg/day) (Sandler et al. 2003; Baron et al. 2003). Aspirin use as a chemopreventive agent is strongly supported by these trails against colorectal carcinogenesis among individuals with a known increased risk as a result of previous disease.

We and others have previously shown that several COX inhibitors, such as indomethacin, piroxicam, aspirin, ibuprofen, and sulindac suppress colon carcinogenesis in AOM-induced F344 rats (Reddy et al. 1993, 1987; Metzger et al. 1984; Narisawa

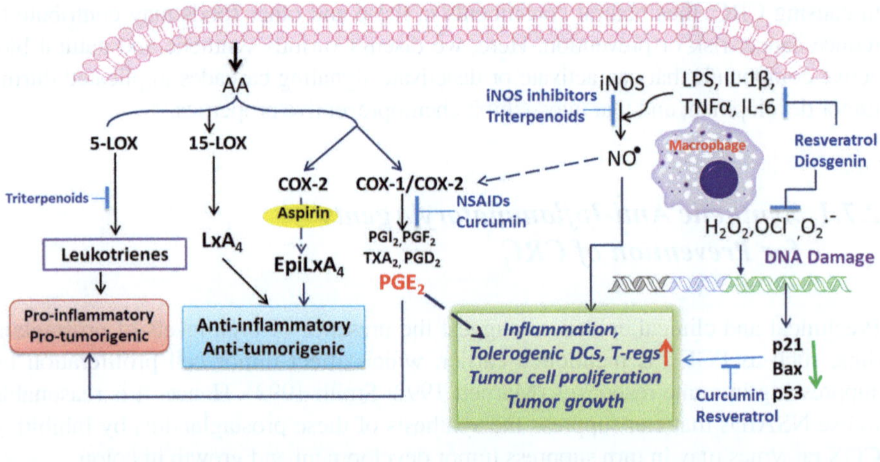

Fig. 2.1 The figure depicts the various pathways observed which initiates inflammation and tumor cell proliferation. Arachidonic acid metabolism leads to formation of both pro-inflammatory and anti-inflammatory metabolites. 5-LOX pathway leads to formation of leukotrienes which are known for their pro-inflammatory and pro-tumorigenic role. Triterpenoids are reported to show inhibitory effects on formation of leukotrienes. COX-2 in the presence of aspirin will lead to formation of epilipoxins (*epiLXA*$_4$), which are anti-inflammatory and anti-tumorigenic in functions. Naturally 5-LOX pathway leads to formation of lipoxins, which show similar functions as that of epiLXA$_4$. COX-1 and COX-2 pathway leads to the formation of eicosanoids, PGI_2, PGF_2, TXA_2, PGD_2, and PGE_2. PGE_2 has been found to play a vital role during inflammation, development of Tregs, formation of tolerogenic DCs, tumor cell proliferation, and growth. NSAIDs and natural agent like curcumin are reported to have inhibitory effects on the formation of eicosanoids. LPS, IL-1β, and TNF-α are known to be involved in formation of nitric oxide (*NO*), and IL-6 is a known inflammatory cytokine involved during tumorigenesis. NO formed can initiate the inflammation and tumor formation by itself or by interacting COX-2 pathway. iNOS inhibitors and triterpenoids are shown to inhibit NO formation, and resveratrol and diosgenin inhibit pro-inflammatory cytokines. The free radical formation by macrophages which can cause DNA damage and eventually tumor cell proliferation by down-regulating p21, p53, and BAX are observed. Curcumin and resveratrol are reported to restore p21, p53, and p53 and inhibit tumor cell proliferation

et al. 1993; Pollard and Luckert 1984; Moorghen et al. 1988). Indomethacin was reported to inhibit tumor growth in chemically induced large-bowel tumors in rats (Kudo et al. 1980). Similar results were observed in other preclinical studies (Pollard and Luckert 1980, 1981; Narisawa et al. 1981). Due to GI toxicities of indomethacin, we developed and tested a potentially less toxic derivative, NO-indomethecin, in AOM-induced carcinoma models. Nitric oxide-releasing non-steroidal anti-inflammatory drugs (NO-NSAID) are promising chemoprevention agents; unlike conventional NSAIDs, they seem to be free of appreciable adverse effects, while they retain the beneficial activities of their parent compounds. NO-indomethecin significantly suppressed AOM-induced tumor multiplicity and incidence in F344 rats (Rao et al. 2006). Its activity is related to suppression of COX, iNOS, and β-catenin levels (Fig. 2.1).

Rigau et al. (1991) have demonstrated that colon mucosal samples from patients on long-term sulindac therapy have a reduced PG-biosynthetic capacity. In a randomized, placebo-controlled, double-blind crossover study in patients with familial adenomatous polyposis (FAP), administration of sulindac at a dose of 300 mg/day for 6–12 months caused disappearance of all polyps (Laybayle et al. 1991). Most of the clinical trials with FAP patients on long-term treatment with sulindac reported a reduction in the number and size of adenomas (Belliveau and Graham 1984; Waddel et al. 1989; Laybayle et al. 1991; Spagnesi et al. 1994; Winde et al. 1993; Giardello et al. 1993). Dietary administration of sulindac inhibited dimethyl hydrazine (DMH)-induced colon tumor incidence and multiplicity in mice (Moorghen et al. 1998; Skinner et al. 1991). In these experiments, sulindac was administered along with DMH throughout the study; however, administration of sulindac to mice seventeen weeks after DMH administration showed no reduction in colon tumor growth or development. Oral administration of sulindac (10 mg/kg) twice daily inhibited DMH-induced primary colon tumor development and growth in rats. Ahnen et al. (1994) showed that dietary administration of sulindac and its metabolite sulindac sulfone significantly inhibited AOM-induced colon carcinogenesis in F344 rats. We found that sulindac was effective at both initiation and postinitiation stages of colon tumor formation in F344 rats (Rao et al. 1995). This study suggested that its inhibitory function may be due to its modulatory effects on AA metabolism. In another study by Suh et al. (2011), the NSAIDs sulindac and naproxen, individually and in combination with atorvastatin, caused significant reduction in AOM-induced colon tumors in F344 rats. The NSAID-fed animals showed reduction in inflammatory markers iNOS and COX-2 as well as in phospho-p65 and in the pro-inflammatory cytokines TNF-α, IL-1β, and interleukin 4 (IL-4). Hence, use of NSAIDs in combination with statins was suggested for retaining efficacy with less/no GI toxicity.

The concern over gastric toxicity associated with aspirin use led to efforts to develop COX-2-specific inhibitors (COXibs such as rofecoxib, celecoxib) (Gupta and Dubois 2001). Available literature provides strong evidence for a role of COX-2 in inflammation and carcinogenesis. Several studies using COX-2 knockout or disrupted genes in mouse models of FAP or in chemically induced colon carcinogenesis in rats indicated that COX-2 selective inhibitors, such as rofecoxib and celecoxib, inhibit formation of intestinal adenomas (Dannenberg et al. 2005; Rao and Reddy 2004; Oshima et al. 1996a, b, 2001; Chulada et al. 2000a, b; Jacoby et al. 2000; Boolbol et al. 1996; Mahmoud et al. 1998; Kawamori et al. 1998; Reddy and Rao 2002). In a clinical trial, FAP patients treated twice daily with 400 or 200 mg celecoxib had 31 and 12 % reduction, respectively, in polyp number (Arber et al. 2006). In this clinical trial, celecoxib, at a dose of 400 mg daily, reduced advanced adenoma formation in the colon by almost 50 % compared with the placebo through a 3-year treatment period (Arbor et al. 2006). Although introduction of COXibs was successful in reducing GI toxicity, these drugs were associated with cardiovascular toxicity due to high selectivity toward COX-2 (Smith et al. 2000; Silverstein et al. 2000; Laine et al. 2003; Bresalier et al. 2005; Nussmeier et al. 2005; Solomon et al. 2005). An initial study indicated possible increases in the incidence of myocardial infarction with use of COXibs (Bombardier et al. 2000). No randomized controlled trials specifically to address the issue of cardiovascular toxicity were conducted; but trials were initiated to test the efficacy of COXibs in the prevention of metachronous colonic polyps (Bresalier et al. 2005; Solomon et al. 2005) and the management of postoperative pain (Nussmeier et al. 2005). The above-mentioned trials suggested that patients using these COX-2 inhibitors were showing cardiovascular events. These observations led to temporary withdrawal of COXibs from the US market in 2004. The findings suggest that this cardiovascular toxicity is specific to this class of drugs; but aspirin and other non-specific COX-2 inhibitors still have potential for chemoprevention of CRC.

In February 2005, the Food and Drug Administration (FDA) Advisory Committee meeting recommended that COXibs remain on the market, but with warnings added to labels (Alberts et al. 2005). The committee agreed that since celecoxib is the least likely to be associated with adverse cardiovascular events, it is the most appropriate COXib to study for the prevention and treatment of cancer. Complicating the risk—benefit evaluation are individual differences in both cancer risk and sensitivity to toxic events. The development of very low non-toxic doses of COXibs or COX and LOX-inhibiting regimens in combination with other agents continues. Licofelone (ML3000) is the first member of a new dual COX/5-LOX inhibitor class and currently is under evaluation as a treatment for osteoarthritis. A multicenter study explored the effects of licofelone in comparison with naproxen as a disease-modifying agent and showed beneficial effects on cartilage. Although phase III trials have been completed successfully, no dates for regulatory submission have been given for this drug. Its safety profile shows fewer GI events than NSAIDs and selective COX-2 inhibitors (Martel-Pelletier et al. 2003; Cicero et al. 2005; Moreau et al. 2005; Bias et al. 2004). We tested licofelone in $APC^{Min/+}$ mice and found it to possess potential chemopreventive properties (Mohammed et al. 2011). The efficacy achieved with licofelone was comparable to or more effective than several NSAIDs and the COX-2-selective inhibitors celecoxib and rofecoxib (Swamy et al. 2006; Jacoby et al. 1996; Rao and Reddy 2004; Rao et al. 2000; Orner et al. 2003). This result suggests that a balanced inhibition of COX and LOX pathways is a better approach to obtain diminished side effects with high efficacy. The beneficial effects of NSAIDs in chemoprevention of CRC suggest that inflammatory mechanisms are playing a vital role in tumor development, with strongest for colorectal cancer. Future work to understand the molecular mechanisms still is needed to establish the chemopreventive potential of NSAIDs for use as a preventive for and treatment of CRC.

2.7.2 Role of iNOS Inhibitors in Prevention of CRC

High NOS activity and high levels of NO are observed in AOM-induced colonic tumors in rats (Rao et al. 1999, 2002), in Crohn's disease (Rachmilewitz et al. 1995) and in ulcerative colitis (Colon et al. 2000). Over-expression of NO was observed in preneoplastic colon lesions and also in human colon adenocarcinomas (Hao et al. 2001; Yagihashi et al. 2000; Lagares-Garcia et al. 2001; Szaleczky et al. 2000). High iNOS levels were observed in colons of animals fed a high-fat diet, suggesting a role of high-fat diets in inducing inflammatory conditions and CRC in humans (Wan et al. 2000). Collectively, these studies support a positive role of iNOS in inducing CRC and use of iNOS-inhibiting agents for suppressing the iNOS activity and its tumorigenic effects (Fig. 2.1).

S,S-1,4-phenylene-*bis*(1,2-ethanediyl)*bis*-isothiourea, PBIT a selective iNOS inhibitor, caused suppression of ACF development in rats by reducing protein levels of j; and iNOS in colonic mucosa (Rao et al. 1999). Kawamori et al. (2000) reported similar results with *L*-nitro arginine methyl ester (L-NAME), an *L*-arginine inhibitor on the development of ACF induced by AOM in rats. Animals that received 100 ppm of L-NAME for 11 weeks showed 32 % inhibition of ACF multiplicity. To increase the potency of PBIT with lower concentrations, a isosteric analog of PBIT, selenium [*S,S′*-1,4-phenylene*bis*(1,2-ethanediyl) *bis*-isothiourea] (Se-PBIT) was developed and tested recently, in colon cancer animal model. We reported chemopreventive properties of Se-PBIT on ACFs induced by AOM in rats (Janakiram et al. 2013). We have studied extensively the role of iNOS inhibitors in colon carcinogenesis (Rao et al. 2002; Rao 2004). We tested iNOS-selective inhibitors individually and in combination with COX inhibitors and found that low-dose combinations of the COX-2 inhibitor celecoxib and the iNOS inhibitor SC-51 inhibited AOM-induced crypt formation in rats (Rao 2004). L-NAME and iNOS-specific inhibitors have been reported to have inhibitory effects on formation of adenomas, adenocarcinomas (Kawamori et al. 2000; Schleiffer et al. 2000), and adenomatous polyps (Ahn and Ohshima 2001). NO signaling cascades also are involved in the migration of tumor cells. More detailed studies into role of NO at different doses and during different stages of tumor development are necessary for design of better iNOS inhibitors for prevention and treatment of CRC.

2.7.3 Natural Anti-Inflammatory Agents for Prevention of CRC

Epidemiologic evidence supports the benefit of changes in dietary and exercise patterns for CRC prevention. Among well-known dietary agents, curcumin has been valued for more than 5,000 years for its medicinal properties and for its warm, peppery flavor. Curcumin is one of the curcuminoids of turmeric. Curcumin is a highly pleiotropic molecule capable of interacting with numerous molecular targets involved in inflammation. It is reported to interact with inflammatory processes by down-regulating COX-2, 5-LOX, iNOS and also production of inflammatory cytokines such as TNF-α, IL-1, -2, -6, -8 and -12, and also macrophage inhibitory protein (MIP), monocytes chemoattractant protein (MCP), and matrix metalloproteinases (MMPs) (Goel et al. 2008; Abe et al.

1999) (Fig. 2.1). Curcumin was found to be effective in reducing colitis induced by 1,4,6-trinitrobenzene sulfonic acid. Ukil et al. (2003) reported reduced levels of NO and O2 radicals and suppression of NF-κB activation in curcumin-treated colonic mucosa. We reported chemopreventive properties of curcumin (2,000 ppm) in inhibiting development of ACF and colon adenocarcinomas in AOM-induced F344 rats (Rao et al. 1995). Dietary administration of curcumin resulted in >50 % inhibition of AOM-induced colon adenocarcinoma incidence and multiplicity. Kawamori et al. (1999) reported a 78 % suppression of progression from adenoma to adenocarcinoma in a preclinical animal model with a high dose (6,000 ppm) of curcumin. Curcumin has been tested in combination with green tea catechins, another class of natural agents, and also in combination with the synthetic COX-2 inhibitor celecoxib for increased efficacy with low doses or to increase its bioavailability for better efficacy (Xu et al. 2010; Shpitz et al. 2006).

Although curcumin is well known for its anti-inflammatory and anti-tumorigenic properties in preclinical animal models, the absorption required for achieving its anti-tumor properties is still a concern. Clinical trials to assess pharmacokinetics, metabolism, and systemic bioavailability in cancer patients are inconclusive. Cheng et al. (2001) conducted a phase 1 clinical trial on cancer patients and reported poor absorption and minimal serum concentrations of curcumin. Another phase 1 study reported similar poor absorption of curcumin in patients (Sharma et al. 2004). However, Garcea et al. (2005) reported pharmacologically efficacious levels of curcumin (12.7 ± 5.7 nmol/g) in both malignant colorectal tissue and normal colorectal tissue (7.7 ± 1.8 nmol/g) from CRC patients, suggesting a potential anti-tumorigenic role for curcumin in CRC. Three other clinical trials have investigated the use of curcumin (curcumin, demethoxycurcumin, or bisdemethoxycurcumin) therapy in patients with established CRC and reported a decrease in carcinogenic embryonic antigen and PGE_2 levels (Sharma et al. 2001, 2004). Another trial of curcumin in CRC patients required high doses (3.6 g daily) to observe any effects on oxidative DNA adducts, and COX-2 markers (Garcea et al. 2005). In that study, no change in COX-2 protein was observed. Additional studies are in progress to develop curcumin formulations, analogs, and tumor site delivery methods to increase bioavailability for prevention and treatment of CRC.

Piperine, the principle bioactive compound of *Piper nigrum* and *Piper longum*, is included in many traditional formulae to enhance the effectiveness of other bioactive compounds, such as curcumin. Piperine has been reported to have immunomodulatory, anti-carcinogenic, anti-asthmatic, stimulatory, hepatoprotective, and anti-inflammatory (Darshan and Doreswamy 2004). It was found to be genotoxic but had no adverse effects when tested for toxicity profile in rats at doses 5–20 times the normal human intake (Bhat and Chandrasekhara 1986; Piyachaturawat et al. 1983). Due to its apolar nature, piperine alters lipid dynamics and it changes the conformation of enzymes in the intestine. Due to its unique properties, it is used in combinations to enhance the bioavailability of the other drugs. Its potential to increase the bioavailability of drugs in humans is of great clinical significance (Bajad et al. 2003). Nalini et al. (2006) reported inhibitory effects of piperine on DMH-induced colon tumors in F344 rats. We reported inhibitory effects of piperine on AOM-induced colon tumors in F344 rats. The potential of piperine to enhance the bioavailability of other potent drugs is an important property that can be exploited to increase the efficacy of agents that inhibit CRC.

Another bioactive molecule available in edible fruits is resveratrol. The chemopreventive function of resveratrol was reported by Jang et al. (1997). They showed that it inhibited cellular events associated with the initiation, promotion, and progression of cancer development. A clinical trial with whole grape extract in patients with colon cancer resulted in reduced the expression of Wnt target genes in normal mucosa with no change in colon tissue (Nguyen et al. 2009). These trial results need more careful evaluation because of lack of control for dietary intake of resveratrol-rich food and the absence of control for ingestion of confounding medications. A second trial in 20 selected histologically confirmed CRC patients administered trans-resveratrol during 8 days prior to surgical resection reported a 5 % ($p = 0.05$) reduction in cell proliferation (Patel et al. 2010). The cell proliferation analysis was carried out preintervention and postintervention with resveratrol in tissue samples. These data suggest achievement of high enough concentrations of resveratrol in the intestinal tissues to show some inhibition of cell proliferation. However, some preclinical and clinical studies suggest that bioavailability of resveratrol is low due to poor absorptions as a result of intestinal metabolism and low activity of ATP-binding cassette (ABC) transporters (Juan et al. 2010, 2012; Alfaras et al. 2010a; Walle 2011; Cottart et al. 2010). In a preclinical animal model in which ACF are induced by DMH, an oral dose of 60 mg/kg resveratrol caused 50 % inhibition in the medial and 48 % inhibition in the distal tumors in rats (Alfaras et al. 2010b). Resveratrol also was observed to have inhibitory effects on mucin-depleted foci (MDFs) with reduction of the number of MDFs by 36 and 53 % in the medial and distal colon, respectively (Alfaras et al. 2010b). It also was found to be effective in long-term preclinical assays with development of adenocarcinomas as an end point. Oral administration of resveratrol (0.2 mg/kg in drinking water) for 100 days showed reduced ACFs and colon carcinogenesis in F344 rats (Tessitore et al. 2000). This reduction probably was due to modulation of Bax and p21, which regulate cell proliferation and apoptosis (Fig. 2.1). Daily administration of 8 mg/kg of trans-resveratrol for 30 weeks in DMH-treated rats resulted in reduction in the incidence and multiplicity of ACFs and also decreased formation of multicrypt (more than 6) ACFs (Sengottuvelan and Nalini 2006). Inhibition of ACFs with 6 or more crypts is an indication of potent chemopreventive efficacy via suppressing the progression of preneoplastic lesions to neoplasia. These results suggest that resveratrol possesses chemopreventive properties and can suppress the progression of preneoplasia to malignant neoplasia in colon. This study also reported inhibitory effects of resveratrol on polyamine synthesis, which is high in neoplastic tissues (Sengottuvelan and Nalini 2006).

Resveratrol also has been evaluated for its anti-tumor activity in genetically modified mice. Resveratrol (0.01 % in drinking water) decreased the number of tumors in the small intestine and completely suppressed tumor formation in the colon of $APC^{Min/+}$ mice (Schneider et al. 2001). In contrast to these results,

Ziegler et al. (2004) reported null results with resveratrol in $APC^{Min/+}$ mice. Even though this study used high doses of resveratrol (4, 20, and 90 mg/kg body weight) in pellet form, no difference was observed in incidence of intestinal tumors. Another Apc min mouse study reported a 27 % decrease in adenoma formation by 60 mg/kg of resveratrol administered in the diet (Sale et al. 2005). This reduction was attributed to decreases (of 58 and 62 % compared with intestinal mucosa from mice on control diet) in PGE_2, which is involved in the maintenance of the malignant phenotype (Sale et al. 2005). Evidence from all of these studies suggests that resveratrol has potential prevention and therapeutic properties and needs further evaluation for its dosage and clinical efficacy in CRC.

Diosgenin, a natural steroidal saponin found predominantly in fenugreek and wild yams, has diverse biological properties (Raju and Mehta 2009). The commercial synthesis of steroid products, such as cortisone, pregnenolone, and progesterone, involves use of diosgenin as a precursor (Raju and Mehta 2009). It is considered safe since it is neither synthesized nor metabolically converted into steroid by-products in the mammalian body. In preliminary studies with human subjects, diosgenin has been found to be effective against hyperglycemia (McAnuff et al. 2005), hypercholesterolemia (Juarez-Oropeza et al. 1987; Son et al. 2007), and hypertriacylglycerolemia (Kwon et al. 2003). Significant anti-inflammatory functions have been demonstrated in relevant animal models. It is used in rats to heal the GI toxicity generated by indomethacin treatment. Its anti-inflammatory role has been explored further by Yamada et al. (1997). Preclinical animal studies with AOM-induced ACFs in F344 rats suggested that diosgenin possesses chemopreventive efficacy in CRC. Administration of 0.1 or 0.05 % diosgenin in the diet during initiation, postinitiation, or promotion stages of colon carcinogenesis dose-dependently decreased ACF formation (Raju et al. 2004). Another study investigated the preventive effects of diosgenin (20, 100, or 500 mg/kg) on AOM/dextran sodium sulfate (DSS)-induced CRC in mice. Diosgenin at very low doses significantly inhibited (53, 46, and 40 %, respectively) colonic mucosal ulcers and dysplastic crypts induced by AOM/DSS treatment and also reduced expression of inflammatory cytokine genes, including IL-1β, IL-6, IL-12b, and TNF-α, which are significantly elevated in the colonic mucosa of mice treated with AOM/DSS (Fig. 2.1). These studies suggest that diosgenin is a potent bioactive molecule possessing both anti-inflammatory and anti-tumorigenic properties that make it ideal for further investigation of its molecular and anti-neoplastic functions in human clinical trials.

Triterpenoids are isolated from various medicinal plants and have been studied for their anti-inflammatory properties. Mostly these compounds are non-toxic and have made their way into cosmetics and health products (Liu 1995). Recently, interest in understanding and elucidating the biological roles of triterpenoids for their hepatoprotective, analgesic, anti-tumor, anti-inflammatory, and immunomodulatory effects is increasing (Mahato and Sen 1997; Liu 1995). These agents are broken down in the gut to release triterpene metabolites, which are integrated into the intestinal cell membranes, absorbed, and lead to modulation of signaling pathways. These molecules inhibit expression of inflammatory genes such as

COX-2, iNOS and various inflammatory cytokines that are known enhancers of carcinogenesis (Janakiram et al. 2008; Rao et al. 2002, Raju et al. 2004) (Fig. 2.1). Recently, triterpene analogs that are more potent than the original parent molecules have been synthesized. Kawamori et al. (1995) found that oleanolic acid (ONA), a crude plant extract of triterpenoid at a dose of 200 ppm, was effective in reducing ACF in the intestine of F344 rats. We reported the anti-neoplastic properties of ONA and the analog 18alpha-olean-12-ene-3 beta-23,28-triol (OT) in AOM-induced ACFs in F344 rats (Janakiram et al. 2008). These triterpenoids significantly suppressed carcinogen-induced colonic preneoplastic lesions at dietary doses of 750 and 1,500 ppm of ONA, and 250 and 500 ppm of OT and without any toxicity. ONA inhibited 52 % of total AOM-induced ACFs and ~66 % of ACF with four or more crypts. OT inhibited up to 48 % of total AOM-induced ACF formation and 60 % of ACF with four or more crypts at very low doses compared with those of ONA. These studies support chemopreventive effects of triterpenoids in CRC and suggest that an in-depth evaluation of these agents in clinical trials should be carried out to assess pharmacokinetics, bioavailability, and anti-neoplastic functions.

Epidemiological, experimental, and clinical studies provide evidence for anti-CRC activity of omega (ω)-3 PUFAs. Evidence from animals and humans suggest that ω-3 PUFAs may play an inhibitory role during different stages of CRC, from primary CRC prevention to "tertiary" prevention after treatment of CRC and advanced metastatic disease. Out of 8 reported clinical studies of ω-3 PUFAs supplementation, 6 reported protective effects. In patients with a previous history of sporadic colorectal adenomas, oral supplementation with ω-3 PUFA has resulted in a 13–70 % reduction in intestinal epithelial cell proliferation as compared to placebo groups (Cockbain et al. 2012). A phase III randomized, double-blind, placebo-controlled trial investigated treatment with eicosapentaenoic acid-free fatty acid (EPA-FFA) in 58 patients with FAP who had previously undergone colectomy and ileorectal anastomosis and showed a 22.4 % reduction in polyp number compared with placebo (West et al. 2010). Colon cancer xenograft studies showed consistent protective effects (40–60 % reduction in xenograft size) in mice supplemented with ω-3 PUFAs as compared to untreated mice (Boudreau et al. 2001; Kato et al. 2002; Calviello et al. 2004). Similar beneficial results were reported from studies with CRC cell allograft tumors (Mund et al. 2007; Cannizzo and Broitman 1989; Togni et al. 2003; Pizato et al. 2005). In spite of these encouraging data, no published studies yet have investigated the anti-neoplastic effect of u-3 PUFAs in patients with primary or metastatic CRC.

Fish and fish oil are rich sources of the ω-3 PUFAs EPA and DHA. The metabolites derived from these PUFAs result in formation of 3-series prostaglandins, which are anti-inflammatory rather than pro-inflammatory and also may possess anti-tumor properties. A report of a switch from 2 series PGE_2 to 3 series PGE_3 was demonstrated in colonic mucosa of rats treated with fish oil (Vanamala et al. 2008). The recently discovered anti-inflammatory lipid mediators RVs and LX derived from EPA and DHA are gaining importance for their anti-neoplastic functions. RVs derived from EPA are called as "E" series. Protectins are also generated from precursors of omega 3-PUFAs. RVs or protectins from DHA, named "D" series, possess anti-inflammatory and immunomodulatory properties. The concentration required for these lipid mediators to exhibit any biological activity is in the nanomolar or picomolar range. Acetylation of aspirin by COX-2 in the presence of EPA results in formation of 5,12,18*R*-trihydroxy-EPA (18*R*-*Rv*E1) (Janakiram et al. 2011) (Fig. 2.1). Ingestion of aspirin and EPA generated 18*R*-*Rv*E1 that was detectable in plasma of healthy volunteers (Oh et al. 2011). The anti-inflammatory role of RvE1 is well documented in a mouse model of DSS-induced colitis; it acts through inhibition of phosphorylation of NF-κB (Ishida et al. 2010). Another study reported a protective role of *Rv*E1 in mouse colitis through induction of intestinal alkaline phosphatase (Campbell et al. 2010). EPA and DHA exhibited protective effects against colitis in a rat model by restoring the number of mature, mucin-filled goblet cells (Arita et al. 2005). Two other studies also reported protective effects of *Rv*E1 against colitis induced by DSS and 2, 4, 6-trinitrobenzene sulfonic acid (Nieto et al. 2002; Ishida et al. 2009).

Lipoxin A_4 (LXA_4) was shown to inhibit neutrophil chemotaxis, adherence, transmigration, and activation during resolution of inflammation and suppression of IL-8 production by epithelia and leukocytes and to cause clearing of neutrophils by up-regulation of monocyte ingestion (Serhan 1997, 2002; Canny et al. 2002). Decreased LXA_4 expression was shown in a DSS-induced colitis model (Gewirtz et al. 2002). Protective effects of LXA_4 analogs were observed in DSS and other chemically induced colitis animal models (Gewirtz et al. 2002; Fiorucci et al. 2001). The protective effects of these analogs are attributed for their LXA_4 receptor-mediated inhibitory effects on pro-inflammatory signaling pathways. 15-epi-LXA_4 is formed in the presence of aspirin; and some of the preventive or therapeutic effects of aspirin-like NSAIDs may be through these 15-*epi*-LX (Claria and Serhan 1995) (Fig. 2.1). The anti-inflammatory functions of these lipid mediators suggest a potential chemopreventive therapeutic strategy for inflammation-related diseases like CRC.

2.8 Conclusions

Epidemiological and clinical literature strongly implicates chronic inflammation in neoplastic diseases, especially in CRC. Different inflammatory molecules and signals play different roles during different stages of CRC development. AA metabolism, via COX-2 and 5-LOX pathways, generates a variety of lipid mediators that affect initiation, growth, and development of CRC. Current evidence from preclinical, clinical, and epidemiological studies supports a positive role for anti-inflammatory agents, particularly NSAIDs as inhibitors of CRC; however, these drugs can have GI and cardiovascular toxicities. Additional studies are needed to design analogs or derivatives of these agents, to manipulate doses and to select appropriate patient populations to provide increased safety without losing efficacy for CRC suppression. It also is important to develop other agents that can balance COX and LOX inhibition, including natural agents like curcumin or synthetic agents like licofelone, to achieve safer toxicity profiles while retaining significant inhibition of CRC. Additional natural bioactive anti-inflammatory compounds are being identified to provide beneficial effects against colitis-induced inflammation and CRC. Many of these agents are well tolerated and may provide safe alternatives to existing, more toxic compounds. Increased consumption of EPA- and DHA-rich foods may reduce inflammation and its related CRC conditions. And other novel lipid mediators, such as LX, RVs and their analogs, need to be evaluated in CRC models for their effects on colon mucosal immunity against development of CRC.

Acknowledgements We want to acknowledge the Grant support NCI-R01-94962; NCI-CN-53300 for the work quoted in this chapter and Dr. Julie Sando for her scientific and language editing of this chapter.

References

Abe Y, Hashimoto S, Horie T (1999) Curcumin inhibition of inflammatory cytokine production by human peripheral blood monocytes and alveolar macrophages. Pharmacol Res 39(1):41–47

Ahn B, Ohshima H (2001) Suppression of intestinal polyposis in Apc (Min/+) mice by inhibiting nitric oxide production. Cancer Res 61:8357–8360

Ahnen D, Hixson L, Alberts D, Bogert C, Einspahr K, Brendel P, Gross N, Paranlea R, Pamukeu R (1994) Sulindac and its sulfone metabolite (FGN-1) both inhibit rat colon carcinogenesis but neither inhibit colonic proliferation. Proc Am Assoc Cancer Res 35:631

Alberts DS et al (2005) What happened to the COXibs on the way to the cardiologist? Cancer Epidemiol. Biomarkers Prev 14:555–556

Alfaras I, Juan ME, Planas JM (2010a) Trans-resveratrol reduces precancerous colonic lesions in dimethylhydrazine-treated rats. J Agric Food Chem 58(13):8104–8110

Alfaras I, Pérez M, Juan ME, Merino G, Prieto JG, Planas JM, Alvarez AI (2010b) Involvement of breast cancer resistance protein (BCRP1/ABCG2) in the bioavailability and tissue distribution of trans-resveratrol in knockout mice. J Agric Food Chem 58(7):4523–4528

Al-Salihi MA, Pearman AT, Doan T, Reichert EC, Rosenberg DW, Prescott SM, Stafforini DM, Topham MK (2009) Transgenic expression of cyclooxygenase-2 in mouse intestine epithelium is insufficient to initiate tumorigenesis but promotes tumor progression. Cancer Lett 273(2):225–232

Arber N, Eagle CJ, Spicak J, Rácz I, Dite P, Hajer J, Zavoral M, Lechuga MJ, Gerletti P, Tang J, Rosenstein RB, Macdonald K, Bhadra P, Fowler R, Wittes J, Zauber AG, Solomon SD, Levin B, PreSAP Trial Investigators (2006) Celecoxib for the prevention of colorectal adenomatous polyps. N Engl J Med 355(9):885–895

Arita M, Yoshida M, Hong S, Tjonahen E, Glickman JN, Petasis NA, Blumberg RS, Serhan CN (2005) Proc Natl Acad Sci 102:7671–7676

Askling J, Dickman PW, Karlen P et al (2001) Family history as a risk factor for colorectal cancer in inflammatory bowel disease. Gastroenterology 120:1356–1362

Atreya I, Atreya R, Neurath MF (2008) NF-kappaB in inflammatory bowel disease. J Intern Med 263:591–596

Atreya I, Neurath MF (2008) Immune cells in colorectal cancer: prognostic relevance and therapeutic strategies. Expert Rev Anticancer Ther 8:561–572

Avis I, Hong SH, Martinez A, Moody T, Choi YH, Trepel J et al (2001) Five-lipoxygenase inhibitors can mediate apoptosis in human breast cancer cell lines through complex eicosanoid interactions. J Fed Am Soc Exp Biol 15:2007–2009

Babbs CF (1990) Free radicals and etiology of colon cancer. Free Rad Biol Med 8:191–200
Bajad S, Coumar M, Khajuria R, Suri OP, Bedi KL (2003) Characterization of a new rat urinary metabolite of piperine by LC/NMR/MS studies. Eur J Pharm Sci 19(5):413–421
Bansal P, Sonnenberg A (1996) Risk factors of colorectal cancer in inflammatory bowel disease. Am J Gastroenterol 91(1):44–48
Baron JA et al (2003) A randomized trial of aspirin to prevent colorectal adenomas. N Engl J Med 348:891–899
Bartosz G (1996) Peroxynitrite mediator of the toxic action of nitric oxide. Acta Biochim Polon 43:645–660
Belliveau P, Graham AM (1984) Mesenteric desmoid tumor in Gardener's syndrome treated by sulindac. Dis Colon Rectum 27:53–54
Bhat BG, Chandrasekhara N (1986) Studies on the metabolism of piperine: absorption, tissue distribution and excretion of urinary conjugates in rats. Toxicology 40(1):83–92
Bias P, Buchner A, Klesser B, Laufer S (2004) The gastrointestinal tolerability of the LOX/COX inhibitor, licofelone, is similar to placebo and superior to naproxen therapy in healthy volunteers: results from a randomized, controlled trial. Am J Gastroenterol 99:611–618
Bombardier C et al VIGOR Study Group (2000) Comparison of upper gastrointestinal toxicity of rofecoxib and naproxen in patients with rheumatoid arthritis. N Engl J Med 343:1520–1528
Boolbol SK, Dannenberg AJ, Chadburn A et al (1996) Cyclooxygenase-2 overexpression and tumor formation are blocked by sulindac in a murine model of familial adenomatous polyposis. Cancer Res 56:2556–2560
Bortuzzo C, Hanif R, Kashfi K, Staiano-Coico L, Shiff SJ, Rigas B et al (1996) The effect of leukotrienes B and selected HETEs on the proliferation of colon cancer cells. Biochimica et Biophysical Acta 1300:240–246
Boudreau MD, Sohn KH, Rhee SH, Lee SW, Hunt JD, Hwang DH (2001) Suppression of tumor cell growth both in nude mice and in culture by n-3 polyunsaturated fatty acids: mediation through cyclooxygenase-independent pathways. Cancer Res 61(4):1386–1391
Bresalier RS et al (2005) Cardiovascular events associated with rofecoxib in a colorectal adenoma chemoprevention trial. N Engl J Med 352:1092–1102
Brown JR, DuBois RN (2005) COX-2: a molecular target for colorectal cancer prevention. J Clin Oncol 23:2840–2855
Byrum RS, Goulet JL, Griffiths RJ, Koller BH (1997) Role of the 5-lipoxygenase-activating protein (FLAP) in murine acute inflammatory responses. J Exp Med 185:1065–1075
Calviello G, Di Nicuolo F, Gragnoli S, Piccioni E, Serini S, Maggiano N, Tringali G, Navarra P, Ranelletti FO, Palozza P (2004) n-3 PUFAs reduce VEGF expression in human colon cancer cells modulating the COX-2/PGE_2 induced ERK-1 and -2 and HIF-1alpha induction pathway. Carcinogenesis 25(12):2303–2310
Campbell EL, MacManus CF, Kominsky DJ, Keely S, Glover LE, Bowers BE, Scully M, Bruyninckx WJ, Colgan SP (2010) Resolvin E1-induced intestinal alkaline phosphatase promotes resolution of inflammation through LPS detoxification. Proc Natl Acad Sci U S A 107(32):14298–14303
Cannizzo F Jr, Broitman SA (1989) Post promotional effects of dietary marine or safflower oils on large bowel or pulmonary implants of CT-26 in mice. Cancer Res 49(15):4289–4294
Canny G, Levy O, Furuta GT, Narravula-Alipati S, Sisson RB, Serhan CN et al (2002) Lipid mediator-induced expression of bactericidal/permeability-increasing protein (BPI) in human mucosal epithelia. Proc Natl Acad Sci 99:3902–3907
Castellone MD, Teramoto H, Gutkind JS (2006) Cyclooxygenase-2 and colorectal cancer chemoprevention: the beta-catenin connection. Cancer Res 66:11085–11088
Cerutti P (1985) Prooxidant states and tumor promotion. Science 227:375–381
Chan AT, Giovannucci EL, Meyerhardt JA et al (2005) Long-term use of aspirin and nonsteroidal anti-inflammatory drugs and risk of colorectal cancer. JAMA 294(8):914–923
Cheng AL, Hsu CH, Lin JK, Hsu MM, Ho YF, Shen TS, Ko JY, Lin JT, Lin BR, Ming-Shiang W, Yu HS, Jee SH, Chen GS, Chen TM, Chen CA, Lai MK, Pu YS, Pan MH, Wang YJ,

Tsai CC, Hsieh CY (2001) Phase I clinical trial of curcumin, a chemopreventive agent, in patients with high-risk or pre-malignant lesions. Anticancer Res 21(4B):2895–2900
Chulada PC, Thompson MB, Mahler JF, Doyle CM, Gaul BW, Lee C, Tiano HF, Morham SG, Smithies O, Langenbach R (2000a) Genetic disruption of Ptgs-1, as well as Ptgs-2, reduces intestinal tumorigenesis in Min mice. Cancer Res 60(17):4705–4708
Chulada PC, Thompson MB, Mahler JF et al (2000b) Genetic disruption of Ptgs-1 as well as Ptgs-2 reduces intestinal tumorigenesis in Min mice. Cancer Res 60:4706–4708
Cicero AF, Derosa G, Gaddi A (2005) Combined lipoxygenase/cyclo-oxygenase inhibition in the elderly: the example of licofelone. Drugs Aging 22:393–403
Claria J, Serhan CN (1995) Aspirin triggers previously undescribed bioactive eicosanoids by human endothelial cell—leukocyte interactions. Proc Natl Acad Sci 92:9475–9479
Clevers H (2004) At the crossroads of inflammation and cancer. Cell 118:671–674
Cockbain AJ, Toogood GJ, Hull MA (2012) Omega-3 polyunsaturated fatty acids for the treatment and prevention of colorectal cancer. Gut 61:135–149
Colon AL, Menchen L, Lizasoain I et al (2000) Inducible nitric oxide synthase activity is expressed not only in inflamed but also in normal colonic mucosa in patients with ulcerative colitis: a potential prognostic marker. Am J Gastroenterol 95:1371–1373
Cottart CH, Nivet-Antoine V, Laguillier-Morizot C, Beaudeux JL (2010) Resveratrol bioavailability and toxicity in humans. Mol Nutr Food Res 54(1):7–16
Crowell JA, Steele VE, Sigman CC, Fay JR (2003) Is inducible nitric oxide synthase a target for chemoprevention? Mol Cancer Ther 2:815–823
Dannenberg AJ, Lippman SM, Mann JR, Subbaramaiah K, Dubois RN (2005) Cyclooxygenase-2 and epidermal growth factor receptor: pharmacologic targets for chemoprevention. J Clin Oncol 23:254–266
Darshan S, Doreswamy R (2004) Patented antiinflammatory plant drug development from traditional medicine. Phytother Res 18(5):343–357
Ding XZ, Iversen P, Cluck MW et al (1999) Lipoxygenase inhibitors abolish proliferation of human pancreatic cancer cells. Biochem Biophys Res Commun 261:218–223
Ding XZ, Tong WG, Adrian TE (2003) Multiple signal pathways are involved in the mitogenic effect of 5(S)- HETE in human pancreatic cancer. Oncology 65:285–294
Dunn GP, Old LJ, Schreiber RD (2004) The immunobiology of cancer immunosurveillance and immunoediting. Immunity 21:137–148
Erdman SE, Sohn JJ, Rao VP et al (2005) CD4CD25 regulatory lymphocytes induce regression of intestinal tumors in ApcMin/ mice. Cancer Res 65:3998–4004
Feagins LA, Souza RF, Spechler SJ (2009) Carcinogenesis in IBD: potential targets for the prevention of colorectal cancer. Nat Rev Gastroenterol Hepatol 6:297–305
Fiorucci S, Meli R, Bucci M, Cirino G (2001) Dual inhibitors of cyclooxygenase and 5-lipoxygenase. A new avenue in anti-inflammatory therapy? Biochem Pharmacol 62:1433–1438
Freedman AN et al (1998) Aspirin use and p53 expression in colorectal cancer. Cancer Detect Prev 22:213–218
Garcea G, Berry DP, Jones DJ, Singh R, Dennison AR, Farmer PB, Sharma RA, Steward WP, Gescher AJ (2005) Consumption of the putative chemopreventive agent curcumin by cancer patients: assessment of curcumin levels in the colorectum and their pharmacodynamic consequences. Cancer Epidemiol Biomarkers Prev 14(1):120–125
Gewirtz AT, Collier-Hyams LS, Young AN, Kucharzik T, Guilford WJ, Parkinson JF et al (2002) Lipoxin A4 analogs attenuate induction of intestinal epithelial proinflammatory gene expression and reduce the severity of dextran sodium sulfate-induced colitis. J Immunol 168(10):5260–5267
Giardello FM, Hamilton SR, Krush AJ, Piantodosi S, Hylind LM, Cleano P, Booker SV, Robinson RC, Offerhaus GJA (1993) Treatment of colonic rectal adenomas with sulindac in familial adenomatous polyposis. N Eng J Med 328:1313–1316
Giovannucci E (1999) The prevention of colorectal cancer by aspirin use. Biomed Pharmacother 53:303–308

Giovannucci E et al (1994) Aspirin use and the risk for colorectal cancer and adenoma in male health professionals. Ann Intern Med 121:241–246

Goel A, Kunnumakkara AB, Aggarwal BB (2008) Curcumin as "Curecumin": from kitchen to clinic. Biochem Pharmacol 75(4):787–809

Goldstein BD, Witz G (1990) Free radicals and carcinogenesis. Free Radic Res Commun 11:3–10

Goulet JL, Snouwaert JN, Latour AM, Coffman TM, Koller BH (1994) Altered inflammatory responses in leukotriene-deficient mice. Proc Natl Acad Sci USA 91(26):12852–12856

Greenberg ER, Baron JA, Freeman DH, Mandel JS, Haile R (1993) Reduced risk of large-bowel adenomas among aspirin users. The Polyp Prevention Study Group. J Natl Cancer Inst 85:912–916

Griffiths RJ, Smith MA, Roach ML, Stock JL, Stam EJ, Milici AJ et al (1997) Collagen-induced arthritis is reduced in 5-lipoxygenase-activating protein-deficient mice. J Exp Med 185:1123–1129

Gupta RA, Dubois RN (2001) Colorectal cancer prevention and treatment by inhibition of cyclooxygenase-2. Nature Rev Cancer 1:11–21

Haklar G, Sayin-Özveri E, Yüksel M, Aktan AÖ, Yalçin AS (2001) Different kinds of reactive oxygen and nitrogen species were detected in colon and breast tumors. Cancer Lett 165(2):219–224

Hammad H, de Heer HJ, Soullie T, Hoogsteden HC, Trottein F, Lambrecht BN (2003) Prostaglandin D_2 inhibits airway dendritic cell migration and function in steady state conditions by selective activation of the D prostanoid receptor 1. J Immunol 171:3936–3940

Hao XP, Pretlow TG, Rao JS, Pretlow TP (2001) Inducible nitric oxide synthase (iNOS) is expressed similarly in multiple aberrant crypt foci and colorectal tumors from the same patients. Cancer Res 61:419–422

Harris RE, Beebe-Donk J, Doss H, Burr D (2005) Aspirin, ibuprofen, and other non-steroidal anti-inflammatory drugs in cancer prevention: a critical review of non-selective COX-2 blockade. Oncol Rep 13:559–583

Hawk ET, Levin B (2005) Colorectal cancer prevention. J Clin Oncol 23:378

Hofseth LJ, Hussain SP, Wogan GN, Harris CC (2003) Nitric oxide in cancer and chemoprevention. Free Radic Biol Med 34:955–968

Hong SH, Avis I, Vos MD, Martinez A, Treston AM, Mulshine JL (1999) Relationship of arachidonic acid metabolizing enzyme expression in epithelial cancer cell lines to the growth effect of selective biochemical inhibitors. Cancer Res 59:2223–2228

Ishida T, Yoshida M, Arita M, Nishitani Y, Nishiumi S, Masuda A et al (2009) Resolvin E1, an endogenous lipid mediator derived from eicosapentaenoic acid, prevents dextran sulfate sodium-induced colitis. Inflammation and Bowel Diseases 16(1):87–95

Ishida T, Yoshida M, Arita M, Nishitani Y, Nishiumi S, Masuda A, Mizuno S, Takagawa T, Morita Y, Kutsumi H, Inokuchi H, Serhan CN, Blumberg RS, Azuma T (2010) Resolvin E1, an endogenous lipid mediator derived from eicosapentaenoic acid, prevents dextran sulfate sodium-induced colitis. Inflamm Bowel Dis 16(1):87–95

Jacoby RF, Marshall DJ, Newton MA, Novakovic K, Tutsch K, Cole CE et al (1996) Chemoprevention of spontaneous intestinal adenomas in APC Min mouse model by the nonsteroidal anti-inflammatory drug piroxicam. Cancer Res 56:710–714

Jacoby RF, Seibert K, Cole CE, Kelloff G, Lubet RA (2000) The cyclooxygenase-2 inhibitor celecoxib is a potent preventive and therapeutic agent in the Min mouse model of adenomatous polyposis. Cancer Res 60:5040–5044

Janakiram NB, Rao CV (2012) iNOS-selective inhibitors for cancer prevention: promise and progress. Future Med. Chem. 4(17):2193–2204

Janakiram NB, Indranie C, Malisetty SV, Jagan P, Steele VE, Rao CV (2008) Chemoprevention of colon carcinogenesis by oleanolic acid and its analog in male F344 rats and modulation of COX-2 and apoptosis in human colon HT-29 cancer cells. Pharm Res 25(9):2151–2157

Janakiram NB, Mohammed A, Rao CV (2011) Role of lipoxins, resolvins, and other bioactive lipids in colon and pancreatic cancer. Cancer Metastasis Rev 30(3–4):507–523

Janakiram NB, Mohammed A, Ravillah D, Choi C-I, Zhang Y, Desai D, Amin S and Rao CV. (2013) Chemopreventive effects of PBI-Se, a selenium-containing analog of PBIT, on AOM-induced aberrant crypt foci in F344 rats. Oncol Rep 30(2):952–960
Jang M, Cai L, Udeani GO, Slowing KV, Thomas CF, Beecher CW, Fong HH, Farnsworth NR, Kinghorn AD, Mehta RG, Moon RC, Pezzuto JM (1997) Cancer chemopreventive activity of resveratrol, a natural product derived from grapes. Science 275(5297):218–220
Juan ME, Alfaras I, Planas JM (2010) Determination of dihydroresveratrol in rat plasma by HPLC. J Agric Food Chem 58(12):7472–7475
Juan ME, Alfaras I, Planas JM (2012) Colorectal cancer chemoprevention by trans-resveratrol. Pharmacol Res 65(6):584–591
Juarez-Oropeza MA, Diaz-Zagoya JC, Rabinowitz JL (1987) In vivo and in vitro studies of hypocholesterolemic effects of diosgenin in rats. Int J Biochem 19(8):679–683
Kato T, Hancock RL, Mohammadpour H, McGregor B, Manalo P, Khaiboullina S, Hall MR, Pardini L, Pardini RS (2002) Influence of omega-3 fatty acids on the growth of human colon carcinoma in nude mice. Cancer Lett 187(1–2):169–177
Kawamori T, Lubet R, Steele VE, Kelloff GJ, Kaskey RB, Rao CV, Reddy BS (1999) Chemopreventive effect of curcumin, a naturally occurring anti-inflammatory agent, during the promotion/progression stages of colon cancer. Cancer Res 59(3):597–601
Kawamori T, Rao CV, Seibert K, Reddy BS (1998) Chemopreventive activity of celecoxib, a specific cyclooxygenase-2 inhibitor, against colon carcinogenesis. Cancer Res 58:409–412
Kawamori T, Takahashi M, Watanabe K et al (2000) Suppression of azoxymethane-induced colonic aberrant crypt foci by a nitric oxide synthase inhibitor. Cancer Lett 148:33–37
Kawamori T, Tanaka T, Hara A, Yamahara J, Mori H (1995) Modifying effects of naturally occurring products on the development of colonic aberrant crypt foci induced by azoxymethane in F344 rats. Cancer Res 55(6):1277–1282
Kudo T, Narisawa T, Abo S (1980) Antitumor activity of indomethacin on methylazoxymethanol-induced large bowel tumors in rats. Gann 71(2):260–264
Kune GA, Kune S, Watson LF (1988) Colorectal cancer risk, chronic illnesses, operations, and medications: case control results from the Melbourne Colorectal Cancer Study. Cancer Res 1988 48:4399–4404. Reprinted Int J Epidemiol 2007 36:951–956
Kwon CS, Sohn HY, Kim SH, Kim JH, Son KH, Lee JS, Lim JK, Kim JS (2003) Anti-obesity effect of Dioscorea nipponica Makino with lipase-inhibitory activity in rodents. Biosci Biotechnol Biochem 67(7):1451–1456
La Vecchia C et al (1977) Aspirin and colorectal cancer. Br J Cancer 76:675–677
Lagares-Garcia JA, Moore RA, Collier B, Heggere M, Diaz F, Qian F (2001) Nitric oxide synthase as a marker in colorectal carcinoma. Am J Surg 67:709–713
Laine L, Wogen J, Yu H (2003) Gastrointestinal health care resource utilization with chronic use of COX-2-specific inhibitors versus traditional NSAIDs. Gastroenterology 125:389–395
Lakatos PL, Lakatos L (2008) Risk for colorectal cancer in ulcerative colitis: changes, causes and management strategies. World J Gastroenterol 14:3937–3947
Laybayle D, Fischer D, Vielh P, Frouhin F, Pariente A, Bories C, Duhamael O, Trousset M, Atti P (1991) Sulindac causes regression of rectal polyps in familial adenomatous polyposis. Gastroenterology 101:635–639
Liu J (1995) Pharmacology of oleanolic acid and ursolic acid. J Ethnopharmacol 49:57–68
Logan RF, Little J, Hawtin PG, Hardcastle JD (1993) Effect of aspirin and non-steroidal anti-inflammatory drugs on colorectal adenomas: case—control study of subjects participating in the Nottingham faecal occult blood screening programme. Br Med J 307:285–289
Mahato SB, Sen S (1997) Advances in triterpenoid research, 1990–1994. Phytochemistry 44(7):1185–1236
Mahmoud NN, Dannenberg AJ, Mestre J et al (1998) Aspirin prevents tumors in a murine model of familial adenomatous polyposis. Medline Surg 124:225–231
Marnett LJ (1992) Aspirin and potential role of prostaglandins in colon cancer. Cancer Res 52:5575–5589

Martel-Pelletier J, Lajeunesse D, Reboul P, Pelletier JP (2003) Therapeutic role of dual inhibitors of 5-LOX and COX, selective and non-selective non-steroidal anti-inflammatory drugs. Ann Rheum Dis 62:501–509

Martinez ME, McPherson RS, Levin B, Annegers JF (1995) Aspirin and other non-steroidal anti-inflammatory drugs and risk of colorectal adenomatous polyps among endoscoped individuals. Cancer Epidemiol Biomarkers Prev 4:703–707

McAnuff MA, Harding WW, Omoruyi FO, Jacobs H, Morrison EY, Asemota HN (2005) Hypoglycemic effects of steroidal sapogenins isolated from Jamaican bitter yam, *Dioscorea polygonoides*. Food Chem Toxicol 43(11):1667–1672

Meira LB, Bugni JM, Green SL et al (2008) DNA damage induced by chronic inflammation contributes to colon carcinogenesis in mice. J Clin Invest 118:2516–2525

Metzger U, Meier J, Uhlschmid G, Weihe H (1984) Influence of various prostglandin synthesis inhibitors on DMH-induced rat colon cancer. Dis Colon Rectum 27:366–369

Mohammed A, Janakiram NB, Li Q, Choi CI, Zhang Y, Steele VE, Rao CV (2011) Chemoprevention of colon and small intestinal tumorigenesis in APCMin/+ Mice by licofelone, a novel dual 5-LOX/COX inhibitor: potential implications for human colon cancer prevention. Cancer Prev Res 4(12):2015–2026

Moorghen M, Ince P, Finney KJ, Sunter JP, Appleton DR, Watson AJA (1988) A protective effect of sulindac against chemically—induced primary colonic tumors in mice. J Pathol 156:341–347

Moorghen M, Orde M, Finney KJ, Appleton DR, Watson AJ (1998) Sulindac enhances cell proliferation in DMH-treated mouse colonic mucosa. Cell Prolif 31:59–70

Moreau M, Daminet S, Martel-Pelletier J, Fernandes J, Pelletier JP (2005) Superiority of the gastroduodenal safety profile of licofelone over rofecoxib, a COX-2 selective inhibitor, in dogs. J Vet Pharmacol Ther 28:81–86

Mund RC, Pizato N, Bonatto S, Nunes EA, Vicenzi T, Tanhoffer R, de Oliveira HH, Curi R, Calder PC, Fernandes LC (2007) Decreased tumor growth in Walker 256 tumor-bearing rats chronically supplemented with fish oil involves COX-2 and PGE_2 reduction associated with apoptosis and increased peroxidation. Prostaglandins Leukot Essent Fatty Acids 76(2):113–120

Murata T, Lin MI, Aritake K et al (2008) Role of prostaglandin D2 receptor DP as a suppressor of tumor hyper-permeability and angiogenesis in vivo. Proc Natl Acad Sci 105(50):20009–20014

Muscat JE, Stellman SD, Wynder EL (1994) Non-steroidal anti-inflammatory drugs and colorectal cancer. Cancer 74:1847–1854

Nalini N, Manju V, Menon VP (2006) Effect of spices on lipid metabolism in 1, 2-dimethylhydrazine-induced rat colon carcinogenesis. J Med Food 9(2):237–245

Nam KT, Oh SY, Ahn B, Kim YB, Jang DD, Yang KH et al (2004) Decreased Helicobacter pylori associated gastric carcinogenesis in mice lacking inducible nitric oxide synthase. Gut 20(53):1250–1255

Narisawa T, Satoh M, Sano M, Takahashi T (1993) Inhibition of initiation and promotionon N-methylnitrosourea-inducedcolon carcinogenesisin rats by nonsteroidal anti-inflammatory agent indomethacin. Carcinogenesis (London) 14:1493–1497

Narisawa T et al (1981) Inhibition of development of methylnitrosourea-induced rat colon tumors by indomethacin treatment. Cancer Res 41:1954–1957

Nguyen AV, Martinez M, Stamos MJ, Moyer MP, Planutis K, Hope C, Holcombe RF (2009) Results of a phase I pilot clinical trial examining the effect of plant-derived resveratrol and grape powder on Wnt pathway target gene expression in colonic mucosa and colon cancer. Cancer Manag Res 1:25–37

Nieto N, Torres MI, Ríos A, Gil A (2002) Dietary polyunsaturated fatty acids improve histological and biochemical alterations in rats with experimental ulcerative colitis. J Nutr 132:11–19

Nussmeier NA et al (2005) Complications of the COX-2 inhibitors parecoxib and valdecoxib after cardiac surgery. N Engl J Med 352:1081–1091

Oh SF, Vickery TW, Serhan CN (2011) Chiral lipidomics of E-series resolvins: aspirin and the biosynthesis of novel mediators. Biochim Biophys Acta 1811(11):737–747

Ohd JF, Nielsen CK, Campbell J, Landberg G, Lofberg H, Sjolander A (2003) Expression of the leukotriene D_4 receptor $CysLT_1$, COX-2, colorectal adenocarcinomas. Gastroenterology 124:57–70

Ohshima H, Bartsch H (1994) Chronic infection and inflammatory processes as cancer risk factors: possible role of NO in carcinogenesis. Mutat Res 305:253–264

Orner GA, Dashwood WM, Blum CA, Daz GD, Li Q, Dashwood RH (2003) Suppression of tumorigenesis in the Apc(Min) mouse: down-regulation of b-catenin signaling by a combination of tea plus sulindac. Carcinogenesis 24:263–267

Oshima M, Dinchuk JE, Kargman SL, Oshima H, Hancock B, Kwong E, Trzaskos JM, Evans JF, Taketo MM (1996a) Suppression of intestinal polyposis in Apc delta 716 knockout mice by inhibition of cyclooxygenase 2 (COX-2). Cell 87(5):803–809

Oshima M, Dinchuk JE, Kargman SL (1996b) Suppression of intestinal polyposis in APCΔ716 knockout mice by inhibition of cyclooxygenase-2 (COX-2). Cell 87:803–809

Oshima M, Murai N, Kargman S et al (2001) Chemoprevention of intestinal polyposis in the APCΔ716 mouse by rofecoxib, a specific cyclooxygenase-2 inhibitor. Cancer Res 61:1733–1740

Patel KR, Brown VA, Jones DJ, Britton RG, Hemingway D, Miller AS, West KP, Booth TD, Perloff M, Crowell JA (2010) Clinical pharmacology of resveratrol and its metabolites in colorectal cancer patients. Cancer Res 70:7392–7399

Peleg II, Maibach HT, Brown SH, Wilcox CM (1994) Aspirin and non-steroidal anti-inflammatory drug use and the risk of subsequent colorectal cancer. Arch Intern Med 154:394–399

Piyachaturawat P, Glinsukon T, Toskulkao C (1983) Acute and subacute toxicity of piperine in mice, rats and hamsters. Toxicol Lett 16(3–4):351–359

Pizato N, Bonatto S, Yamazaki RK, Aikawa J, Nogata C, Mund RC, Nunes EA, Piconcelli M, Naliwaiko K, Curi R, Calder PC, Fernandes LC (2005) Ratio of n6 to n-3 fatty acids in the diet affects tumor growth and cachexia in Walker 256 tumor-bearing rats. Nutr Cancer 53(2):194–201

Pollard M, Luckert PH (1980) Indomethacin treatment of rats with dimethylhydrazine-induced intestinal tumors. Cancer Treat Rep 64:1323–1327

Pollard M, Luckert PH (1984) Effect of piroxicam on primary intestinal tumors induced in rats by *N*-methylnitrosourea. Cancer Left 25:117–121

Pollard M, Luckert PH (1981) Treatment of chemically-induced intestinal cancers with indomethacin. Proc Soc Exp Biol Med 167:161–164

Qiao L, Kozoni V, Tsioulias GJ, Koutsos MI, Hanif R, Shiff SJ et al (1995) Selected eicosanoids increase the proliferation rate of human colon carcinoma cell lines and mouse colonocytes in vivo. Biochim et Biophys Acta 1258:215–223

Rachmilewitz D, Stamler JS, Bachwich D, Karmeli F, Ackerman Z, Podolsky DK (1995) Enhanced colonic nitric oxide generation and nitric oxide synthase activity in ulcerative colitis and Crohn's disease. Gut 36:718–723

Raju J, Mehta R (2009) Cancer chemopreventive and therapeutic effects of diosgenin, a food saponin. Nutr Cancer 61(1):27–35

Raju J, Patlolla JM, Swamy MV, Rao CV (2004) Diosgenin, a steroid saponin of Trigonella foenum graecum (Fenugreek), inhibits azoxymethane-induced aberrant crypt foci formation in F344 rats and induces apoptosis in HT-29 human colon cancer cells. Cancer Epidemiol Biomarkers Prev 13(8):1392–1398

Rao CV (2004) Nitric Oxide signaling in colon cancer chemoprevention. Mut Res 555:107–119

Rao CV, Cooma I, Rodriguez JG, Simi B, El-Bayoumy K, Reddy BS (2000) Chemoprevention of familial adenomatous polyposis development in the APC(min) mouse model by 1, 4-phenylene bis(methylene) selenocyanate. Carcinogenesis 21:617–621

Rao CV, Cooma I, Simi B, Manning PT, Connor JR, Reddy BS (2002) Chemopreventive properties of a selective inducible nitric oxide synthase inhibitor in colon carcinogenesis,

administered alone or in combination with celecoxib, a selective cyclooxygenase-2 inhibitor. Cancer Res 62:165–170
Rao CV, Kawamori T, Hamid R, Reddy BS (1999) Chemoprevention of colonic aberrant crypt foci by an inducible nitric oxide synthase—selective inhibitor. Carcinogenesis 20:641–644
Rao CV, Reddy BS, Steele VE, Wang CX, Liu X, Ouyang N, Patlolla JM, Simi B, Kopelovich L, Rigas B (2006) Nitric oxide-releasing aspirin and indomethacin are potent inhibitors against colon cancer in azoxymethane-treated rats: effects on molecular targets. Mol Cancer Ther 6:1530–1538
Rao CV, Reddy BS (2004) NSAIDs and chemoprevention. Curr Cancer Drug Targets 4:29–42
Rao CV, Rivenson A, Simi B, Zang E, Kelloff G, Steele V, Reddy BS (1995) Chemoprevention of colon carcinogenesis by sulindac, a nonsteroidal anti-inflammatory agent. Cancer Res 55:1464–1472
Reddy BS, Maruyama H, Kelloff G (1987) Dose-related inhibition of colon carcinogenesis by dietary piroxicam, a nonsteroidal anti-inflammatory drug, during different stages of rat colon tumor development. Cancer Res 47:5340–5346
Reddy BS, Rao CV, Rivenson A, Kelloff G (1993) Inhibitory effect of aspirin on azoxymethane-induced colon carcinogenesis in F344 rats. Carcinogenesis (London) 14:1493–1497
Reddy BS, Rao CV (2002) Novel approaches for colon cancer prevention by COX-2 inhibitors. J Environ Pathol Toxicol Oncol 21:155–164
Rigau J, Pique JM, Rubio E, Planas R, Tarrech JM, Bordas JM (1991) Effect of long-term sulindac therapy on colonic polyposis. Ann Intern Med 115:952–954
Sale S, Tunstall RG, Ruparelia KC, Potter GA, Steward WP, Gescher AJ (2005) Comparison of the effects of the chemopreventive agent resveratrol and its synthetic analog trans 3, 4, 5, 4′-tetramethoxystilbene (DMU-212) on adenoma development in the Apc(Min+) mouse and cyclooxygenase-2 in human-derived colon cancer cells. Int J Cancer 115(2):194–201
Sandler RS et al (2003) A randomized trial of aspirin to prevent colorectal adenomas in patients with previous colorectal cancer. N Engl J Med 348:883–890
Schleiffer R, Duranton B, Gossé F, Bergmann C, Raul F (2000) Nitric oxide synthase inhibition promotes carcinogen-induced preneoplastic changes in the colon of rats. Nitric Oxide 4(6):583–589
Schneider Y, Duranton B, Gossé F, Schleiffer R, Seiler N, Raul F (2001) Resveratrol inhibits intestinal tumorigenesis and modulates host-defense-related gene expression in an animal model of human familial adenomatous polyposis. Nutr Cancer 39(1):102–107
Schreinemachers DM, Everson RB (1994) Aspirin use and lung, colon, and breast cancer incidence in a prospective study. Epidemiology 5:138–146
Sengottuvelan M, Nalini N (2006) Dietary supplementation of resveratrol suppresses colonic tumour incidence in 1, 2-dimethylhydrazine-treated rats by modulating biotransforming enzymes and aberrant crypt foci development. Br J Nutr 96(1):145–153
Serhan CN (1997) Lipoxins and novel aspirin-triggered 15-epi-lipoxins (ATL). Prostaglandins 53:107–137
Serhan CN (2002) Lipoxins and aspirin-triggered 15-epilipoxin biosynthesis: an update and role in anti-inflammation and pro-resolution. Prostaglandins Other Lipid Mediat 68–69:4333–4455
Sharma RA, Euden SA, Platton SL, Cooke DN, Shafayat A, Hewitt HR, Marczylo TH, Morgan B, Hemingway D, Plummer SM, Pirmohamed M, Gescher AJ, Steward WP (2004) Phase I clinical trial of oral curcumin: biomarkers of systemic activity and compliance. Clin Cancer Res 10(20):6847–6854
Sharma RA, McLelland HR, Hill KA, Ireson CR, Euden SA, Manson MM, Pirmohamed M, Marnett LJ, Gescher AJ, Steward WP (2001) Pharmacodynamic and pharmacokinetic study of oral Curcuma extract in patients with colorectal cancer. Clin Cancer Res 7:1894–1900
Shpitz B, Giladi N, Sagiv E, Lev-Ari S, Liberman E, Kazanov D, Arber N (2006) Celecoxib and curcumin additively inhibit the growth of colorectal cancer in a rat model. Digestion 74(3–4):140–144
Silverstein FE et al (2000) Gastrointestinal toxicity with celecoxib vs nonsteroidal anti-inflammatory drugs for osteoarthritis and rheumatoid arthritis: the CLASS study: a randomized controlled trial. Celecoxib long-term arthritis safety study. JAMA 284:1247–1255

Skinner SA, Penney AG, O'Brien PE (1991) Sulindac inhibits the rate of growth and appearance of colon tumor in the rat Arch Surg 126:1094–1096

Smalley WE, DuBois RN (1997) Colorectal cancer and nonsteroidal anti-inflammatory drugs. Adv Pharmacol 39:1–20

Smith WL, DeWitt DL, Garavito RM (2000) Cyclooxygenases: structural, cellular, and molecular biology. Ann Rev Biochem 69:145–182

Smith WL (1992) Prostanoid biosynthesis and mechanisms of action. Am J Physiol 263:F181–F191

Solomon SD et al (2005) Cardiovascular risk associated with celecoxib in a clinical trial for colorectal adenoma prevention. N Engl J Med 352:1071–1080

Son IS, Kim JH, Sohn HY, Son KH, Kim JS, Kwon CS (2007) Antioxidative and hypolipidemic effects of diosgenin, a steroidal saponin of yam (Dioscorea spp.), on high-cholesterol fed rats. Biosci Biotechnol Biochem 71(12):3063–3071

Spagnesi MT, Tonelli F, Dolara P, Caderni G, Valanzano R, Anastasi A, Bianchini F (1994) Rectal proliferation and polyp occurrence in patients with familial adenomatous polyposis after sulindac treatment. Gastroenterology 106:362–366

Suh N, Reddy BS, DeCastro A, Paul S, Lee HJ, Smolarek AK, So JY, Simi B, Wang CX, Janakiram NB, Steele V, Rao CV (2011) Combination of atorvastatin with sulindac or naproxen profoundly inhibits colonic adenocarcinomas by suppressing the p65/b-catenin/cyclin D1 signaling pathway in rats. Cancer Prev Res 4:1895–1902

Suh O, Mettlin C, Petrelli NJ (1993) Aspirin use, cancer, and polyps of the large bowel. Cancer 72:1171–1177

Swamy MV, Patlolla JM, Steele VE, Kopelovich L, Reddy BS, Rao CV (2006) Chemoprevention of familial adenomatous polyposis by low doses of atorvastatin and celecoxib given individually and in combination to APCMin mice. Cancer Res 66:7370–7377

Szaleczky E, Pronai L, Nakazawa H, Tulassay Z (2000) Evidence of in vivo peroxynitrite formation in patients with colorectal carcinoma, higher plasma nitrate/nitrite levels, and lower protection against oxygen free radicals. J Clin Gastroenterol 30:47–51

Tamir S, Tannenbaus SR (1996) The role of nitric oxide in carcinogenic process. Biochim Biophys Acta 1288:F31–F36

Tenesa A, Dunlop MG (2009) New insights into the aetiology of colorectal cancer from genome-wide association studies. Nat Rev Genet 10:353–358

Tessitore L, Davit A, Sarotto I, Caderni G (2000) Resveratrol depresses the growth of colorectal aberrant crypt foci by affecting bax and p21 (CIP) expression. Carcinogenesis 21(8):1619–1622

Thun MH, Namboodiri MM, Heath CW (1991) Aspirin use and reduced risk of fatal colon cancer. N Eng J Med 325:1593–1596

Togni V, Ota CC, Folador A, Júnior OT, Aikawa J, Yamazaki RK, Freitas FA, Longo R, Martins EF, Calder PC, Curi R, Fernandes LC (2003) Cancer cachexia and tumor growth reduction in Walker 256 tumor-bearing rats supplemented with N-3 polyunsaturated fatty acids for one generation. Nutr Cancer 46(1):52–58

Tong WG, Ding XZ, Talamonti MS, Bell RH, Adrian TE (2005) LTB4 stimulates growth of human pancreatic cancer cells via MAPK and PI-3 kinase pathways. Biochem Biophys Res Commun 335:949–956

Trebino CE, Stock JL, Gibbons CP, Naiman BM, Wachtmann TS, Umland JP, Pandher K, Lapointe JM, Saha S, Roach ML, Carter D, Thomas NA, Durtschi BA, McNeish JD, Hambor JE, Jakobsson PJ, Carty TJ, Perez JR, Audoly LP (2003) Impaired inflammatory and pain responses in mice lacking an inducible prostaglandin E synthase. Proc Natl Acad Sci USA 100:9044–9049

Ukil A, Maity S, Karmakar S, Datta N, Vedasiromoni JR, Das PK (2003) Curcumin, the major component of food flavour turmeric, reduces mucosal injury in trinitrobenzene sulphonic acid-induced colitis. Br J Pharmacol 139:209–218

Vanamala J, Glagolenko A, Yang P, Carroll RJ, Murphy ME, Newman RA, Ford JR, Braby LA, Chapkin RS, Turner ND, Lupton JR (2008) Dietary fish oil and pectin enhance colonocyte apoptosis in part through suppression of PPAR delta/PGE_2 and elevation of PGE_3. Carcinogenesis 29(4):790–796

Velayos FS, Loftus EV, Jess T, Harmsen WS, Bida J, Zinsmeister AR, Tremaine WJ, Sandborn WJ (2006) Predictive and protective factors associated with colorectal cancer in ulcerative colitis: a case-control study. Gastroenterol 130:1941–1949

Waddel RW, Ganser GF, Cerise EJ, Loughry RW (1989) Sulindac for polyposis of the colon. Am J Surg 157:175–179

Waldner MJ, Neurath MF (2008) Cytokines in colitis associated cancer: potential drug targets? Inflamm Allergy Drug Targets 7:187–194

Walle T (2011) Bioavailability of resveratrol. Ann NY Acad Sci 1215:9–15

Wan G, Kato N, Watanabe H (2000) High fat diet elevates the activity of inducible nitric oxide synthase and 1, 2 dimethyl-hydrazine induced aberrant crypt foci in colon of rats. Oncolo Rep 7:391–395

Wang D, Dubois RN (2006) Review prostaglandins and cancer. Gut 55(1):115–122

West NJ, Clark SK, Phillips RKS, Hutchinson JM, Leicester RJ, Belluzzi A, Hull MA (2010) Eicosapentaenoic acid reduces rectal polyp number and size in familial adenomatous polyposis. Gut. doi:10.1136/gut.2009.200642

Westbrook AM, Wei B, Braun J, Schiestl RH (2009) Intestinal mucosal inflammation leads to systemic genotoxicity in mice. Cancer Res 69:4827–4834

Winde G, Gumbinger HG, Osswald H, Kemper F, Bunte H (1993) The NSAID sulindac reverses rectal adenomas in colectomized patients with familial adenomatous polyposis: clinical results of a dose finding study on rectal sulindac administration. Int J Colorect Dis 8:13–17

Xu G, Ren G, Xu X, Yuan H, Wang Z, Kang L, Yu W, Tian K (2010) Combination of curcumin and green tea catechins prevents dimethylhydrazine-induced colon carcinogenesis. Food Chem Toxicol 48(1):390–395. doi:10.1016/j.fct.2009.10.027. Epub 25 Oct 2009

Xu W, Liu L, Charles IG (2002) Microencapsulated iNOS-expressing cells cause tumor suppression in mice. FASEB J 16:213–215

Yagihashi N, Kasajima H, Sugai S et al (2000) Increased in situ expression of nitric oxide synthase in human colorectal cancer. Virchows Arch 436:109–114

Yamada T, Hoshino M, Hayakawa T, Ohhara H, Yamada H, Nakazawa T, Inagaki T, Iida M, Ogasawara T, Uchida A, Hasegawa C, Murasaki G, Miyaji M, Hirata A, Takeuchi T (1997) Dietary diosgenin attenuates subacute intestinal inflammation associated with indomethacin in rats. Am J Physiol 273(2):G355–G364

Ziegler CC, Rainwater L, Whelan J, McEntee MF (2004) Dietary resveratrol does not affect intestinal tumorigenesis in Apc(Min/+) mice. J Nutr 134(1):5–10

Chapter 3
The Role of Inflammation in Inflammatory Breast Cancer

Tamer M. Fouad, Takahiro Kogawa, James M. Reuben and Naoto T. Ueno

Abstract Inflammatory breast cancer (IBC) is the most aggressive form of breast cancer. Despite extensive study, whether inflammation contributes to the tumorigenicity or aggressiveness of IBC remains largely unknown. In this chapter, we will review the potential role played by inflammation in IBC based on the results of in vitro, in vivo, and patient studies. Current evidence suggests that several major inflammatory signaling pathways are constitutively active in IBC and breast cancer. Among them, the NF-κB, COX-2, and JAK/STAT signaling systems seem to play a major role in the tumorigenesis of IBC. Inflammatory molecules such as interleukin-6, tumor necrosis factor alpha (TNF-α), and gamma interferon have been shown to contribute to malignant transformation in preclinical studies of IBC, while transforming growth factor-β, interleukins 8 and 1β, as well as TNF-α appear to play a role in proliferation, survival, epithelial–mesenchymal transition, invasion, and metastasis. In this chapter, we also describe work thus far involving inhibitors of inflammation in the development of prevention and treatment strategies for IBC.

T. M. Fouad · T. Kogawa · N. T. Ueno (✉)
Department of Breast Medical Oncology, Morgan Welch Inflammatory Breast Cancer Research Program and Clinic, The University of Texas MD Anderson Cancer Center, 1515 Holcombe Blvd., Unit 1354, Houston, TX 77030, USA
e-mail: nueno@mdanderson.org

J. M. Reuben
Department of Hematopathology, Morgan Welch Inflammatory Breast Cancer Research Program and Clinic, The University of Texas MD Anderson Cancer Center, Houston, TX, USA

T. M. Fouad
Department of Medical Oncology, The National Cancer Institute, Cairo University, Cairo, Egypt

B. B. Aggarwal et al. (eds.), *Inflammation and Cancer*, Advances in Experimental Medicine and Biology 816, DOI: 10.1007/978-3-0348-0837-8_3, © Springer Basel 2014

3.1 Introduction

Breast cancer is the second most common cancer, following skin cancer, among women in America. The American Cancer Society estimates that there will be 232,670 new cases of breast cancer among women in the United States in 2014 (ACS 2014). It is also the second leading cause of death from cancer in women, approximately with 40,000 predicted deaths for 2014. Inflammatory breast cancer (IBC) is the most aggressive form of breast cancer. Although it accounts for an estimated incidence rate of up to 5 % of breast cancers (Anderson et al. 2005; Hance et al. 2005; Jaiyesimi et al. 1992), IBC is responsible for a disproportionate 8–10 % of all breast cancer-related deaths (Hance et al. 2005).

The word "inflammatory" was first applied to the IBC subtype of breast cancer by Haagensen (1971). His description was based on certain presenting features that are unique to this subgroup of patients. IBC presents with rapid onset of breast erythema occupying at least one-third of the breast, accompanied by breast edema leading to the characteristic peau d'orange appearance of the skin. Other features include breast enlargement, pain, and tenderness. Approximately 50 % of patients do not present with a palpable mass or radiographic evidence of cancer (Ueno et al. 1997; Yang et al. 2008). Almost all IBC patients present with lymph node metastasis at the time of diagnosis, and approximately 30 % present with distant metastasis (Jaiyesimi et al. 1992; Li et al. 2011).

For diagnosing IBC, consensus guidelines recommend at a minimum a core biopsy to enable detection of invasive carcinoma and to allow marker study (hormone receptors and HER2). A skin punch biopsy to confirm the presence of dermal lymphatic invasion, one of the hallmarks of IBC, is also strongly recommended in suspected cases (Dawood et al. 2011).

Treatment of IBC, as for other types of breast cancer, involves a multidisciplinary approach that includes surgery, radiation therapy, and medical oncology. Patients are stratified according to extent of disease and the molecular subtype. This approach has been associated with a significant reduction in cancer-related mortality (Ueno et al. 1997; Kesson et al. 2012). Currently, the most active anti-cancer agents include anthracycline and taxanes, in addition to anti-HER2 therapy and endocrine therapy. However, compared with other types of breast cancer, treating IBC has proved to be more challenging mainly because of its rapidly aggressive nature combined with the lack of effective targeting therapy.

Despite extensive study, whether inflammation contributes to the tumorigenicity or aggressiveness of IBC remains unknown. In this chapter, we will review the potential role played by inflammation in IBC based on the results of in vitro, in vivo, and patient studies. We will also describe work thus far involving inhibitors of inflammation in the prevention and treatment of IBC.

3.2 Inflammatory Signaling Pathways Associated with IBC

Several intrinsic pathways driven by oncogenes or tumor suppressor genes have been shown to activate the expression of inflammation-related programs in both IBC and breast cancer in general. These pathways are described below.

NF-κB The nuclear factor of kappaB (NF-κB) family of sequence-specific transcription, known to play a critical role in inflammation and the innate immune response, has recently been implicated in tumorigenesis. It is ubiquitously expressed in all cell types, where, in most cases, it is maintained in an inactive state in the cytoplasm bound to a class of inhibitory proteins known as IκBs (inhibitors of κB). Activation of NF-κB occurs by a variety of stimuli and is regulated in normal cells via two main pathways, the classical (canonical) pathway and the alternative (non-canonical) pathway (Prasad et al. 2010). Both pathways involve kinase-dependent degradation of inhibitory molecules to release NF-κB, but they differ in the inhibitory molecule involved, the activated kinases, and the types of NF-κB proteins as well as the stimuli that trigger them. Upon activation, NF-κB is transported to the nucleus, where it upregulates the expression of target genes that are responsible for a wide variety of effects, including the inflammatory and immune response, proliferation, cell–matrix adhesion, chemotaxis, and angiogenesis (Shostak and Chariot 2011).

In a variety of cancers, including breast cancer, NF-κB undergoes persistent (constitutive) activation (Nakshatri et al. 1997). Laere et al. (2005) performed a genome-wide expression profile using a cDNA microarray to compare IBC and non-IBC tissue samples. The authors reported that an unusually high number of NF-κB target genes were differentially overexpressed in IBC versus non-IBC. In a similar study, the mRNA expression levels of 60 NF-κB-related genes were compared in IBC versus non-IBC samples using real-time quantitative RT-PCR. The authors reported that approximately 60 % of NF-κB-related genes were upregulated in the IBC samples compared to non-IBC samples. The resulting five-gene molecular signature was matched with patient outcomes; it included two genes that are regulated by NF-κB (Lerebours et al. 2008). Collectively, these studies confirm the importance of NF-κB in IBC and its contribution to the aggressive phenotype of IBC.

In a recent study, El-Shinawi et al. (2013) examined the association between evidence of human cytomegalovirus (HCMV) infection in the serum and tissue of IBC and non-IBC patients and whether HCMV was associated with NF-κB activation in IBC. The authors reported significantly higher levels of serum HCMV IgG as well as higher levels of HCMV DNA in the tumor tissue of IBC patients. Infected IBC samples also had enhanced NF-κB/p65 signaling compared to non-IBC controls (El-Shinawi et al. 2013). While these findings suggest an association between IBC and HCMV could exist, the authors noted that the evidence is not conclusive. If the results are confirmed, they may help explain the higher incidence of IBC in some geographic areas (Soliman et al. 2011).

Several studies have suggested complex cross talk between NF-κB and estrogen receptor (ER) in IBC as well as in breast cancer in general. In a separate study, Van Laere et al. reported that NF-κB activation in IBC tumors was associated with ER downregulation, which was linked to both EGFR and/or HER2 overexpression and MAPK hyperactivation (Laere et al. 2007). Additionally, ER seems to be capable of inhibiting both the constitutive and the inducible activation of NF-κB in a dose-dependent manner (Biswas et al. 2004). On the other hand, studies also seem to suggest that in ER-positive patients, cross talk between ER and NF-κB occurs that may either be transrepressive or positive (Kalaitzidis and Gilmore 2005). Theoretically, this could explain how in luminal B subtypes and some ER-positive IBC patients, resistance to hormonal therapy and poorer outcome could result from positive cross talk between NF-κB and ER leading to enhanced ER-mediated expression of genes involved in cell proliferation, survival, and resistance.

COX family The cyclooxygenase (COX) family of enzymes consists of two members, COX-1 and COX-2. Both enzymes catalyze the conversion of arachidonic acid to prostanoids and are also responsible for the generation of eicosanoid products, which are important mediators of pain and inflammation. Tissue upregulation of COX-2 can be triggered by several stimuli, including growth factors and oncogenes (Williams et al. 1999). Aberrant activation of COX/prostaglandin signaling is common in many cancers, especially in colon cancer, where COX-2 is overexpressed in 85 % of tumors (Brown and DuBois 2005). This has also been the case with breast cancer; enzyme levels have been found to be increased in 40 % of breast tumor tissues examined (Yoshimura et al. 2003).

Several studies have documented the role that the PTGS2 gene, which encodes COX-2, plays in cell proliferation, invasion, angiogenesis, and metastasis (Wang and Dubois 2004; Menter et al. 2010). Overexpression of COX-2 in breast cancer correlates with a more aggressive breast cancer profile that is characterized by higher proliferation rates, larger tumors, higher pathologic grade, hormone receptor negativity, and HER2 overexpression (Ristimaki et al. 2002; Subbaramaiah et al. 2002). Compared with non-IBC tumors, the PTGS2 gene is differentially overexpressed in IBC, and it is identified as a key component in the molecular signature for IBC (Laere et al. 2005, 2007). Moreover, prostaglandin E2 (PGE2), which is a product of COX-2 enzymatic activity, is known to be upregulated in primary IBC tumors and metastatic lesions (Robertson et al. 2008). These findings emphasize the role of the COX-2 pathway in IBC and its potential use as a target for disease prevention and treatment.

JAK/STAT signaling The JAK/STAT signaling system is the main pathway for a variety of cytokines, including interferon and interleukins (e.g. IL-6), as well as growth factors or other chemical messengers. Depending on both the context and the integrity of the pathway, JAK/STAT signaling can stimulate proliferation and cell migration versus differentiation and apoptosis (Rawlings et al. 2004).

STAT3 is known to be constitutively activated in >50 % of breast cancers and tumor-derived cell lines (Garcia et al. 1997; Diaz et al. 2006). Using small interfering RNA (siRNA) to block STAT3 in both cell culture and xenograft models of breast cancer, investigators were able to show increased apoptosis through the Fas-mediated intrinsic apoptotic pathway, as well as reduced expression of the transmembrane molecule B-cell lymphoma-extra large (Bcl-xL), which promotes survival (Kunigal et al. 2009). Additionally, constitutive activation of STAT led to accelerated mammary tumorigenesis and increased metastatic potential in cancer cells expressing ErbB2 (Barbieri et al. 2010). Moreover, ablation of STAT3 resulted in inhibition of anchorage-independent growth of breast cancer cells, thus limiting their metastatic potential. More recently, however, it was found that JAK2/STAT3 appears to be necessary for growth and survival of tumor cells expressing the cancer stem cell (CSC) phenotype (Ma et al. 2011). More recently, investigators were able to induce cell death in SUM149 IBC tumor spheres by inhibiting STAT3 activation in a dose-dependent manner using a novel JAK2 inhibitor (Ma et al. 2011).

In summary, current evidence suggests that several major inflammatory signaling pathways are constitutively active in IBC and breast cancer. Among them, the NF-κB, COX-2, and JAK/STAT signaling systems seem to play a major role in the tumorigenesis of IBC. Blocking these pathways may prove to be a promising therapeutic strategy owing to their multiple roles in promoting cancer cell survival and metastasis.

3.3 Role of Inflammatory Molecules in the Development of IBC: Evidence From In Vitro Studies

3.3.1 Role of Inflammatory Molecules in Malignant Transformation

Accumulating DNA mutations play a causal role in the process of malignant transformation. Oncogenic insults may result in activation of oncogenes, loss of tumor suppressor genes, or the constitutive activation of membrane receptors or lead to the alteration of critical cellular processes such as the cell cycle or apoptosis (Hanahan and Weinberg 2000). In this setting, inflammation may contribute to carcinogenesis through the activation of the DNA damage response system in response to major oncogenic insults (Martin et al. 2011; Hartman et al. 2011). Moreover, viral infections, such as human papillomavirus (HPV), whose genome has been detected in breast cancer tissue, may also cause DNA damage, resulting in activation of the DNA damage response pathway, and stimulate the formation of a pro-inflammatory tumor microenvironment (Moody and Laimins 2009; Kan et al. 2005).

Interleukin-6 (IL-6), which is overexpressed in the SUM149 preclinical model of IBC (Golen et al. 2000), plays a potent role in malignant transformation. IL-6 was able to convert a non-transformed mammary epithelial cell line (MCF-10A) to the transformed state in 24–36 h (Iliopoulos et al. 2009, 2010).

Additionally, HER2 overexpression, which is known to occur in up to 60 % of IBC tumors and 25 % of non-IBC tumors, is associated with poor outcome (Guerin et al. 1989; Kallioniemi et al. 1991). HER2 amplification was associated with marked increase in IL-6 in breast cancer cells and induced STAT3 activation, suggesting a HER2-IL-6-STAT3 signaling pathway could play a critical role in tumorigenesis (Hartman et al. 2011).

On the other hand, cancer stem cells (CSCs), also known as tumor-initiating cells, are highly tumorigenic cells and are enriched in IBC tumors as well as in preclinical models of IBC (Laere et al. 2010; Charafe-Jauffret et al. 2010; Xiao et al. 2008). IL-6 acts as a growth factor for CSCs and is sufficient to convert non-stem cancer cells to CSCs (Iliopoulos et al. 2011). IL-6 gene expression was found to promote self-renewal, as well as invasive potential, in both normal and MCF-7-derived spheroids (Sansone et al. 2007). IL-6 is also at the center of epigenetic regulation of stem cells (D'Anello et al. 2010; Hodge et al. 2005). IL-6 thus plays a critical role in mediating the epigenetic switch that involves NF-κB and STAT3 and links inflammation to cell transformation (Iliopoulos et al. 2009, 2010).

Additional inflammatory signaling involved in the regulation of CSCs includes the tumor necrosis factor alpha (TNF-α) and gamma interferon (IFN-γ) pathways, both of which are upregulated in breast CSCs (Murohashi et al. 2010). Both cytokines are also able to activate the NF-κB pathway (Cheshire and Baldwin 1997; Hayden and Ghosh 2008; Matsumoto et al. 2005). Treatment with the chemokine IL-8 resulted in increased mammosphere formation, whereas IL-8 receptor/CXCR1 blockade depleted the breast CSC population both in vitro and in xenografts (Murohashi et al. 2010; Charafe-Jauffret et al. 2009; Ginestier et al. 2010). Expression of CCL5/RANTES was also found to be upregulated in breast CSC populations (Murohashi et al. 2010).

3.3.2 Role of Inflammatory Molecules in the Survival of IBC Cells

One of the hallmarks of cancer cells is their capacity to acquire resistance to apoptotic signals (Hanahan and Weinberg 2000). Transforming growth factor (TGF)-β is a pro-apoptotic cytokine that normally induces cell cycle arrest in the early phases of tumorigenesis. The mechanisms by which cancer cells escape the inhibitory effects of TGF-β are not fully understood but may include inactivating mutations or homozygous deletions(Kaklamani et al. 2003; Pasche et al. 2004; Dunning et al. 2003) or upregulation in oncogenic expression (Zhang et al. 2003). Once the pro-apoptotic functions of TGF-β are subverted, its tumorigenic potential becomes unhindered, thus stimulating growth, invasion, and angiogenesis (Biswas et al. 2007; Lei et al. 2002).

Likewise, although TNF-α promotes apoptosis in MCF-7 cells (Simstein et al. 2003), a process similar to TGF-β subverts the pro-apoptotic effect of TNF-α (Rivas et al. 2008). HER2 amplification, which is present in up to 60 % of IBC patients, was shown to confer resistance to TNF-α-induced apoptosis in breast cancer cell lines mainly through an Akt/NF-κB anti-apoptotic cascade (Zhou et al. 2000). Likewise, increased expression of claudin-1 was able to reverse TNF-α-induced apoptosis in the MCF-7 breast cancer cell line (Liu et al. 2012). These studies suggest that there are multiple pathways by which breast cancer cells can overcome TNF-α-induced apoptosis, thus promoting cancer cell survival and unleashing the tumorigenic potential of TNF-α.

Using mastectomy samples from patients with either invasive or non-invasive breast cancer as well as tissue from benign controls, both IL-6 protein levels and IL-6 receptor levels, were correlated with tissue levels of B-cell lymphoma 2 (Bcl-2) and Bcl-2-associated X (Bax) proteins (Garcia-Tunon et al. 2005). A higher proportion of malignant samples, compared with benign controls, were positive for IL-6, Bcl-2, and Bax by immunohistochemistry. The more invasive samples had a more intense immunoreaction for Bcl-2 than did benign lesions. In addition, infiltrating tumors that were positive for IL-6 were also positive for Bcl-2 with a high degree of correlation between immunoreaction intensities of both antibodies (Garcia-Tunon et al. 2005). These results, along with others, suggest that IL-6 plays a central role in protecting cancer cells against apoptosis as well as the regulation of survival in CSCs via several pathways, including the canonical JAK/STAT3 pathway, and by direct action on Bcl-2 family gene products (Iliopoulos et al. 2011; Hinohara and Gotoh 2010; Heinrich et al. 2003).

3.3.3 Role of Inflammatory Molecules in the Proliferation of IBC Cells

Cancer is fundamentally a disease of inappropriate cell division and proliferation. Cytokines can enhance growth through their interaction with growth factors, e.g., ER, and transcriptional pathways such as IL-6/JAK/STAT3. An in vitro study comparing ER-positive to ER-negative breast cancer cell lines reported higher levels of IL-6-mediated STAT3 phosphorylation in ER-negative versus ER-positive cells. Upon exposure of MCF-7 ER-positive cells to IL-6, tumor cell growth rates were enhanced by >two-fold (Sasser et al. 2007).

IL-1β is a major proinflammatory cytokine that is known to contribute to tumor proliferation, angiogenesis, and local invasion (Apte et al. 2006). Higher IL-1β levels in breast cancer tissue or serum were correlated with more aggressive disease and poorer outcome (Goldberg and Schwertfeger 2010). However, the interaction between IL-1β and ER in tumor growth in breast cancer has been less understood with evidence supporting transcriptional activation of ER by IL-1β (Speirs et al. 1999). A recent study suggested that IL-1 secretion in breast cancer may be regulated by estradiol in vivo and that its release may be inhibited by antiestrogen therapy (Abrahamsson et al. 2012).

TNF-α, a potent suppressor of proliferation in normal cells, was found to enhance proliferation in the T47D breast cancer cell line through an NF-κB-dependent pathway (Rubio et al. 2006). Proliferating cells were found to express high levels of cyclin D1 (Rivas et al. 2008). Furthermore, the addition of a specific NF-κB inhibitor, Bay 11-7082, was able to block TNF-α-induced tumor promotion and cyclin D1 expression. Additional in vitro studies on MCF-7 cells demonstrated the capacity of TNF-α to upregulate several genes associated with cancer proliferation (Yin et al. 2009). Alternatively, TNF-α can interact with ER as well as other transcription factors in an NF-κB-independent manner to regulate genes that are important for proliferation in breast cancer (Gloire et al. 2006).

3.3.4 Role of Inflammatory Molecules in the Invasion, Metastasis, and Angiogenesis of IBC Cells

Cancer cell progression is a multistep process that involves the acquisition of several characteristics that include epithelial–mesenchymal transition (EMT), cell invasion, migration, intra- and extravasation, and angiogenesis. EMT is the process by which cancer cells lose epithelial properties such as cell polarity and cell-to-cell contact and acquire mesenchymal (fibroblastic) characteristics. This process confers malignant properties such as invasiveness and motility and is essential for cancer cells to metastasize (Thiery 2002; Thiery et al. 2009).

IBC gene expression profiles have revealed the activation of specific stem-cell-related pathways that contribute to the activation of NF-κB, which in turn induces EMT (Laere et al. 2010). Recently, investigators were able to reproduce EMT in IBC cells using a three-dimensional culture system. IBC cells exhibited a reduction in epithelial markers (E-cadherin) and overexpression of mesenchymal marker vimentin. Investigators were able to inhibit EMT by blocking the EGFR pathway using an EGFR tyrosine kinase inhibitor, erlotinib (Zhang et al. 2009).

Overexpression of TGF-β has been associated with several tumors and correlates with aggressive features (Derynck et al. 2001). TGF-β plays a central role in the induction of EMT (Moustakas and Heldin 2007). It inhibits expression of E-cadherin (Xu et al. 2009) and is associated with reduced levels of claudins and occludins, as well as tight-junction degradation (Moustakas and Heldin 2007). Moreover, TGF-β1 induces expression of Mdm2, which results in the destabilization of p53, a critical step in the EMT of breast cancer that is associated with advanced disease (Araki et al. 2010).

In tissue samples of human breast cancers, high levels of TGF-β1 mRNA were associated with increased angiogenesis as measured by microvessel density, features that are common in IBC (de Jong et al. 1998). TGF-β is known to trigger the expression of vascular endothelial growth factor (VEGF) as well as act as a chemo-attractant for monocytes, which in turn release angiogenic factors (Yang and Moses 1990; Ashcroft 1999). Furthermore, TGF-β is also able to induce cell migration through the expression of matrix metalloproteases MMP-2 and MMP-9 (Hagedorn et al. 2001). The results of these studies suggest that TGF-β exerts a broad range of effects that confer invasiveness and metastasis through its regulation of EMT and cell motility (Docherty et al. 2006; Yang et al. 2006).

Higher levels of IL-6 in the SUM149 IBC model have been attributed to regulation by RhoC GTPase, which plays a role in the development of the invasive/angiogenic phenotype of IBC (Golen et al. 2000). In turn, IL-6 activates multiple effectors involved in the process of invasion and metastasis (Heinrich et al. 2003; Tawara et al. 2011). Sullivan et al. (2009) observed that IL-6 induced EMT as well as enhanced invasiveness of MCF-7 cancer cells. Furthermore, IL-6 produced by fibroblasts or stromal adipocytes derived from breast tissue or from metastatic sites promoted invasion in MCF-7 cells (Studebaker et al. 2008; Walter et al. 2009).

The chemokine IL-8 is another inflammatory molecule that is differentially expressed in IBC tumors (Laere et al. 2005, 2007). IL-8 production is amplified in metastatic breast cancer lesions and plays a key role in tumor progression, invasion, and angiogenesis (Freund et al. 2004; Yao et al. 2007; Lin et al. 2004). A similar effect can be seen with increased tumor and serum levels of IL-1β, which were associated with invasiveness in ER-negative breast tumors (Goldberg and Schwertfeger 2010). In ER-positive tumors, IL-1β was found to promote EMT changes as well as cell migration, invasion, angiogenesis, and metastasis (Franco-Barraza et al. 2010; Wang et al. 2005).

Studies in MCF-7 breast cancer cells have also shown TNF-α to promote the expression of a panel of genes that are known to be associated with invasion and metastasis (Yin et al. 2009). Moreover, the chemokine receptor CXCR4 and its ligand CXCL12 (stromal cell-derived factor-1 alpha) are differentially expressed in IBC tumors and are known to regulate interactions between tumor cells and the microenvironment that are critical for the development of organ-specific metastasis (Cabioglu et al. 2007; Clezardin 2011).

3.4 Role of Inflammatory Molecules in the Development of IBC: Evidence From In Vivo Studies

One of the challenges facing IBC research is the development of preclinical models that accurately recapitulate the aggressiveness of the disease. Currently, there is a need for better immunocompetent mouse models of IBC that allow assessment of the molecular and inflammatory mechanisms underlying the disease and the development of effective therapeutic targets.

In a recent study that looked at the role of NF-κB signaling in conferring self-renewal to breast cancer cells, three types of IBC SUM149 cells were prepared and injected into the mammary fat pads of nude mice. These included cells expressing IκBα-SR at low or high density or an empty vector (Kendellen et al. 2013). Investigators assessed self-renewal by measuring the ability of cells when injected at limiting dilutions to establish primary tumors. Cells with deficient NF-κB signaling produced smaller tumors at a much later onset compared to those with empty vector, whereas the low density of SUM149 cells expressing IκBα-SR did not form tumors. The ability to self-renew appears to require both intact canonical and non-canonical NF-κB pathways (Kendellen et al. 2013). This demonstrates the importance of NF-κB for tumorigenesis in xenograft models.

Cyclooxygenase-2 (COX-2) is over-expressed in mammary tumors derived from rodent models of breast cancer. Enhanced COX-2 expression was found to be sufficient to induce mammary gland tumorigenesis in the mouse mammary tumor virus (MMTV)/COX-2 transgenic mouse strain, thus providing evidence for its in vivo oncogenicity (Liu et al. 2001). Additionally, mammary gland involution after weaning was delayed in the transgenic animals compared to controls, suggesting that apoptosis suppression was also involved (Liu et al. 2001).

Studies have also demonstrated that tumor formation in these models can be suppressed either pharmacologically by using anti-inflammatory drugs, including COX inhibitors, or through genetic ablation (Howe 2007; Howe et al. 2001; Howe et al. 2005). COX inhibitors were also evaluated in HER2/neu transgenic mice, which are also ER negative. Celecoxib administration was able to significantly delay tumor formation in the animal model (Howe et al. 2002; Lanza-Jacoby et al. 2003).

To examine the consequences of knocking out COX-2, investigators adopted an approach used in intestinal cancer models (Oshima et al. 1996), by crossing COX-2 knockout mice with mammary tumor virus/neu deletion mutant (MMTV/NDL) mice and comparing tumor multiplicity to HER2/neu transgenic mice that were COX-2 wild type, heterozygous, and null (Howe et al. 2005). Tumor multiplicity and size were significantly reduced in COX-2 knockout mice (heterozygous and null) compared to controls (Howe et al. 2005). Additionally, the authors observed that COX-2 null animals were associated with reduced expression in several angiogenesis factors, which led to a reduction in mammary blood vessel formation. Together, these studies suggest that an intact COX-2 pathway is both necessary and sufficient for the induction of tumorigenesis.

Similarly, the tumorigenicity of TGF-β was assessed by developing a doxycycline-inducible triple transgenic mice model in which doxycycline can be used to induce TGF-β1 expression in polyomavirus middle T antigen (PyVmT) transformed mammary tumors (Muraoka-Cook et al. 2004). TGF-β1 stimulation resulted in rapidly accelerated metastatic progression with >ten-fold increase in lung metastases in as little as 2 weeks. Antisense-mediated inhibition of TGF-β1 resulted in decreased cell motility, survival, anchorage-independent growth, tumorigenicity, and metastasis. Similarly, Criswell et al. looked at the role of TGF-β type III receptors in inducing EMT, cancer cell motility, and invasion of metastatic cancer cells through a similar transgenic model (Criswell et al. 2008).

To address the role of IL-6 in cancer proliferation, investigators looked at whether expression of IL-6 in MCF-7 cells would alter tumor growth rates in immunocompromised mice. Xenografts expressing IL-6 underwent rapid engraftment and expansion relative to MCF-7 xenografts that did not express IL-6 (Sasser et al. 2007). On the other hand, using siRNA to knock down STAT3 expression in nude mice, investigators were able to suppress breast cancer cell growth compared with controls. pRNAi-STAT3 also led to downregulation of STAT3 and Bcl-xL, as well as upregulation of Fas and induction of apoptosis via expression of cleaved caspase-3 (Kunigal et al. 2009; Matthews et al. 2007).

3.5 Evidence From Patients for the Role of Inflammation in IBC

The rarity of IBC as a disease has not allowed the role of inflammation to be systematically examined in clinical studies involving IBC patients; however, numerous clinical reports and observational studies have addressed the role of inflammation in breast cancer in general.

C-reactive protein (CRP) is an acute-phase protein that is considered the classic marker of systemic inflammation. CRP levels in plasma are known to rise rapidly in response to acute inflammation (Black et al. 2004; Casas et al. 2008; Gabay and Kushner 1999), but have also been found to be moderately increased in chronic inflammatory disease (Hirschfield and Pepys 2003). Large epidemiologic studies have suggested a correlation between high circulating levels of CRP and the risk of developing cancer. This observation has not been demonstrated for breast cancer, however. The Women's Health Study measured baseline plasma CRP levels for 27,919 healthy women aged 45 years or older. After a mean follow-up of 10 years, 892 patients had developed breast cancer; results showed no association between increased CRP levels and the risk of developing breast cancer (Zhang et al. 2007).

Likewise, in a Danish general population study, 10,408 individuals had their CRP levels measured at baseline and were observed for up to 16 years. During follow-up, 1,624 went on to develop cancer, and 998 patients died. Increased CRP levels were associated with an increased risk of cancer of any type and possibly an increased risk of colorectal cancer and lung cancer, but not breast cancer (Allin et al. 2009).

On the other hand, high CRP levels were found to be associated with poor prognosis in several types of cancer, including breast cancer. Allin et al. (2011) looked at CRP levels at baseline in 2,910 breast cancer patients. Higher CRP levels were found to be associated with larger tumor size, development of distant metastases, and poor prognosis. More importantly, the authors reported that breast cancer was the leading cause of death in this cohort, thus excluding the possibility that the outcome was confounded by risk of cardiac disease, for which CRP is an established risk factor (Allin et al. 2011).

Ristimaki and colleagues analyzed the expression of COX-2 protein using immunohistochemistry in tissue specimens of 1,576 patients with breast cancer (Ristimaki et al. 2002). Increased levels were found in approximately 40 % of breast tumors and were associated with shorter distant metastasis-free survival. Tumors with COX-2 expression were associated with negative hormone receptor status as well as the presence of HER2 amplification and axillary nodal metastasis. Additional unfavorable features associated with COX-2 increase include larger tumor size, higher histological grade, high Ki-67 proliferation rates, higher p53 expression, and ductal type histology. However, the differences in outcome between patients with increased COX-2 protein and those without was even more pronounced in patients with more favorable prognostic characteristics, such as ER positivity, low p53 expression, and no HER-2 amplification.

The preclinical model of IBC, a disease known for its aggressive course, expressed increased levels of IL-6 and IL-8 (Golen et al. 2000). High levels of IL-6 were reported to be associated with poorer response to therapy in patients with metastatic breast cancer (Zhang and Adachi 1999). This was confirmed in the clinical setting; breast cancer patients were found to have higher serum levels of IL-6 than do healthy women (Kozlowski et al. 2003; Jiang et al. 2000). Two studies looked at IL-6 in different tumor stages and found higher levels of IL-6 were correlated to advanced cancer stage (Jablonska et al. 2001; Lyons et al. 2011). Others looked at how serum levels correlated with recurrence and outcome in the metastatic setting (Nishimura et al. 2000; Bozcuk et al. 2004; Salgado et al. 2003). One study analyzed the association between IL-6 serum levels and response to therapy as designated by the Response Evaluation Criteria in Solid Tumors (RECIST); higher levels were associated with poor objective response to therapy (Zhang and Adachi 1999).

Similarly, TGF-β levels in plasma in breast cancer patients were found to be increased and predictive of lymph node and distant metastasis (Ivanovic et al. 2009; Yu et al. 2010). Additionally, increased levels of IL-1β in the tumor and in the serum of ER-negative breast tumors were correlated with tumor invasiveness and poor outcome (Studebaker et al. 2008). The production of IL-8 in ER-positive breast cancer patients was associated with shorter relapse-free survival (Freund et al. 2003). Furthermore, increased circulating levels of TNF-α were correlated with increased lymph node metastasis and breast cancer stage (Sheen-Chen et al. 1997).

3.6 Inhibitors of Inflammation for the Prevention and Treatment of IBC

Management of IBC consists of tri-modality therapy: neoadjuvant chemotherapy, then modified radical mastectomy, followed by locoregional radiotherapy. Prior to the era of multimodality therapy, the 5-year overall survival rate was less than 5 % (Robbins et al. 1974). In a more recent study, patients who received all components of tri-modality therapy achieved an overall survival rate at 5 years of 51 %, versus 24 % for patients who did not receive all three components (Bristol et al. 2008).

One of the biggest challenges in the treatment of IBC thus far has been the lack of clinically relevant treatment targets. In a retrospective analysis, 316 IBC patients were assigned according to ER and HER2 status into four groups: ER positive (33 %), ER positive/HER2 positive (12 %), HER2 positive (26 %), and triple negative (29 %) (Li et al. 2011). The triple-negative subtype was found to predict the worst overall survival and high recurrence rates. Hence, the search for potential treatment targets has become a priority in particular for patients with triple-negative IBC. One promising tactic has been to target the inflammatory pathways in the adjuvant setting or in combination with systemic therapy (Pierga et al. 2010; Agrawal and Fentiman 2008).

Pan et al. looked at the activity of tetrathiomolybdate, a copper chelator, in tumors derived from SUM149 IBC cells. Tetrathiomolybdate was shown to effectively suppress angiogenesis and motility in IBC cell line tumors through its inhibitory effects on NF-κB signaling (Pan et al. 2002, 2003). This was accompanied by reduced levels of VEGF, basic fibroblast growth factor (bFGF), IL-6, IL-1α, and IL-8, as well as decreased tumor volume (Pan et al. 2002). Another compound that is known to inhibit the NF-κB pathway is pyrrolidinedithiocarbamate (Zhou et al. 2008). Inhibition of the NF-κB pathway, which is upregulated in IBC, is one of the most promising areas of research.

The chemokine CXCR4/CXCL12 receptor/ligand pair has been observed to promote angiogenesis as well as confer survival on CSCs (Duda et al. 2011; Greenfield et al. 2010). The CXCR4 antagonist, CTCE 9908, in combination with paclitaxel, was evaluated in a SUM149 preclinical model of triple-negative IBC

(Singh et al. 2010). CTCE-9908 as a single agent inhibited skeletal metastases but failed to prevent primary tumor growth or pulmonary metastasis.

Owing to their unacceptable cardiotoxicity, the use of selective COX-2 inhibitors has been limited despite initial enthusiasm regarding promising epidemiologic results and their anti-cancer activities (Psaty and Furberg 2005; Graham et al.2005). Interest has instead shifted to searching for alternative COX-2-targeted agents. One such target is the family of prostanoid receptors, particularly EP4, that bind with PGE2, which is a product of COX-2 (Jones et al. 2009). EP4 was found to mediate invasion and metastasis in both inflammatory and non-IBCs, and EP3 suppressed angiogenesis in IBC tumors (Robertson et al. 2008, 2010). None of the available EP4 antagonists have yet been tested in cancer patients.

Apricoxib is a novel selective COX inhibitor analog that is currently under evaluation in breast cancer in combination with lapatinib and capecitabine in the treatment of HER2/neu-positive advanced breast cancer (Health NIo 2001). Tranilast is another compound under investigation and is known as a potent inhibitor of PGE2. It was shown to suppress tumorigenesis in both xenograft mammary tumors and human triple-negative breast cancer cells (Chakrabarti et al. 2009; Subramaniam et al. 2010, 2011).

Another agent under evaluation in breast cancer is fish oil. Fish oils contain the omega-3 fatty acids docosahexaenoic acid (DHA) and eicosapentaenoic acid (EPA), which ultimately lead to the inhibition of inflammation in the body (Weaver et al. 2009). This is suspected to occur through inhibition of COX/PGE2 production (Wendel and Heller 2009).

Recently, a new role for statins as a preventive agent against cancer has emerged. Recent evidence has suggested that in addition to their lipid-lowering effects, statins exert powerful anti-inflammatory effects by acting on multiple inflammatory gene pathways (Jain and Ridker 2005). The anti-cancer effects of statins have also been linked to the mevalonate pathway, which in turn leads to the inhibition of many downstream growth factors (Nielsen et al. 2012). Large observational studies have pointed toward the potential role this pathway has against cancer in general as well as breast cancer specifically (Nielsen et al. 2012; Ahern et al. 2011). Brewer et al. have also addressed the potential role of statins in improving the survival of patients with IBC (Brewer et al. 2012).

Curcumin is the principal derivative of turmeric, the popular Indian spice and a member of the ginger family. Various preclinical studies have looked into its role in breast cancer as a chemosensitizer and radiosensitizer to agents such as doxorubicin, 5-fluorouracil, and paclitaxel (Goel and Aggarwal 2010). Curcumin is a known potent inhibitor of NF-κB, STAT3, and COX-2 as well as other growth factors and anti-apoptotic proteins (Goel and Aggarwal 2010).

3.7 Conclusions and Future Directions

Current evidence supports that inflammation plays a central role in the process of tumor formation in IBC at various levels. Several important inflammatory gene pathways are differentially upregulated in IBC and contribute to the formation of a pro-inflammatory feedback loop that is critical for malignant transformation (Hartman et al. 2011). On the other hand, downstream cytokines and chemokines are involved at every step of tumorigenesis/carcinogenesis, including initiation, transformation, proliferation, cancer cell survival, invasion, angiogenesis, and metastasis. Several pharmacological compounds that target the inflammatory signaling pathways are currently being tested in the laboratory and in the clinical setting. There is a demand for better immunocompetent IBC mouse models for more accurate in vivo testing and drug development. Proteomic analysis of IBC offers the opportunity to conduct a quantitative and functional evaluation of protein activity in the various signaling networks involved (Chen et al. 2002). It allows assessment of posttranslational modifications, complementing gene expression studies in IBC (Bichsel et al. 2001). New approaches such as high-throughput screening may help identify novel agents that inhibit key signaling pathways. Ultimately, the clinical role of targeting inflammation in IBC needs to be tested prospectively.

Acknowledgments Grant Support: State of Texas Rare and Aggressive Breast Cancer Research Program Grant.

References

Abrahamsson A, Morad V, Saarinen NM, Dabrosin C (2012) Estradiol, tamoxifen, and flaxseed alter IL-1beta and IL-1Ra levels in normal human breast tissue in vivo. J Clin Endocrinol Metab 97(11):E2044–E2054

ACS (2014) Cancer facts and figures 2014. American Cancer Society, Atlanta, GA. Accessed 25 Mar 2014

Agrawal A, Fentiman IS (2008) NSAIDs and breast cancer: a possible prevention and treatment strategy. Int J Clin Pract 62(3):444–449

Ahern TP, Pedersen L, Tarp M et al (2011) Statin prescriptions and breast cancer recurrence risk: a Danish nationwide prospective cohort study. J Natl Cancer Inst 103(19):1461–1468

Allin KH, Bojesen SE, Nordestgaard BG (2009) Baseline C-reactive protein is associated with incident cancer and survival in patients with cancer. J Clin Oncol: Off J Am Soc Clin Oncol 27(13):2217–2224

Allin KH, Nordestgaard BG, Flyger H, Bojesen SE (2011) Elevated pre-treatment levels of plasma C-reactive protein are associated with poor prognosis after breast cancer: a cohort study. Breast Cancer Res 13(3):R55

Anderson WF, Schairer C, Chen BE, Hance KW, Levine PH (2005) Epidemiology of inflammatory breast cancer (IBC). Breast Dis 22:9–23

Apte RN, Krelin Y, Song X et al (2006) Effects of micro-environment- and malignant cell-derived interleukin-1 in carcinogenesis, tumour invasiveness and tumour-host interactions. Eur J Cancer 42(6):751–759

Araki S, Eitel JA, Batuello CN et al (2010) TGF-beta1-induced expression of human Mdm2 correlates with late-stage metastatic breast cancer. J Clin Investig 120(1):290–302

Ashcroft GS (1999) Bidirectional regulation of macrophage function by TGF-beta. Microbes Infect/Ins Pasteur 1(15):1275–1282

Barbieri I, Pensa S, Pannellini T et al (2010) Constitutively active Stat3 enhances neu-mediated migration and metastasis in mammary tumors via upregulation of cten. Cancer Res 70(6):2558–2567

Bichsel VE, Liotta LA, Petricoin EF 3rd (2001) Cancer proteomics: from biomarker discovery to signal pathway profiling. Cancer J 7(1):69–78

Biswas DK, Shi Q, Baily S et al (2004) NF-kappa B activation in human breast cancer specimens and its role in cell proliferation and apoptosis. Proc Natl Acad Sci USA 101(27):10137–10142

Biswas S, Guix M, Rinehart C et al (2007) Inhibition of TGF-beta with neutralizing antibodies prevents radiation-induced acceleration of metastatic cancer progression. J Clin Investig 117(5):1305–1313

Black S, Kushner I, Samols D (2004) C-reactive Protein. J Biol Chem 279(47):48487–48490

Bozcuk H, Uslu G, Samur M et al (2004) Tumour necrosis factor-alpha, interleukin-6, and fasting serum insulin correlate with clinical outcome in metastatic breast cancer patients treated with chemotherapy. Cytokine 27(2–3):58–65

Brewer TM, Masuda H, Iwamoto T et al (2012) Statin use and improved survival outcome in primary inflammatory breast cancer: retrospective cohort study. Paper presented at: CTRC-AACR: san antonio breast cancer symposium, 4–8 Dec 2012, San Antonio, TX

Bristol IJ, Woodward WA, Strom EA et al (2008) Locoregional treatment outcomes after multimodality management of inflammatory breast cancer. Int J Radiat Oncol Biol Phys 72(2):474–484

Brown JR, DuBois RN (2005) COX-2: a molecular target for colorectal cancer prevention. J Clin Oncol: Official J Am Soc Clin Oncol 23(12):2840–2855

Cabioglu N, Gong Y, Islam R et al (2007) Expression of growth factor and chemokine receptors: new insights in the biology of inflammatory breast cancer. Ann Oncol: Off J Eur Soc Med Oncol/ESMO 18(6):1021–1029

Casas JP, Shah T, Hingorani AD, Danesh J, Pepys MB (2008) C-reactive protein and coronary heart disease: a critical review. J Intern Med 264(4):295–314

Chakrabarti R, Subramaniam V, Abdalla S, Jothy S, Prud'homme GJ (2009) Tranilast inhibits the growth and metastasis of mammary carcinoma. Anti-Cancer Drugs 20(5):334–345

Charafe-Jauffret E, Ginestier C, Iovino F et al (2009) Breast cancer cell lines contain functional cancer stem cells with metastatic capacity and a distinct molecular signature. Cancer Res 69(4):1302–1313

Charafe-Jauffret E, Ginestier C, Iovino F et al (2010) Aldehyde dehydrogenase 1-positive cancer stem cells mediate metastasis and poor clinical outcome in inflammatory breast cancer. Clin Cancer Res: Off J Am Assoc Cancer Res 16(1):45–55

Chen G, Gharib TG, Huang CC et al (2002) Discordant protein and mRNA expression in lung adenocarcinomas. Mol Cell Proteomics 1(4):304–313

Cheshire JL, Baldwin AS Jr (1997) Synergistic activation of NF-kappaB by tumor necrosis factor alpha and gamma interferon via enhanced I kappaB alpha degradation and de novo I kappaB beta degradation. Mol Cell Biol 17(11):6746–6754

Clezardin P (2011) Therapeutic targets for bone metastases in breast cancer. Breast Cancer Res: BCR 13(2):207

Criswell TL, Dumont N, Barnett JV, Arteaga CL (2008) Knockdown of the transforming growth factor-beta type III receptor impairs motility and invasion of metastatic cancer cells. Cancer Res 68(18):7304–7312

D'Anello L, Sansone P, Storci G et al (2010) Epigenetic control of the basal-like gene expression profile via Interleukin-6 in breast cancer cells. Mol Cancer 9:300

Dawood S, Merajver SD, Viens P et al (2011) International expert panel on inflammatory breast cancer: consensus statement for standardized diagnosis and treatment. Ann Oncol: Official J Eur Soc Med Oncol/ESMO 22(3):515–523

de Jong JS, van Diest PJ, van der Valk P, Baak JP (1998) Expression of growth factors, growth-inhibiting factors, and their receptors in invasive breast cancer. II: Correlations with proliferation and angiogenesis. J Pathol 184(1):53–57

Derynck R, Akhurst RJ, Balmain A (2001) TGF-beta signaling in tumor suppression and cancer progression. Nat Genet 29(2):117–129

Diaz N, Minton S, Cox C et al (2006) Activation of stat3 in primary tumors from high-risk breast cancer patients is associated with elevated levels of activated SRC and survivin expression. Clin Cancer Res: Off J Am Assoc Cancer Res 12(1):20–28

Docherty NG, O'Sullivan OE, Healy DA et al (2006) TGF-beta1-induced EMT can occur independently of its proapoptotic effects and is aided by EGF receptor activation. Am J Physiol: Ren Physiol 290(5):F1202–F1212

Duda DG, Kozin SV, Kirkpatrick ND, Xu L, Fukumura D, Jain RK (2011) CXCL12 (SDF1alpha)-CXCR4/CXCR7 pathway inhibition: an emerging sensitizer for anticancer therapies? Clin Cancer Res: Off J Am Assoc Cancer Res 17(8):2074–2080

Dunning AM, Ellis PD, McBride S et al (2003) A transforming growth factorbeta1 signal peptide variant increases secretion in vitro and is associated with increased incidence of invasive breast cancer. Cancer Res 63(10):2610–2615

El-Shinawi M, Mohamed HT, El-Ghonaimy EA et al (2013) Human cytomegalovirus infection enhances NF-kappaB/p65 signaling in inflammatory breast cancer patients. PLoS ONE 8(2):e55755

Franco-Barraza J, Valdivia-Silva JE, Zamudio-Meza H et al (2010) Actin cytoskeleton participation in the onset of IL-1beta induction of an invasive mesenchymal-like phenotype in epithelial MCF-7 cells. Arch Med Res 41(3):170–181

Freund A, Chauveau C, Brouillet JP et al (2003) IL-8 expression and its possible relationship with estrogen-receptor-negative status of breast cancer cells. Oncogene 22(2):256–265

Freund A, Jolivel V, Durand S et al (2004) Mechanisms underlying differential expression of interleukin-8 in breast cancer cells. Oncogene 23(36):6105–6114

Gabay C, Kushner I (1999) Acute-phase proteins and other systemic responses to inflammation. New Engl J Med 340(6):448–454

Garcia R, Yu CL, Hudnall A et al (1997) Constitutive activation of Stat3 in fibroblasts transformed by diverse oncoproteins and in breast carcinoma cells. Cell Growth Differ: Mol Biol J Am Assoc Cancer Res 8(12):1267–1276

Garcia-Tunon I, Ricote M, Ruiz A, Fraile B, Paniagua R, Royuela M (2005) IL-6, its receptors and its relationship with bcl-2 and bax proteins in infiltrating and in situ human breast carcinoma. Histopathology 47(1):82–89

Ginestier C, Liu S, Diebel ME et al (2010) CXCR1 blockade selectively targets human breast cancer stem cells in vitro and in xenografts. J Clin Investig 120(2):485–497

Gloire G, Dejardin E, Piette J (2006) Extending the nuclear roles of IkappaB kinase subunits. Biochem Pharmacol 72(9):1081–1089

Goel A, Aggarwal BB (2010) Curcumin, the golden spice from Indian saffron, is a chemosensitizer and radiosensitizer for tumors and chemoprotector and radioprotector for normal organs. Nutr Cancer 62(7):919–930

Goldberg JE, Schwertfeger KL (2010) Proinflammatory cytokines in breast cancer: mechanisms of action and potential targets for therapeutics. Curr Drug Targets 11(9):1133–1146

Graham DJ, Campen D, Hui R et al (2005) Risk of acute myocardial infarction and sudden cardiac death in patients treated with cyclo-oxygenase 2 selective and non-selective non-steroidal anti-inflammatory drugs: nested case-control study. Lancet 365(9458):475–481

Greenfield JP, Cobb WS, Lyden D (2010) Resisting arrest: a switch from angiogenesis to vasculogenesis in recurrent malignant gliomas. J Clin Investig 120(3):663–667

Guerin M, Gabillot M, Mathieu MC et al (1989) Structure and expression of c-erbB-2 and EGF receptor genes in inflammatory and non-inflammatory breast cancer: prognostic significance. Int J Cancer: J Int du Cancer 43(2):201–208

Haagensen C (1971) Diseases of the breast, 2nd edn. Saunders, Philadelphia

Hagedorn HG, Bachmeier BE, Nerlich AG (2001) Synthesis and degradation of basement membranes and extracellular matrix and their regulation by TGF-beta in invasive carcinomas (review). Int J Oncol 18(4):669–681

Hanahan D, Weinberg RA (2000) The hallmarks of cancer. Cell 100(1):57–70

Hance KW, Anderson WF, Devesa SS, Young HA, Levine PH (2005) Trends in inflammatory breast carcinoma incidence and survival: the surveillance, epidemiology, and end results program at the National Cancer Institute. J Natl Cancer Inst 97(13):966–975

Hartman ZC, Yang XY, Glass O et al (2011) HER2 overexpression elicits a proinflammatory IL-6 autocrine signaling loop that is critical for tumorigenesis. Cancer Res 71(13):4380–4391

Hayden MS, Ghosh S (2008) Shared principles in NF-kappaB signaling. Cell 132(3):344–362
Health NIo (2001) APRiCOT-B: Study to Evaluate Apricoxib in Combination With Lapatinib and Capecitabine in the Treatment of HER2/Neu+ Breast Cancer (TP2001-202). http://clinicaltrials.gov/show/NCT00657137. Accessed on 4 Apr 2013
Heinrich PC, Behrmann I, Haan S, Hermanns HM, Muller-Newen G, Schaper F (2003) Principles of interleukin (IL)-6-type cytokine signalling and its regulation. Biochem J 374(Pt 1):1–20
Hinohara K, Gotoh N (2010) Inflammatory signaling pathways in self-renewing breast cancer stem cells. Curr Opin Pharmacol 10(6):650–654
Hirschfield GM, Pepys MB (2003) C-reactive protein and cardiovascular disease: new insights from an old molecule. QJM: Monthly J Assoc Phys 96(11):793–807
Hodge DR, Peng B, Cherry JC et al (2005) Interleukin 6 supports the maintenance of p53 tumor suppressor gene promoter methylation. Cancer Res 65(11):4673–4682
Howe LR (2007) Inflammation and breast cancer, cyclooxygenase/prostaglandin signaling and breast cancer. Breast Cancer Res: BCR 9(4):210
Howe LR, Subbaramaiah K, Brown AM, Dannenberg AJ (2001) Cyclooxygenase-2: a target for the prevention and treatment of breast cancer. Endocr Relat Cancer 8(2):97–114
Howe LR, Subbaramaiah K, Patel J et al (2002) Celecoxib, a selective cyclooxygenase 2 inhibitor, protects against human epidermal growth factor receptor 2 (HER-2)/neu-induced breast cancer. Cancer Res 62(19):5405–5407
Howe LR, Chang SH, Tolle KC et al (2005) HER2/neu-induced mammary tumorigenesis and angiogenesis are reduced in cyclooxygenase-2 knockout mice. Cancer Res 65(21):10113–10119
Iliopoulos D, Hirsch HA, Struhl K (2009) An epigenetic switch involving NF-kappaB, Lin28, Let-7 MicroRNA, and IL6 links inflammation to cell transformation. Cell 139(4):693–706
Iliopoulos D, Jaeger SA, Hirsch HA, Bulyk ML, Struhl K (2010) STAT3 activation of miR-21 and miR-181b-1 via PTEN and CYLD are part of the epigenetic switch linking inflammation to cancer. Mol Cell 39(4):493–506
Iliopoulos D, Hirsch HA, Wang G, Struhl K (2011) Inducible formation of breast cancer stem cells and their dynamic equilibrium with non-stem cancer cells via IL6 secretion. Proc Natl Acad Sci USA 108(4):1397–1402
Ivanovic V, Dedovic-Tanic N, Milovanovic Z et al (2009) Quantification of transforming growth factor beta 1 levels in metastatic axillary lymph node tissue extracts from breast cancer patients: a new specimen source. Anal Quant Cytol Histol/Int Acad Cytol Am Soc Cytol 31(5):288–295
Jablonska E, Kiluk M, Markiewicz W, Piotrowski L, Grabowska Z, Jablonski J (2001) TNF-alpha, IL-6 and their soluble receptor serum levels and secretion by neutrophils in cancer patients. Arch Immunologiae et Ther Exp 49(1):63–69
Jain MK, Ridker PM (2005) Anti-inflammatory effects of statins: clinical evidence and basic mechanisms Nature reviews. Drug Discov 4(12):977–987
Jaiyesimi IA, Buzdar AU, Hortobagyi G (1992) Inflammatory breast cancer: a review. J Clin Oncol: Off J Am Soc Clin Oncol 10(6):1014–1024
Jiang XP, Yang DC, Elliott RL, Head JF (2000) Reduction in serum IL-6 after vacination of breast cancer patients with tumour-associated antigens is related to estrogen receptor status. Cytokine 12(5):458–465
Jones RL, Giembycz MA, Woodward DF (2009) Prostanoid receptor antagonists: development strategies and therapeutic applications. Br J Pharmacol 158(1):104–145
Ma LZ, Walgren B, Clayton RA, Burkholder JR (2011) T.P. LY2784544, a small molecule JAK2 inhibitor, induces apoptosis in inflammatory breast cancer spheres through targeting IL-6-JAK-STAT3 pathway. Paper presented at: Proceedings of the annual meeting of the American Association for Cancer Research; 2–6 Apr 2011, Orlando
Kaklamani VG, Hou N, Bian Y et al (2003) TGFBR1*6A and cancer risk: a meta-analysis of seven case-control studies. J Clin Oncol: Off J Am Soc Clin Oncol 21(17):3236–3243
Kalaitzidis D, Gilmore TD (2005) Transcription factor cross-talk: the estrogen receptor and NF-kappaB. Trends Endocrinology and Metabolism: TEM 16(2):46–52
Kallioniemi OP, Holli K, Visakorpi T, Koivula T, Helin HH, Isola JJ (1991) Association of c-erbB-2 protein over-expression with high rate of cell proliferation, increased risk of

visceral metastasis and poor long-term survival in breast cancer. I J Cancer: J Int du Cancer 49(5):650–655
Kan CY, Iacopetta BJ, Lawson JS, Whitaker NJ (2005) Identification of human papillomavirus DNA gene sequences in human breast cancer. Br J Cancer 93(8):946–948
Kendellen MF, Bradford JW, Lawrence CL, Clark KS, Baldwin AS (2013) Canonical and non-canonical NF-kappaB signaling promotes breast cancer tumor-initiating cells. Oncogene, 11 Mar 2013
Kesson EM, Allardice GM, George WD, Burns HJ, Morrison DS (2012) Effects of multidisciplinary team working on breast cancer survival: retrospective, comparative, interventional cohort study of 13,722 women. BMJ 344:e2718
Kozlowski L, Zakrzewska I, Tokajuk P, Wojtukiewicz MZ (2003) Concentration of interleukin-6 (IL-6), interleukin-8 (IL-8) and interleukin-10 (IL-10) in blood serum of breast cancer patients. Rocz Akad Med Bialymst 48:82–84
Kunigal S, Lakka SS, Sodadasu PK, Estes N, Rao JS (2009) Stat3-siRNA induces Fas-mediated apoptosis in vitro and in vivo in breast cancer. Int J Oncol 34(5):1209–1220
Lanza-Jacoby S, Miller S, Flynn J et al (2003) The cyclooxygenase-2 inhibitor, celecoxib, prevents the development of mammary tumors in Her-2/neu mice. Cancer Epidemiol Biomarkers Prev 12(12):1486–1491
Lei X, Bandyopadhyay A, Le T, Sun L (2002) Autocrine TGFbeta supports growth and survival of human breast cancer MDA-MB-231 cells. Oncogene 21(49):7514–7523
Lerebours F, Vacher S, Andrieu C et al (2008) NF-kappa B genes have a major role in inflammatory breast cancer. BMC Cancer 8:41
Li J, Gonzalez-Angulo AM, Allen PK et al (2011) Triple-negative subtype predicts poor overall survival and high locoregional relapse in inflammatory breast cancer. Oncologist 16(12):1675–1683
Lin Y, Huang R, Chen L et al (2004) Identification of interleukin-8 as estrogen receptor-regulated factor involved in breast cancer invasion and angiogenesis by protein arrays. Int J Cancer. J Int du Cancer 109(4):507–515
Liu CH, Chang SH, Narko K et al (2001) Overexpression of cyclooxygenase-2 is sufficient to induce tumorigenesis in transgenic mice. J Biol Chem 276(21):18563–18569
Liu Y, Wang L, Lin XY et al (2012) Anti-apoptotic effect of claudin-1 on TNF-alpha-induced apoptosis in human breast cancer MCF-7 cells. Tumour Biol 33(6):2307–2315
Lyons TR, O'Brien J, Borges VF et al (2011) Postpartum mammary gland involution drives progression of ductal carcinoma in situ through collagen and COX-2. Nat Med 17(9):1109–1115
Martin OA, Redon CE, Dickey JS, Nakamura AJ, Bonner WM (2011) Para-inflammation mediates systemic DNA damage in response to tumor growth. Communicative Integr Biol 4(1):78–81
Matsumoto G, Namekawa J, Muta M et al (2005) Targeting of nuclear factor kappaB Pathways by dehydroxymethylepoxyquinomicin, a novel inhibitor of breast carcinomas: antitumor and antiangiogenic potential in vivo. Clin Cancer Res 11(3):1287–1293
Matthews JR, Watson SM, Tevendale MC, Watson CJ, Clarke AR (2007) Caspase-dependent proteolytic cleavage of STAT3alpha in ES cells, in mammary glands undergoing forced involution and in breast cancer cell lines. BMC Cancer 7:29
Menter DG, Schilsky RL, DuBois RN (2010) Cyclooxygenase-2 and cancer treatment: understanding the risk should be worth the reward. Clinical Cancer Res 16(5):1384–1390
Moody CA, Laimins LA (2009) Human papillomaviruses activate the ATM DNA damage pathway for viral genome amplification upon differentiation. PLoS Pathog 5(10):e1000605
Moustakas A, Heldin CH (2007) Signaling networks guiding epithelial-mesenchymal transitions during embryogenesis and cancer progression. Cancer Sci 98(10):1512–1520
Muraoka-Cook RS, Kurokawa H, Koh Y et al (2004) Conditional overexpression of active transforming growth factor beta1 in vivo accelerates metastases of transgenic mammary tumors. Cancer Res 64(24):9002–9011
Murohashi M, Hinohara K, Kuroda M et al (2010) Gene set enrichment analysis provides insight into novel signalling pathways in breast cancer stem cells. Br J Cancer 102(1):206–212
Nakshatri H, Bhat-Nakshatri P, Martin DA, Goulet RJ Jr, Sledge GW Jr (1997) Constitutive activation of NF-kappaB during progression of breast cancer to hormone-independent growth. Mol Cell Biol 17(7):3629–3639

Nielsen SF, Nordestgaard BG, Bojesen SE (2012) Statin use and reduced cancer-related mortality. New Engl J Med 367(19):1792–1802

Nishimura R, Nagao K, Miyayama H et al (2000) An analysis of serum interleukin-6 levels to predict benefits of medroxyprogesterone acetate in advanced or recurrent breast cancer. Oncology 59(2):166–173

Oshima M, Dinchuk JE, Kargman SL et al (1996) Suppression of intestinal polyposis in Apc delta716 knockout mice by inhibition of cyclooxygenase 2 (COX-2). Cell 87(5):803–809

Pan Q, Kleer CG, van Golen KL et al (2002) Copper deficiency induced by tetrathiomolybdate suppresses tumor growth and angiogenesis. Cancer Res 62(17):4854–4859

Pan Q, Bao LW, Merajver SD (2003) Tetrathiomolybdate inhibits angiogenesis and metastasis through suppression of the NFkappaB signaling cascade. Mol Cancer Res 1(10):701–706

Pasche B, Kaklamani V, Hou N et al (2004) TGFBR1*6A and cancer: a meta-analysis of 12 case-control studies. J Clin Oncol 22(4):756–758

Pierga JY, Delaloge S, Espie M et al (2010) A multicenter randomized phase II study of sequential epirubicin/cyclophosphamide followed by docetaxel with or without celecoxib or trastuzumab according to HER2 status, as primary chemotherapy for localized invasive breast cancer patients. Breast Cancer Res Treat 122(2):429–437

Prasad S, Ravindran J, Aggarwal BB (2010) NF-kappaB and cancer: how intimate is this relationship. Mol Cell Biochem 336(1–2):25–37

Psaty BM, Furberg CD (2005) COX-2 inhibitors–lessons in drug safety. New Engl J Med 352(11):1133–1135

Rawlings JS, Rosler KM, Harrison DA (2004) The JAK/STAT signaling pathway. J Cell Sci 117(Pt 8):1281–1283

Ristimaki A, Sivula A, Lundin J et al (2002) Prognostic significance of elevated cyclooxygenase-2 expression in breast cancer. Cancer Res 62(3):632–635

Rivas MA, Carnevale RP, Proietti CJ et al (2008) TNF alpha acting on TNFR1 promotes breast cancer growth via p42/P44 MAPK, JNK, Akt and NF-kappa B-dependent pathways. Exp Cell Res 314(3):509–529

Robbins GF, Shah J, Rosen P, Chu F, Taylor J (1974) Inflammatory carcinoma of the breast. Surg Clin North Am 54(4):801–810

Robertson FM, Simeone AM, Mazumdar A et al (2008) Molecular and pharmacological blockade of the EP4 receptor selectively inhibits both proliferation and invasion of human inflammatory breast cancer cells. J Exp Ther Oncol 7(4):299–312

Robertson FM, Simeone AM, Lucci A, McMurray JS, Ghosh S, Cristofanilli M (2010) Differential regulation of the aggressive phenotype of inflammatory breast cancer cells by prostanoid receptors EP3 and EP4. Cancer 116(11):2806–2814

Rubio MF, Werbajh S, Cafferata EG et al (2006) TNF-alpha enhances estrogen-induced cell proliferation of estrogen-dependent breast tumor cells through a complex containing nuclear factor-kappa B. Oncogene 25(9):1367–1377

Salgado R, Junius S, Benoy I et al (2003) Circulating interleukin-6 predicts survival in patients with metastatic breast cancer. Int J Cancer: J Int du Cancer 103(5):642–646

Sansone P, Storci G, Tavolari S et al (2007) IL-6 triggers malignant features in mammospheres from human ductal breast carcinoma and normal mammary gland. J Clin Investig 117(12):3988–4002

Sasser AK, Sullivan NJ, Studebaker AW, Hendey LF, Axel AE, Hall BM (2007) Interleukin-6 is a potent growth factor for ER-alpha-positive human breast cancer. FASEB J: Off Publ Fed Am Soc Exp Biol 21(13):3763–3770

Sheen-Chen SM, Chen WJ, Eng HL, Chou FF (1997) Serum concentration of tumor necrosis factor in patients with breast cancer. Breast Cancer Res Treat 43(3):211–215

Shostak K, Chariot A (2011) NF-kappaB, stem cells and breast cancer: the links get stronger. Breast Cancer Res: BCR 13(4):214

Simstein R, Burow M, Parker A, Weldon C, Beckman B (2003) Apoptosis, chemoresistance, and breast cancer: insights from the MCF-7 cell model system. Exp Biol Med 228(9):995–1003

Singh B, Cook KR, Martin C et al (2010) Evaluation of a CXCR4 antagonist in a xenograft mouse model of inflammatory breast cancer. Clin Exp Metastasis 27(4):233–240

Soliman AS, Kleer CG, Mrad K et al (2011) Inflammatory breast cancer in North Africa: comparison of clinical and molecular epidemiologic characteristics of patients from Egypt, Tunisia, and Morocco. Breast Dis 33(4):159–169

Speirs V, Kerin MJ, Newton CJ et al (1999) Evidence for transcriptional activation of ERalpha by IL-1beta in breast cancer cells. Int J Oncol 15(6):1251–1254

Studebaker AW, Storci G, Werbeck JL et al (2008) Fibroblasts isolated from common sites of breast cancer metastasis enhance cancer cell growth rates and invasiveness in an interleukin-6-dependent manner. Cancer Res 68(21):9087–9095

Subbaramaiah K, Norton L, Gerald W, Dannenberg AJ et al (2002) Cyclooxygenase-2 is overexpressed in HER-2/neu-positive breast cancer: evidence for involvement of AP-1 and PEA3. J Biol Chem 277(21):18649–18657

Subramaniam V, Chakrabarti R, Prud'homme GJ, Jothy S (2010) Tranilast inhibits cell proliferation and migration and promotes apoptosis in murine breast cancer. Anti-Cancer Drugs 21(4):351–361

Subramaniam V, Ace O, Prud'homme GJ, Jothy S (2011) Tranilast treatment decreases cell growth, migration and inhibits colony formation of human breast cancer cells. Exp Mol Pathol 90(1):116–122

Sullivan NJ, Sasser AK, Axel AE et al (2009) Interleukin-6 induces an epithelial-mesenchymal transition phenotype in human breast cancer cells. Oncogene 28(33):2940–2947

Tawara K, Oxford JT, Jorcyk CL (2011) Clinical significance of interleukin (IL)-6 in cancer metastasis to bone: potential of anti-IL-6 therapies. Cancer Manag Res 3:177–189

Thiery JP (2002) Epithelial-mesenchymal transitions in tumour progression. Nat Rev Cancer 2(6):442–454

Thiery JP, Acloque H, Huang RY, Nieto MA (2009) Epithelial-mesenchymal transitions in development and disease. Cell 139(5):871–890

Ueno NT, Buzdar AU, Singletary SE et al (1997) Combined-modality treatment of inflammatory breast carcinoma: twenty years of experience at M. D. Anderson Cancer Center. Cancer Chemother Pharmacol 40(4):321–329

van Golen KL, Wu ZF, Qiao XT, Bao L, Merajver SD (2000) RhoC GTPase overexpression modulates induction of angiogenic factors in breast cells. Neoplasia 2(5):418–425

Van Laere S, Van der Auwera I, Van den Eynden GG et al (2005) Distinct molecular signature of inflammatory breast cancer by cDNA microarray analysis. Breast Cancer Res Treat 93(3):237–246

Van Laere SJ, Van der Auwera I, Van den Eynden GG et al (2007) NF-kappaB activation in inflammatory breast cancer is associated with oestrogen receptor downregulation, secondary to EGFR and/or ErbB2 overexpression and MAPK hyperactivation. Br J Cancer 97(5):659–669

Van Laere S, Limame R, Van Marck EA, Vermeulen PB, Dirix LY (2010) Is there a role for mammary stem cells in inflammatory breast carcinoma?: a review of evidence from cell line, animal model, and human tissue sample experiments. Cancer 116(11 Suppl):2794–2805

Walter M, Liang S, Ghosh S, Hornsby PJ, Li R (2009) Interleukin 6 secreted from adipose stromal cells promotes migration and invasion of breast cancer cells. Oncogene 28(30):2745–2755

Wang D, Dubois RN (2004) Cyclooxygenase-2: a potential target in breast cancer. Semin Oncol 31(1 Suppl 3):64–73

Wang FM, Liu HQ, Liu SR, Tang SP, Yang L, Feng GS (2005) SHP-2 promoting migration and metastasis of MCF-7 with loss of E-cadherin, dephosphorylation of FAK and secretion of MMP-9 induced by IL-1beta in vivo and in vitro. Breast Cancer Res Treat 89(1):5–14

Weaver KL, Ivester P, Seeds M, Case LD, Arm JP, Chilton FH (2009) Effect of dietary fatty acids on inflammatory gene expression in healthy humans. J Biol Chem 284(23):15400–15407

Wendel M, Heller AR (2009) Anticancer actions of omega-3 fatty acids–current state and future perspectives. Anti-Cancer Agents Med Chem 9(4):457–470

Williams CS, Mann M, DuBois RN (1999) The role of cyclooxygenases in inflammation, cancer, and development. Oncogene 18(55):7908–7916

Xiao Y, Ye Y, Yearsley K, Jones S, Barsky SH (2008) The lymphovascular embolus of inflammatory breast cancer expresses a stem cell-like phenotype. Am J Pathol 173(2):561–574

Xu J, Lamouille S, Derynck R (2009) TGF-beta-induced epithelial to mesenchymal transition. Cell Res 19(2):156–172

Yang EY, Moses HL (1990) Transforming growth factor beta 1-induced changes in cell migration, proliferation, and angiogenesis in the chicken chorioallantoic membrane. J Cell Biol 111(2):731–741

Yang Y, Pan X, Lei W, Wang J, Song J (2006) Transforming growth factor-beta1 induces epithelial-to-mesenchymal transition and apoptosis via a cell cycle-dependent mechanism. Oncogene 25(55):7235–7244

Yang WT, Le-Petross HT, Macapinlac H et al (2008) Inflammatory breast cancer: PET/CT, MRI, mammography, and sonography findings. Breast Cancer Res Treat 109(3):417–426

Yao C, Lin Y, Chua MS et al (2007) Interleukin-8 modulates growth and invasiveness of estrogen receptor-negative breast cancer cells. Int J Cancer: J Int du Cancer 121(9):1949–1957

Yin Y, Chen X, Shu Y (2009) Gene expression of the invasive phenotype of TNF-alpha-treated MCF-7 cells. Biomed Pharmacotherapie 63(6):421–428

Yoshimura N, Sano H, Okamoto M et al (2003) Expression of cyclooxygenase-1 and -2 in human breast cancer. Surg Today 33(11):805–811

Yu Y, Wang Y, Ren X et al (2010) Context-dependent bidirectional regulation of the MutS homolog 2 by transforming growth factor beta contributes to chemoresistance in breast cancer cells. Mol Cancer Res 8(12):1633–1642

Zhang GJ, Adachi I (1999) Serum interleukin-6 levels correlate to tumor progression and prognosis in metastatic breast carcinoma. Anti-Cancer Res 19(2B):1427–1432

Zhang F, Lundin M, Ristimaki A et al (2003) Ski-related novel protein N (SnoN), a negative controller of transforming growth factor-beta signaling, is a prognostic marker in estrogen receptor-positive breast carcinomas. Cancer Res 63(16):5005–5010

Zhang SM, Lin J, Cook NR et al (2007) C-reactive protein and risk of breast cancer. J Natl Cancer Inst 99(11):890–894

Zhang D, LaFortune TA, Krishnamurthy S et al (2009) Epidermal growth factor receptor tyrosine kinase inhibitor reverses mesenchymal to epithelial phenotype and inhibits metastasis in inflammatory breast cancer. Clin Cancer Res: Off J Am Assoc Cancer Res 15(21):6639–6648

Zhou BP, Hu MC, Miller SA et al (2000) HER-2/neu blocks tumor necrosis factor-induced apoptosis via the Akt/NF-kappaB pathway. J Biol Chem 275(11):8027–8031

Zhou J, Zhang H, Gu P, Bai J, Margolick JB, Zhang Y (2008) NF-kappaB pathway inhibitors preferentially inhibit breast cancer stem-like cells. Breast Cancer Res Treat 111(3):419–427

Chapter 4
The Role of Inflammation in Brain Cancer

James L. Sowers, Kenneth M. Johnson, Charles Conrad, Joel T. Patterson and Lawrence C. Sowers

Abstract Malignant brain tumors are among the most lethal of human tumors, with limited treatment options currently available. A complex array of recurrent genetic and epigenetic changes has been observed in gliomas that collectively result in derangements of common cell signaling pathways controlling cell survival, proliferation, and invasion. One important determinant of gene expression is DNA methylation status, and emerging studies have revealed the importance of a recently identified demethylation pathway involving 5-hydroxymethylcytosine (5hmC). Diminished levels of the modified base 5hmC is a uniform finding in glioma cell lines and patient samples, suggesting a common defect in epigenetic reprogramming. Within the tumor microenvironment, infiltrating immune cells increase oxidative DNA damage, likely promoting both genetic and epigenetic changes that occur during glioma evolution. In this environment, glioma cells are selected that utilize multiple metabolic changes, including changes in the metabolism of the amino acids glutamate, tryptophan, and arginine. Whereas altered metabolism can promote the destruction of normal tissues, glioma cells exploit these changes to promote tumor cell survival and to suppress adaptive immune

J. L. Sowers · K. M. Johnson · L. C. Sowers (✉)
Department of Pharmacology and Toxicology, The University of Texas Medical Branch (UTMB), Galveston, TX, USA
e-mail: lasowers@utmb.edu

J. L. Sowers
Combined MD-PhD Program, UTMB, Galveston, TX, USA

C. Conrad
Department of Neuro-Oncology, The University of Texas MD Anderson Cancer Center, Houston, TX, USA

J. T. Patterson
Department of Surgery, Division of Neurosurgery, UTMB, Galveston, TX, USA

L. C. Sowers
Department of Internal Medicine, Division of Oncology, UTMB, Galveston, TX, USA

B. B. Aggarwal et al. (eds.), *Inflammation and Cancer*, Advances in Experimental Medicine and Biology 816, DOI: 10.1007/978-3-0348-0837-8_4,

responses. Further understanding of these metabolic changes could reveal new strategies that would selectively disadvantage tumor cells and redirect host antitumor responses toward eradication of these lethal tumors.

4.1 Malignant Tumors of the Central Nervous System: Focus on Glioblastoma

4.1.1 WHO Classification of CNS Tumors

Tumors of the central nervous system (CNS) were first classified by the World Health Organization (WHO) on the basis of histopathology, clinical, and diagnostic criteria in 1979. In 1993, immunohistochemical criteria were added, and in 2000, some genetic profiles, epidemiological data, clinical signs and symptoms, imaging, and other predictive factors were added to the classification. As of 2007, additional types had been added, creating an array of more than 130 tumor types and subtypes (Louis et al. 2007; Huttner 2012). The WHO grading scale is based upon histology and includes a "malignancy scale" useful in predicting biological behavior and in selecting treatment strategies. Of the "gliomas," Grade I tumors have low proliferative potential and include all pilocytic astrocytomas and generally can be cured surgically. Grade II tumors demonstrate some infiltration and are likely to recur following surgery. Grade III tumors demonstrate evidence of malignancy, and patients with these tumors generally receive radiation and chemotherapy. Grade IV tumors are malignant, mitotically active and are likely to show evidence of necrosis and vascular proliferation. Grade IV tumors progress rapidly, usually with fatal outcome. CNS tumors can be classified broadly as gliomas, including astrocytomas, oligodendrogliomas, and ependymomas, or non-glial tumors, including meningiomas, pituitary tumors, and medulloblastoma.

Glioblastoma multiforme, a Grade IV tumor, is the most common primary malignant brain tumor diagnosed in the USA and is recognized for its aggressive growth, recurrence, resistance to therapy, and short median survival (Fig. 4.1). As glioblastomas account for approximately 80 % of malignant brain tumors (CBTRUS 2011), they will be the focus of this review on inflammation and brain cancer. Glioblastomas primarily affect adults with a peak incidence between 40 and 70 years. Most glioblastomas arise in older individuals as primary tumors (primary glioblastoma) in the cerebral hemispheres and demonstrate microvascular proliferation and necrosis. A smaller number (<10 %) likely arose from tumors of a lower grade in younger patients that progressed (secondary glioblastoma) (Huttner 2012).

Current treatment strategies include surgical resection, radiation therapy, and chemotherapy, primarily with the alkylating agent temozolomide.

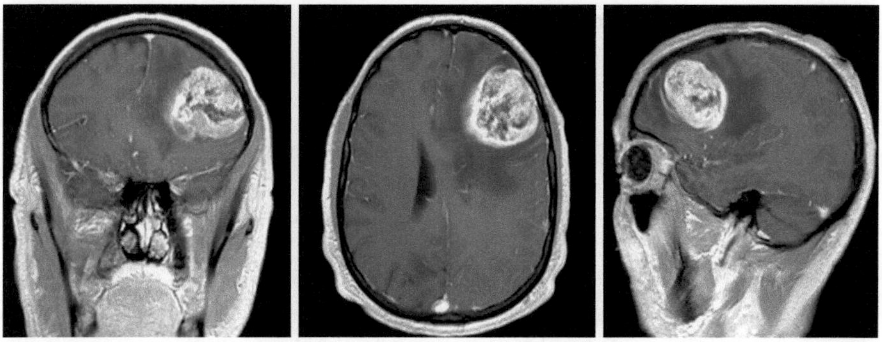

Fig. 4.1 Example of patient with GBM. T1-weighted gadolinium enhanced magnetic resonance images demonstrating a left frontal tumor with mass effect. Pathology is consistent with glioblastoma multiforme

4.1.2 Genetic Changes Driving Glioblastoma

The intricate landscape of brain tumors defined by histology becomes more complicated as histologically similar tumors are further subdivided by the identification of recurrent mutations. Somatic mutations have been identified in glioblastoma in multiple genes, and these mutations are observed in a significant percentage of tumors including *TP53* (42 %), *PTEN* (33 %), *NF1* (21 %), epidermal growth factor receptor (*EGFR*) (18 %), *RB1* (11 %), *PIK3R1* (10 %), and *PIK3CA* (7 %) (Dunn et al. 2012). Current efforts are directed at understanding the significance of these mutations within the context of cell signaling "networks," which could substantially reduce the complexity and increase understanding of the biological properties of glioblastomas (Dunn et al. 2012; Cancer Genome Atlas Research Network 2008; Huse and Holland 2010). To date, three critical signaling pathways have been identified in glioblastoma in which at least one member of each pathway is altered (Fig. 4.2). The pathways include the RTK/RAS/PI3K pathway, altered in 88 % of glioblastomas, the p53 pathway, mutated in 87 %, and the RB pathway, mutated in 78 % (Cancer Genome Atlas Research Network 2008). The majority of glioblastomas have defects in all three pathways that promote cell proliferation, enhance cell survival, and circumvent cell cycle checkpoints, senescence, and apoptosis.

4.1.2.1 The RTK/RAS/PI3K Pathway

The receptor tyrosine kinase (RTK) signaling pathway is initiated by ligand binding to one of several membrane-bound RTKs, initiating a signaling cascade that ultimately promotes or inhibits cellular proliferation, migration, and survival

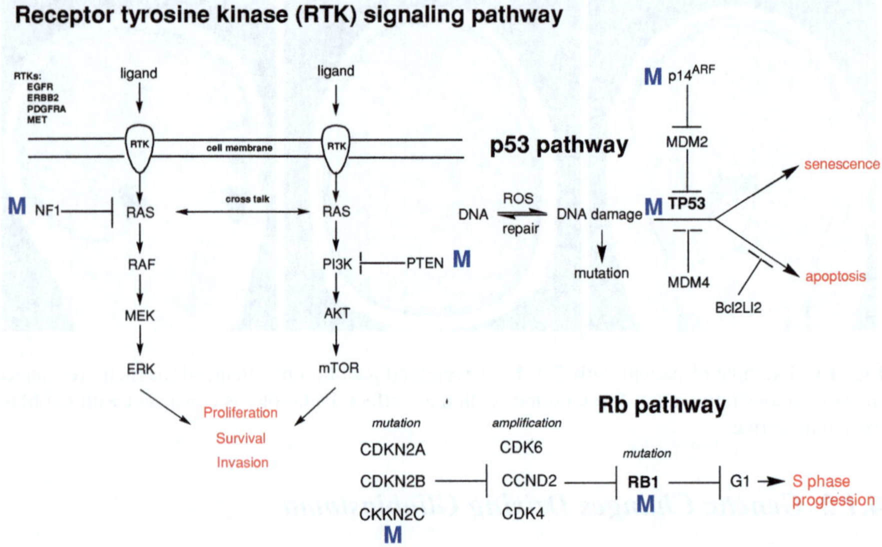

Fig. 4.2 Signaling pathways dysregulated in glioblastoma. A *blue M* indicates protein activities known to be transcriptionally silenced in gliomas

(Rajasekhar et al. 2003; Aksamitiene et al. 2011; Chen et al. 2012). Members of the RTK family significant in glioblastoma include amplification of *EGFR, EGFRvIII ERBB2, PDGFRA*, and *MET.* The binding of ligands to these membrane receptors stimulates the intrinsic tyrosine kinase activity of the RTK, leading to receptor autophosphorylation and activation of Ras by GTP binding. The RAS signaling kinase cascade can then proceed down the RAS/PI3K/PTEN/AKT/mTOR or the RAS/RAF/MEK/ERK pathways. Ultimately, either a series of transcription factors are activated that promote transcription of a subset of genes, or existing mRNAs are differentially recruited into polysomes. Although these pathways are often presented as being discrete, substantial cross talk occurs, creating a complicated signaling network.

Under normal conditions, these signaling pathways allow a cell to communicate with its environment and to respond appropriately. Changes in protein levels or mutations in key genes can result in the disruption of normal signaling. In glioblastoma, signaling through these pathways is often perturbed by amplification or mutation of the RTK member, EGFR. Mutations or amplification in other RTKs are less frequently observed. The neurofibromatosis 1 (NF1) and PTEN (phosphatase and tensin homolog deleted on chromosome 10) gene products act as regulators of each arm of this pathway, and both are known to be mutated or deleted in a substantial number of glioblastomas. Loss or alteration of these regulators results in partial or complete loss of regulation of the signaling pathway. Mutations in RAS, PI3K, or other members of the network could result in constitutive activation of the signaling cascade.

4.1.2.2 The p53 Pathway

The TP53 gene product is an important tumor suppressor that reduces the number of mutant cells in a population by directing cells with substantial DNA damage toward senescence or apoptosis through transcription-dependent or -independent mechanisms. The TP53 gene is frequently mutated in human tumors and is the most frequently mutated gene in glioblastoma. Protein levels of p53 are regulated by the mouse double minute 2 homolog (MDM2) and double minute 4 protein (MDM4) ubiquitin ligases, which mark p53 for proteosomal degradation, as well as inhibit p53-mediated transcriptional activation. The amplification of either of these ubiquitin ligases can diminish p53 levels and thus abrogate p53 function. Another member of the p53 network is $p14^{Arf}$ transcribed from an alternate reading frame of the CDNK2A locus that inhibits MDM2; therefore, deletion or mutation of $p14^{Arf}$ would result in increased MDM2 levels and increased p53 degradation (Riemenschneider et al. 1999; Zheng et al. 2008; Stegh and DePinho 2011).

4.1.2.3 The RB Pathway

The retinoblastoma (RB) tumor suppressor gene controls cellular proliferation by sequestering the E2F family of transcription factors, originally identified as factors binding to the E2 adenovirus promoter. In this pathway, mitogenic signals are able to induce the cyclin-dependent kinases (CDK4/6) to phosphorylate Rb in a pRB-E2F dimer, thereby releasing E2F. The activity of the CDKs is modulated by the p16 tumor suppressor gene (CDKN2). Loss or mutation of p16 would then result in loss of control over Rb phosphorylation, causing constitutive E2A activation and cell cycle progression. The loss or mutation of p16, pRB, or the amplification of the CDKs is observed in most glioblastomas (Ueki et al. 1996; Chow et al. 2011).

4.1.2.4 Coupling Common Defects in Glioblastoma for New Therapy Development

As each of the three pathways above is functionally altered in the majority of glioblastomas, developing therapies based upon defects in multiple pathways might provide significant targeting and selectivity for glioblastoma treatment. In many glioblastomas (~78 %), the RB pathway is inoperative due to a defect in one of the constitutive components, thereby abrogating the control of entry into the cell cycle. In many glioblastomas, the EGFR gene is mutated, and a frequent mutation resulting from the deletion of exons 2–7 generates the mutant RTK, EGFRvIII. Overexpression of either wild type or EGFRvIII facilitates greater signaling through this pathway and increased cell proliferation, survival, and migration of the tumor cells.

Wild-type adenoviruses similarly exploit the critical role of pRB upon infection of human cells by expressing the virally encoded E1A protein. This protein binds to pRB, releasing E2F and allowing progression of quiescent cells into the cell cycle, therefore promoting viral replication. An oncolytic adenovirus has been engineered in which a 24 base pair deletion has been inserted into the E1A region (Δ24). This virus will replicate only in RB-deficient cells, resulting in cell lysis (Fueyo et al. 2000). Adenovirus normally binds to the coxsackie and adenovirus receptor (CAR) present on the surface of some human cells. However, a mutation can be created that prevents binding to this receptor. In its place, an RGD-4C peptide coding sequence has been inserted, effectively retargeting the adenovirus to cells that express integrins $\alpha v\beta 3,5$, which are frequently upregulated in a number of high-grade tumors including glioblastoma (Piao et al. 2009). Thus, the combined Δ24-RGD oncolytic adenovirus will selectively destroy glioblastoma tumor cells with defects in the RB pathway and increased expression in integrins. Clinical trials are currently underway with this viral vector approach.

4.1.3 Epigenetic Changes in Glioblastoma

In addition to somatic mutations, human tumors frequently have simultaneous heritable epigenetic changes including DNA methylation (5-methylcytosine, 5mC) patterns, histone modifications, and noncoding RNAs (miRNA) (Berger et al. 2009). Changes in DNA methylation patterns have been studied frequently in human tumors, including glioblastoma. Aberrant cytosine methylation patterns can result in the inappropriate expression of tumor suppressor genes or in the transcriptional silencing of tumor suppressor genes.

In normal human cells, cytosine residues in DNA can be enzymatically methylated in the 5-position of the pyrimidine ring by methyltransferases using S-adenosylmethionine as the methyl donor (Razin and Riggs 1980; Chen and Riggs 2011; You and Jones 2012) (Fig. 4.3). In humans, three methyltransferases have been identified: DNMT1, DNMT3A, and DNMT3B. Once established, methylation patterns can be heritably transmitted to progeny cells following DNA replication because the DNMT1 maintenance methyltransferase preferentially methylates hemimethylated CpG dinucleotides on the progeny strand following DNA replication (Herring et al. 2009).

Methylated DNA sequences can then modulate expression of surrounding genes by blocking the binding of some transcription factors or by enhancing the binding of proteins containing a methyl-binding domain, referred to as methyl-binding proteins (MBPs). MBPs, including MeCP2, bind to symmetrically methylated sequences with one hundred times greater affinity over unmethylated sequences (Lao et al. 2010). The MBPs recruit histone-modifying enzymes, including the histone deacetylases which modify histone proteins, resulting in a compact chromatin structure inaccessible to transcription factors (Bird and Wolffe 1999; Klose and Bird 2006).

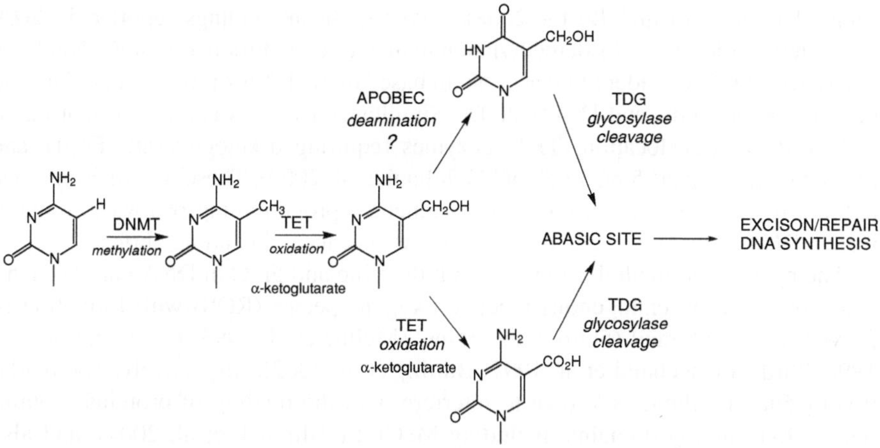

Fig. 4.3 Dynamic methylation and demethylation of DNA

In glioblastoma tumor cells, several genes are frequently methylated (Nakamura et al. 2001; Costello et al. 1996; Bello and Resy 2006; Cecener et al. 2012; Martinez et al. 2009; Di Vinci et al. 2012; Lorent et al. 2008; Martinez and Esteller 2010; Martinez 2012; Alelu-Paz et al. 2012). Many of the genes frequently mutated in glioblastoma can also be silenced by aberrant methylation, and therefore, hypermethylation can conspire with genetic mutations in disrupting critical signaling pathways as shown in Fig. 4.2. Aberrant methylation of additional genes could also have important consequences influencing treatment choices. One such gene is O^6-methylguanine methyltransferase (MGMT) which encodes a DNA repair protein that removes alkyl groups from the O^6 position of guanine in DNA. One of the few chemotherapy agents shown to have activity in glioblastoma is the alkylating agent temozolomide, which forms such an adduct with guanine in DNA (Esteller et al. 2000; Weller et al. 2010). In cells where MGMT is expressed, the guanine-temozolamide adducts can be repaired; however, in the absence of MGMT, the adduct is persistent and blocks DNA replication. In clinical trials, patients who have tumors in which the MGMT gene is methylated show substantially greater responses than those with unmethylated MGMT (Esteller et al. 2000).

4.1.4 Defects in Epigenetic Reprogramming: A New Paradigm in Glioblastoma

Cytosine methylation patterns are established during cellular differentiation, and once formed, these patterns can be heritably transmitted to progeny cells. However, biological evidence for changes in methylation patterns in differentiated cells led to several different proposed mechanisms for active methylation later found to be irreproducible (Ooi and Bestor 2008). Two significant findings reported in 2009 redirected studies on DNA demethylation to an oxidation product of 5mC, 5hmC. In one study, 5hmC was identified as a "sixth base" in the DNA of mammalian Purkinji neurons (Kriaucionis and Heintz 2009). Simultaneously, it was reported that mammalian 10–11 translocation (TET) enzymes requiring α-ketoglutarate, Fe(II), and oxygen could convert 5mC to 5hmC (Tahiliani et al. 2009). These reports have since led to a flood of reports on potential epigenetic reprogramming pathways in mammalian DNA with demonstrated defects in human cancer, including glioblastoma.

The pyrimidine methyl groups of both thymine and 5mC in DNA can be chemically oxidized by endogenous reactive oxygen species (ROS) with formation of 5-hydroxymethyluracil (5hmU) and 5hmC (Mellac et al. 1993; Privat and Sowers 1996; Tardy-Planechaud et al. 1997; Burdzy et al. 2002), respectively. The oxidation of 5mC to 5hmC is known to interfere with the binding of proteins containing methyl-binding domains, including MeCP2 (Valinluck et al. 2004), and also with methyl-directed methylation of hemimethylated DNA by methyltransferases, including mammalian DNMT1 (Valinluck and Sowers 2007). This confirms earlier suggestions that 5hmC might be an intermediate in a DNA demethylation pathway (Rusmintratip and Sowers 2000). Potential mechanisms are currently being explored for downstream events in the processing of 5hmC, including enzymatic deamination to 5hmU, followed by removal by the thymine-DNA glycosylase (TDG) (Guo et al. 2011; Cortellino et al. 2011), and further enzymatic oxidation by TET family members to 5-formylcytosine (5foC) and 5-carboxylcytosine (5caC), also removed by TDG (He et al. 2011).

Recent studies have measured 5hmC levels in both normal brain tissues and in tumors by both liquid chromatography mass spectrometry (LC-MS) and localization by immunohistochemistry (IHC). In the mouse tissue, 5mC is found in all tissues, with the highest levels in neurons within the CNS (Munzel et al. 2010; Globisch et al. 2010; Munzel et al. 2011). In human adult and embryonic tissues, the highest levels of 5hmC are found in terminally differentiated cells. Less differentiated cells and stem cell compartments had lower 5hmC levels (Haffner et al. 2011). In the normal adult brain, 5hmC is abundant in cells of the cortex and white matter; however, reduced levels are found in gliomas, with lower levels in tumors of higher grade (Kraus et al. 2012; Orr et al. 2012). In adult GBM, low 5hmC levels are related to reduced survival (Orr et al. 2012), suggesting that the formation and metabolism of 5hmC represent critical events in the development of GBM and might reveal future treatment strategies. It is as yet unknown if 5hmC functions primarily as an intermediate in a 5mC demethylation pathway or if 5hmC might have an independent function in modulating specific DNA–protein interactions with currently unidentified proteins (Yildirim et al. 2011).

It is as yet unknown what metabolic events result in the loss of 5hmC, though several mechanisms are under investigation (Fig. 4.3). A convergence between 5hmC formation and glioblastoma somatic mutation has been shown for the isocitrate dehydrogenase gene (IDH1/2). IDH mutations (Sahm et al. 2011; Xu et al. 2011; Jin et al. 2011; Liu et al. 2012) are frequently found in secondary glioblastomas, although rarely in primary tumors. The IDH gene product converts isocitrate to α-ketoglutarate either in mitochondria (IDH1) or in the cytosol (IDH2), and α-ketoglutarate is a required cofactor for the Tet-mediated conversion of 5mC to 5hmC. Several IDH mutations have been identified; however, a R132H mutation results in a protein that consumes α-ketoglutarate, reducing it to 2-hydroxyglutarate, an inhibitor of Tet-mediated 5mC oxidation. The role of IDH mutations in glioblastoma is as yet unclear because only a subset of tumors harbors IDH mutations. However, 5hmC levels are low or undetectable in most tumor cells and glioma patient samples. Other mechanisms have been identified that could interfere with 5hmC formation, including mutations in Tet genes (Mohr et al. 2011), promoter methylation and transcriptional silencing (Kim et al. 2011), and exclusion of Tet from the nucleus (Muller et al. 2012). The role of 2-hydroxyglutarate in IDH mutant cells is also unclear as 2-hydroxyglutarate inhibition is not exclusive to the Tet family. Several dioxygenases, including histone demethylases (Xiao et al. 2012) and the hypoxia-inducible factor (HIF) prolyl hydroxylase (PHD) in the HIF-1α hypoxia signaling pathway are inhibited by 2-hydroxyglutarate (Reitman and Yan 2010).

Hypermethylation of a subset of genes at CpG dinucleotides has been identified in several human tumors, and this phenomenon has been identified as a CpG island methylator phenotype, or CIMP (Noushmehr et al. 2010; Shinawi et al. 2013). The CIMP phenotype has been associated with the common IDH R132H mutation. A greater number of methylated CpG islands are found in tumor cells derived from long-term survivors, as opposed to short-term survivors, suggesting that the IDH mutation diminishes tumor survival. As the hypermethylation observed in CIMP is associated with IDH mutations, this phenotype is more likely a defective "demethylation" phenotype, as opposed to a methylator phenotype.

4.2 Inflammation and Glioblastoma Initiation and Progression

4.2.1 The Inflammatory Microenvironment of Glioblastoma

The tumor microenvironment in glioblastoma is influenced by many cell types, including infiltrative inflammatory cells, cells with stem-like properties, cells with neural, glial, and myeloid markers, as well as some cells undergoing necrosis. Rapid tumor growth results in both hypoxia and aberrant vascular proliferation as well as the infiltration of immune cells including macrophages, eosinophils, neutrophils, and T lymphocytes. Signaling pathways among these various cell types are complex, involving numerous cytokines that function in both a paracrine and autocrine manner resulting in aberrant activation or suppression of multiple signaling pathways. While these multiple interacting components likely facilitate tissue repair following injury, the presence of activated inflammatory cells and the release of inflammatory mediators promote tumor proliferation, angiogenesis, and invasion and likely contribute to the molecular evolution of the tumor cells

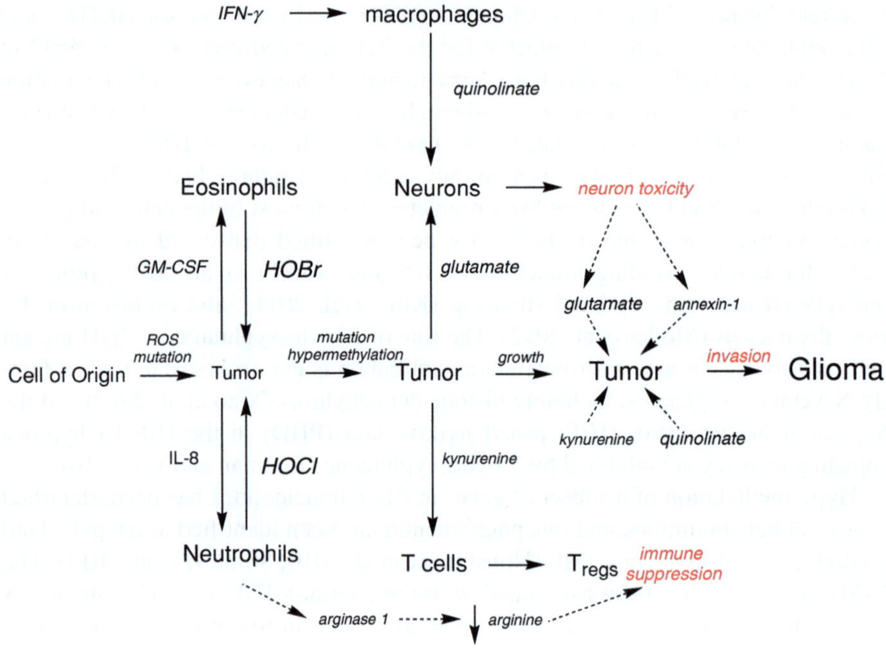

Fig. 4.4 Inflammation cascade and cross talk in glioblastoma

(Rossi et al. 1987; Fossati et al. 1999; Murat et al. 2009; Charles and Holland 2010; Yang et al. 2011; Sen 2011; Huysentruyt et al. 2011; Curran and Bertics 2012; Charles et al. 2012). Interactions in the tumor microenvironment are presented diagrammatically in Fig. 4.4.

4.2.2 Inflammation, Oxidative DNA Damage, and Repair

While cytokine signaling within the tumor microenvironment promotes tumor growth and invasion, how might the inflammatory environment contribute to the array of genetic and epigenetic changes commonly seen in gliomas? Although inflammation has been strongly implicated in the development of cancer (Balkwill and Mantovani 2001), the molecular basis for this association is as yet unclear. While cellular communication between tumor and inflammatory cells is accomplished primarily by soluble mediators that bind with high affinity and specificity to membrane receptors, much of innate immunity is based upon the production of reactive oxidizing chemicals that function well as antimicrobial agents but cause collateral damage to host cells as well. When stimulated by cytokines, macrophages release superoxide ($O_2^{\cdot}$) and hydrogen peroxide (H_2O_2) through an NADPH-dependent oxidative burst. Macrophages also generate nitric oxide (NO), an important signaling molecule in modulating vascular tone, which can combine with O_2 to form peroxynitrite (ONOO-). Neutrophils and eosinophils can combine H_2O_2 with halogens to generate hypochlorous acid (HOCl) and hypobromous acid (HOBr). These reactive oxygen, nitrogen, and halogen species can react with lipids, proteins, and nucleic acids to form a complicated array of reaction products. Numerous DNA adducts have been identified that can induce polymerase (PARP) miscoding, resulting in genetic mutations (Lewis and Adams 1987; Ames et al. 1995; Lonkar and Dedon 2011).

Among the many mutagenic DNA oxidation damage products known to form, 8-oxo-2'-deoxyguanosine (8-oxodG) has been most extensively studied. While oxidative DNA damage occurs in all metabolically active cells, levels of 8-oxodG in glioblastoma tissues are reported to be roughly twice those found in normal brain tissues. The increase in oxidation is accompanied by a reduction in total antioxidant capacity (Tuzgen et al. 2007). Increased 8-oxodG in GBM tissues is associated with increases in the phosphorylated histone H2AX (γH2AX) and induction of a DNA damage response that signals to p53 (Bartkova et al. 2010). While in the tumor microenvironment, ROS from outside of the cell can contribute to increased DNA damage, and molecular alterations within the cell can also increase oxidative stress. Glioblastoma cells with the common EGFRvIII mutation have increased 8-oxodG and upregulate DNA repair genes in response to increased DNA damage (Nitta et al. 2010). Presumably, increased signaling through EGFR results in increased oxidative stress, increased DNA damage, and further promotes genetic instability.

Single-base oxidative damage like 8-oxodG is repaired by the base excision-repair (BER) pathway. Although glioblastoma cells likely experience enhanced oxidative damage within the tumor microenvironment, the levels of multiple glycosylases of the BER pathway are significantly downregulated in astrocytoma Grades II to IV. Expression of the OGG1 glycosylase involved in 8-oxodG repair is reduced by more than an order of magnitude (Jiang et al. 2006). Interestingly, patients with high EGFR expression and low relative BER capacity had longer survival times (Nitta et al. 2010), suggesting that the relationship between DNA damage and repair in glioma might extend beyond tumor initiation and could suggest targets for selective chemotherapy.

4.2.3 *Inflammation, DNA Damage, and Genetic Mutations in Glioblastoma*

Among the many genes often mutated in glioblastoma, the p53 gene is the most frequently mutated and has been studied the most extensively. The most prevalent mutations in p53 of brain tumors are single-base changes, with ~85 % simple substitutions (Greenblatt et al. 1994). Among these, transition mutations (GC to AT or AT to GC) comprise ~65 % of the substitutions. A significant number (~30 %) of the GC to AT transitions are within a CpG dinucleotide, and CpG dinucleotides in the p53 gene are generally methylated (Tornaletti and Pfeifer 1995). Therefore, a significant number of p53 mutations arise from the hydrolytic deamination of 5mC to thymine, a base change that is difficult to repair. The spectrum of single-base mutations found in the p53 gene outside of CpG dinucleotides in brain tumors is consistent with cycles of endogenous damage and repair cycles.

The T-G mispair formed by hydrolytic deamination of 5-methylcytosine can be repaired by four human glycosylases: UNG2, SMUG1, MBD4, and TDG (Vasovcak et al. 2012). Failure to repair the T-G mispair would result in the observed GC to AT transition mutations frequently observed at p53 CpG sites in glioblastoma. The TDG glycosylase might be of particular importance as it is involved in epigenetic reprogramming/demethylation as previously discussed (Fig. 4.3), and TDG expression is apparently regulated by p53 (da Costa et al. 2012) and is essential for maintaining epigenetic stability (Cortázar et al. 2011). The TDG glycosylase represents an intersection between p53 mutation and epigenetic reprogramming in glioblastoma.

4.2.4 Inflammation Induced Epigenetic Changes in Glioblastoma

Aberrant hypermethylation of the promoter regions of multiple genes has been demonstrated in glioblastoma, as well as several other human tumors as discussed above. However, the mechanisms leading to hypermethylation are as yet unknown. Inflammation has long been associated with cancer development, yet a mechanistic link has been difficult to identify. Inflammation-mediated ROS can induce multiple forms of DNA damage; however, most forms of DNA damage inhibit the binding of MBPs and block enzymatic methylation. It has been recently discovered that some forms of inflammation-mediated DNA damage might supply such a link (Whiteman et al. 1997).

The tumor microenvironment in glioblastoma promotes the infiltration of immune cells, including eosinophils and neutrophils. Upon activation, both initiate an oxidative burst that generates H_2O_2, HOBr, and HOCl (Lonkar and Dedon 2011). DNA damage products include both 5-chlorocytosine (5ClC) and 5-bromocytosine (5BrC) (Whiteman et al. 1997; Winterbourn and Kettle 2000; Kang and Sowers 2008). Both 5ClC and 5BrC have been shown in in vitro studies to mimic 5mC and to act as fraudulent epigenetic signals (Valinluck et al. 2005; Lao et al. 2009, 2010; Valinluck and Sowers 2007). Therefore, inflammation-mediated formation of either 5ClC or 5BrC could account in part for the aberrant hypermethylation in glioblastoma. Halogenated cytosine residues have been identified in human T cells (Badouard et al. 2005), in inflamed human sinus tissues (Seiberling et al. 2012), and in a mouse model of inflammation-mediated colon cancer (Mangerich et al. 2012).

Halogenated cytosine bases have not yet been measured in glioblastoma or normal brain tissues. Myeloperoxidase (MPO) converts H_2O_2 to HOCl, which in turn can generate 5ClC (Lonkar and Dedon 2011). MPO concentrations in both tumor tissue and in plasma are significantly higher in glioblastoma patients versus control (Atukeren et al. 2010). Elevated MPO levels have been measured inside tumors and in peritumoral cerebrum using a gadolinium-based MRI method in rodent gliomas (Kleijn et al. 2011). Although MPO is likely derived from infiltrating neutrophils, it has been reported that astrocytes can aberrantly express MPO in a mouse model of Alzheimer's disease (Maki et al. 2009). Further studies examining halogenated DNA bases in human glioblastoma are warranted.

4.3 Cross Talk Between Glioblastoma Cells and Infiltrating Immune Cells

4.3.1 Neutrophils and Neuroinflammation

Emerging evidence indicates that astrocytes and neutrophils interact with one another in a normal process of neuroinflammatory homeostasis. Following injury or infection in the brain, neutrophils and other peripheral immune cells infiltrate the brain parenchyma. Through interacting with normal astrocytes in the brain, infiltrating immune cells can destroy infectious agents, eliminate necrotic tissues, and stimulate tissue repair. Recent studies in mice have revealed some interacting pathways (Xie et al. 2010). Neutrophils undergo spontaneous apoptosis to limit inflammatory damage mediated by ROS, including HOCl generated by MPO. Direct contact between neutrophils and astrocytes may prolong neutrophil survival and reduce necrosis, which results in the dumping of matrix metalloproteinases (MMPs) and MPO into the tissues. The antimicrobial activity of neutrophils requires an NADPH-dependent oxidative burst generating H_2O_2, followed by MPO-mediated conversion to HOCl. Cell–cell contact between astrocytes and neutrophils can decrease both the production of ROS in neutrophils and the release of MPO by neutrophils (Xie et al. 2010).

4.3.2 Signaling with Neutrophils in the Tumor Microenvironment

While neutrophils may interact effectively with normal brain cells in destroying invading pathogens or promoting tissue turnover and repair, HOCl generated by neutrophils is indiscriminate in its chemical reactivity and can damage the DNA of normal cells, including astrocytes, promoting both genetic and epigenetic changes as described previously. MPO-positive neutrophils are frequently identified within human glioma tissues; though their role in tumor initiation and progression has not yet been established. The presence of neutrophils increases with tumor grade, as approximately 85 % of Grade IV gliomas samples show significant infiltration

(Fossati et al. 1999), suggest an increasingly mutagenic tumor microenvironment. In addition, circulating WBC counts increase in glioma patients, due primarily to increased circulating neutrophils (Fossati et al. 1999). Several interactions between glioma cells and neutrophils are discussed below.

4.3.2.1 TNF-α → IL-8 → Neutrophils

Several pathways have been identified for communication between neutrophils and gliomas. Glioma cells can attract neutrophils by secreting interleukin-8 (IL-8), a member of the CXC chemokine family (CXCL8) that is defined by its ability to direct the migration of neutrophils as well as other inflammatory cells. The CXCL8 ligand interacts with the CXCR1 and CXCR2 receptors found on neutrophils (Brat et al. 2005). Although the IL-8 present in the complex tumor samples could be attributed to macrophages, glioblastoma cells lines also have been shown to produce IL-6 and IL-8, especially when stimulated by TNF-α, IL-2, and IL-β (Tada et al. 1993).

4.3.2.2 Annexin1 → Neutrophils

Human neutrophils, as well as glioma cells, express formylpeptide receptor (FPR), a G-protein-coupled chemoattractant receptor (GPCR) that binds N-formyl-methionyl-leucyl-phenylalanine (fMLF), a product of gram-negative bacteria (Huang et al. 2008). Necrotic human glioblastoma cells are also known to release Annexin 1, which is chemotactic for neutrophils and also stimulates glioma growth via the formyl peptide receptor 1 (FPR1) (Yang et al. 2011).

4.3.2.3 Hypoxia → OPN → Neutrophil

In hypoxic areas of tumors, HIF-1α mediates the upregulation of osteopontin (OPN) expression, an arginine–glycine–aspartate (RGD)-containing glycophosphoprotein. Tumor-derived OPN also facilitates the influx of neutrophils into glioblastoma, likely by interacting with the α9β1 integrin, which is highly expressed on neutrophils (Atai et al. 2010).

4.3.3 Signaling with Eosinophils in the Tumor Microenvironment

In 1967, it was demonstrated that glioblastoma cells, cocultured with eosinophils, promoted eosinophil survival (Ciembroniewicz and Kolar 1967). It has since been established that the infiltration of eosinophils into glioblastoma is mediated by tumor-derived granulocyte macrophage colony-stimulating factor (GM-CSF). TNF-α increases tumor cell GM-CSF production, which is reversed by dexamethasone.

Eosinophils stimulated with GM-CSF release TGF-α, a ligand that can promote glioma proliferation via the EGF receptor (Curran and Bertics 2012; Curran et al. 2011).

4.3.3.1 GM-CSF → Eosinophils and Neutrophils

Human gliomas produce both granulocyte colony-stimulating factor (G-CSF) and GM-CSF ligands as well as receptors for these ligands. G-CSF and GM-CSF are important factors that control the proliferation and activation of granulocytes. The presence of both ligands and receptors in advanced stage tumors suggests both paracrine and autocrine functions (Curran et al. 2011; Mueller et al. 1999; Revoltella et al. 2011).

Several previous studies have shown an inverse relationship between atopic disease and risk for glioblastoma (Linos et al. 2007). As the eosinophil has been identified as an effector cell in the pathophysiology of atopic disease (Curran and Bertics 2012), eosinophils may also be responsible for destroying glioblastoma at an early stage. The possibility that eosinophils might be responsible for both initiating tumor formation via DNA damage, and in eliminating glioblastoma cells through inflammatory responses suggest that the interactions between infiltrating immune cells and normal brain cells must be carefully orchestrated. It is known that some chemical carcinogens at low levels can be mutagenic, but at higher levels are cytotoxic.

4.4 Activation of Tryptophan Metabolism in the Tumor Microenvironment

4.4.1 The Kynurenine Pathway

Tryptophan is an essential amino acid that serves as a building block for protein synthesis but also functions as a precursor for other biochemical mediators including serotonin. Tryptophan also undergoes metabolism through the kynurenine pathway (Fig. 4.5), ultimately generating quinolinic acid needed for the synthesis of nicotinamide adenine dinucleotide (NAD^+). Several of the metabolites formed along this pathway, including kynurenine, kynurenic acid, and quinolinic acid, have activities that can result in neuroprotection or pathophysiology. Several reviews have been published on the role of the kynurenine pathway in the brain (Guillemin et al. 2001; Schwarcz and Pellicciari 2012; Guillemin et al. 2007; Schwarcz et al. 2012; Adams et al. 2012; Vécsei et al. 2013).

The kynurenine pathway is triggered by inflammatory cytokines found in the glioma tumor microenvironment including IFN-α, IFN-γ, TNF-α, TGF-β, IL-4, and IL-23 (Mándi and Vécsei 2012). These cytokines induce the first enzyme of the kynurenine pathway, indoleamine 2,3-dioxygenase (IDO), which converts tryptophan to kynurenine. However, induction of the enzymes along the kynurenine pathway can be both cytokine and cell-type specific. In human mesenchymal stem cells, both IFN-β and IFN-γ upregulate expression of mRNAs for all of the enzymes along

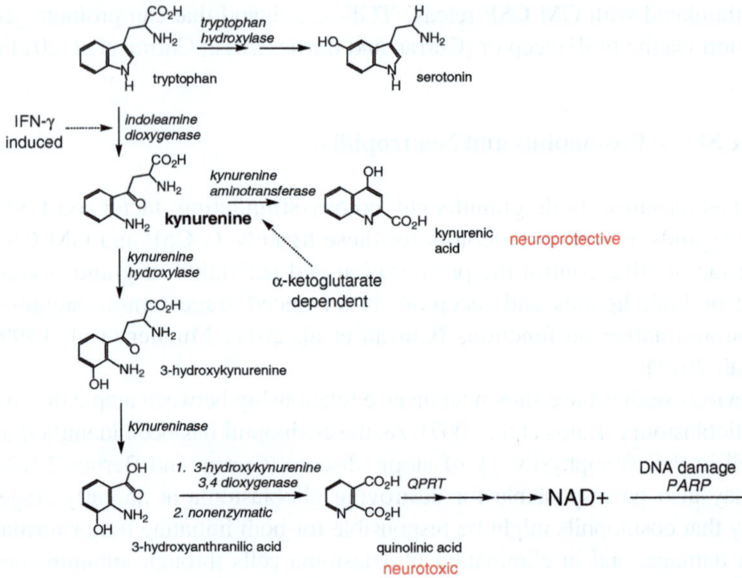

Fig. 4.5 The kynurenine pathway

the pathway, and IFN-γ upregulates all pathway enzymes substantially in macrophages. In contrast, in mouse neural stem cells, IFN-g upregulates the initiating enzyme, IDO, kynurenine aminotransferase that converts kynurenine to kynurenic acid, and quinolinate phosphoribosyltransferase (QPRT) that converts quinolinic acid to nicotinic acid ribonucleotide, a necessary substrate for (NAD^+) synthesis (Croitoru-Lamoury et al. 2011). Astrocytes lack kynurenine hydroxylase, such that activation of the kynurenine pathway in these cells generates kynurenine and kynurenic acid, but not quinolinic acid (Guillemin et al. 2001).

The upregulation of some, but not all of the kynurenine pathway enzymes in neurons suggests that some of the initial metabolites including kynurenine and kynurenic acid could be beneficial to neurons, but that quinolinic acid is not. However, quinolinic acid generated by other cells might be utilized as a substrate for replenishing (NAD^+) in neurons. Therefore, examining the kynurenine pathway within the context of the inflammatory tumor microenvironment might provide important clues not revealed by examining the same pathway in a single cell type in isolation.

4.4.2 The Biological Activity of Kynurenine

The first metabolite of the kynurenine pathway is kynurenine. In addition to serving as an intermediate along this pathway, the emerging role of kynurenine in modulation of inflammation is only beginning to be recognized. As with astrocytes, human malignant glioma cells in culture increase expression of IDO when stimulated with IFN-γ. In contrast, 3-hydroxyanthranilate 3,4-dioxygenase (3HAO) is not induced so that glioma cells could produce kynurenine and kynurenic acid, but not quinolinic acid. Glioma cells could potentially utilize exogenous quinolinic acid produced by other cells for (NAD^+) synthesis (Miyazaki et al. 2009). Recent clinical studies have demonstrated that IDO expression levels in resected glioma specimens are inversely correlated with patient survival (Wainwright et al. 2012; Mitsuka et al. 2013).

While induction of IDO activity could deplete tryptophan, resulting in inhibition of cellular replication, activation of the kynurenine pathway more likely decreases patient survival by inducing immunosuppression. Within the tumor microenvironment, kynurenine could be generated by multiple cells including tumor cells and macrophages. Prior studies have demonstrated that T-cell function could be modulated through the aryl hydrocarbon receptor (AhR) present on T cells and that environmental chemicals such as 2,3,7,8 tetrachlorobenzo-p-dioxin (TCDD, dioxin) could activate formation of regulatory T cells (Treg) while inhibiting natural killer cells (Stevens et al. 2009). However, emerging studies have revealed that kynurenine is an endogenous ligand for the AhR and has a similar immunomodulatory effect on T cells (Nguyen et al. 2010; Opitz et al. 2011). While the effect of kynurenine on T-cell function is likely part of an immunomodulatory feedback loop needed for the maintenance of homeostasis, its impact on tumor growth, evasion of immune regulation, and patient survival may be profound.

Many cell types express the AhR, including glioma cells. AhR expression at both the mRNA and protein levels has been observed in both glioma cell lines and in primary cells. Activation of the AhR has been shown to promote glioma cell proliferation and invasion through upregulation of TGF-β (Gramatzki et al. 2009). In human lung cancer cells, TCDD has been shown to activate the AhR that binds directly to the nuclear factor erythroid 2 p45-related factor (NRF2) promoter, resulting in the expression of the NRF2 transcription factor (Tsay et al. 2013). Expression of the NRF2 transcription factor in human U251 glioma cells results in both multidrug resistance and proliferation, as well as upregulation of MMP9 (matrix metalloproteinase 9), an enzyme involved in degradation of the extracellular matrix (Pan et al. 2012).

Inflammation within the glioblastoma tumor microenvironment induces production of kynurenine, which has a potent immunomodulatory effect on T cells and can promote glioma cell proliferation and invasion in a paracrine and autocrine manner. Inhibition of kynurenine production via inhibition of IDO is therefore a potentially important therapeutic target that could result in inhibition of Treg induction, as well as inhibit a shift from a TH1 response to a TH2 response (Mándi and Vécsei 2012; Miyazaki et al. 2009; Stevens et al. 2009). IDO inhibitors include the tryptophan analog 1-methyl L-tryptophan (Miyazaki et al. 2009), as well as the antiviral agent acyclovir (Söderlund et al. 2010). Interestingly, acyclovir has previously been shown to inhibit human glioblastoma cells in culture (Kominsky et al. 2010); however, the mechanism has not yet been clarified.

4.4.3 The Biological Activity of Kynurenic Acid

Once formed, kynurenine many be oxidized to 3-hydroxykynurenine and then on to quinolinic acid. Alternatively, kynurenine can be converted to kynurenic acid (KYNA) by kynurenine aminotransferase. KYNA is an antagonist of the glutamate-gated ion channel receptors found in the human brain: the *N*-methyl-D-aspartate (NMDA), α-amino-3-hydroxy-5-methyl-4-isoxazolepropionic acid (AMPA), and kainate receptors (Birch et al. 1988). KYNA is also a noncompetitive inhibitor of the α7-nicotinic acetylcholine receptor, as well as an endogenous ligand for an orphan G-protein-coupled receptor, GPR35. KYNA is considered to be neuroprotective because it inhibits glutamate excitotoxicity by inhibiting the glycine site of the NMDA receptor. However, the IC_{50} for KYNA at the glycine site of the NMDA receptor is approximately 8 μM (Passera et al. 2011), yet concentrations of KYNA rise from only 1 nM to approximately 5 nM in the cerebrospinal fluid of humans with tick-borne encephalitis (Holtze et al. 2012). This suggests that KYNA might be of limited value in protecting from glutamate excitoxicity. However, plasma KYNA levels rise to near 1 μM in patients with inflammatory bowel disease (Forrest et al. 2002). KYNA could be generated by multiple cells within the tumor microenvironment, yet KYNA formation would be limited in glioblastoma cells carrying an IDH mutation because a required cofactor for kynurenine aminotransferase is α-ketoglutarate (Passera et al. 2011), which is depleted in glioma cells carrying an IDH mutation.

KYNA stimulates the proliferation of human glioblastoma cells in vitro and unexpectedly inhibits the release of fibroblast growth factor (FGF-1); however, the mechanism connecting these events is unknown (Barth et al. 2009). KYNA can also bind to the GPR35 orphan receptor and induce adhesion of human monocytes via β1 and β2 integrins at millimolar concentration (Barth et al. 2009).

4.4.4 The Biological Activity of Quinolinic Acid

4.4.4.1 Quinolinic Acid is Neurotoxic

The metabolism of tryptophan along the kynurenine pathway generates quinolinic acid that can be utilized to replenish NAD^+ in cells following oxidative DNA damage and PARP activation. However, quinolinic acid is also an agonist of the NMDA receptor present on neurons and potentially can induce excitotoxic death. In experimental rat brain tumors, quinolinic acid immunoreactivity is observed in and around tumors; however, the positive cells were primarily macrophages and microglia (Moffett et al. 1997). This finding is consistent with expression of all enzymes along the pathway expressed in macrophages and microglia, but not in astrocytes or neurons. Glioblastoma cells in culture (U373GM) produce significant amounts of kynurenine upon incubation with IFN-γ, but do not produce quinolinate (Saito et al. 1993; Heyes et al. 1996).

Quinolinate can induce neuronal death both in vitro and in vivo (Schwarcz et al. 1983; Bordelon et al. 1999; Moroni 1999; Chiarugi et al. 2001; Leaver et al. 2012). Injection of small amounts of quinolinate, (60 nmol) into the striatum is frequently used to model excitotoxic neurodegeneration in rodents (Leaver et al. 2012). The loss of neuronal cells, but not glial cells, is observed around the injection site four days after injection (Schwarcz et al. 1983). Although quinolinate can induce neuron toxicity, quinolinate is only a weak agonist for the NMDA receptor glutamate-binding site. Concentrations of quinolinate have been measured as high as 7.3 μM by in vivo microdialysis in the brains of gerbils following intrastriatal infusion of lipopolysaccharide, which is 10–100 fold higher than control levels (Beagles et al. 1998). Nanomolar quinolinate levels have been measured in the CSF of patients with hepatitis C treated with IFN-α (Raison et al. 2010). However, activation of the NMDA receptor requires millimolar quinolinate concentrations (Obrenovitch 2001). The mechanism of quinolinate neurotoxicity is therefore as yet unresolved and might involve additional potentiating factors or longer time of exposure (Chiarugi et al. 2001; Stone and Behan 2007).

4.4.4.2 Quinolinic Acid Supports Glioma Survival and Proliferation

Quinolinate generated by activate macrophages could promote the survival and proliferation of glioma cells by serving as a precursor for NAD^+. NAD^+ is essential for ATP synthesis, intracellular calcium homeostasis, and DNA repair. In the inflammatory microenvironment, oxidative damage to DNA triggers a DNA damage response, including activation of PARP which consumes NAD^+. PARP-1 protein is usually not present in normal neurons, but human primary glioblastoma tissues uniformly have positive immunohistochemical staining for PARP-1 (Galia et al. 2012). Because NAD^+ is essential for many biochemical reactions, depletion of NAD^+ can induce cell death.

Experimental studies have shown that quinolinate promotes the proliferation of glioma cells in culture, and that exogenous quinolinate can increase intracellular NAD^+ levels (Grant and Kapoor 1998; Braidy et al. 2009). The inhibition of NAD^+ synthesis sensitizes glioma cells to the cytotoxic activity of temozolamide, suggesting future directions for combination chemotherapy (Watson et al. 2009; Goellner et al. 2011). Oxidative stress, temozolomide, and irradiation induce QPRT expression in gliomas, and QPRT levels are increased in higher grade tumors. Whereas quinolinic acid generated by microglia and macrophages can be toxic to neurons, glioma cells can exploit quinolinate generated by other cells for the regeneration of NAD^+. Increased expression of QPRT confers resistance and results in poorer patient prognosis (Sahm et al. 2013).

4.5 The Role of Glutamate in the Tumor Microenvironment

4.5.1 Excessive Glutamate is Toxic to Neurons

Glutamate is the main excitatory neurotransmitter in the mammalian central nervous system. Glutamate binding to NMDA, AMPA, and kainate receptors mediates synaptic transmission largely through an increase in Na^+ permeability, and glutamate can also bind to metabotropic glutamate receptors that induce signaling through multiple second messenger pathways. Glutamate concentrations near synapses are maintained at very low concentrations (low micromolar) by reuptake by specific glutamate transporters, and nearby glial cells that convert glutamate to glutamine. In contrast to normal glial cells, glioma cells release rather than take up glutamate, and glutamate released by glioma cells cocultured with neurons activates the neuronal NMDA receptor, causing Na^+ influx and excitotoxic cell death. The release of glutamate by glioma cells is proposed as an explanation for seizures, common in glioma patients (de Groot and Sontheimer 2011).

The tissue concentration of glutamate in the brain is approximately 10 mM, however, most of this is intracellular. The concentration of extracellular glutamate in the brain is estimated to be only 0.6 μM. Damage to neurons is expected when extracellular glutamate exceeds 5 μM (Lipton and Rosenberg 1994). Peritumoral glutamate levels have been measured in glioma patients by microdialysis and have been found to exceed 100 μM (Ye and Sontheimer 1999; Marcus et al. 2010). Therefore, once a sufficient number of glioma cells dump glutamate into the tumor microenvironment to kill a few neurons, those neurons will dump intracellular glutamate, resulting in a cascade of damage to surrounding neurons.

4.5.2 Excessive Glutamate Facilitates Glioma Cell Survival and Proliferation

Although glutamate is excitotoxic to neurons, glioma cells not only have a much higher threshold for glutamate damage, but glutamate binding to glioma-specific receptors can also promote glioma cell proliferation. Multiple groups have recently reported that glioma cells and glioblastoma-derived brain tumor initiating cells (BTICs) have Ca^{2+} permeable AMPA receptors. AMPA receptors are tetrameric and are composed of GluR1 through GluR4 subunits, and GluR2-lacking receptors are Ca^{2+} permeable. AMPA receptors on BTICs are comprised of GluR1 and GluR4 subunits (Oh et al. 2012), whereas AMPA receptors on the glioblastoma cell line U87MG contain the GluR2 subunit and are Ca^{2+} impermeable (Ekici et al. 2012). Human surgical glioma tissues contain Ca^{2+} permeable AMPA receptors, and glutamate activation promotes cell growth and mobility (Lyons et al. 2007) by activation of the Akt pathway (Ishiuchi et al. 2007; Schunemann et al. 2010).

4.6 Arginine Metabolism in the Tumor Microenvironment

4.6.1 Arginine is Important in the Human Immune Response

L-arginine is converted to L-citrulline with the release of NO by NO synthase. Macrophages within the tumor environment can generate NO, which has potent antimicrobial and tumoricidal activity (Bogdan 2001; Munder 2009). NO can also combine with O_2 to produce peroxynitrite ($ONOO^-$). Peroxynitrite can react with nucleic acids to produce mutagenic 8-nitroguanine adducts (Hiraku 2010).

4.6.2 Arginine Metabolism by Neutrophil-Derived Arginase

In glioblastoma patients, degranulation of neutrophils generates high levels of arginase. Arginase converts L-arginine to L-ornithine and urea, thereby depleting L-arginine needed for NO generation. Therefore, neutrophil degranulation within the tumor microenvironment diminishes macrophage-mediated antitumor activity (Sippel et al. 2011). Further, depletion of local L-arginine could inhibit the proliferation of T cells, resulting in T-cell dysfunction, which can be reversed by L-arginine supplementation (Sippel et al. 2011).

4.7 Summary, Conclusions, and Future Directions

At the time of presentation, high-grade gliomas are aggressive tumors that display aberrant vascularization with infiltrating immune cells creating a heterogeneous tumor microenvironment. Multiple recurrent genetic and epigenetic abnormalities are observed in glioma cells that converge on several key signaling pathways involved in tumor cell survival, proliferation, and invasion. Despite the significant increases in understanding of the molecular changes found in glioma cells, current therapy options remain focused on surgical resection, radiation therapy, and chemotherapy with the alkylating agent temozolomide, and survival is still measured in months.

Very little is currently known about agents or events that might drive the genetic and epigenetic changes leading to the evolution of high-grade glioma, and it is unknown if the multitude of observed changes must occur in a particular sequence. It is likely that initial metabolic changes within tumor initiating cells increase intracellular oxidative stress, leading to increased oxidative DNA damage. Increased DNA damage, coupled with diminished DNA repair could then drive subsequent mutations. Within the inflammatory tumor microenvironment, reactive oxygen, nitrogen and halogen species contributed by activated macrophages, neutrophils, and eosinophils likely contribute to further mutations and epigenetic changes as glioma cells progress.

The genetic and epigenetic changes in glioma cells account for the survival, proliferation, and invasion of tumors. Yet, these changes alter cellular metabolism in ways that could be exploited for the future development of targeted chemotherapy focused against metabolism. Altered metabolism within the tumor cells is also coupled to changes within the tumor environment that influence the impact of the glioma cells on normal neurons and immune cells. Although a multitude of genetic and epigenetic changes can be found in glioma cells, a uniform finding in glial tumors is the absence of the modified DNA base, 5hmC. This recently identified modified base is believed to be an intermediate in an enzymatic demethylation pathway required for epigenetic reprogramming. The uniform loss of 5hmC in glioma cells lines and human tissues suggests a common defect central to gliomagenesis.

Emerging studies indicate that metabolic activity of three amino acids, glutamate, tryptophan, and arginine, and these metabolic alterations have profound effects on glioma progression. Whereas normal glial cells sequester glutamate, maintaining low extracellular levels, glioma cells export glutamate that is excitotoxic to neurons. Subsequent neuronal death results in further increases in extracellular glutamate, promoting a cascade of neuron loss and tissue destruction. In contrast with normal neurons, glutamate drives glioma progression by binding to glutamate AMPA receptors, activating cell signaling pathways that drive proliferation.

Tissue destruction results in increases in inflammatory mediators including IFN-γ. Inflammatory cytokines upregulate enzymes of tryptophan metabolism within the kynurenine pathway. In most cell types, including glioma cells, IFN-γ upregulates the first enzyme of this pathway, IDO, which converts tryptophan to kynurenine. Kynurenine binds to the AhR on T cells diminishing antitumor T-cell responses and promoting the formation of Tregs. Activation of the entire kynurenine pathway in macrophages results in the conversion of tryptophan to quinolinic acid. Although quinolinic acid is toxic to human neurons, and is commonly used in experimental models of excitotoxic neurodegeneration, quinolinic acid promotes glioma cell survival and proliferation. Increased oxidative stress within glioma cells results in increased DNA damage which in turn results in upregulation of PARP-1 and consumption of NAD^+. Diminished NAD^+ levels can lead to energy failure and cellular death; however, quinolinic acid generated by other cells can serve as a precursor for NAD^+ synthesis in glioma cells.

Chemoattractants generated within the tumor microenvironment are able to facilitate the invasion of neutrophils. Reactive molecules from activated neutrophils can lead to further tissue destruction and glioma mutagenesis. Neutrophil degranulation also dumps arginase 1, which converts arginine to ornithine. Diminished arginine concentrations reduce macrophage-generated NO and profoundly suppress T-cell immune responses. Through both tryptophan and arginine metabolic pathways, inflammation within the tumor microenvironment promotes immunosuppression and promotes tumor evolution.

Substantial further studies are required to understand the complex interactions between the multiple cell types associated with gliomas, as well as how genetic and epigenetic changes within glioma cells are both likely induced by the inflammatory environment and exploited by glioma cells to promote tumor cell survival with collateral damage to normal tissues. Studying tumor cells in isolation may provide targets for metabolic intervention and future chemotherapy development. However, a more complete understanding of the complex interactions between the tumor cells and surrounding normal tissues could lead to strategies to redirect the host response against these rapidly growing and lethal human tumors.

References

Adams S, Braidy N, Bessede A, Brew BJ, Grant R, Teo C, Guillemin GJ (2012) The kynurenine pathway in brain tumor pathogenesis. Cancer Res 72:5649–5657

Aksamitiene E, Kiyatkin A, Kholodenko BN (2011) Cross-talk between mitogenic Ras/MAPK and survival PI3K/Akt pathways: a fine balance. Biochem Soc Trans 40:139–146

Alelu-Paz R, Ashour N, Gonzalez-Corpas A, Ropero S (2012) DNA methylation, histone modifications, and signal transduction pathways: a close relationship in malignant gliomas pathophysiology. J Signal Transduct 1–8

Ames BN, Gold LS, Willett WC (1995) The causes and prevention of cancer. Proc Natl Acad Sci USA 92:5258–5265

Atai NA, Bansal M, Lo C, Bosman J, Tigchelaar W, Bosch KS, Jonker A, De Witt Hamer PC, Troost D, McCulloch CA, Everts V, Van Noorden CJ, Sodek J (2010) Osteopontin is upregulated and associated with neutrophil and macrophage infiltration in glioblastoma. Immunology 132:39–48

Atukeren P, Kemerdere R, Kacira T, Hanimoglu H, Ozlen F, Yavuz B, Tanriverdi T, Gumustas K, Canbaz B (2010) Expressions of some vital molecules: glioblastoma multiforme versus normal tissues. Neurol Res 32:492–501

Badouard C, Masuda M, Nishino H, Cadet J, Favier A, Ravanat JL (2005) Detection of chlorinated DNA and RNA nucleosides by HPLC coupled to tandem mass spectrometry as potential biomarkers of inflammation. J Chromatogr B Analyt Technol Biomed Life Sci 827:26–31

Balkwill F, Mantovani A (2001) Inflammation and cancer: back to Virchow? Lancet 357:539–545

Barth MC, Ahluwalia N, Anderson TJ, Hardy GJ, Sinha S, Alvarez-Cardona JA, Pruitt IE, Rhee EP, Colvin RA, Gerszten RE (2009) Kynurenic acid triggers firm arrest of leukocytes to vascular endothelium under flow conditions. J Biol Chem 284:19189–19195

Bartkova J, Hamerlik P, Stockhausen MT, Ehrmann J, Hlobilkova A, Laursen H, Kalita O, Kolar Z, Poulsen HS, Broholm H, Lukas J, Bartek J (2010) Replication stress and oxidative damage contribute to aberrant constitutive activation of DNA damage signalling in human gliomas. Oncogene 29:5095–5102

Beagles KE, Morrison PF, Heyes MP (1998) Quinolinic acid in vivo synthesis rates, extracellular concentrations, and intercompartmental distributions in normal and immune-activated brain as determined by multiple-isotope microdialysis. J Neurochem 70:281–291

Bello MJ, Resy JA (2006) The p53/Mdm2/p14ARF cell cycle control pathway genes may be inactivated by genetic and epigenetic mechanisms in gliomas. Cancer Genet Cytogenet 164:172–173

Berger SL, Kouzarides T, Shiekhattar R, Shilatifard A (2009) An operational definition of epigenetics. Genes Dev 23:781–783

Birch PJ, Grossman CJ, Hayes AG (1988) Kynurenate and FG9041 have both competitive and non-competitive antagonist actions at excitatory amino acid receptors. Eur J Pharmacol 151:313–315

Bird AP, Wolffe AP (1999) Methylation-induced repression—belts, braces, and chromatin. Cell 99:451–454

Bogdan C (2001) Nitric oxide and the immune response. Nat Immunol 2:907–916

Bordelon YM, Mackenzie L, Chesselet MF (1999) Morphology and compartmental location of cells exhibiting DNA damage after quinolinic acid injections into rat striatum. J Comp Neurol 412:38–50

Braidy N, Grant R, Brew BJ, Adams S, Jayasena T, Guillemin GJ (2009) Effects of kynurenine pathway metabolites on intracellular NAD synthesis and cell death in human primary astrocytes and neurons. Int J Tryptophan Res 2:61–69

Brat DJ, Bellail AC, Van Meir EG (2005) The role of interleukin-8 and its receptors in gliomagenesis and tumoral angiogenesis. Neuro Oncol 7:122–133

Burdzy A, Noyes KT, Valinluck V, Sowers LC (2002) Synthesis of stable-isotope enriched 5-methylpyrimidines and their use as probes of base reactivity in DNA. Nucleic Acids Res 30:4068–4074

Cancer Genome Atlas Research Network (2008) Comprehensive genomic characterization defines human glioblastoma genes and core pathways. Nature 455:1061–1068

CBTRUS (2011) Statistical report: primary brain and central nervous system tumors diagnosed in the United States in 2004–2007. http://www.cbtrus.org/2011-NPCR-SEER/WEB-0407-Report-3-3-2011.pdf

Cecener G, Tunca B, Egeli U, Bekar A, Tezcan G, Erturk E, Bayram N, Tolunay S (2012) The promoter hypermethylation status of GATA6, MGMT and FHIT in glioblastoma. Cell Mol Neurobiol 32:237–244

Charles N, Holland EC (2010) The perivascular niche microenvironment in brain tumor progression. Cell Cycle 9:3012–3021

Charles NA, Holland EC, Gilbertson R, Glass R, Kettenmann H (2012) The brain tumor microenvironment. Glia 60:502–514

Chen ZX, Riggs AD (2011) DNA methylation and demethylation in mammals. J Biol Chem 286:18347–18353

Chen J, McKay RM, Parada LF (2012) Malignant glioma: lessons from genomics, mouse models, and stem cells. Cell 149:36–47

Chiarugi A, Calvani M, Meli E, Traggiai E, Moroni F (2001a) Synthesis and release of neurotoxic kynurenine metabolites by human monocyte-derived macrophages. J Neuroimmunol 120:190–198

Chiarugi A, Meli E, Moroni F (2001b) Similarities and differences in the neuronal death processes activated by 3OH-kynurenine and quinolinic acid. J Neurochem 77:1310–1318

Chow LM, Endersby R, Zhu X, Rankin S, Qu C, Zhang J, Broniscer A, Ellison DW, Baker SJ (2011) Cooperativity within and among Pten, p53 and Rb pathways induces high-grade astrocytoma in adult brain. Cancer Cell 19:305–316

Ciembroniewicz J, Kolar O (1967) Eosinophilic response in glioblastoma tissue culture after addition of autologous lymphocytes. Science 157:1054–1055

Cortázar D, Kunz C, Selfridge J, Lettieri T, Saito Y, MacDougall E, Wirz A, Schuermann D, Jacobs AL, Siegrist F, Steinacher R, Jiricny J, Bird A, Schär P (2011) Embryonic lethal phenotype reveals a function of TDG in maintaining epigenetic stability. Nature 470:419–423

Cortellino S, Xu J, Sannai M, Moore R, Caretti E, Cigliano A, Le Coz M, Devarajian K, Wessels A, Soprano D, Abramowitz LK, Bartolomei MS, Rambow F, Bassi MR, Fanciulli M, Renner C, Klein-Szanto AJ, Matsumoto Y, Kobi D, Davidson I, Alberti C, Larue L, Bellacosa A (2011) Thymine DNA glycosylase is essential for active DNA demethylation by linked deamination-base excision repair. Cell 146:67–79

Costello JF, Berger MS, Huang HS, Cavenee WK (1996) Silencing of p16/CDKN2 expression in human gliomas by methylation and chromatin condensation. Cancer Res 56:2405–2410

Croitoru-Lamoury J, Lamoury FM, Caristo M, Suzuki K, Walker D, Takikawa O, Taylor R, Brew BJ (2011) Interferon-γ regulates the proliferation and differentiation of mesenchymal stem cells via activation of indoleamine 2,3 dioxygenase (IDO). PLoS One 16:e14698

Curran CS, Bertics PJ (2012) Eosinophils in glioblastoma biology. J Neuroinflammation 9:11

Curran CS, Evans MD, Bertics PJ (2011) GM-CSF production by glioblastoma cells has a functional role in eosinophil survival, activation, and growth factor production for enhanced tumor cell proliferation. J Immunol 187:1254–1263 da Costa NM, Hautefeuille A, Cros MP, Melendez ME, Waters T, Swann P, Hainaut P, Pinto LF (2012) Transcriptional regulation of thymine DNA glycosylase (TDG) by the tumor suppressor protein p53. Cell Cycle 11:4570–4578

de Groot J, Sontheimer H (2011) Glutamate and the biology of gliomas. Glia 59:1181–1189

Di Vinci A, Casciano I, Marasco E, Banelli B, Ravetti GL, Borzi L, Brigati C, Forlani A, Dorcaratto A, Allemanni G, Zona G, Spaziante R, Gohlke H, Gardin G, Merlo DF, Mantovani V, Romani M (2012) Quantitative methylation analysis of HOXA3, 7, 9, and 10 genes in glioma: association with tumor WHO grade and clinical outcome. J Cancer Res Clin Oncol 138:35–47

Dunn GP, Rinne ML, Wykosky J, Genovese G, Quayle SN, Dunn IF, Agarwalla PK, Chheda MG, Campos B, Wang A, Brennan C, Ligon KL, Furnari F, Cavenee WK, Depinho RA, Chin L, Hahn WC (2012) Emerging insights into the molecular and cellular basis of glioblastoma. Genes Dev 26:756–784

Ekici M, Keim A, Rössler OG, Hohl M, Thiel G (2012) Chromatin structure and expression of the AMPA receptor subunit Glur2 in human glioma cells: major regulatory role of REST and Sp1. J Cell Biochem 113:528–543

Esteller M, Garcia-Foncillas J, Andion E, Goodman SN, Hidalgo OF, Vanaclocha V, Baylin SB, Herman JG (2000) Inactivation of the DNA-repair gene MGMT and the clinical response of gliomas to alkylating agents. N Engl J Med 343:1350–1354

Forrest CM, Youd P, Kennedy A, Gould SR, Darlington LG, Stone TW (2002) Purine, kynurenine, neopterin and lipid peroxidation levels in inflammatory bowel disease. J Biomed Sci 9:436–442

Fossati G, Ricevuti G, Edwards SW, Walker C, Dalton A, Rossi ML (1999) Neutrophil infiltration into human gliomas. Acta Neuropathol 98:349–354

Fueyo J, Gomez-Mazano C, Alemany R, Lee PS, McDonnell TJ, Mitlianga P, Shi Y, Levin VA, Yung WK, Kyritsis AP (2000) A mutant oncolytic adenovirus targeting the Rb pathway produces anti-glioma effect in vivo. Oncogene 19:2–12

Galia A, Calogero AE, Condorelli R, Fraggetta F, La Corte A, Ridolfo F, Bosco P, Castiglione R, Salemi M (2012) PARP-1 protein expression in glioblastoma multiforme. Eur J Histochem 56:e9

Globisch D, Munzel M, Muller M, Michalkas S, Wagner M, Koch S, Bruckl T, Biel M, Carell T (2010) Tissue distribution of 5-hydroxymethylcytosine and search for active demethylation intermediates. PLoS One 5:e15367

Goellner EM, Grimme B, Brown AR, Lin YC, Wang XH, Sugrue KF, Mitchell L, Trivedi RN, Tang JB, Sobol RW (2011) Overcoming temozolomide resistance in glioblastoma via dual inhibition of NAD+ biosynthesis and base excision repair. Cancer Res 71:2308–2317

Gramatzki D, Pantazis G, Schittenhelm J, Tabatabai G, Köhle C, Wick W, Schwarz M, Weller M, Tritschler I (2009) Aryl hydrocarbon receptor inhibition downregulates the TGF-beta/smad pathway in human glioblastoma cells. Oncogene 28:2593–2605

Grant RS, Kapoor V (1998) Murine glial cells regenerate NAD, after peroxide-induced depletion, using either nicotinic acid, nicotinamide, or quinolinic acid as substrates. J Neurochem 70:1759–1763

Greenblatt MS, Bennett WP, Hollstein M, Harris CC (1994) Mutations in the p53 tumor suppressor gene: clues to cancer etiology and molecular pathogenesis. Cancer Res 54:4855–4878

Guillemin GJ, Kerr SJ, Smythe GA, Smith DG, Kapoor V, Armati PJ, Croitoru J, Brew BJ (2001) Kynurenine pathway metabolism in human astrocytes: a paradox for neuronal protection. J Neurochem 78:842–853

Guillemin GJ, Cullen KM, Lim CK, Smythe GA, Garner B, Kapoor V, Takikawa O, Brew BJ (2007) Characterization of the kynurenine pathway in human neurons. J Neurosci 27:12884–12892

Guo JU, Su Y, Zhong C, Ming GL, Song H (2011) Hydroxylation of 5-methylcytosine by TET1 promotes active DNA demethylation in the adult brain. Cell 145:423–434

Haffner MC, Chaux A, Meeker AK, Esopi DM, Gerber J, Pellakuru LG, Toubaji A, Argani P, Iacobuzio-Donahue C, Nelson WG, Netto GJ, De Marzo AM, Yegnasubramanian S (2011) Global 5-hydroxymethylcytosine content is significantly reduced in tissue stem/progenitor cell compartments and in human cancers. Oncotarget 2:627–637

He YF, Li BZ, Li Z, Liu P, Wang Y, Tang Q, Ding J, Jia Y, Chen Z, Li L, Sun Y, Li X, Dai Q, Song CX, Zhang K, He C, Xu GL (2011) Tet-mediated formation of 5-carboxylcytosine and its excision by TDG in mammalian DNA. Science 333:1303–1307

Herring JL, Rogstad DK, Sowers LC (2009) Enzymatic methylation of DNA in cultured human cells studied by stable isotope incorporation and mass spectrometry. Chem Res Toxicol 22:1060–1068

Heyes MP, Achim CL, Wiley CA, Major EO, Saito K, Markey SP (1996) Human microglia convert l-tryptophan into the neurotoxin quinolinic acid. Biochem J 320:595–597

Hiraku Y (2010) Formation of 8-nitroguanine, a nitrative DNA lesion, in inflammation-related carcinogenesis and its significance. Environ Health Prev Med 15:63–72

Holtze M, Mickienė A, Atlas A, Lindquist L, Schwieler L (2012) Elevated cerebrospinal fluid kynurenic acid levels in patients with tick-borne encephalitis. J Intern Med 272:394–401

Huang J, Chen K, Gong W, Zhou Y, Le Y, Bian X, Wang JM (2008) Receptor "hijacking" by malignant glioma cells: a tactic for tumor progression. Cancer Lett 267:254–261

Huse JT, Holland EC (2010) Targeting brain cancer: advances in the molecular pathology of malignant glioma and medulloblastoma. Nat Rev Cancer 10:319–331

Huttner A (2012) Overview of primary brain tumors. Pathologic classification, epidemiology, molecular biology, and prognostic markers. Hematol Oncol Clin North Am 26:715–732

Huysentruyt LC, Akgoc Z, Seyfried TN (2011) Hypothesis: are neoplastic macrophages/microglia present in glioblastoma multiforme? ASN Neuro 3:183–193

Ishiuchi S, Yoshida Y, Sugawara K, Aihara M, Ohtani T, Watanabe T, Saito N, Tsuzuki K, Okado H, Miwa A, Nakazato Y, Ozawa S (2007) Ca2+-permeable AMPA receptors regulate growth of human glioblastoma via Akt activation. J Neurosci 27:7987–8001

Jiang Z, Hu J, Li X, Jiang Y, Zhou W, Lu D (2006) Expression analyses of 27 DNA repair genes in astrocytoma by TaqMan low-density array. Neurosci Lett 409:112–117

Jin SG, Jiang Y, Qui R, Rauch TA, Wang Y, Schackert G, Krex D, Lu Q, Pfeifer GP (2011) 5-Hydroxymethylcytosine is strongly depleted in human cancers but its levels do not correlate with IDH1 mutations. Cancer Res 71:7360–7365

Kang JI, Sowers LC (2008) Examination of hypochlorous acid-induced damage to cytosine residues in a CpG dinucleotide in DNA. Chem Res Toxicol 21:1211–1218

Kim YH, Pierscianek D, Mittlebronn M, Vital A, Mariani L, Hassleblatt M, Oghaki H (2011) TET2 promoter methylation in low-grade diffuse gliomas lacking IDH1/2 mutations. J Clin Pathol 64:850–852

Kleijn A, Chen JW, Buhrman JS, Wojtkiewicz GR, Iwamoto Y, Lamfers ML, Stemmer-Rachamimov AO, Rabkin SD, Weissleder R, Martuza RL, Fulci G (2011) Distinguishing inflammation from tumor and peritumoral edema by myeloperoxidase magnetic resonance imaging. Clin Cancer Res 17:4484–4493

Klose RJ, Bird AP (2006) Genomic DNA methylation: the mark and its mediators. Trends Biochem Sci 31:89–97

Kominsky SL, Subramaniam PS, Johnson HM, Torres BA (2010) Inhibitory effects of IFN-gamma and acyclovir on the glioblastoma cell cycle. J Interferon Cytokine Res 20:463–469

Kraus TF, Globisch D, Wagner M, Eigenbrod S, Widmann D, Munzel M, Muller M, Pfaffender T, Hackner B, Feiden W, Schuller U, Carell T, Kretzschmar HA (2012) Low values of 5-hydroxymethylcytosine (5hmC), the "sixth base", are associated with anaplasia in human brain tumors. Int J Cancer 131:1577–1590

Kriaucionis S, Heintz N (2009) The nuclear DNA base 5-hydroxymethylcytosine is present in Purkinje neurons and the brain. Science 324:929–930

Lao VV, Herring JL, Kim CH, Darwanto A, Soto U, Sowers C (2009) Incorporation of 5-chlorocytosine into mammalian DNA results in heritable gene silencing and altered cytosine methylation patterns. Carcinogenesis 30:886–893

Lao VV, Darwanto A, Sowers LC (2010) Impact of base analogues within a CpG dinucleotide on the binding of DNA by the methyl-binding domain of MeCP2 and methylation by DNMT1. Biochemistry 49:10228–10236

Leaver KR, Reynolds A, Bodard S, Guilloteau D, Chalon S, Kassiou M (2012) Effects of translocator protein (18 kDa) ligands on microglial activation and neuronal death in the quinolinic-acid-injected rat striatum. ACS Chem Neurosci 3:114–119

Lewis JG, Adams DO (1987) Inflammation, oxidative DNA damage, and carcinogenesis. Environ Health Perspect 76:19–27

Linos E, Raine T, Alonso A, Michaud D (2007) Atopy and risk of brain tumors: a meta-analysis. J Natl Cancer Inst 99:1544–1550

Lipton SA, Rosenberg PA (1994) Excitatory amino acids as a final common pathway for neurologic disorders. N Engl J Med 330:613–622

Liu Y, Jiang W, Liu J, Zhao S, Xiong J, Mao Y, Wang Y (2012) IDH1 mutations inhibit multiple α-ketoglutarate-dependent dioxygenase activities in astroglioma. J Neurooncol 109:253–260

Lonkar P, Dedon PC (2011) Reactive species and DNA damage in chronic inflammation: reconciling chemical mechanisms and biological fates. Int J Cancer 128:1999–2009

Lorent A, Mueller W, Urdangarin E, Lazcoz P, Lass U, von Deimling A, Castresana JS (2008) RASSF1A, BLU, NORE1A, PTEN, and MGMT expression and promoter methylation in gliomas and glioma cell lines and evidence of deregulated expression of de novo DNMTs. Brain Pathol 19:279–292

Louis DN, Ohgaki H, Wiestler OD, Cavenee WK, Burger PC, Jouvet A, Scheithauer BW, Kleihues P (2007) The 2007 WHO classification of tumors of the central nervous system. Acta Neuropathol 114:97–109

Lyons SA, Chung WJ, Weaver AK, Ogunrinu T, Sontheimer H (2007) Autocrine glutamate signaling promotes glioma cell invasion. Cancer Res 167:9463–9471

Maki RA, Tyurin VA, Lyon RC, Hamilton RL, DeKosky ST, Kagan VE, Reynolds WF (2009) Aberrant expression of myeloperoxidase in astrocytes promotes phospholipid oxidation and memory deficits in a mouse model of Alzheimer disease. J Biol Chem 284:3158–3169

Mándi Y, Vécsei L (2012) The kynurenine system and immunoregulation. J Neural Transm 119:197–209

Mangerich A, Knutson CG, Parry NM, Muthupalani S, Ye W, Prestwich E, Cui L, McFaline JL, Mobley M, Ge Z, Taghizadeh K, Wishnok JS, Wogan GN, Fox JG, Tannenbaum SR, Dedon PC (2012) Infection-induced colitis in mice causes dynamic and tissue-specific changes in stress response and DNA damage leading to colon cancer. Proc Natl Acad Sci USA 109:E1820–E1829

Marcus HJ, Carpenter KL, Price SJ, Hutchinson PJ (2010) In vivo assessment of high-grade glioma biochemistry using microdialysis: a study of energy-related molecules, growth factors and cytokines. J Neurooncol 97:11–23

Martinez R (2012) Beyond genetics in glioma pathways: the ever-increasing crosstalk between epigenomic and genomic events. J Signal Transduct 1–9

Martinez R, Esteller M (2010) The DNA methylome of glioblastoma multiforme. Neurobiol Dis 39:40–46

Martinez R, Martin-Subero JI, Rohde V, Kirsch M, Alaminos M, Fernandez AF, Ropero S, Schackert G, Esteller M (2009) A microarray-based DNA methylation study of glioblastoma multiforme. Epigenetics 4:255–264

Mellac S, Fazakerley GV, Sowers LC (1993) Structures of base pairs with 5-(hydroxymethyl)-2'-deoxyuridine in DNA determined by NMR spectroscopy. Biochemistry 32:7779–7786

Mitsuka K, Kawataki T, Satoh E, Asahara T, Horikoshi T, Kinouchi H (2013) Expression of indoleamine 2,3-dioxygenase and correlation with pathological malignancy in gliomas. Neurosurgery. 19 Feb 2013 (Epub ahead of print)

Miyazaki T, Moritake K, Yamada K, Hara N, Osago H, Shibata T, Akiyama Y, Tsuchiya M (2009) Indoleamine 2,3-dioxygenase as a new target for malignant glioma therapy: laboratory investigation. J Neurosurg 111:230–237

Moffett JR, Els T, Espey MG, Walter SA, Streit WJ, Namboodiri MA (1997) Quinolinate immunoreactivity in experimental rat brain tumors is present in macrophages but not in astrocytes. Exp Neurol 144:287–301

Mohr F, Dohner K, Buske C, Rawat VP (2011) TET genes: new players in DNA demethylation and important determinants for stemness. Exp Hematol 39:272–281

Moroni F (1999) Tryptophan metabolism and brain function: focus on kynurenine and other indole metabolites. Eur J Pharmacol 375:87–100

Mueller MM, Herold-Mende CC, Riede D, Lange M, Steiner HH, Fusenig NE (1999) Autocrine growth regulation by granulocyte colony-stimulating factor and granulocyte macrophage colony-stimulating factor in human gliomas with tumor progression. Am J Pathol 155:1557–1567

Muller T, Gessi M, Waha A, Isselstein LJ, Luxen D, Freihoff D, Freihoff J, Becker A, Simon M, Hammes J, Denkhaus D, Zur Muhlen A, Pietsch T, Waha A (2012) Nuclear exclusion of TET1 is associated with loss of 5-hydroxymethylcytosine in IDH1 wild-type gliomas. Am J Pathol 181:675–683

Munder M (2009) Arginase: an emerging key player in the mammalian immune system. Br J Pharmacol 158:638–651

Munzel M, Globisch D, Bruckl T, Wagner M, Welzmiller V, Michalkis S, Muller M, Biel M, Carell T (2010) Quantification of the sixth DNA base hydroxymethylcytosine in the brain. Angew Chem Int Ed Engl 49:5375–5377

Munzel M, Globisch D, Carell T (2011) 5-hydroxymethylcytosine, the sixth base of the genome. Angew Chem Int Ed Engl 50:6460–6468

Murat A, Migliavacca E, Hussain SF, Heimberger AB, Desbaillets I, Hamou MF, Ruegg C, Stupp R, Delorenzi M, Hegi ME (2009) Modulation of angiogenic and inflammatory response in glioblastoma by hypoxia. PLoS One 4:e5947

Nakamura M, Yonekawa Y, Kleihues P, Ohgaki H (2001) Promoter methylation of the RB1 gene in glioblastomas. Lab Invest 81:77–820

Nguyen NT, Kimura A, Nakahama T, Chinen I, Masuda K, Nohara K, Fujii-Kuriyama Y, Kishimoto T (2010) Aryl hydrocarbon receptor negatively regulates dendritic cell immunogenicity via a kynurenine-dependent mechanism. Proc Natl Acad Sci USA 107:19961–19966

Nitta M, Kozono D, Kennedy R, Stommel J, Ng K, Zinn PO, Kushwaha D, Kesari S, Inda MD, Wykosky J, Furnari F, Hoadley KA, Chin L, DePinho RA, Cavenee WK, D'Andrea A, Chen CC (2010) Targeting EGFR induced oxidative stress by PARP1 inhibition in glioblastoma therapy. PLoS One 5:e10767

Noushmehr H, Weisenberger DJ, Diefes K, Phillips HS, Pujara K, Berman BP, Pan F, Pelloski CE, Sulman EP, Bhat KP, Verhaak RG, Hoadley KA, Hayes DN, Perou CM, Schmidt HK, Ding L, Wilson RK, Van Den Berg D, Shen H, Bengtsson H, Neuvial P, Cope LM, Buckley J, Herman JG, Baylin SB, Laird PW, Aldape K, The Cancer Genome Atlas Research Network (2010) Identification of a CpG island methylator phenotype that defines a distinct subgroup of glioma. Cancer Cell 17:510–522

Obrenovitch TP (2001) Quinolinic acid accumulation during neuroinflammation. Does it imply excitotoxicity? Ann NY Acad Sci 939:1–10

Oh MC, Kim JM, Safaee M, Kaur G, Sun MZ, Kaur R, Celli A, Mauro TM, Parsa AT (2012) Overexpression of calcium-permeable glutamate receptors in glioblastoma derived brain tumor initiating cells. PLoS One 7:e47846

Ooi SK, Bestor TH (2008) The colorful history of active DNA demethylation. Cell 133:1145–1148

Opitz CA, Litzenburger UM, Sahm F, Ott M, Tritschler I, Trump S, Schumacher T, Jestaedt L, Schrenk D, Weller M, Jugold M, Guillemin GJ, Miller CL, Lutz C, Radlwimmer B, Lehmann I, von Deimling A, Wick W, Platten M (2011) An endogenous tumour-promoting ligand of the human aryl hydrocarbon receptor. Nature 478:197–203

Orr BA, Haffner MC, Nelson WG, Yegnasubramanian S, Eberhart CG (2012) Decreased 5-hydroxymethylcytosine is associated with neural progenitor phenotype in normal brain and shorter survival in malignant glioma. PLoS One 7:e41036

Pan H, Wang H, Zhu L, Mao L, Qiao L, Su X (2012) The role of Nrf2 in migration and invasion of human glioma cell U251. World Neurosurg. 7 Nov 2011 (Epub ahead of print)

Passera E, Campanini B, Rossi F, Casazza V, Rizzi M, Pellicciari R, Mozzarelli A (2011) Human kynurenine aminotransferase II–reactivity with substrates and inhibitors. FEBS J 278:1882–1900

Piao Y, Jiang H, Alemany R, Krasnykh V, Marini FC, Xu J, Alonso MM, Conrad CA, Aldape KD, Gomez-Manzano C, Fueyo J (2009) Oncolytic adenovirus retargeted to delta-EGFR induces selective antiglioma activity. Cancer Gene Ther 16:256–265

Privat E, Sowers LC (1996) Photochemical deamination and demethylation of 5-methylcytosine. Chem Res Toxicol 9:745–750

Raison CL, Dantzer R, Kelley KW, Lawson MA, Woolwine BJ, Vogt G, Spivey JR, Saito K, Miller AH (2010) CSF concentrations of brain tryptophan and kynurenines during immune stimulation with IFN-alpha: relationship to CNS immune responses and depression. Mol Psychiatry 15:393–403

Rajasekhar VK, Viale A, Socci ND, Wiedmann M, Hu X, Holland EC (2003) Oncogenic Ras and Akt signaling contribute to glioblastoma formation by differential recruitment of existing mRNAs to polysomes. Mol Cell 12:889–901

Razin A, Riggs AD (1980) DNA methylation and gene function. Science 210:604–610

Reitman ZJ, Yan H (2010) Isocitrate dehydrogenase 1 and 2 mutations in cancer: alterations at a crossroads of cellular metabolism. J Natl Cancer Inst 102:932–941

Revoltella RP, Menicagli M, Campani D (2011) Granulocyte-macrophage colony-stimulating factor as an autocrine survival-growth factor in human gliomas. Cytokine 57:347–359

Riemenschneider MJ, Buschges R, Wolter M, Reifenberger J, Bostrom J, Kraus JA, Schlegel U, Reifenberger G (1999) Amplification and overexpression of the MDM4 (MDMX) gene from 1q32 in a subset of malignant gliomas without TP53 mutation or MDM2 amplification. Cancer Res 59:6091–6096

Rossi ML, Hughes JT, Esri MM, Coakham HB, Brownell DB (1987) Immunohistological study of mononuclear cell infiltrate in malignant gliomas. Acta Neurpathol 74:269–277

Rusmintratip V, Sowers LC (2000) An unexpectedly high excision capacity for mispaired 5-hydroxymethyluracil in human cell extracts. Proc Natl Acad Sci USA 97:14183–14187

Sahm F, Capper D, Pusch S, Balss J, Koch A, Langhans CD, Okun JG, von Deimling A (2011) Detection of 2-hydroxyglutarate in formalin-fixed paraffin-embedded glioma specimens by gas chromatography/mass spectrometry. Brain Path 22:1–6

Sahm F, Oezen I, Opitz CA, Radlwimmer B, von Deimling A, Ahrendt T, Adams S, Bode HB, Guillemin GJ, Wick W, Platten M (2013) The endogenous tryptophan metabolite and NAD+ precursor quinolinic acid confers resistance of gliomas to oxidative stress. Cancer Res. 2 Apr 2013 (Epub ahead of print)

Saito K, Chen CY, Masana M, Crowley JS, Markey SP, Heyes MP (1993) 4-Chloro-3-hydroxyanthranilate, 6-chloro tryptophan and norharman attenuate quinolinic acid formation by interferon-gamma-stimulated monocytes (THP-1 cells). Biochem J 291:11–14

Schunemann DP, Grivicich I, Regner A, Leal LF, de Araújo DR, Jotz GP, Fedrigo CA, Simon D, da Rocha AB (2010) Glutamate promotes cell growth by EGFR signaling on U-87MG human glioblastoma cell line. Pathol Oncol Res 16:285–293

Schwarcz R, Pellicciari R (2012) Manipulation of brain kynurenines: glial targets, neuronal effects, and clinical opportunities. J Pharmacol Exp Ther 303:1–10

Schwarcz R, Whetsell WO Jr, Mangano RM (1983) Quinolinic acid: an endogenous metabolite that produces axon-sparing lesions in rat brain. Science 219:316–318

Schwarcz R, Bruno JP, Muchowski PJ, Wu HQ (2012) Kynurenines in the mammalian brain: when physiology meets pathology. Nat Rev Neurosci 13:465–477

Seiberling KA, Church CA, Herring J, Sowers LC (2012) Epigenetics of chronic rhinosinusitis and the role of the eosinophil. Int Forum Allergy Rhinol 2:80–84

Sen E (2011) Targeting inflammation-induced transcription factor activation: an open frontier for glioma therapy. Drug Discov Today 16:1044–1051

Shinawi T, Hill VK, Krex D, Schackert G, Gentle D, Morris MR, Wei W, Cruickshank G, Maher ER, Latif F (2013) DNA methylation profiles of long- and short-term glioblastoma survivors. Epigenetics 8:149–156

Sippel TR, White J, Nag K, Tsvankin V, Klaassen M, Kleinschmidt-DeMasters BK, Waziri A (2011) Neutrophil degranulation and immunosuppression in patients with GBM: restoration of cellular immune function by targeting arginase I. Clin Cancer Res 17:6992–7002

Söderlund J, Erhardt S, Kast RE (2010) Acyclovir inhibition of IDO to decrease tregs as a glioblastoma treatment adjunct. J Neuroinflammation 7:44

Stegh AH, DePinho RA (2011) Beyond effector caspase inhibition: Bcl2L12 neutralizes p53 signaling in glioblastoma. Cell Cycle 10:33–38

Stevens EA, Mezrich JD, Bradfield CA (2009) The aryl hydrocarbon receptor: a perspective on potential roles in the immune system. Immunology 127:299–311

Stone TW, Behan WM (2007) Interleukin-1beta but not tumor necrosis factor-alpha potentiates neuronal damage by quinolinic acid: protection by an adenosine A2A receptor antagonist. J Neurosci Res 85:1077–1085

Tada M, Suzuki K, Yamakawa Y, Sawamura Y, Sakuma S, Abe H, van Meir E, de Tribolet N (1993) Human glioblastoma cells produce 77 amino acid interleukin-8 (IL-8(77)). J Neurooncol 16:25–34

Tahiliani M, Koh KP, Shen Y, Pastor WA, Bandukwala H, Brudno Y, Agarwal S, Iyer LM, Liu DR, Aravind L, Rao A (2009) Conversion of 5-methylcytosine to 5-hydroxymethylcytosine in mammalian DNA by MML partner TET1. Science 324:930–935

Tardy-Planechaud S, Fujimoto J, Lin SS, Sowers LC (1997) Solid phase synthesis and restriction endonuclease cleavage of oligooxynucleotides containing 5-(hydroxymethyl)-cytosine. Nucleic Acids Res 25:553–559

Tornaletti S, Pfeifer GP (1995) Complete and tissue-independent methylation of CpG sites in the p53 gene: implications for mutations in human cancers. Oncogene 10:1493–1499

Tsay JJ, Tchou-Wong KM, Greenberg AK, Pass H, Rom WN (2013) Aryl hydrocarbon receptor and lung cancer. Anticancer Res 33:1247–1256

Tuzgen S, Hanimoglu H, Tanriverdi T, Kacira T, Sanus GZ, Atukeren P, Dashti R, Gumustas K, Canbaz B, Kaynar MY (2007) Relationship between DNA damage and total antioxidant capacity in patients with glioblastoma multiforme. Clin Oncol 19:177–181

Ueki K, Ono Y, Henson JW, Efird JT, von Demling A, Louis DN (1996) CDKN2/p16 or RB alterations occur in the majority of glioblastomas and are inversely correlated. Cancer Res 56:150–153

Valinluck V, Sowers LC (2007a) Endogenous cytosine damage products alter the site selectivity of human DNA maintenance methyltransferase DNMT1. Cancer Res 67:946–950

Valinluck V, Sowers LC (2007b) Inflammation-mediated cytosine damage: a mechanistic link between inflammation and the epigenetic alterations in human cancers. Cancer Res 67:5583–5586

Valinluck V, Tsai HH, Rogstad DK, Burdzy A, Bird A, Sowers LC (2004) Oxidative damage to methyl-CpG sequences inhibits the binding of the methyl-CpG binding domain (MBD) of methyl-CpG binding protein 2 (MeCP2). Nuleic Acids Res 32:4100–4108

Valinluck V, Liu P, Kang JI Jr, Burdzy A, Sowers LC (2005) 5-halogenated pyrimidine lesions within a CpG sequence context mimic 5-methylcytosine by enhancing the binding of the methyl-CpG-binding domain of methyl-CpG-binding protein 2 (MeCP2). Nucleic Acids Res 33:3057–3064

Vasovcak P, Krepelova A, Menigatti M, Puchmajerova A, Skapa P, Augustinakova A, Amann G, Wernstedt A, Jiricny J, Marra G, Wimmer K (2012) Unique mutational profile associated with a loss of TDG expression in the rectal cancer of a patient with a constitutional PMS2 deficiency. DNA Repair 11:616–623

Vécsei L, Szalárdy L, Fülöp F, Toldi J (2013) Kynurenines in the CNS: recent advances and new questions. Nat Rev Drug Discov 12:64–82

Wainwright DA, Balyasnikova IV, Chang AL, Ahmed AU, Moon KS, Auffinger B, Tobias AL, Han Y, Lesniak MS (2012) IDO expression in brain tumors increases the recruitment of regulatory T cells and negatively impacts survival. Clin Cancer Res 18:6110–6121

Watson M, Roulston A, Bélec L, Billot X, Marcellus R, Bédard D, Bernier C, Branchaud S, Chan H, Dairi K, Gilbert K, Goulet D, Gratton MO, Isakau H, Jang A, Khadir A, Koch E, Lavoie

M, Lawless M, Nguyen M, Paquette D, Turcotte E, Berger A, Mitchell M, Shore GC, Beauparlant P (2009) The small molecule GMX1778 is a potent inhibitor of NAD+ biosynthesis: strategy for enhanced therapy in nicotinic acid phosphoribosyltransferase 1-deficient tumors. Mol Cell Biol 29:5872–5888

Weller M, Stupp R, Reifenberger G, Brandes AA, van den Bent MJ, Wick W, Hegi ME (2010) MGMT promoter methylation in malignant gliomas: ready for personalized medicine? Nat Rev Neurol 6:39–51

Whiteman M, Jenner A, Halliwell B (1997) Hypochlorous acid-induced base modifications in isolated calf thymus DNA. Chem Res Toxicol 10:1240–1246

Winterbourn CC, Kettle AJ (2000) Biomarkers of myeloperoxidase-derived hypochlorous acid. Free Radical Biol Med 29:403–409

Xiao M, Yang H, Xu W, Ma S, Lin H, Zhu H, Liu L, Liu Y, Yang C, Xu Y, Zhao S, Ye D, Xiong Y, Guan KL (2012) Inhibition of α-KG-dependent histone and DNA demethylases by fumarate and succinate that are accumulated in mutations of FH and SDH tumor suppressor. Genes Dev 26:1326–1338

Xie L, Poteet EC, Li W, Scott AE, Liu R, Wen Y, Ghorpade A, Simpkins JW, Yang SH (2010) Modulation of polymorphonuclear neutrophil functions by astrocytes. J Neuroinflammation 7:1–15

Xu W, Yang H, Liu Y, Yang Y, Wang P, Kim SH, Ito S, Yang C, Wang P, Xiao MT, Liu LX, Jiang WQ, Liu J, Zhang JY, Wang B, Frye S, Zhang Y, Xu YH, Lei QY, Guan KL, Zhao SM, Xiong Y (2011) Oncometabolite 2-hydroxyglutarate is a competitive inhibitor of α-ketoglutarate-dependent dioxygenases. Cancer Cell 19:17–30

Yang I, Han SJ, Sughrue ME, Tihan T, Parsa AT (2011a) Immune cell infiltrate differences in pilocytic astrocytoma and glioblastoma: evidence of distinct immunological microenvironments that reflect tumor biology. J Neurosurg 115:505–511

Yang Y, Liu Y, Yao X, Ping Y, Jiang T, Liu Q, Xu S, Huang J, Mou H, Gong W, Chen K, Bian X, Wang JM (2011b) Annexin 1 released by necrotic human glioblastoma cells stimulates tumor cell growth through the formyl peptide receptor 1. Am J Pathol 179:1504–1512

Ye ZC, Sontheimer H (1999) Glioma cells release excitotoxic concentrations of glutamate. Cancer Res 59:4383–4391

Yildirim O, Li R, Hung JH, Chen PB, Dong X, Ee LS, Weng Z, Rando OJ, Fazzio TG (2011) Mbd3/NURD complex regulates expression of 5-hydroxymethylcytosine marked genes in embryonic stem cells. Cell 147:1498–1510

You JS, Jones PA (2012) Cancer genetics and epigenetics: two sides of the same coin? Cancer Cell 22:9–20

Zheng H, Ying H, Yan H, Kimmelman AC, Hiller DJ, Chen AJ, Perry SR, Tonon G, Chu GC, Ding Z, Stommel JM, Dunn KL, Wiedemeyer R, You MJ, Brennan C, Wang YA, Ligon KL, Wong WH, Chin L, DePinho RA (2008) p53 and Pten control neural and glioma stem/progenitor cell renewal and differentiation. Nature 455:1129–1134

Chapter 5
The Role of Inflammation in Head and Neck Cancer

Marcelo Bonomi, Alexis Patsias, Marshall Posner and Andrew Sikora

Abstract Cancer-related inflammation is considered the "seventh hallmark of cancer"; numerous studies demonstrate that tumors develop and progress within inflammatory diseases. Central to the development of cancer are genetic changes that endow these cancer cells with many of the hallmarks of cancer, such as self-sufficient growth and resistance to anti-growth and pro-death signals. However, while the genetic changes that occur within cancer cells themselves, such as activated oncogenes or dysfunctional tumor suppressors, are responsible for many aspects of cancer development, they are not sufficient. Tumor promotion and progression are dependent on ancillary processes involving cells of the tumor environment that are not necessarily cancerous themselves. Infiltration of immune cells facilitates tumor development through the production of factors that promote carcinogenesis and by enabling tumors to evade the host immune response. Small molecules including cytokines, chemokines, and growth factors play key roles in both inflammation and cancer by promoting proliferation, angiogenesis, and carcinogenesis and by recruiting immune cells. The extracellular matrix is altered in inflammation and provides structural support to developing tumors. Hypoxia is a common state in cancers and inflamed tissues which causes DNA damage and induces tumorigenic factors. Finally, tissue vasculature is a vital part of its microenvironment, supplying oxygen, nutrients, and growth factors to rapidly dividing cells and providing a mechanism for metastatic spread. This review will discuss the reflexive relationship between cancer and inflammation with particular focus on how by considering the role of inflammation in physiologic processes such as the maintenance of tissue

M. Bonomi (✉)
Head and Neck Oncology Program, Wake Forest School of Medicine, Winston-Salem, North Carolina, USA
e-mail: mbonomi@wakehealth.edu

A. Patsias · M. Posner · A. Sikora
Head and Neck Oncology Program, Mount Sinai School of Medicine, New York, USA

M. Posner
e-mail: marshall.posner@mssm.edu

B. B. Aggarwal et al. (eds.), *Inflammation and Cancer*, Advances in Experimental Medicine and Biology 816, DOI: 10.1007/978-3-0348-0837-8_5, © Springer Basel 2014

homeostasis and repair may provide a logical framework for understanding the connection between the inflammatory response and cancer. The cells and molecules outlined here represent potential targets for the treatment of head and neck cancer.

5.1 Introduction

Head and neck squamous cell carcinoma (HNSCC) originates in the mucosa of 5 major anatomic subsites: the oral cavity, oropharynx, larynx, hypopharynx, and nasopharynx. It is the sixth most common cancer worldwide, with approximately 650,000 new cases reported annually. Aggravating factors are tobacco smoking, alcohol consumption, betel chewing, and human papilloma virus (HPV) infection (Curado and Hashibe 2009). In the United States, there were 49,000 new cases in 2010, with 11,000 deaths (Jemal et al. 2010). Despite the overall decreased incidence of HNSCC in the United States over the past 3 decades, researchers have observed a significant increase in the incidence of squamous cell malignancies of the base of tongue, and tonsil, particularly in young-to-middle-age patients likely due to rising incidence of HPV-associated HNSCC (Shiboski et al. 2005).

Despite treatment advances in multimodality therapy with surgery, radiotherapy, and chemotherapy, 5-year survival is still poor for patients with locoregionally advanced disease (Forastiere et al. 2003; Posner et al. 2007; Vermorken et al. 2007).

The genetic alteration of cells in wide preneoplastic fields (field cancerization) results in locoregional recurrence and second primary cancer. Half of all individuals still die from their disease. The characterization of the mechanisms involved in the metastasis formation and the identification of markers allowing identifying patients with biologically aggressive tumors is of great interest for the effective management of HNSCC patients.

Cigarette smoke (CS) causes considerable morbidity and mortality by inducing cancer, chronic lung and vascular diseases, and oral disease. Despite the well-recognized risks associated with smoking, the habit remains unacceptably prevalent. Several toxins present in CS have immune modulatory effects. CS also contains trace amounts of microbial cell components, including bacterial lipopolysaccharide. These and other CS constituents induce chronic inflammation at mucosal surfaces and modify host responses to exogenous antigens. Mucosal damage from chronic tobacco and alcohol exposure has been well characterized, both in terms of its clinicopathologic course and the underlying molecular derangements responsible for tumor development. Premalignant lesions, including leukoplakia and erythroplakia, progress to invasive carcinomas along a well-described pathologic sequence (Perez-Ordonez et al. 2006).

Molecular events that undergird this process include increasing cytogenic abnormalities, inactivation of tumor suppressor genes, and changes in intracellular signaling pathways that induce cellular immortalization. The effects of CS on immunity are far-reaching and complex; both pro-inflammatory and suppressive effects may be induced. The net effect of CS on immunity depends on many variables, including the dose and type of tobacco, the route, and chronicity of exposure, and the presence of other factors at the time of immune cell stimulation, such as Toll receptor ligands or other inflammatory mediators. CS impairs innate defenses against pathogens, modulates antigen presentation, and promotes autoimmunity. CS also impairs immunity in the oral cavity and promotes gingival and periodontal disease and oral cancer. The recognition of specific mechanisms by which CS affects host immunity is an important step toward elucidating mechanisms of tobacco-induced disease and may identify novel therapeutic approaches for the management of smoking-related diseases (Lee et al. 2012).

Human papilloma virus-related oropharyngeal carcinoma (HPVOPC) clinically behaves differently than tobacco- and alcohol-induced HNSCC. Inflammation and immunosuppression are likely to also play a critical role in HPVOPC. These patients tend to present at a younger age, and without a history of excessive tobacco or alcohol use. Overall, HPVOPC patients also have better outcomes, with tumors more responsive to both surgical and non-surgical therapies and a lower risk of dying from disease. The relationship of HPVOP to inflammation remains largely unexplored (Chung and Gillison 2009; Ang et al. 2010).

5.2 Inflammatory Signaling Pathways Associated with Head and Neck Cancer

There are several genetic alterations associated with chronic inflammation in HNSCC. Inactivation of tumor suppressor genes through homozygous deletion, point mutations, and epigenetic alterations such as hypermethylation fuels the neoplastic process. For instance, a common genetic alteration in 70–80 % of dysplastic squamous cells and HNSCC tumors is the loss of chromosome 9p21, a region that contains cyclin-dependent kinase inhibitor 2A (CDKN2A), encodes tumor suppressor genes p16 and p14, and is involved in the G1 phase cell-cycle regulation. Loss of 3p, a locus with tumor suppressor phenotype, is another common genetic event seen early in dysplasia (Perez-Ordonez et al. 2006). Inactivation of p16 is a frequent event witnessed in >80 % of tumor specimens. Similarly, loss of heterozygosity of 17p—the region encoding tumor suppressor p53—is extremely common (Reed et al. 1996). It has been found that half of all tumor specimens from patients with HNSCC contain p53 mutations. Notably, disruption of TP53—the genetic locus on 17p giving rise to p53—has been associated with reduced survival after surgical therapy for HNSCC (Poeta et al. 2007).

Telomerase, an enzyme active in germ line cells but normally quiescent in somatic cells, has been shown to be overexpressed in 90 % of HNSCC cells. Telomerase is responsible for maintaining genomic stability by protecting chromosomal ends, especially in rapidly dividing cells; its activity in malignant cells enables evasion of apoptosis and contributes to cellular immortality (McCaul et al. 2002). Altered intracellular signaling also facilitates neoplastic development in HNSCC, including activation of oncogenic pathways downstream of the epidermal growth factor receptor (EGFR) and other molecular pathways.

HPV inactivates the same pathways via direct viral effects. The HPV is a circular, double-stranded DNA virus that encompasses many different subtypes, with HPV-16 and HPV-18 being the most common oncogenic variants in HPVOPC. Using in situ hybridization, HPV-16 DNA has been found in up to 72 % of oropharyngeal cancer specimens where this association remains the highest (D'Souza et al. 2007). On a molecular level, HPV gains access to the intracellular compartment of mucosal squamous cells and integrates into host DNA. The integrated virus subsequently expresses oncoproteins E6 and E7, which act synergistically to target the tumor suppressor genes p53 and pRb for ubiquitin-mediated intracellular degradation, resulting in genomic instability and oncogenic transformation as the normal cell-cycle regulatory points are inactivated (Chung and Gillison 2009).

Experimental tumor model studies show that non-steroidal anti-inflammatory drugs (NSAIDs) impair the growth and development of HNSCC, indicating potential as a chemopreventive agent. Furthermore, regular use of NSAIDs and aspirin has been shown to reduce the risk of other cancers.

Biologically, NSAIDs act as non-specific inhibitors for the pro-inflammatory cyclooxygenase enzymes (COX-1 and COX-2), which are involved in the conversion of arachidonic acid (AA) to prostaglandins (PG). COX-1 is present in most tissues and is involved in the production of PGs required for many normal physiologic functions, while COX-2 is found only in a limited number of cell types and is induced by stimulatory factors implicated with inflammation and many cancers.

Overexpression of COX-2 and PGs have been reported in a variety of cancer sites, including HNSCC, with increased levels reported in both tumor tissue and adjacent epithelium in HNSCC but not normal epithelium. Studies also suggest a correlation between COX-2 expression and head and neck tumor size and prognosis, with higher expression correlating with poorer outcome (Wilson et al. 2011). The downstream actions of PGs, such as increased cell proliferation, cell mobility and invasion, neo-angiogenesis, and the inhibition of apoptosis, are known to play important roles in cancer development. The mechanism by which NSAIDs inhibit tumor development is not clearly understood, although it is thought that they may act through the inhibition of COX-2 and consequently the synthesis of PGs and their pro-cancerous downstream effects (Wilson et al. 2011).

It has been shown that the EGFR and COX-2 have an important role in the biology of HNSCC. Overexpression of COX-2 is associated with a poor prognosis in HNSCC, and COX-2 inhibitors have demonstrated synergy when combined with EGFR inhibitors in preclinical models (Chen et al. 2004; Chung et al. 2011). Inflammatory mediators can promote epithelial–mesenchymal transition (EMT), a process by which epithelial cells lose their cell polarity and cell–cell adhesion, and gain migratory and invasive properties to become mesenchymal cells. This process is responsible for the increase resistance to EGFR-TKIs in HNSCC. These studies provide a strong rationale for combining a COX-2 inhibitor with an EGFR TKI (Kao et al. 2011).

Recent advances in the understanding of the oncogenesis of HNSCC have revealed multiple deregulated signaling pathways. Transforming growth factor-β (TGF-β) and PTEN/PI3K/Akt/mTOR pathways are among the most frequently altered signaling routes. Both pathways have central roles in numerous cellular processes, including metabolism, cell growth, apoptosis, survival, and differentiation, which ultimately contribute to HNSCC progression (Molinolo et al. 2009).

NF-κB is a pleiotropic transcription factor which plays a role in both innate and adaptive immunity and is required for the expression of several pro-inflammatory factors. Chronic inflammation is often a key factor in cancer development. As the head and neck area is prone to exposure to factors causing irritation and inflammation of the squamous epithelium, it might therefore be plausible that chronic inflammation also might be a major cause for the development of HNSCC. It has been shown that NF-κB and its pro-inflammatory target genes are activated in HNSCC cell lines and tumor specimens. Blocking NF-κB function in HNSCC greatly reduces tumor growth and decreases the expression of IL-6 and IL-8 along with many other cytokines and chemokines associated with the pro-inflammatory state (Kross et al. 2010).

Cytokines are soluble proteins that play an important role in the initiation and maintenance of inflammatory and immune responses as well as intercellular cross talking. Cytokines regulate immunity, inflammation, and hematopoiesis, and this family of proteins includes interleukins (ILs), interferons (IFNs), tumor necrosis factors (TNFs), and growth factors. They are typically divided into two categories: pro-inflammatory (e.g., IL-1, IL-6, IL-8, TNF-α, and IFN-γ) and anti-inflammatory [e.g., IL-4, IL-10, TGF-β, and vascular endothelial growth factor (VEGF)]. They bind to receptors and transducer signals via second messengers to control growth, differentiation, and activation of cells (Wang et al. 2009). It has been shown that high levels of cytokines and growth factors may have a role in the development of different cancers (Wang et al. 2009). High levels of IL-1a, IL-6, IL-8, granulocyte macrophage colony stimulating factor (GM-CSF), growth-regulated oncogene-(a) GRO1, VEGF, and hepatocyte gowth factor (HGF) have been involved in the development of HNSCC (Lee et al. 2007). It is also important to notice that altered levels of cytokines and growth factors can predict response to therapy and high levels of pro-inflammatory cytokines are associated with poor outcomes in patients undergoing chemoradiation treatments for HNSCC (Allen et al. 2007).

Interleukin-6 (IL-6) is a multifunctional cytokine synthesized in response to stimuli such as infection and trauma by a variety of cells such as macrophages, neutrophils, keratinocytes, fibroblasts, and endothelial cells. IL-6 cell signals are transmitted through a receptor expressed in a wide range of target cell types. In addition to this, a soluble IL-6 receptor (sIL-6R) enables to widen the repertoire of cells responsive to IL-6 (Jones et al. 2001). IL-6 is able to stimulate a number of biologic processes including antibody (and probable autoantibody) production, activation of T cells, B cell differentiation, increase in acute-phase proteins, hematopoiesis, induction of angiogenesis, vascular permeability, and osteoclast differentiation (Ridker et al. 1997; Nibali et al. 2012). It is also a strong stimulator of hepcidin, a liver-produced hormone that regulates intestinal iron absorption (Hohaus et al. 2010), potentially contributing to sideropenic anemia in chronic inflammation. IL-6 activity in inflammation is considered double-edged, acting both as anti-inflammatory (e.g., down-regulation of neutrophil recruitment and pro-inflammatory cytokine expression) (Xing et al. 1998) but also as pro-inflammatory (e.g., induction of acute-phase reactants by the liver) in chronic diseases (Jones et al. 2001). IL-6 is also believed to have growth factor properties regarding the development and progression of many types of cancers (Nishimoto 2010).

5.3 Role of Inflammatory Molecules in the Invasion, Metastasis and Angiogenesis of Head and Neck Cancer Cells

Epidemiologic and experimental evidence supports the concept that chronic inflammation promotes the development and progression of cancers. Because inflammation is a complex process involving many effector cells and mediators, it is likely that inflammation facilitates tumor progression through multiple mechanisms (Balkwill and Mantovani 2001).

The initiation of an epithelial-to-mesenchymal transition (EMT) is required for tumor dissemination to occur. E-cadherin has a key role in epithelial intercellular adhesion and its down-regulation is a hallmark of EMT, which is associated with invasion, metastasis, and poor prognosis. EMT is the major mechanism responsible for mediating invasiveness and metastasis of epithelial cancers. E-cadherin transcriptional repressors have a role in the inflammation-induced promotion of EMT in HNSCC, which is mediated by COX-2. Levels of COX-2 and its catalytic product PGE2 are increased in HNSCC (Buchanan et al. 2003; Dannenberg and Subbaramaiah 2003; Cooper et al. 2004). PGE2 can stimulate cell proliferation, motility, and angiogenesis while inhibiting apoptosis and immune surveillance (Buchanan et al. 2003; Cooper et al. 2004). COX-2-derived PGE2 may also promote metastasis by stimulating EMT and cell invasion (Dohadwala et al. 2006). It has been reported that PGE2 is transported or passed through the cell membrane via pro-staglandin-specific transporters, including the pro-staglandin transporter (PGT, an influx transporter). Intratumoral PGE2 levels depend not only upon the rate of production, but also on the rate of degradation. Inactivation of PGE2 located in the developing tumor microenvironment has been suggested to occur by a two-step model (Haddad et al. 2009). The first step is mediated by the PGT, which engages carrier-mediated membrane transport of pro-staglandins, including PGE2, PGF2a, and PGD2, from the extracellular milieu to the cytoplasm (Haddad et al. 2009). This transporter belongs to the organic anion superfamily of transporting polypeptides that contain 12 transmembrane spanning domains. The second step of PGE2 inactivation occurs in the cytoplasm, where 15-hydroxyprostaglandin dehydrogenase (15-PGDH) catabolizes and thus inactivates PGE2 (Haddad et al. 2009). Studies have shown that 15-PGDH expression is frequently reduced in several other epithelial cancers as well, (Ichikawa et al. 1996; Holla et al. 2008) suggesting that abnormalities in catabolism of PGE2 may have an important role in the development of these cancers.

During the process of tumor dissemination, tumor cells lose their epithelial characteristics [inhibition of E-cadherin (Cdh1)] to the profit of mesenchymal properties (expression of Snail1 and increased migratory abilities), allowing them to invade blood and lymphatic systems and establish new colonies in distant organs (Thiery et al. 2009). Other inflammatory mediators in addition to COX-2 have been shown to modulate EMT. Indeed in HNSCC cell lines, IL-1β was reported to stimulate Snail1 and inhibit Cdh1 expression (John et al. 2009). Among inflammatory actors, IL-32 was reported to modulate cytokine expression and to be up-regulated by TNF-α, IL-1β and IL-6 (Shioya et al. 2007; Kim et al. 2005). IL-8 and GRO1 serve as chemoattractants for neutrophils, monocytes, and endothelial cells, which are all major constituents of the inflammatory and angiogenesis response, and their expression promotes aggressive growth and metastasis (Van Waes 2007). In addition, IL-1 and IL-6 are potent inducers of HGF production by stromal cells, such as fibroblasts, further enhancing IL-8 and VEGF expression (Worden et al. 2005). Several cytokines and growth factors also activate signal pathways that promote the malignant phenotype. TNF-α, IL-1, HGF, and their receptors promote activation of the mitogen-activated protein kinase-activator protein-1 (MAPK-AP-1), nuclear factor-kappa B (NF-κB), and phosphatidylinositol-3 kinase (PI3K)/Akt pathways (Van Waes 2007). Epidermal growth factor (EGF) and IL-6 activate signal transducer and activating transcription factor-3 (STAT3) in HNSCC cells (Lee et al. 2008).

An increasing number of studies have recently focused on the role of cytokine networks, including IL-6, in the pathogenesis and progression of oral malignancy. In particular, clinical studies reported elevation of IL-6 levels in serum and saliva of patients with oral and other cancers of the head and neck compared with age-matched control subjects and their significant relation with staging and response to therapy (Chen et al. 1999; Bigbee et al. 2007). The expression of IL-6 and IL-8 genes was shown, via large-scale gene expression profiling on laser-captured microdissected oral cancer and normal oral epithelial cells, to be uniquely associated with HNSCC (Alevizos et al. 2001). IL-6 seems to contribute to oral cancer pathogenesis through different mechanisms and biologic processes. An in vitro study showed that IL-6 can stimulate HNSCC cells to enhanced secretion of matrix metalloproteinases 1 and 9, which play a major role in infiltrative growth, metastasis, and neo-angiogenesis (Sundelin et al. 2005). IL-6 may also modulate a variety of keratinocytes pathways including cell growth, survival, and differentiation. In particular, IL-6 has been shown to stimulate proliferation of cultured human keratinocytes in psoriatic skin (Nibali et al. 2012). Furthermore, IL-6 can activate transcription factors such as signal transducer and activator of transcription (STAT)-1 and STAT-3, which in turn have been observed in various tumors (Hirano et al. 2000). A recent study showed that IL-6 can also promote tumorigenesis by causing DNA hypomethylation as well as aberrant promoter hypermethylation changes, which can lead to epigenetic changes in gene expression of HNSCC cells (Gasche et al. 2011). Furthermore, in vitro studies demonstrated that oral keratinocytes can produce IL-6 in response to a number of environmental factors well known to increase oral cancer risk such as areca nut and tobacco smoking (Jeng et al. 2003). Indeed, biopsies from individuals with oral submucous fibrosis showed increased expression of IL-6 in the epithelium and underlying inflammatory infiltrate, as well as in peripheral blood mononuclear cells (Haque et al. 2000).

IL-32 is one of the cytokines with pro-inflammatory activities implicated in inflammatory disorders, such as rheumatoid arthritis, mycobacterium tuberculosis infections, and inflammatory bowel disease (Shioya et al. 2007; Heinhuis et al. 2011). On a retrospective study of 65 patients with HNSCC, it was shown that patients with tumors expressing high amounts of IL32 had a worse disease-free survival and overall survival in comparison with individuals with weak IL32 tumor expression. In addition, in vitro data linked IL32 expression to metastatic potential (Guenin et al. 2013). The inverse correlation between IL32 and p53 expression found in this study was also found in patients with hepatocarcinoma (Kang et al. 2012). The increased p53 expression induced by IL-32 inhibition could originate from the loss of Snail1 which would not be able to form a complex with p53 leading to its degradation through a transcription-independent mechanism (Lee et al. 2009). Alternatively, IL-32 inhibition was reported to decrease NF-κB which is a well-described p53 inhibitor and an activator of Snail1 expression (Gurova et al. 2005; Tergaonkar and Perkins 2007; Zhang et al. 2011). Therefore, IL-32 down-regulation might allow p53 re-expression through NF-κB and Snail1 inhibition (Kim et al. 2011). We can speculate that IL32 plays a pivotal role in tumor responses to inflammatory mediators and enhances cell invasiveness properties through a nuclear NF-κB/Snail1 axis in which intermediary actors have to be identified. This is supported by its nuclear localization found in the more aggressive tumors (Guenin et al. 2013).

TGF-β belongs to a superfamily of multifunctional cytokines that regulate cell proliferation, differentiation, migration, adhesion, and apoptosis, thereby influencing important physiologic processes such as embryonic development, immune function, and carcinogenesis (Derynck and Zhang 2003; Massague 2008). The three mammalian TGF-β isoforms, TGF-β1, TGF-β2, and TGF-β3, exert their functions through a cell-surface receptor complex composed of type I (TGFBR1) and type II (TGFBR2) serine/threonine kinase receptors. Upon ligand binding, TGFBR2 recruits and phosphorylates TGFBR1, which in turn phosphorylates Smad2 or Smad3. Phosphorylated Smad2 or Smad3 binds to Smad4, and then, these complexes translocate from the cytoplasm into the nucleus. This results in the transcriptional activation of TGF-β-responsive genes that mediate the effects of TGF-β at the cellular level. In addition to Smad-mediated signaling, receptor activation also induces other downstream targets, including Ras, RhoA, TAK1 (TGF-β-activated kinase-1), MEKK1, PI3K, and PP2A, to produce the full spectrum of TGF-β response (Moustakas and Heldin 2009; Zhang 2009).

The effects of TGF-β signaling on carcinogenesis largely depend on the tissue of origin and the tumor type. In most types of human cancer, TGF-β has a paradoxical role in cancer development by way of functioning as a tumor suppressor during the early stages (Engle et al. 1999) and as a tumor promoter during the later stages (Piek and Roberts 2001; Tang et al. 2003). Several reports have noted that mutations and polymorphisms of TGFBR1 and Smads are associated with HNSCC, (Chen et al. 2001; Xie et al. 2003; Pasche et al. 2005) suggesting that TGF-β functions as a potent tumor suppressor. However, it is not clear whether alterations in TGF-β signaling act alone or in concert with alterations in other pathways to promote a pro-oncogenic phenotype in advanced late-stage HNSCC.

As noted above, The PI3K/Akt pathway is important for suppressing apoptosis, and promoting cell growth and proliferation. In HNSCC, hyper activation of PI3K can be induced by mutations or by enhanced activity of its upstream activators, including the activation of Ras oncoproteins or inactivation of phosphatase and tensin homolog (PTEN) deleted on chromosome 10 (Molinolo et al. 2009). PTEN is a potent tumor suppressor gene and a negative regulator of the PI3K/Akt pathway. As PTEN mutations were identified in 0–16 % of HNSCCs, loss of PTEN expression was observed in 29 % of tongue cancers and loss of heterozygosity of the PTEN locus was identified in 40 % of HNSCCs (Henderson et al. 1998; Shao et al. 1998; Lee et al. 2001). Additionally, 47 % of HNSCC cases showed at least one molecular alteration in the PI3K/Akt pathway, including PI3 KCA and AKT2 amplification, p110α overexpression and PTEN protein down-regulation. This suggests the critical role of the PTEN/PI3K/Akt signaling pathways in the carcinogenesis of HNSCC (Pedrero et al. 2005). It seems that there may be negative cross talk between the TGF-β tumor suppressor and the PI3K/Akt pathways (Bian et al. 2012). It was shown that defects in the TGF-β and PI3K/Akt signaling pathways are common in human HNSCCs. Activation of the PI3K/Akt pathway due to PTEN deletion initiates tumor formation by increasing proliferation in the head and neck epithelia. However, PTEN deletion alone is not sufficient to induce invasive HNSCC due to the induction of premature senescence by p-Akt in the presence of the tumor suppressor TGF-β. In combination with the additional loss of TGFBR1, which blocks tumor inhibition by TGF-β signaling, premalignant cells cannot undergo cellular senescence and will progress into cancer cells (Bian et al. 2012).

Studies on a 2cKO mouse model showed that TGFBR1 and PTEN work collaboratively in suppressing tumor progression. The loss of TGFBR1/PTEN function is associated with increased cell proliferation, loss of apoptosis, and increase levels of Cyclin D1 (CCND1) in head and neck cancer (Bian et al. 2012).

The multifunctional cytokine TGF-B has different effects in premalignant and malignant cells. In epithelial cells, TGF-B has a tumor-suppressor effect via its autocrine interaction with other signaling pathways. On the other hand, in tumor cells, TGF-B increases tumor proliferation via its paracrine effects which include but not limited to inflammation, angiogenesis, and escape form immunosurveillance (De Wever and Mareel 2003).

The interaction between different pathways, transcription factors, and multifuncitonal cytokines is far more complex than previously thought. For instance, in a head and neck mouse model, it was recently shown that the deletion of TGFBR1/PTEN is associated with the activation of the NF-kB pathway. As a result of this interaction, several genes that are associated with an inflammatory state are also over-expressed (i.e., Cxcl1, Cxcl5, Ptgs2). This pro-inflammatory state is responsible for the recruitment of myeloid-derived suppressor cells

(MDSCs), which increases the angiogenesis and immune suppressive state within the tumor stroma (Bian et al. 2012). The disruption of the TGF-B signaling pathway can lead to similar findings (Lu et al. 2006; Bierie et al. 2008). These data support the concept that the tumor stroma has a pivotal role in the development and progression of head and neck cancer (Bian et al. 2012).

Neuroblast differentiation-associated protein AHNAK, also known as desmoyokin, is a protein that in humans is encoded by the AHNAK gene. AHNAK was originally identified in 1989 (in bovine muzzle epidermal cells) and named desmoyokin due to its localization pattern (that resembled a yoke) in the desmosomal plaque. It is a protein of exceptionally large size (700 kDa) that is expressed in a variety of cell types (Shtivelman et al. 1992). This protein has the ability to shuttle between various subcellular compartments. For instance, it has been shown that AHNAK can translocate from the cytoplasm to the plasma membrane of keratinocytes in a manner dependent on Ca^{2+} and protein kinase C (Hashimoto et al. 1995). Furthermore, AHNAK was shown to contain a nuclear export signal (NES) sequence which allowed it to be excluded from the nuclei of epithelial cells following cell–cell contact and activation of protein kinase B, respectively (Sussman et al. 2001). At functional level, AHNAK was shown to be involved in various cellular processes, including calcium regulation and organization of the actin cytoskeleton (Haase et al. 1999; Gentil et al. 2001). In tumor cells, AHNAK was recently found to be essential for pseudopodia formation and tumoral migration/invasion (Shankar et al. 2010). Other recent studies proposed that the AHNAK gene might be involved in mutagenic transformation of colon epithelial cells and thus carcinogenesis (Tanaka et al. 2008). It is well established that solid tumors display an inflammatory microenvironment characterized by large numbers of tumor-infiltrating immune cells (Coussens and Werb 2002). Within this microenvironment, the immune cells of the host are reprogrammed by the tumor cells to acquire pro-tumoral activities. Although less characterized than tumor-associated macrophages (TAMs) or tumor-infiltrating lymphocytes (TILs), tumor-infiltrating neutrophils are emerging as important players in the pathophysiology of cancer. Within the tumor tissue, neutrophils can modulate several cellular processes which may ultimately lead to tumor progression. Neutrophils were shown to modulate angiogenesis in several murine tumor models (Nozawa et al. 2006; Jablonska et al. 2010; Bekes et al. 2011) and were recently associated with angiogenesis progression in hepatocellular carcinoma patients (Kuang et al. 2011). Further studies showed that neutrophils could directly modulate the biology and functions of tumor cells by promoting their migration, invasion or proliferation (Gregory and Houghton 2011).

There is an association of high numbers of tumor-infiltrating neutrophils with advanced disease and poor clinical outcome in patients with different types of cancer, such as renal cancer, hepatocellular cancer, non-small-cell lung carcinoma (NSCLC), or melanoma (Dumitru et al. 2012).

In head and neck cancer patients, it was demonstrated that a high neutrophilic infiltration of the tumor tissue was correlated with high tumor stage and poor survival (Trellakis et al. 2011). In vitro studies indicated a direct interaction between neutrophils and head and neck cancer cells by showing that neutrophils were primed by the tumor cells to release pro-inflammatory factors, which promoted tumoral migration in a feedback manner (Dumitru et al. 2011, 2012). Selected soluble inflammatory mediators, such as cytokines, chemokines, and metabolites of the AA pathway, have been found to change the function and differentiation of immune cells (Lin and Karin 2007). Among these molecules, macrophage migration inhibitory factor (MIF) is emerging as an important regulator of inflammation in cancer (Bucala and Donnelly 2007). A number of studies found that high levels of MIF in the tumor tissues or serum of patients with different types of cancer were associated with advanced disease and poor clinical outcome (Grieb et al. 2010). It was also demonstrated that overexpression of tumoral MIF was associated with poor overall survival in patients with orohypopharyngeal cancer (Dumitru et al. 2011). More importantly, MIF was identified as one of the missing links in the tumor-neutrophil interaction and showed that head and neck cancer cells released MIF which subsequently enhanced the pro-inflammatory functions of neutrophils to promote tumoral migration (Dumitru et al. 2011). AHNAK overexpression is associated with poor survival in these patients. Interestingly, in patients with HNSCC, it was found that high levels of AHNAK together with high MIF expression or high neutrophilic infiltration, respectively, were strongly associated with poor survival. Synchronous high levels of MIF and tumor-infiltrating neutrophils had stronger predictor values over the individual markers as well. Finally, patients with high levels of all three markers displayed the shortest survival in the entire patient cohort (Dumitru et al. 2013). These findings suggest that AHNAK might cooperate with MIF and/or neutrophils to enhance progression of HNSCC. There is data regarding direct interactions between HNSCC-derived MIF and neutrophils both in vitro and in vivo. It was shown that HNSCC-derived MIF enhanced neutrophil chemotaxis in vitro and that tumoral MIF levels correlated with the neutrophilic infiltration in tissues from orohypopharyngeal carcinoma patients (Dumitru et al. 2011). Since MIF is a known ligand for CXCR2, one of the major chemokine receptors on neutrophils, (Bernhagen et al. 2007) MIF-mediated recruitment might be a critical mechanism for infiltration of HNC tissues by neutrophils. It was further demonstrated that HNC-derived MIF stimulated neutrophils to release large amounts of pro-inflammatory factors, among which CCL4 and MMP9 (Dumitru et al. 2011). Neutrophils enhance the motility, migration, and invasion of tumor cells via—not fully identified—soluble factors and molecular mechanisms (Dumitru et al. 2012). Interestingly, AHNAK was recently linked to regulation of tumoral migration/invasion. It seems that AHNAK is essential for rearrangement of the actin cytoskeleton and pseudopodia formation (Shankar et al. 2010).

HPV-HNSCC differs from tobacco-related head and neck cancers in several ways. The patients tend to be younger in age, lack a significant tobacco and/or alcohol history, and have improved clinical outcomes. The virus-related tumors arise from the deep crypts within the lymphoid tissue of the tonsil and base of tongue and the majority can be distinguished from tobacco-related HNSCC by the characteristic infiltration of lymphocytes in the stroma and tumor nests. Nevertheless, despite this profound inflammatory response, HPV-HNSCCs are able to evade immune surveillance, persist, and grow (Gillison et al. 2008).

Various mechanisms have been proposed for the resistance of human solid tumors to immune recognition and obliteration, including the recruitment of regulatory T cells, MDSCs, and local secretion of inhibitory cytokines. Recent evidence suggests that tumors develop physiologic mechanisms of tissue protection from inflammatory destruction via up-regulation of immune inhibitory ligands. Antigen-induced activation and proliferation of T cells are regulated by the temporal expression of both co-stimulatory and co-inhibitory receptors and their cognate ligands (Topalian et al. 2012).

In the context of cancer, in which immune responses are directed against antigens specifically or selectively expressed by tumor cells, these immune checkpoints can represent major obstacles to the generation and maintenance of clinically meaningful anti-tumor immunity. CTLA-4 and programmed cell death-1 (PD-1) are two such checkpoint receptors being actively targeted in the clinic (Lyford-Pike et al. 2013).

It has been shown that in HPV-HNSCCs that are highly infiltrated with lymphocytes, PD-L1 expression on both tumor cells and CD68(+) TAMs is geographically localized to sites of lymphocyte fronts, whereas the majority of CD8þ TILs express high levels of PD-1, the inhibitory PD-L1 receptor. Significant levels of mRNA for IFN-γ, a major cytokine inducer of PD-L1 expression, were found in HPV(+) PD-L1(+) tumors. These findings support the role of the PD-1: PD-L1 interaction in creating an "immune-privileged" site for initial viral infection and subsequent adaptive immune resistance once tumors are established and suggest a rationale for therapeutic blockade of this pathway (Lyford-Pike et al. 2013).

5.4 Role of Inflammatory Molecules in the Development of Head and Neck Cancer: Evidence from In Vivo Studies

Chronic inflammation is frequently associated with malignant growth and is thought to promote and enhance tumor progression, although the mechanisms which regulate this relationship remain elusive (Coussens and Werb 2002). It has been reported that interleukin (IL)-1β promoted tumor progression by enhancing the accumulation of MDSCs and hypothesized that inflammation leads to cancer through the production of MDSCs which inhibit tumor immunity (Bunt et al. 2006) if inflammation-induced MDSCs promote tumor progression by blocking anti-tumor immunity, then a reduction in inflammation should reduce MDSC levels and delay tumor progression; whereas an increase in inflammation should increase MDSC levels and hasten tumor progression (Dinarello 1996). This hypothesis was tested by using the 4T1 mammary carcinoma and IL-1 receptor (IL-1R)–deficient mice which have a reduced potential for inflammation, and IL-1R antagonist–deficient mice, which have an increased potential for inflammation. Consistent with the initial hypothesis, IL-1R–deficient mice have a delayed accumulation of MDSC and reduced primary and metastatic tumor progression. Accumulation of MDSCs and tumor progression are partially restored by IL-6, indicating that IL-6 is a downstream mediator of the IL-1B-induced expansion of MDSC. In contrast, excessive inflammation in IL-1R antagonist-deficient mice promotes the accumulation of MDSC and produces MDSC with enhanced suppressive activity. These results show that immune suppression by MDSC and tumor growth are regulated by the inflammatory milieu and support the hypothesis that the induction of suppressor cells which down-regulate tumor immunity is one of the mechanisms linking inflammation and cancer (Bunt et al. 2007).

The potential role of TGFBR1/PTEN in development of head and neck cancer was studied in the 2cKO mouse model. It was found that deletions of TGFBR1/PTEN are associated with tumor cells with a proliferative and invasive phenotype. Interestingly, the nonmalignant epithelial cells of the head and neck area also revealed and enhanced proliferation pattern, loss of apoptosis, and increased expression of CCND1 (Bian et al. 2012). The effects of TGF-B was shown to have different effects on premalignant and malignant cells. On premalignant cells, TGF-B exerts tumor-suppression effects through its autocrine interaction with other signaling pathways. The effect of TGF-B on tumor cells is exert by its paracrine activity and is associated with an aggressive tumor phenotype and a pro-inflammatory state (De Wever and Mareel 2003). There is increasing evidence that the tumor micro-environment has an important role in cancer development and tumor progression. For instance, deletions of TGFBR/PTEN in the mouse head and epithelium are associated with activation of the NF-kB pathway, the generation of a pro-inflammatory stroma. As a result of all these events, there is a recruitment of MDSC's and increase angiogenesis, and an immuno-suppressive state of the tumor micro-environment that facilitates the proliferative and infiltrating pattern of head and neck tumor cells (Bian et al. 2012; Lu et al. 2006; Bierie et al. 2008)

5.5 Evidence from Patients for the Role of Inflammation in Head and Neck Cancer

It is well established that high levels of pro-inflammatory cytokines play a role in the development of HNSCC (Wang et al 2009). In clinical practice, it has been shown that low levels of cytokines and growth factors are associated with response to therapy and high levels are associated with poor outcomes in patients with HNSCC receiving chemotherapy and radiation. (Allen et al. 2007).

It has been shown that there is a significant reduction in HNC risk with aspirin use, with the strongest protective effect for laryngeal cancers. A subanalysis in individuals with information on alcohol use revealed an increasing reduction in HNC risk, albeit non-significant, with aspirin use among participants with increasing alcohol use. The exact mechanism by which this may be occurring is uncertain. Ethanol found in alcohol has been reported to act as a local irritant potentially leading to localized inflammation, which may possibly explain the observed reduction in HNC in aspirin users who consume alcohol.

In patients with HPV-related oropharyngeal cancer, there is some evidence to suggest an up-regulation of COX-2 in HPV-infected tissues, and this might explain the reduction in HNSCC in this patient population (Wilson et al. 2013). However, the chemopreventive effect of aspirin and NSAIDs cannot be explained by the inhibition of pro-staglandin synthesis alone, since several NSAIDs have anti-proliferative effects in cells without COX activity. High aspirin doses induce apoptosis through COX-independent mechanisms, by regulating several different targets—e.g., ALOX15, a pro-apoptotic gene PAWR, and an anti-apoptotic gene BCL2L1. Additionally, NSAIDs including aspirin also induce apoptosis by the activation of caspases, the activation of p38 MAP kinase, release of mitochondrial cytochrome c, and activation of the ceramide pathway. These effects might not be universal to all cell types and the range of doses of aspirin needed in such COX-independent pathways could be higher than for the inhibition of COX-2 (Elwood et al. 2009). Celecoxib, in conjunction with erlotinib and reirradiation, was shown to be a feasible and clinically active regimen in a population of patients with recurrent HNSCC who had a poor prognosis (Kao et al. 2011). However, the majority of data suggest a limited role for celecoxib in head and neck cancer therapy, either due to toxicity or lack of efficacy (Dannenberg and Subbaramaiah 2003; Jaeckel et al. 2001). Celecoxib was ineffective in controlling oral premalignant lesions in a recent randomized controlled trial (Papadimitrakopoulou et al. 2008). COX-2 inhibition has a chemopreventive effect, but its application as a treatment of HNSCC in a clinical setting still requires further research to overcome its limited anticancer effects (Kim et al. 2010).

Apricoxib is a selective COX-2 inhibitor with preclinical data showing analgesic, anti-inflammatory, and anti-tumor effects. Apricoxib plus erlotinib was tested in a phase I study in non-small-cell lung cancer and was found to be well tolerated with a 60 % disease control rate (Reckamp et al. 2011). In addition to reversing EMT via inhibition of COX-2, Apricoxib up-regulates 15-prostaglandin dehydrogenase and the PGT, thereby reducing the levels of active PGE2 by both suppressing its synthesis and increasing its catabolism (St John et al. 2012). Treatment of HNSCC cells with Apricoxib also causes greater up-regulation of E-cadherin expression and down-regulation of vimentin, as compared to celecoxib treatment. This has significant implications for targeted chemoprevention and anticancer therapy because E-cadherin expression has been implicated as a marker of sensitivity to EGFR TKI (St John et al. 2012). Studies have shown that EGFR and COX-2 have an important role in the biology of HNSCC. Overexpression of COX-2 is associated with a poor prognosis in HNSCC, and COX-2 inhibitors have demonstrated synergy when combined with EGFR inhibitors in preclinical models (Chen et al. 2004; Chung et al. 2011). Inflammatory mediators can promote EMT and increase resistance to EGFR-TKIs in HNSCC. These studies provide a strong rationale for combining a COX-2 inhibitor with an EGFR TKI.

In patients with HPVOPC, the PD-1: PD-L1 pathway plays a role in both persistence of HPV infection (through expression of PDL1in the tonsillar crypt epithelium—the site of initial infection) as well as resistance to immune elimination during malignant progression. Given the high levels of membranous PD-L1 expression within the tumors, recent studies support a rationale for administering PD-1/PD-L1-targeted therapy to the HPVOPC patient population (Topalian et al. 2012).

5.6 Conclusions and Future Directions

In conclusion, current evidence supports the concept that chronic inflammation promotes the development and progression of cancer. Because inflammation is a complex process involving many effector cells and mediators, it is likely that inflammation facilitates tumor progression through multiple mechanisms that are not yet fully understood. Tumor promotion and progression are dependent on physiologic responses provided by supportive tissues of the tumor environment but that are not necessarily cancerous themselves. Infiltration of immune cells facilitates tumor development through production of factors that promote carcinogenesis and by enabling tumors to evade the host immune response. Small molecules including cytokines, chemokines, and growth factors play key roles in both inflammation and cancer by promoting proliferation, angiogenesis, and carcinogenesis and by recruiting immune cells. Many of these physiologic processes and small molecules are potential targets with anti-neoplastic activity.

From in vitro and in vivo data, it seems that in the future, the use of different molecules that can affect one of the inflammatory pathways at different levels (i.e., co-administration of EGFR and STAT inhibitors) or different pathways at different levels (i.e., COX-2 inhibitors, NF-κB, and STAT inhibitors) will probably be needed to improve the anti-neoplastic activity of these molecules.

The role of the PD-1: PD-L1 interaction in creating an "immune-privileged" site for initial viral infection and subsequent adaptive immune resistance once tumors are established supports the rationale for therapeutic blockade of this pathway in patients with HPVOPC.

References

Alevizos I, Mahadevappa M, Zhang X, Ohyama H, Kohno Y, Posner M et al (2001) Oral cancer in vivo gene expression profiling assisted by laser capture microdissection and microarray analysis. Oncogene 20(43):6196–6204

Allen C, Duffy S, Teknos T, Islam M, Chen Z, Albert PS et al (2007) Nuclear factor-kappaB-related serum factors as longitudinal biomarkers of response and survival in advanced oropharyngeal carcinoma. Clin Cancer Res Off J Am Assoc Cancer Res 13(11):3182–3190

Ang KK, Harris J, Wheeler R, Weber R, Rosenthal DI, Nguyen-Tan PF et al (2010) Human papillomavirus and survival of patients with oropharyngeal cancer. New Engl J Med 363(1):24–35

Balkwill F, Mantovani A (2001) Inflammation and cancer: back to Virchow? Lancet 357(9255):539–545

Bekes EM, Schweighofer B, Kupriyanova TA, Zajac E, Ardi VC, Quigley JP et al (2011) Tumor-recruited neutrophils and neutrophil TIMP-free MMP-9 regulate coordinately the levels of tumor angiogenesis and efficiency of malignant cell intravasation. Am J Pathol 179(3):1455–1470

Bernhagen J, Krohn R, Lue H, Gregory JL, Zernecke A, Koenen RR et al (2007) MIF is a non-cognate ligand of CXC chemokine receptors in inflammatory and atherogenic cell recruitment. Nat Med 13(5):587–596

Bian Y, Hall B, Sun ZJ, Molinolo A, Chen W, Gutkind JS et al (2012) Loss of TGF-beta signaling and PTEN promotes head and neck squamous cell carcinoma through cellular senescence evasion and cancer-related inflammation. Oncogene 31(28):3322–3332

Bierie B, Stover DG, Abel TW, Chytil A, Gorska AE, Aakre M et al (2008) Transforming growth factor-beta regulates mammary carcinoma cell survival and interaction with the adjacent microenvironment. Cancer Res 68(6):1809–1819

Bigbee WL, Grandis JR, Siegfried JM (2007) Multiple cytokine and growth factor serum biomarkers predict therapeutic response and survival in advanced-stage head and neck cancer patients. Clin Cancer Res Off J Am Assoc Cancer Res 13(11):3107–3108

Bucala R, Donnelly SC (2007) Macrophage migration inhibitory factor: a probable link between inflammation and cancer. Immunity 26(3):281–285

Buchanan FG, Wang D, Bargiacchi F, DuBois RN (2003) Prostaglandin E2 regulates cell migration via the intracellular activation of the epidermal growth factor receptor. J Biol Chem 278(37):35451–35457

Bunt SK, Sinha P, Clements VK, Leips J, Ostrand-Rosenberg S (2006) Inflammation induces myeloid-derived suppressor cells that facilitate tumor progression. J Immunol (Baltimore, Md 1950) 176(1):284–290

Bunt SK, Yang L, Sinha P, Clements VK, Leips J, Ostrand-Rosenberg S (2007) Reduced inflammation in the tumor microenvironment delays the accumulation of myeloid-derived suppressor cells and limits tumor progression. Cancer Res 67(20):10019–10026

Chen Z, Malhotra PS, Thomas GR, Ondrey FG, Duffey DC, Smith CW et al (1999) Expression of proinflammatory and proangiogenic cytokines in patients with head and neck cancer. Clin Cancer Res Off J Am Assoc Cancer Res 5(6):1369–1379

Chen T, Yan W, Wells RG, Rimm DL, McNiff J, Leffell D et al (2001) Novel inactivating mutations of transforming growth factor-beta type I receptor gene in head-and-neck cancer metastases. Int J Cancer 93(5):653–661 (Journal international du cancer)

Chen Z, Zhang X, Li M, Wang Z, Wieand HS, Grandis JR et al (2004) Simultaneously targeting epidermal growth factor receptor tyrosine kinase and cyclooxygenase-2, an efficient approach to inhibition of squamous cell carcinoma of the head and neck. Clin Cancer Res Off J Am Assoc Cancer Res 10(17):5930–5939

Chung CH, Gillison ML (2009) Human papillomavirus in head and neck cancer: its role in pathogenesis and clinical implications. Clin Cancer Res Off J Am Assoc Cancer Res 15(22):6758–6762

Chung JH, Rho JK, Xu X, Lee JS, Yoon HI, Lee CT et al (2011) Clinical and molecular evidences of epithelial to mesenchymal transition in acquired resistance to EGFR-TKIs. Lung Cancer (Amst Neth) 73(2):176–182

Cooper JS, Pajak TF, Forastiere AA, Jacobs J, Campbell BH, Saxman SB et al (2004) Postoperative concurrent radiotherapy and chemotherapy for high-risk squamous-cell carcinoma of the head and neck. New Eng J Med 350(19):1937–1944

Coussens LM, Werb Z (2002) Inflammation and cancer. Nature 420(6917):860–867

Curado MP, Hashibe M (2009) Recent changes in the epidemiology of head and neck cancer. Curr Opin Oncol 21(3):194–200

Dannenberg AJ, Subbaramaiah K (2003) Targeting cyclooxygenase-2 in human neoplasia: rationale and promise. Cancer Cell 4(6):431–436

De Wever O, Mareel M (2003) Role of tissue stroma in cancer cell invasion. J Pathol 200(4):429–447

Derynck R, Zhang YE (2003) Smad-dependent and Smad-independent pathways in TGF-beta family signalling. Nature 425(6958):577–584

Dinarello CA (1996) Biologic basis for interleukin-1 in disease. Blood 87(6):2095–2147

Dohadwala M, Yang SC, Luo J, Sharma S, Batra RK, Huang M et al (2006) Cyclooxygenase-2-dependent regulation of E-cadherin: prostaglandin E(2) induces transcriptional repressors ZEB1 and snail in non-small cell lung cancer. Cancer Res 66(10):5338–5345

D'Souza G, Kreimer AR, Viscidi R, Pawlita M, Fakhry C, Koch WM et al (2007) Case-control study of human papillomavirus and oropharyngeal cancer. New Engl J Med 356(19):1944–1956

Dumitru CA, Gholaman H, Trellakis S, Bruderek K, Dominas N, Gu X et al (2011) Tumor-derived macrophage migration inhibitory factor modulates the biology of head and neck cancer cells via neutrophil activation. Int J Cancer 129(4):859–869 (Journal international du cancer)

Dumitru CA, Moses K, Trellakis S, Lang S, Brandau S (2012a) Neutrophils and granulocytic myeloid-derived suppressor cells: immunophenotyping, cell biology and clinical relevance in human oncology. Cancer Immunol Immunoth (CII) 61(8):1155–1167

Dumitru CA, Fechner MK, Hoffmann TK, Lang S, Brandau S (2012b) A novel p38-MAPK signaling axis modulates neutrophil biology in head and neck cancer. J Leukoc Biol 91(4):591–598

Dumitru CA, Bankfalvi A, Gu X, Zeidler R, Brandau S, Lang S (2013) AHNAK and inflammatory markers predict poor survival in laryngeal carcinoma. PLoS One 8(2):e56420

Elwood PC, Gallagher AM, Duthie GG, Mur LA, Morgan G (2009) Aspirin, salicylates, and cancer. Lancet 373(9671):1301–1309

Engle SJ, Hoying JB, Boivin GP, Ormsby I, Gartside PS, Doetschman T (1999) Transforming growth factor beta1 suppresses nonmetastatic colon cancer at an early stage of tumorigenesis. Cancer Res 59(14):3379–3386

Forastiere AA, Goepfert H, Maor M, Pajak TF, Weber R, Morrison W et al (2003) Concurrent chemotherapy and radiotherapy for organ preservation in advanced laryngeal cancer. New Engl J Med 349(22):2091–2098

Gasche JA, Hoffmann J, Boland CR, Goel A (2011) Interleukin-6 promotes tumorigenesis by altering DNA methylation in oral cancer cells. Int J Cancer 129(5):1053–1063

Gentil BJ, Delphin C, Mbele GO, Deloulme JC, Ferro M, Garin J et al (2001) The giant protein AHNAK is a specific target for the calcium- and zinc-binding S100B protein: potential implications for Ca2+ homeostasis regulation by S100B. J Biol Chem 276(26):23253–23261

Gillison ML, D'Souza G, Westra W, Sugar E, Xiao W, Begum S et al (2008) Distinct risk factor profiles for human papillomavirus type 16-positive and human papillomavirus type 16-negative head and neck cancers. J Natl Cancer Inst 100(6):407–420

Gregory AD, Houghton AM (2011) Tumor-associated neutrophils: new targets for cancer therapy. Cancer Res 71(7):2411–2416

Grieb G, Merk M, Bernhagen J, Bucala R (2010) Macrophage migration inhibitory factor (MIF): a promising biomarker. Drug News Perspect 23(4):257–264

Guenin S, Mouallif M, Hubert P, Jacobs N, Krusy N, Duray A et al (2013) Interleukin-32 expression is associated with a poorer prognosis in head and neck squamous cell carcinoma. Mol Carcinog

Gurova KV, Hill JE, Guo C, Prokvolit A, Burdelya LG, Samoylova E et al (2005) Small molecules that reactivate p53 in renal cell carcinoma reveal a NF-kappaB-dependent mechanism of p53 suppression in tumors. Proc Natl Acad Sci USA 102(48):17448–17453

Haase H, Podzuweit T, Lutsch G, Hohaus A, Kostka S, Lindschau C et al (1999) Signaling from beta-adrenoceptor to L-type calcium channel: identification of a novel cardiac protein kinase A target possessing similarities to AHNAK. FASEB 13(15):2161–2172

Haddad Y, Choi W, McConkey DJ (2009) Delta-crystallin enhancer binding factor 1 controls the epithelial to mesenchymal transition phenotype and resistance to the epidermal growth factor receptor inhibitor erlotinib in human head and neck squamous cell carcinoma lines. Clin Cancer Res 15(2):532–542

Haque MF, Meghji S, Khitab U, Harris M (2000) Oral submucous fibrosis patients have altered levels of cytokine production. J Oral Pathol Med 29(3):123–128

Hashimoto T, Gamou S, Shimizu N, Kitajima Y, Nishikawa T (1995) Regulation of translocation of the desmoyokin/AHNAK protein to the plasma membrane in keratinocytes by protein kinase C. Exp Cell Res 217(2):258–266

Heinhuis B, Koenders MI, van Riel PL, van de Loo FA, Dinarello CA, Netea MG et al (2011) Tumour necrosis factor alpha-driven IL-32 expression in rheumatoid arthritis synovial tissue amplifies an inflammatory cascade. Ann Rheum Dis 70(4):660–667

Henderson YC, Wang E, Clayman GL (1998) Genotypic analysis of tumor suppressor genes PTEN/MMAC1 and p53 in head and neck squamous cell carcinomas. Laryngoscope 108(10):1553–1556

Hirano T, Ishihara K, Hibi M (2000) Roles of STAT3 in mediating the cell growth, differentiation and survival signals relayed through the IL-6 family of cytokine receptors. Oncogene 19(21):2548–2556

Hohaus S, Massini G, Giachelia M, Vannata B, Bozzoli V, Cuccaro A et al (2010) Anemia in Hodgkin's lymphoma: the role of interleukin-6 and hepcidin. J Clin Oncol 28(15):2538–2543

Holla VR, Backlund MG, Yang P, Newman RA, DuBois RN (2008) Regulation of prostaglandin transporters in colorectal neoplasia. Cancer Prev Res (Philadelphia, Pa) 1(2):93–99

Ichikawa A, Sugimoto Y, Negishi M (1996) Molecular aspects of the structures and functions of the prostaglandin E receptors. J Lipid Mediat Cell Signal 14(1–3):83–87

Jablonska J, Leschner S, Westphal K, Lienenklaus S, Weiss S (2010) Neutrophils responsive to endogenous IFN-beta regulate tumor angiogenesis and growth in a mouse tumor model. J Clin Invest 120(4):1151–1164

Jaeckel EC, Raja S, Tan J, Das SK, Dey SK, Girod DA et al (2001) Correlation of expression of cyclooxygenase-2, vascular endothelial growth factor, and peroxisome proliferator-activated receptor delta with head and neck squamous cell carcinoma. Arch Otolaryngol Head Neck Surg 127(10):1253–1259

Jemal A, Siegel R, Xu J, Ward E (2010) Cancer statistics, 2010. CA Cancer J Clin 60(5):277–300

Jeng JH, Wang YJ, Chiang BL, Lee PH, Chan CP, Ho YS et al (2003) Roles of keratinocyte inflammation in oral cancer: regulating the prostaglandin E2, interleukin-6 and TNF-alpha production of oral epithelial cells by areca nut extract and arecoline. Carcinogenesis 24(8):1301–1315

John MAS, Dohadwala M, Luo J, Wang G, Lee G, Shih H et al (2009) Proinflammatory mediators upregulate snail in head and neck squamous cell carcinoma. Clin Cancer Res 15(19):6018–6027

Jones KG, Brull DJ, Brown LC, Sian M, Greenhalgh RM, Humphries SE et al (2001) Interleukin-6 (IL-6) and the prognosis of abdominal aortic aneurysms. Circulation 103(18):2260–2265

Kang YH, Park MY, Yoon DY, Han SR, Lee CI, Ji NY et al (2012) Dysregulation of overexpressed IL-32alpha in hepatocellular carcinoma suppresses cell growth and induces apoptosis through inactivation of NF-kappaB and Bcl-2. Cancer Lett 318(2):226–233

Kao J, Genden EM, Chen CT, Rivera M, Tong CC, Misiukiewicz K et al (2011) Phase 1 trial of concurrent erlotinib, celecoxib, and reirradiation for recurrent head and neck cancer. Cancer 117(14):3173–3181

Kim SH, Han SY, Azam T, Yoon DY, Dinarello CA (2005) Interleukin-32: a cytokine and inducer of TNFalpha. Immunity 22(1):131–142

Kim YY, Lee EJ, Kim YK, Kim SM, Park JY, Myoung H et al (2010) Anti-cancer effects of celecoxib in head and neck carcinoma. Mol Cells 29(2):185–194

Kim NH, Kim HS, Li XY, Lee I, Choi HS, Kang SE et al (2011) A p53/miRNA-34 axis regulates Snail1-dependent cancer cell epithelial-mesenchymal transition. J Cell Biol 195(3):417–433

Kross KW, Heimdal JH, Aarstad HJ (2010) Mononuclear phagocytes in head and neck squamous cell carcinoma. Eur Arch Otorhinolaryngol 267(3):335–344

Kuang DM, Zhao Q, Wu Y, Peng C, Wang J, Xu Z et al (2011) Peritumoral neutrophils link inflammatory response to disease progression by fostering angiogenesis in hepatocellular carcinoma. J Hepatol 54(5):948–955

Lee JI, Soria JC, Hassan KA, El-Naggar AK, Tang X, Liu DD et al (2001) Loss of PTEN expression as a prognostic marker for tongue cancer. Arch Otolaryngol Head Neck Surg 127(12):1441–1445

Lee TL, Yang XP, Yan B, Friedman J, Duggal P, Bagain L et al (2007) A novel nuclear factor-kappaB gene signature is differentially expressed in head and neck squamous cell carcinomas in association with TP53 status. Clin Cancer Res 13(19):5680–5691

Lee TL, Yeh J, Friedman J, Yan B, Yang X, Yeh NT et al (2008) A signal network involving coactivated NF-kappaB and STAT3 and altered p53 modulates BAX/BCL-XL expression and promotes cell survival of head and neck squamous cell carcinomas. Int J Cancer 122(9):1987–1998

Lee SH, Lee SJ, Jung YS, Xu Y, Kang HS, Ha NC et al (2009) Blocking of p53-Snail binding, promoted by oncogenic K-Ras, recovers p53 expression and function. Neoplasia (NY) 11(1):22–31 (6p following)

Lee J, Taneja V, Vassallo R (2012) Cigarette smoking and inflammation: cellular and molecular mechanisms. J Dent Res 91(2):142–149

Lin WW, Karin M (2007) A cytokine-mediated link between innate immunity, inflammation, and cancer. J Clin Invest 117(5):1175–1183

Lu SL, Herrington H, Reh D, Weber S, Bornstein S, Wang D et al (2006) Loss of transforming growth factor-beta type II receptor promotes metastatic head-and-neck squamous cell carcinoma. Genes Dev 20(10):1331–1342

Lyford-Pike S, Peng S, Young GD, Taube JM, Westra WH, Akpeng B et al (2013) Evidence for a role of the PD-1:PD-L1 pathway in immune resistance of HPV-associated head and neck squamous cell carcinoma. Cancer Res 73(6):1733–1741

Massague J (2008) TGFbeta in cancer. Cell 134(2):215–230

McCaul JA, Gordon KE, Clark LJ, Parkinson EK (2002) Telomerase inhibition and the future management of head-and-neck cancer. Lancet Oncol 3(5):280–288

Molinolo AA, Amornphimoltham P, Squarize CH, Castilho RM, Patel V, Gutkind JS (2009) Dysregulated molecular networks in head and neck carcinogenesis. Oral Oncol 45(4–5):324–334

Moustakas A, Heldin CH (2009) The regulation of TGFbeta signal transduction. Dev (Cambridge, Engl) 136(22):3699–3714

Nibali L, Fedele S, D'Aiuto F, Donos N (2012) Interleukin-6 in oral diseases: a review. Oral Dis 18(3):236–243

Nishimoto N (2010) Interleukin-6 as a therapeutic target in candidate inflammatory diseases. Clin Pharmacol Ther 87(4):483–487

Nozawa H, Chiu C, Hanahan D (2006) Infiltrating neutrophils mediate the initial angiogenic switch in a mouse model of multistage carcinogenesis. Proc Natl Acad Sci USA 103(33):12493–12498

Papadimitrakopoulou VA, William WN Jr, Dannenberg AJ, Lippman SM, Lee JJ, Ondrey FG et al (2008) Pilot randomized phase II study of celecoxib in oral premalignant lesions. Clin Cancer Res 14(7):2095–2101

Pasche B, Knobloch TJ, Bian Y, Liu J, Phukan S, Rosman D et al (2005) Somatic acquisition and signaling of TGFBR1*6A in cancer. JAMA 294(13):1634–1646

Pedrero JM, Carracedo DG, Pinto CM, Zapatero AH, Rodrigo JP, Nieto CS et al (2005) Frequent genetic and biochemical alterations of the PI 3-K/AKT/PTEN pathway in head and neck squamous cell carcinoma. Int J Cancer 114(2):242–248

Perez-Ordonez B, Beauchemin M, Jordan RC (2006) Molecular biology of squamous cell carcinoma of the head and neck. J Clin Pathol 59(5):445–453

Piek E, Roberts AB (2001) Suppressor and oncogenic roles of transforming growth factor-beta and its signaling pathways in tumorigenesis. Adv Cancer Res 83:1–54

Poeta ML, Manola J, Goldwasser MA, Forastiere A, Benoit N, Califano JA et al (2007) TP53 mutations and survival in squamous-cell carcinoma of the head and neck. New Engl J Med 357(25):2552–2561

Posner MR, Hershock DM, Blajman CR, Mickiewicz E, Winquist E, Gorbounova V et al (2007) Cisplatin and fluorouracil alone or with docetaxel in head and neck cancer. New Engl J Med 357(17):1705–1715

Reckamp K, Gitlitz B, Chen LC, Patel R, Milne G, Syto M et al (2011) Biomarker-based phase I dose-escalation, pharmacokinetic, and pharmacodynamic study of oral apricoxib in combination with erlotinib in advanced nonsmall cell lung cancer. Cancer 117(4):809–818

Reed AL, Califano J, Cairns P, Westra WH, Jones RM, Koch W et al (1996) High frequency of p16 (CDKN2/MTS-1/INK4A) inactivation in head and neck squamous cell carcinoma. Cancer Res 56(16):3630–3633

Ridker PM, Cushman M, Stampfer MJ, Tracy RP, Hennekens CH (1997) Inflammation, aspirin, and the risk of cardiovascular disease in apparently healthy men. New Engl J Med 336(14):973–979

Shankar J, Messenberg A, Chan J, Underhill TM, Foster LJ, Nabi IR (2010) Pseudopodial actin dynamics control epithelial-mesenchymal transition in metastatic cancer cells. Cancer Res 70(9):3780–3790
Shao X, Tandon R, Samara G, Kanki H, Yano H, Close LG et al (1998) Mutational analysis of the PTEN gene in head and neck squamous cell carcinoma. Int J Cancer 77(5):684–688
Shiboski CH, Schmidt BL, Jordan RC (2005) Tongue and tonsil carcinoma: increasing trends in the U.S. population ages 20–44 years. Cancer 103(9):1843–1849
Shioya M, Nishida A, Yagi Y, Ogawa A, Tsujikawa T, Kim-Mitsuyama S et al (2007) Epithelial overexpression of interleukin-32 alpha in inflammatory bowel disease. Clin Exp Immunol 149(3):480–486
Shtivelman E, Cohen FE, Bishop JM (1992) A human gene (AHNAK) encoding an unusually large protein with a 1.2-microns polyionic rod structure. Proc Natl Acad Sci USA 89(12):5472–5476
St John MA, Wang G, Luo J, Dohadwala M, Hu D, Lin Y et al (2012) Apricoxib upregulates 15-PGDH and PGT in tobacco-related epithelial malignancies. Br J Cancer 107(4):707–712
Sundelin K, Roberg K, Grenman R, Hakansson L (2005) Effects of cytokines on matrix metalloproteinase expression in oral squamous cell carcinoma in vitro. Acta Otolaryngol 125(7):765–773
Sussman J, Stokoe D, Ossina N, Shtivelman E (2001) Protein kinase B phosphorylates AHNAK and regulates its subcellular localization. J Cell Biol 154(5):1019–1030
Tanaka M, Jin G, Yamazaki Y, Takahara T, Takuwa M, Nakamura T (2008) Identification of candidate cooperative genes of the Apc mutation in transformation of the colon epithelial cell by retroviral insertional mutagenesis. Cancer Sci 99(5):979–985
Tang B, Vu M, Booker T, Santner SJ, Miller FR, Anver MR et al (2003) TGF-beta switches from tumor suppressor to prometastatic factor in a model of breast cancer progression. J Clin Invest 112(7):1116–1124
Tergaonkar V, Perkins ND (2007) p53 and NF-kappaB crosstalk: IKKalpha tips the balance. Mol Cell 26(2):158–159
Thiery JP, Acloque H, Huang RY, Nieto MA (2009) Epithelial-mesenchymal transitions in development and disease. Cell 139(5):871–890
Topalian SL, Hodi FS, Brahmer JR, Gettinger SN, Smith DC, McDermott DF et al (2012) Safety, activity, and immune correlates of anti-PD-1 antibody in cancer. New Engl J Med 366(26):2443–2454
Trellakis S, Bruderek K, Dumitru CA, Gholaman H, Gu X, Bankfalvi A et al (2011) Polymorphonuclear granulocytes in human head and neck cancer: enhanced inflammatory activity, modulation by cancer cells and expansion in advanced disease. Int J Cancer 129(9):2183–2193
Van Waes C (2007) Nuclear factor-kappaB in development, prevention, and therapy of cancer. Clin Cancer Res Off J Am Assoc Cancer Res 13(4):1076–1082
Vermorken JB, Remenar E, van Herpen C, Gorlia T, Mesia R, Degardin M et al (2007) Cisplatin, fluorouracil, and docetaxel in unresectable head and neck cancer. New Engl J Med 357(17):1695–1704
Wang F, Arun P, Friedman J, Chen Z, Van Waes C (2009) Current and potential inflammation targeted therapies in head and neck cancer. Curr Opin Pharmacol 9(4):389–395
Wilson JC, Anderson LA, Murray LJ, Hughes CM (2011) Non-steroidal anti-inflammatory drug and aspirin use and the risk of head and neck cancer: a systematic review. Cancer Causes Control (CCC) 22(5):803–810
Wilson JC, Murray LJ, Hughes CM, Black A, Anderson LA (2013) Non-steroidal anti-inflammatory drug and aspirin use and the risk of head and neck cancer. Br J Cancer 108(5):1178–1181
Worden B, Yang XP, Lee TL, Bagain L, Yeh NT, Cohen JG et al (2005) Hepatocyte growth factor/scatter factor differentially regulates expression of proangiogenic factors through Egr-1 in head and neck squamous cell carcinoma. Cancer Res 65(16):7071–7080

Xie W, Bharathy S, Kim D, Haffty BG, Rimm DL, Reiss M (2003) Frequent alterations of Smad signaling in human head and neck squamous cell carcinomas: a tissue microarray analysis. Oncol Res 14(2):61–73

Xing Z, Gauldie J, Cox G, Baumann H, Jordana M, Lei XF et al (1998) IL-6 is an antiinflammatory cytokine required for controlling local or systemic acute inflammatory responses. J Clin Invest 101(2):311–320

Zhang YE (2009) Non-Smad pathways in TGF-beta signaling. Cell Res 19(1):128–139

Zhang K, Zhaos J, Liu X, Yan B, Chen D, Gao Y et al (2011) Activation of NF-B upregulates Snail and consequent repression of E-cadherin in cholangiocarcinoma cell invasion. Hepatogastroenterology 58(105):1–7

Chapter 6
The Role of Inflammation in Pancreatic Cancer

Simone Hausmann, Bo Kong, Christoph Michalski, Mert Erkan and Helmut Friess

Abstract Pancreatic ductal adenocarcinoma (PDAC) is a devastating disease with an extremely poor prognosis. Inflammatory processes have emerged as key mediators of pancreatic cancer development and progression. In genetically engineered mouse models, induction of pancreatitis accelerates PDAC development, and patients with chronic pancreatitis are known to have a higher risk of developing pancreatic cancer. In recent years, much effort has been given to identify the underlying mechanisms that contribute to inflammation-induced tumorigenesis. Many inflammatory pathways have been identified and inhibitors have been developed in order to prevent cancer development and progression. In this chapter, we discuss the role of inflammatory pathways in the initiation and progression of pancreatic cancer as well as the role of inhibitors used in treatment and prevention of pancreatic cancer.

6.1 Introduction: Clinical Aspects and Current Therapy Options in Pancreatic Ductal Adenocarcinoma

A relationship between inflammation and cancer was hypothesized by Rudolph Virchow back in the 1850s (Balkwill and Mantovani 2001). Dvorak (1986) later described tumors as "wounds that do not heal", where microenvironment-derived growth-promoting factors sustain the survival and proliferation of initiated cells. It is known that chronic persistent inflammatory conditions are associated with cancer in many organs, such as ulcerative colitis and colon carcinoma, Barrett's

S. Hausmann · B. Kong · C. Michalski · M. Erkan · H. Friess (✉)
Department of Surgery, Klinikum rechts der Isar, Technische Universität München, Ismaningerstrasse 22, 81675 Munich, Germany
e-mail: helmut@friess.cc; helmut.friess@chir.med.tu-muenchen.de; helmut.friess@tum.de

B. B. Aggarwal et al. (eds.), *Inflammation and Cancer*, Advances in Experimental Medicine and Biology 816, DOI: 10.1007/978-3-0348-0837-8_6, © Springer Basel 2014

esophagus and esophageal cancer, hepatitis and liver cancer. The fibroinflammatory stroma of chronic pancreatitis resembles that of pancreatic cancer, and patients with familial chronic pancreatitis have a 26-fold increased risk of developing pancreatic cancer compared with the normal population—probably owing to chronic inflammation (Lowenfels et al. 1993). In this chapter, key pathways involved in this multifaceted interaction between inflammatory cells and pancreatic cancer are summarized.

6.1.1 Incidence and Survival

Pancreatic ductal adenocarcinoma is the fourth deadly cancer worldwide with an age-adjusted incidence rate of 12.1 per 100,000 men and woman per year (Siegel et al. 2013). It is estimated that in the United States, 45,220 patients will be diagnosed with pancreatic cancer in 2013 (Siegel et al. 2013). With a five-year survival rate of only 6 % and 38,460 estimated deaths in 2013, its incidence and mortality rates are almost identical (Siegel et al. 2013). Despite intensive research to prolong the survival of pancreatic cancer patients, little has been achieved, and like thirty years ago, surgery remains to be the only therapy option to cure some and provide the best palliation for many patients (Winter et al. 2012). However, only 15–20 % of the patients are initially candidates for surgical resection (Winter et al. 2012). Unfortunately, with the conventional non-surgical therapy options such as radiotherapy and chemotherapy, the survival of pancreatic cancer patients can only be prolonged for a couple of weeks to a few months (Moore et al. 2007; Michl and Gress 2013).

6.1.2 Current Therapy Options

The poor prognosis of pancreatic cancer patients is mostly due to late diagnosis and the absence of effective therapy options. Considering that three quarters of patients are not candidates for surgery at the time of first diagnosis, the most commonly employed therapy consists of radio- and chemotherapy. In the last decade, gemcitabine-based chemotherapy became the reference treatment since studies comparing gemcitabine with 5-fluorouracil showed similar survival advantages but better quality of life with the former (Neoptolemos et al. 2010). Different combinations of gemcitabine with other cytotoxic drugs could not improve the survival of patients significantly compared to gemcitabine treatment alone. Even the highly toxic regimen Folfirinox, consisting of irinotecan, oxaliplatin, 5-fluorouracil and folinic acid, resulted in a median survival of less than one year in patients with advanced pancreatic cancer (Conroy et al. 2011). Many targeted agents, including angiogenesis inhibitors, which have shown success in the preclinical setting, failed to prolong survival of pancreatic cancer patients in the clinical setting (Erkan et al. 2012). The only FDA approved targeted agent Erlotinib (a tyrosine kinase inhibitor that acts on human epidermal growth factor receptor type 1 [HER1/EGFR]) is no exception. This agent only increases median survival from 5.91 months (gemcitabine and placebo) to 6.24 months (gemcitabine and erlotinib) in patients with advanced pancreatic cancer (Moore et al. 2007).

Recently, the abundant fibrotic stroma of pancreatic cancer is shown to form a mechanical barrier for the effective delivery of chemotherapeutic agents. This observation has led to the emergence of anti-fibrotic therapies which appear to be effective in the preclinical setting. For example, the inhibition of the hedgehog signaling pathway in a genetically engineered mouse model of pancreatic cancer showed a better penetrance of the tumor with gemcitabine and a longer survival of the mice (Olive et al. 2009). However, the first phase II trial (IPI-926-03) has to be stopped after interim analysis due to increased mortality in the therapy arm (Erkan 2013a). These results hint that the problem in pancreatic cancer is multifaceted, and a successful therapy should aim at correcting several defects at genetic, epigenetic, and microenvironmental levels.

6.2 Inflammatory Signaling Pathways Associated with Pancreatic Cancer

6.2.1 The NFκB Signaling Pathway as Key Modulator of Inflammation-Induced Carcinogenesis

The transcription factor nuclear factor κB is a key regulator of inflammatory processes and therefore plays an important role in the development of pancreatitis and pancreatic carcinogenesis (DiDonato et al. 2012). NFκB belongs to a family of proteins sharing the Rel homology domain (RHD), which can bind to DNA either as hetero- or homodimers. There are 5 NFκB/Rel family members, p65 (RelA), c-Rel, Rel-B, and the precursor proteins NFκB1 (p105/p50) and NFκB2 (p100/p52), which form homo- or heterodimers (Karin et al. 2002). In the pancreas, the p65/p50 heterodimer is the predominant form of NFκB (Han et al. 2001). In the healthy pancreas, the NFκB signaling pathway is inactivated, and the abovementioned regulatory subunits are kept in the cytoplasm by interaction to the IκB family of inhibitory proteins, which include IκB-α, IκB-β, IκB-γ, IκB-ε, Bcl-3, p105/NFκB1, and p100/NFκB2 (Beg and Baldwin 1993; Thompson et al. 1995; Baldwin 1996; Verma et al. 1995). Due to microbial and viral infections as well as pro-inflammatory cytokines, the IκB kinase (IKK) complex gets activated and phosphorylates the IκB proteins at two conserved serine residues (Ling et al. 1998). The IKK complex consists of the two catalytic active protein kinases IKKα and IKKβ and the regulatory subunit IKKγ which is also called NEMO (Israel 2010). By phosphorylation of the inhibitory proteins, IκB gets targeted for ubiquitination and subsequent degradation by the 26S proteasomal system (Chen et al. 1995).

After the separation from the inhibitory protein IκB, the subunits can translocate to the nucleus, bind to κB-sequences within promoter regions and regulate the transcription of different genes involved in survival, inflammation as well as its own inhibitor IκB-α (Pahl 1999; Hayden and Ghosh 2011).

In many studies, it could be shown that the NFκB pathway is activated in early stages of pancreatitis and enhances the pro-inflammatory response through the activation of anti-apoptotic and inflammatory genes (Gukovsky et al. 1998; Steinle et al. 1999; Karin 1998). In a recent paper published by Huang and colleagues, it was demonstrated that the level of NFκB correlates with the severity of acute pancreatitis. Furthermore, the group displayed that long periods of activated NFκB in pancreatic acinar cells lead to a chronic pancreatitis characterized by severe pancreatic damage, immune cell infiltration, and fibrosis (Huang et al. 2013). Another group showed that the deletion of the IκB kinase IKK2 in all pancreatic epithelial cells prevented the formation of PanIN lesions in $Pdx^{Cre/+}$; $LSL\text{-}Kras^{G12D/+}$ mice (Maniati et al. 2011) thus indicating that the NFκB pathway plays an important role in the carcinogenesis of pancreatic cancer.

6.2.2 TheIL-6–STAT3 Axis and its Importance in Development of Pancreatic Cancer

The signal transducer and activator of transcription 3 (STAT3) is known to be an important regulator of stem cell renewal, cancer cell survival as well as inflammation. In the normal pancreas, STAT3 is inactive and located in the cytoplasm (Lee and Hennighausen 2005). In inflammatory conditions as well as in PDAC, however, STAT3 gets activated by phosphorylation on a tyrosine residue. Subsequent dimerization and translocation to the nucleus lead to the transcription of many target genes involved in inflammation and stem cell renewal (Shuai et al. 1993, 1994; Frank 2007; Bromberg and Darnell 2000). In inflammatory conditions, growth factors and cytokines such as IL-6 activate the Janus-activated kinase (JAK) family of tyrosine kinases that in return phosphorylate STAT proteins on their tyrosine residue (Zhong et al. 1994). Other tyrosine kinases such as src have also been reported to activate STAT proteins (Cao et al. 1996). The importance of STAT3 in the process of pancreatic cancer was recently shown by Miyatsuka et al. (2006) who proved that STAT3 is essential for the development of acinar-to-ductal metaplasia (ADM), an early event in the pathogenesis of pancreatic cancer. Furthermore, STAT3 was shown to be important for fostering progression of pancreatic cancer at different stages in mouse models and pancreatic cancer cell lines (Corcoran et al. 2011). The group of Hebrok additionally showed that the inflammatory mediator STAT3 contributes to PDAC initiation by promoting pancreatic cancer precursor lesions and support of cell proliferation and metaplasia-associated inflammation (Fukuda et al. 2011). In line, Lesina et al. (2011) showed that inhibition of IL-6 or STAT3 can reduce PanIN progression and diminishes the development of PDAC. These results from in vitro and in vivo studies emphasize the importance of the IL-6–STAT3 axis in the initiation as well as progression of pancreatic cancer.

6.2.3 The Role of Toll-like Receptors in Pancreatic Cancer

Toll-like receptors (TLRs) belong to the pattern recognition receptors and are mainly expressed on innate immune cells as well as on neoplastic tissues (Huang et al. 2008). Ligands for the Toll-like receptors include conserved patterns of bacterial and viral origin also referred to as pathogen-associated molecular patterns (PAMPs) as well as damage-associated molecular patterns (DAMPs). A recent paper published by Ochi et al. (2012) showed that the TLR7 is not only overexpressed in the epithelial compartment in pancreatic cancer but also in the tumor stroma in mice and humans. Using a mouse model of pancreatic cancer ($p48^{Cre/+}$; $Kras^{G12D/+}$), the group showed that TLR7 ligation accelerated the development of pancreatic cancer and inhibition of TLR7 was able to inhibit pancreatic tumorigenesis. The activation of TLR7 induced STAT3 activation and interacted with Notch, canonical NFκB, and MAP kinase pathways. Another group showed that the inflammatory substance lipopolysaccharide (LPS) which activates TLR4 increased the invasive behavior of pancreatic cancer cell lines Panc-1 and AsPC-1 through the activation of the NFκB signaling pathway. These results demonstrate the interplay between TLR4 and NFκB signaling may be one of the pathways linking inflammation and PDAC progression in vitro (Ikebe et al. 2009).

6.2.4 TGF-β Signaling Pathway

TGF-β is an anti-inflammatory cytokine which plays an important role in cell growth, apoptosis, and differentiation of cells and often correlates with advanced tumor stage (Patterson and Padgett 2000; Lu et al. 1997; Daroqui et al. 2012). Under normal conditions, TGF-β has suppressive effects on tumorigenesis through inhibition of cell growth and promotion of apoptosis. Upon ligand binding, the TGF-β type I and TGF-β type II receptors heterodimerize and the type II receptor phosphorylates the receptor I kinase domain. The signal cascade is further forwarded by phosphorylation of SMAD proteins which is performed only by the type I receptor (Massague et al. 2000). The activated SMAD proteins then translocate into the nucleus and activate the transcription of target genes that mediate the tumor-suppressive effects. In pancreatic cancer, the role of the TGF-β signaling pathway is well established (Friess et al. 1993a). Like in many cancers, the TGF-β signaling is impaired in pancreatic cancer leading to tumor-promoting effects such as increased cell growth, survival of cancer cells, invasion and metastasis as well as decreased survival of pancreatic cancer patients (Friess et al. 1993a, b). For many pancreatic cancer cell lines, it has been shown that SMAD4 is deleted or that the cancer cells have defects in TGF-β receptors (Villanueva et al. 1998). TGF-β has been shown to play an important role in the development and progression of chronic pancreatitis. In a study in which TGF-β signaling in the mouse pancreas was inhibited, the mice showed a stronger response to cerulein-mediated pancreatitis which was characterized by severe pancreatic edema, immune cell infiltration, hyperactivation of B and T cells and antibodies against pancreatic acinar cells (Hahm et al. 2000). Due to the important role of TGF-β in development and progression of pancreatitis, it has become an interesting drug target. In the recent years, several TGF-β receptor kinase inhibitors have been developed and have shown promising results in in vitro and in vivo experiments.

6.3 Role of Inflammatory Molecules in the Development of Pancreatic Cancer: Evidence from In Vitro Studies

6.3.1 Role of Inflammatory Molecules in the Transformation of Pancreatic Cancer Cells

Disturbances of pancreatic tissue homeostasis through various mechanisms lead commonly to a fibroinflammatory response in the pancreas. If there is an imbalance of the inflammatory reaction, chronic pancreatitis can ensue, which in the long term may enable transformation of premalignant cells to a malignant state. Apart from loss of tumor suppressor genes and deregulation of genes controlling the cell cycle, cytokines have been shown to contribute to the malignant transformation of cells. Moreover, during the typical fibroinflammation seen in chronic pancreatitis, microenvironmental factors, specifically hypoxia, acidosis, and reactive oxygen species, are also shown to induce genetic instability in the epithelial cells (Gillies et al. 2012).

6.3.1.1 The Role of the Cytokine TNF-α and the EGFR Signaling in the Transformation of Pancreatic Cancer Cells

In response to acinar damage, the expression of the cytokine tumor necrosis factor alpha (TNF-α) is induced. In human pancreatic cancer cell lines, it could be shown that the treatment of these cell lines with TNF-α was able to induce the expression of epidermal growth factor receptor (EGFR) and its ligand, transforming growth factor α (TGF-α) (Schmiegel et al. 1993). In vitro studies by Means et al.

the further demonstrated the importance of the EGFR signaling pathway in the transformation of acinar cells toward a malignant phenotype. Treatment of wild-type acinar cells with TGF-α resulted in transformation of acinar cells into a ductal phenotype which was accompanied by loss of acinar markers and expression of ductal markers like cytokeratin 19 (Means et al. 2005).

6.3.1.2 The Influence of the Cytokine IL-1α on Transformation of Pancreatic Cancer Cells

Another cytokine that plays an important role in the malignant transformation of pancreatic cells is the pro-inflammatory cytokine interleukin-1α (IL-1α). In a study by Sawai and colleagues, it could be shown that IL-1α enhanced proliferation, adhesion, and migration of the pancreatic cancer cell lines BxPC3, Capan-2, and SW1990. These changes were explained by the upregulation of the integrin subunit α_6 as well as by alterations of the urokinase plasminogen activator (uPA) and urokinase plasminogen activator receptor (uPAR) expression, which are both known to be upregulated in pancreatic cancer and play a role in disease progression (Cantero et al. 1997). Furthermore, IL-1α induced the activation of Ras and the downstream ERK signaling pathway (Sawai et al. 2006). By using an integrin α_6 antibody, the IL-1α-mediated effects could be abolished indicating that IL-1α mediates its effects through the integrin signaling pathway. Another study demonstrated that forced expression of IL-1α in the pancreatic cancer cell line MiaPaCa-2 activated NFκB expression, uPA as well as vascular endothelial growth factor (VEGF) and IL-8. Due to these changes in the expression profile, the non-metastatic cell line MiaPaCa-2 showed an invasive behavior in in vitro as well as in an orthotopic mouse model (Melisi et al. 2009).

6.3.2 Role of Inflammatory Molecules in Survival of Pancreatic Cancer Cells

6.3.2.1 NFκB and IL-6 Induce Anti-Apoptotic Genes

Resistance to apoptosis is one of the hallmarks of cancer and promotes tumor growth and metastasis (Hanahan and Weinberg 2000). In pancreatic cancer, the key regulator of inflammatory processes NFκB contributes to apoptosis resistance of pancreatic cancer cells (Liptay et al. 2003; Greten et al. 2002). Different studies showed that NFκB has anti-apoptotic effects on pancreatic cancer cells by activating different downstream target genes. In several pancreatic cancer cell lines, NFκB- and STAT3-dependent upregulation of the anti-apoptotic gene BcL-xL was demonstrated. However, this is not the only mechanism by which

NFκB exerts its anti-apoptotic effects. Several studies were able to show that NFκB is also involved in the regulation of cyclin D1 expression (Yamamoto and Gaynor 2001). In a recent study, it was shown that downregulation of the NFκB subunit p65 in pancreatic cancer cells leads to a subsequent downregulation of the pro-apoptotic gene BcL-2 as well as to the cell cycle gene cyclin D1 leading to growth inhibition of the pancreatic cancer cell line BxPC-3 (Kong et al. 2010). Another study showed that blocking the EGFR pathway in the pancreatic cancer cell line MDA Panc-28 resulted in a decreased NFκB binding activity as well as a reduced expression of the pro-apoptotic gens BcL-xL and Bfl-1 (Sclabas et al. 2003). The pro-inflammatory cytokine IL-6 was also shown to contribute to survival of pancreatic cancer cells by upregulating BcL-2 and BcL-xL. This effect could be reverted by the use of an IL-6 antibody (Miyamoto et al. 2001).

6.3.3 *Role of Inflammatory Molecules in the Proliferation of Pancreatic Cancer Cells*

6.3.3.1 The Cytokines IL-4, IL-6, and IL-8 have Proliferative Effects on Pancreatic Cancer Cells

Cytokines are found abundantly in the fibroinflammatory microenvironment of pancreatic cancer. The pro-inflammatory cytokine IL-6 was shown to affect pancreatic cancer cell proliferation in vitro by activating the STAT3 signaling pathway (Friess et al. 1999; Huang et al. 2010). In a recent study, it could be demonstrated that IL-6 induces the release of Th2-type cytokines as well as activates the ERK2 signaling pathway in pancreatic cancer cells. These results indicate that IL-6 signaling creates a tumor environment which promotes the development of pancreatic cancer by Th2-driven events as well as by upregulating cell proliferation-related genes (Feurino et al. 2007). Another cytokine that has a major role in promoting proliferation of pancreatic cancer cells is IL-8. The pancreatic cancer cell line Capan-1 has been identified to secret IL-8 as well as its receptor CXCR2. When IL-8 was inhibited using an IL-8 antibody, growth of Capan-1 cells was inhibited (Takamori et al. 2000). Another study showed that IL-8 inhibition in the cell line Hup-T4 via IL-8 antisense oligonucleotides also reduced the cell growth (Miyamoto et al. 1998). Additionally, IL-4 was identified to influence pancreatic cancer cell growth since pancreatic cancer cells as well as pancreatic cancer tissue show a high upregulation of the IL-4 receptor (Kawakami et al. 2001). In vitro studies displayed that the anti-inflammatory cytokine IL-4 significantly enhances the tumor growth of different pancreatic cell lines (AsPC-1, Colo-357, Capan-1, Panc-1). Moreover, the ablation of IL-4 in cell culture showed a reduced tumor growth, confirming the proliferative effect of IL-4 on pancreatic tumor cells (Prokopchuk et al. 2005).

6.3.4 *Role of Inflammatory Molecules in the Invasion, Metastasis, and Angiogenesis of Pancreatic Cancer Cells*

6.3.4.1 The Pro-inflammatory Cytokine Interleukin-1α Plays an Important Role in Invasion and Metastasis of Pancreatic Cancer Cells

Many inflammatory molecules have been indicated to play a role in invasion, metastasis, and angiogenesis of PDAC. One of these is the pro-inflammatory cytokine IL-1α which is produced by pancreatic cancer cells. In recent studies, it could be demonstrated that IL-1α promotes proliferation, adhesion, and migration of the pancreatic cancer cell lines BxPC-3, SW1990, and Capan-2 through the upregulation of the integrin subunits α_6 and β_1 and the uPAR. The above-mentioned effects are associated with the activation of RAS and the downstream ERK signaling pathway. By using inhibitory antibodies against α6, β1, and uPA, the group showed that the activation of the ERK signaling as well as proliferation, adhesion, and migration of pancreatic cancer cell lines was prevented (Sawai et al. 2006). In an additional study, it was elucidated that IL-1α produced by pancreatic cancer cells is able to induce the expression of hepatocyte growth factor (HGF) by fibroblasts (Xu et al. 2010). In co-culture experiments with pancreatic cancer cells and fibroblasts, the group showed not only the IL-1α-dependent expression of HGF by fibroblasts but also an increased invasive and proliferative behavior of pancreatic cancer cells as well as of human umbilical vein endothelial cells (HUVECs). This can be explained by binding of HGF to its receptor c-met/HGF on the surface of pancreatic cancer cells and thus fostering the observed behavior of pancreatic cancer cells (Xu et al. 2010). Another study demonstrated that forced expression of IL-1α in the pancreatic cancer cell line MiaPaCa-2 activated the NFκB signaling pathway as assessed by an increase in NFκB downstream targets. As a result of the forced expression of IL-1α and subsequent NFκB activation, the cells gained an invasive phenotype. However, when the NFκB pathway was inactivated by the expression of a dominant negative IκB protein, the metastatic behavior was prevented. The same behavior of the cells was observed when IL-1α was silenced in the metastatic pancreatic cancer cell line L3.6pl, indicating that IL-1α-induced NFκB expression is contributing to the metastatic phenotype of pancreatic cancer cells (Melisi et al. 2009).

6.3.4.2 The Pro-Inflammatory Cytokines TNF-α, IL-6, and IL-1β are Important for the Survival, Metastasis of Cancer Cells, and Escape from Immune Surveillance

In many cancer types, the pro-inflammatory cytokine IL-1β has been indicated to influence metastasis and tumor growth (Apte et al. 2006). IL-1β together with IL-1α belongs to the IL-1 family and has been shown to induce the expression of pro-inflammatory genes such as cyclooxygenase-2 (COX-2), inducible NO synthetase (iNOS), and IL-6. Pancreatic cancer cell lines treated with recombinant IL-1β revealed that the cancer cells stimulated with IL-1β showed a strong invasive behavior, whereas extracellular matrix adhesion was not influenced (Greco et al. 2005).

The NFκB pathway has been shown to have an important impact on survival of pancreatic cancer cells through the upregulation of anti-apoptotic genes such as BcL-XL. Several studies showed that inhibition of NFκB in human pancreatic cancer cells resulted in increased apoptosis of cancer cells. Different mechanisms contributing to the anti-apoptotic effects of NFκB in pancreatic cancer cells have been described. In a paper by Sclabas and colleagues, EGFR-dependent NFκB activation was analyzed (Sclabas et al. 2003). Therefore, the EGF receptor was blocked in the human pancreatic cancer cell line MDA Panc-28 using an anti-EGFR monoclonal antibody which resulted in decreased NFκB activity as well as a diminished expression of the apoptotic genes BcL-XL and BfL-1. Furthermore, the group was able to show a significant increase in apoptosis of MDA Panc-28 cells when they were treated with the EGFR monoclonal antibody and gemcitabine together (Sclabas et al. 2003). The results of this study indicate that signaling through the EGF receptor can induce NFκB signaling and subsequently influence apoptosis of pancreatic cancer cells in vitro. Another study showed that silencing of NFκB had an effect on gemcitabine-sensitive pancreatic cancer cell lines BxPC3, L3.6pl, and CFPAC-1 alone or in combination with gemcitabine. However, if NFκB was silenced in gemcitabine-resistant pancreatic cancer cell lines (MPanc-96, Panc-1, MiaPaCa-2), no effect on apoptosis could be detected (Pan et al. 2008). Therefore, inhibition of NFκB may only be a therapeutic advantage for a subset of pancreatic cancer patients.

6.3.4.3 TGF-β Mediates Invasiveness of Pancreatic Cancer Cells

In normal epithelial cells, TGF-β functions as inhibitor of cell growth (Logsdon et al. 1992). The same effects can be observed in early stages of cancer and in some pancreatic cancer cell lines such as Colo-357 (Kleeff and Korc 1998). However, at late stages of cancer, the cells are not responsive to the growth inhibitory effects due to mutations of downstream molecules such as SMADs or the expression of TGF-β signaling inhibitors (Kleeff et al. 1999a, b), and hence TGF-β functions as tumor-supporting factor. Treatment of the pancreatic cancer cell lines Panc-1 and IMIM-PC1 with recombinant TGF-β increased the invasiveness of these cells. The invasive behavior of Panc-1 and IMIM-PC1 could be completely abolished by using a neutralizing TGF-β antibody. Furthermore, the treatment of cells with TGF-β upregulated the matrix metalloproteinase 2 (MMP2) and the uPA system and thus mediated the invasive behavior of Panc-1 and IMIM-PC1 (Ellenrieder et al. 2001). Another study analyzed the pancreatic cancer cell lines Panc-1, BxPC3, and MiaPaCa in regard to stimulation of TGF-β and found out that the pancreatic cancer cell lines had a defective response to the TGF-β stimulation as determined by 3[H]thymidine incorporation and TGF-β-sensitive reporter assays.

Furthermore, no correlation of the unresponsiveness to TGF-β and TGF-β type I and II receptor or Smad2 and Smad3 was identified. However, when Smad4 was introduced into the cell line BxPC3 which has a homologous deletion of SMAD4, it restored the responsiveness to TGF-β, indicating that Smad4 plays a crucial role in the loss of TGF-β responsiveness at least in some pancreatic cancer cells (Simeone et al. 2000). The role of SMAD4 in mediating TGF-β effects was further confirmed by a study by Chow et al. The group showed that TGF-β facilitates motility and invasiveness of the pancreatic cancer cell lines BxPC3 and Capan-1 through inhibition of PTEN expression and activation of NFκB. However, when SMAD4 expression was restored in BxPC3 and Capan-1 cells, the invasive behavior was prevented due to the inhibited activation of NFκB pathway (Chow et al. 2010).

6.3.4.4 IL-6 and IL-8 Induce Angiogenesis by Activating Vascular Endothelial Growth Factor

In a variety of tumors, IL-8 is known to contribute to the regulation of tumor growth, invasion, and angiogenesis (Strieter et al. 1995). In head and neck cancer, IL-8 was identified as an autocrine growth factor and it could be shown that IL-8 expression leads to cancer cell survival and tumor growth. IL-8 expression was induced by IL-1α-dependent activation of the transcription factors NFκB and AP-1 which in turn promoted survival of head and neck squamous cell carcinoma cells in vitro (Wolf et al. 2001). Similarly, in pancreatitis and pancreatic cancer, an upregulation of IL-8 can be detected which correlates with an increase in angiogenesis and metastatic behavior of cells (Farrow et al. 2004). In fact, many pancreatic cancer cell lines produce a mixture of pro- and anti-angiogenic substances. Their dominant effect on angiogenesis remains mostly inhibitory (Erkan et al. 2009). IL-8 belongs to the pro-angiogenic factors produced by pancreatic cancer cell lines. In vitro, HUVEC co-cultured with some other pancreatic cancer cells show an increase in proliferation and angiogenesis (Matsuo et al. 2004). Moreover, the human pancreatic cancer cell line Panc-1 shows an increased metastatic behavior when stimulated with exogenous IL-8 (Kuwada et al. 2003). Recent studies revealed that the observed angiogenic effect mediated by IL-8 is in part due to induction of VEGF and neuropilin-2 produced by pancreatic cancer cells (Li et al. 2008).

Another important cytokine involved in mediating angiogenesis in pancreatic cancer cell lines is IL-6. A recent study showed that the IL-6 levels are increased in different pancreatic cancer cell lines such as BxPC-3, MiaPaCa-2, Panc-1, and PaCa-2 compared to human pancreatic ductal epithelium cells. Further investigations showed that similar to IL-8, IL-6 also induced expression of VEGF and neuropilin-1 supporting angiogenesis and metastasis of pancreatic cancer cells (Feurino et al. 2007). Both IL-8 and IL-6 activate the MAP kinase pathway. This could be demonstrated by an increase in ERK2 phosphorylation when Panc-1 cells were stimulated with IL-8 or IL-6. Through the activation of this signaling pathway, proliferation of pancreatic cancer cells is fostered and thus progression of pancreatic cancer in enhanced.

6.4 Role of Inflammatory Molecules in the Development of Pancreatic Cancer: Evidence from In Vivo Studies

6.4.1 STAT3 Contributes to Pancreatic Ductal Adenocarcinoma Initiation and Progression

Not only in vitro studies were able to show that the inflammatory mediator STAT3 is linked with pancreatic precursor lesion formation, but also in vivo studies demonstrated the role of STAT3 in the development of preneoplastic lesions (Corcoran et al. 2011; Fukuda et al. 2011; Lesina et al. 2011; Li et al. 2011). Corcoran et al. (2011) showed that STAT3 is necessary both for the development of precursor lesions [i.e., ADM, pancreatic intraepithelial neoplasia (PanIN)], and progression to PDAC. Fukuda et al. (2011) confirmed that STAT3, which is overexpressed in epithelial cells after cerulein-induced inflammation in a KrasG12D mouse model, helps to initiate tumor development and progression. Blocking of STAT3 has led to attenuation of precursor lesion formation and proliferation as well as increased apoptosis, proving the contribution of STAT3 to cancer initiation. Moreover, the group also identified that the loss of epithelial STAT3 leads to a reduced inflammatory cell infiltration as well as decreased expression of inflammatory cytokines. These results indicate that STAT3 not only has an influence on the proliferative, dedifferentiated state of the epithelial cells but also contributes to inflammatory processes associated with metaplasia (Fukuda et al. 2011). Lesina et al. (2011) observed the same events but additionally identified the myeloid compartment to secrete the pro-inflammatory cytokine IL-6 which leads to the activation of STAT3 in the pancreas and fosters the development and progression of PanIN lesions. The identification of this mechanism strengthens the role of the microenvironment in the development of PDAC and was also shown to be valid for human PDAC by analyzing human PDAC specimen and patient data. Therefore, the results of these studies indicate STAT3 as a potential therapeutic target for preventing inflammation-induced development of PDAC at an early stage.

6.5 Clinical Evidence on the Role of Fibroinflammation in Pancreatic Cancer

Inflammation has early been indicated to play a major role in pancreatic cancer development. Similarities between the fibroinflammatory stroma (Fig. 6.1) composition in chronic pancreatitis and pancreatic cancer emphasize the pathogenetic link between them (Chu et al. 2007). Inflammatory cells such as macrophages, mast cells, neutrophils, dendritic cells, B and T lymphocytes as well as activated PSC have all been described in the stroma of pancreatic cancer. However, only

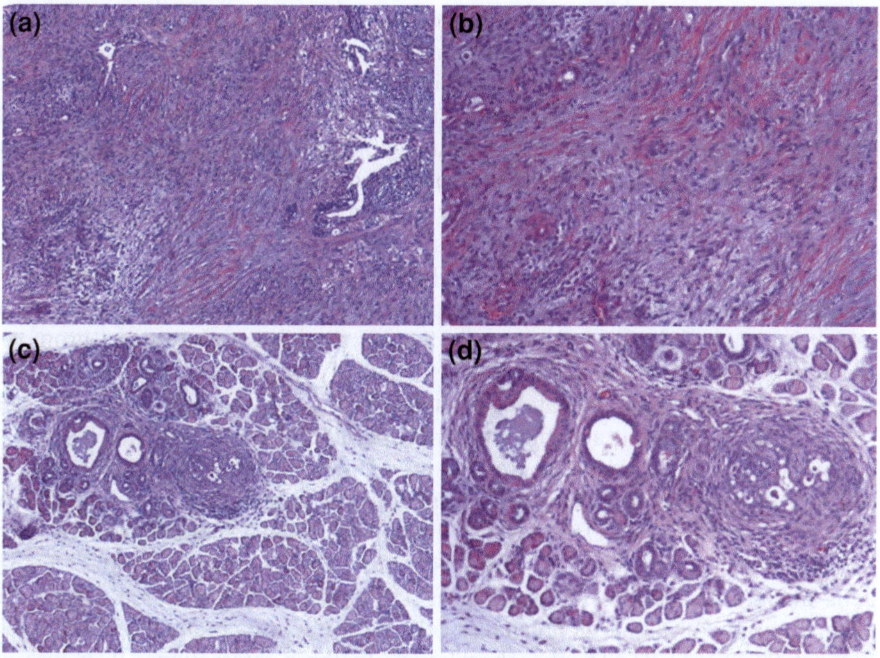

Fig. 6.1 Hematoxylin + Eosin staining of human and murine tissues depicting the fibroinflammatory stroma. **a** (50×) and **b** (100×) tissue from a pancreatic cancer patient showing the strong inflammatory stroma. **c** (50×) and **d** (100×) tissue of a mouse overexpressing the oncogene Kras under the control of the pancreas-specific promoter p48. Precancerous lesions develop which are surrounded by a strong stromal response with concomitant immune cell infiltration

a few experimental studies exploited the functional role of immune cells in the biology of PDAC. Most of these studies rely on correlation analysis which needs further confirmation using functional analysis as well as animal experiments. For example, studies on mast cells show that they foster neoangiogenesis (Esposito et al. 2002, 2004) and that there is a positive correlation between the number of mast cells in the pancreatic fibroinflammatory stroma and angiogenesis. To such extent that the number of mast cells correlates positively with the occurrence of metastasis and negatively with survival of patients with PDAC (Esposito et al. 2002, 2004). Epidemiologic studies show that inflammation significantly increases the risk of pancreatic cancer development. Importantly, these studies reveal that the elevated risk was independent of gender, ethnicity, and type of pancreatitis (Lowenfels et al. 1993; Malka et al. 2002). A recently conducted study identified inflammatory monocytes to play a role in survival of pancreatic cancer patients. The study revealed that monocytes in the peripheral blood are negatively correlated with the survival of pancreatic cancer patients, whereas a low amount of peripheral monocytes showed an increased survival of pancreatic cancer patients with a resected tumor (Sanford et al. 2013). It is also shown that

M2 macrophages which are characterized by a high expression of the cytokines IL-4 and IL-10 are associated with large tumor size and shortened survival time in pancreatic cancer patients indicating the important role of inflammatory cells in the survival of pancreatic cancer patients (Yoshikawa et al. 2012). Furthermore, elevated serum levels of the cytokine IL-6 have been found in pancreatic cancer patients compared to healthy individuals and chronic pancreatitis patients. These increased serum levels correlated with tumor size as well as liver metastases in pancreatic cancer patients (Talar-Wojnarowska et al. 2009; Okada et al. 1998). Lesina et al. (2011) highlighted the importance of IL-6 in pancreatic cancer development and progression by identifying myeloid cells to produce IL-6 which is responsible for activating the STAT3 signaling pathway that promotes the progression of precancerous lesions. Recently, it was also shown that IL-6 produced by pancreatic stellate cells enhances myeloid-derived suppressor cell (MDSC) differentiation and function from peripheral blood mononuclear cells, which promotes an immunosuppressive microenvironment in PDAC (Mace et al. 2013). PSC supernatants promoted peripheral blood mononuclear cells differentiation into an MDSC (CD11b+CD33+) phenotype and a subpopulation of polymorphonuclear CD11b+CD33+CD15+ cells. The resulting CD11b+CD33+ cells functionally suppressed autologous T lymphocyte proliferation. Culture of normal peripheral blood mononuclear cells with PSC supernatants led to STAT3 but not STAT1 or STAT5 phosphorylation. In these interactions, IL-6 was an important mediator as its neutralization inhibited PSC supernatant-mediated STAT3 phosphorylation and MDSC differentiation. Moreover, chemical inhibition of STAT3 abrogated PSC supernatant-mediated MDSC differentiation, PSC viability, and reduced autocrine IL-6 production, indicating these processes are STAT3 dependent. These results identify a novel role for PSC in driving immune escape in pancreatic cancer and extend the evidence that STAT3 acts as a driver of stromal immunosuppression to enhance its interest as a therapeutic target (Mace et al. 2013).

In the last decade, the fibroinflammatory stroma/desmoplasia, produced by the activated pancreatic stellate cells, has attracted attention as it forms a physical barrier for the effective delivery of therapeutic agents. There is also considerable amount of evidence stemming from in vitro and animal experiments that PSC and various ECM components support tumor growth by various mechanisms such as promoting tumor growth, creating apoptosis resistance, creating a niche for cancer stem cells, enabling immune escape of cancer cells, modulation of angiogenesis, facilitation of metastatic spread, and increasing therapy resistance (Erkan 2013b). Moreover, depletion of the desmoplastic stroma of the PDAC has led to better chemotherapy delivery and drug response in Kras-based genetic mouse models confirming the previous observations (Olive et al. 2009; Jacobetz et al. 2013; Provenzano et al. 2012). Although anti-fibrotic therapy appears as a new hope in the treatment of PDAC, it is not for certain that this fibrotic reaction is exclusively pro-tumorigenic as there is also evidence that various stromal components can as well be protective (see below).

6.6 Inhibitors of Inflammation for the Prevention and Treatment of Pancreatic Cancer

Currently, there is not enough clinical evidence to support the routine usage of anti-inflammatory drugs to improve outcome in pancreatic cancer patients. Some under-powered studies show partial benefit when anti-inflammatory therapy (i.e., COX-2 inhibition) is added to conventional chemotherapy (Lipton et al. 2010). Similarly, there is some circumstantial evidence that anti-inflammatory drugs reduce the risk of malignant pancreatic lesions. Below, some experimental data are reported.

6.6.1 *TGF-β Receptor Kinase Inhibitors*

As mentioned above, in normal cells, TGF-β exerts tumor-suppressive functions by inhibiting proliferation and inducing apoptosis. However, in many cancers including pancreatic cancer, TGF-β levels increase significantly and can support tumor growth, angiogenesis, invasion, and metastasis. Therefore, small molecular inhibitors have been developed to block TGF-β function and to inhibit these tumor-promoting effects. In a preclinical study, the TGF-β receptor kinase inhibitor SD-208 was investigated using the human pancreatic cell line Panc-1. The study demonstrated that the TGF-β receptor kinase inhibitor was able to inhibit invasion of Panc-1 cells in vitro. Moreover, the study revealed that the use of SD-208 in a xenograft mouse model reduced the size of the primary tumor and diminished the incidence of metastasis (Gaspar et al. 2007). Another study tested an inhibitor against the TGF-β receptors I and III (LY2109761). In cell culture experiments, the inhibitor was able to prevent migration, invasion, and induced anoikis in soft agar experiments. In further in vivo studies, LY2109761 in combination with gemcitabine was able to decrease the tumor burden in an orthotopic mouse model, prolonged the survival, and reduced liver metastases in these mice (Melisi et al. 2008). These promising results from in vitro and in vivo studies implicate that TGF-β receptor kinase inhibitors may serve as therapeutic agents in prevention of metastasis of pancreatic cancer.

6.6.2 *Cyclooxygenase-2 Inhibitors*

Cyclooxygenase (COX) and 5-lipoxygenase are the main regulators of the arachidonic acid metabolism and have been shown to be dysregulated in pancreatic cancer (Hennig et al. 2002, 2005; Ding et al. 2001). COX-2, which is a prostaglandin synthetase, catalyzes the conversion of arachidonic acid into prostaglandin G2. In the pancreas, COX-2 expression is induced by inflammatory cytokines, growth factors, and mitogenic stimuli and was shown to be overexpressed in pancreatic cancer

(Yip-Schneider et al. 2000). By supporting proliferation, invasion, and angiogenesis of pancreatic cancer cells, COX-2 contributes to the aggressive phenotype of PDAC (Chu et al. 2003; Ito et al. 2004; Eibl et al. 2003). Hermanova et al. (2008) found a different expression pattern in normal, premalignant, malignant pancreatic tissue indicating the important role of COX-2 in the progression of precancerous lesions. Treatment of pancreatic cancer cell lines displaying a high COX-2 expression such as BxPC-3 with gemcitabine and celecoxib (COX-2 inhibitor) showed a significantly inhibition of growth and enhanced apoptosis compared to gemcitabine treatment alone. However, in pancreatic cancer cell lines with low COX-2 expression, no such effect could be observed (El-Rayes et al. 2004). In vivo studies using COX-2 inhibitors in $Pdx^{Cre/+}$; $LSL\text{-}Kras^{G12D/+}$ mice which recapitulate all steps of pancreatic cancer development also demonstrated a decreased pancreatic tumor growth as well as a delay in the progression from precancerous lesions into pancreatic cancer (Funahashi et al. 2007; Eibl et al. 2005). In a study by Guerra and colleagues, mice were treated with the COX-1/2 inhibitor sulindac for a period of 3 months after induction of pancreatitis by the cholecystokinin analog cerulein for 3 months. Histology showed that the pancreata of these mice were almost normal with the exception of few areas displaying atrophy and immune cells (Guerra et al. 2011). Interestingly, sulindac hardly reduced low-grade lesions, but a significant reduction of high-grade lesions and PDAC could be observed. These results stress the importance of inflammation in the progression of early lesions to PDAC development.

Following these promising results in cell culture and mouse models, selective COX-2 inhibitors were developed for phase II studies. In a trial with patients suffering of advanced or metastatic pancreatic adenocarcinoma, treatment with gemcitabine and an additional daily oral dose of celecoxib twice a day was performed. However, the results of this study were disappointing since the additional administration of celecoxib did not improve the clinical outcome (Dragovich et al. 2008). Another phase II trial involving patients with unresectable pancreatic cancer radiotherapy combined with uracil/tegafur plus leucovorin and celecoxib did not show a response and moreover the patients showed gastrointestinal toxicity. Therefore, treatment of patients with a locally advanced pancreatic tumor cannot be advised as standard therapy (Morak et al. 2011). Despite the promising effects of COX-2 inhibitors in vitro and in mouse models, so far there is no promising treatment for pancreatic cancer patients with COX-2 inhibitors.

6.6.3 Inhibition of NFκB

The NFκB signaling pathway has been shown to play multitudes of roles in the development of pancreatic cancer as well as in metastatic spread due to its role in controlling proliferation, apoptosis, and angiogenesis. Therefore, inhibition of NFκB expression is a promising therapeutic target to reduce tumor growth and metastasis formation in pancreatic cancer patients. In vitro studies showed that inhibition of NFκB signaling in combination with gemcitabine resulted in decreased angiogenesis, proliferation, and induction of apoptosis of BxCP-3 and Panc-1 cells (Kong et al. 2010). The same anti-tumor effects could be observed when NFκB activity was inhibited in a human pancreatic cancer cell line and subsequently implanted into the pancreas of nude mice (Xiong et al. 2004). Due to these promising in vitro and in vivo results, pharmacological NFκB inhibitors have been developed and investigated in clinical studies. One of them is the proteasome inhibitor bortezomib which was analyzed in a clinical trial with metastatic pancreatic cancer patients. In this trial, 44 enrolled patients received bortezomib alone, and 43 patients were treated with bortezomib and gemcitabine. However, the results of this study revealed that the treatment with bortezomib and the treatment with the combination of bortezomib and gemcitabine did not have a better outcome for metastatic pancreatic cancer patients compared to gemcitabine treatment alone (Alberts et al. 2005). Despite of the promising results of bortezomib in in vitro experiments, this NFκB inhibitor does not have an effect on metastatic pancreatic cancer patients. Therefore, further substances need to be developed to target pancreatic cancer development and chemoresistance.

6.6.4 Anti-Fibrotic Therapies

Recently, the abundant fibrotic stroma, produced by the activated pancreatic stellate cells, has attracted attention as it might form a physical barrier for the effective delivery of therapeutic agents. There is a considerable amount of evidence stemming from in vitro and animal experiment that PSC and various ECM components support tumor growth by various mechanisms such as promoting tumor growth, creating apoptosis resistance, creating a niche for cancer stem cells, enabling immune escape of cancer cells, modulation of angiogenesis, facilitation of metastatic spread, and increasing therapy resistance (Erkan 2013b). In line with these observations, depletion of the desmoplastic stroma of the PDAC has led to better chemotherapy delivery and drug response in Kras-based genetic mouse models (Conroy et al. 2011; Erkan et al. 2012; Olive et al. 2009). Taken together, anti-fibrotic therapy appears as a new hope in the treatment of PDAC. However, as of today, data from clinical studies are largely missing. However, as a proof of principle, Von Hoff et al. (2011) used in a phase I/II trial nanoparticle albumin-bound (nab) paclitaxel (to deplete the stroma in PDAC) alone and in combination with gemcitabine and showed that through depletion of the stroma, higher concentrations of gemcitabine can be delivered in the tumor.

Despite the initial hope mostly stemming from the success achieved in genetic mouse models of PDAC, the clinical reality seems to be more complex. As mentioned above, the first trial using an inhibitor of sonic hedgehog signaling to deplete the stroma of PDAC (IPI-926-03 trial, http://www.clinicaltrials.gov/) has been stopped due to increased mortality in the treatment arm. Currently, several other trials are recruiting patients where various forms of anti-fibrotic therapies are applied concomitantly with conventional therapies. The results of these trials will help understanding whether nonselective anti-fibrotic therapy would improve the results of conventional therapies (Erkan 2013b). Nonetheless, judging by the results of the above-mentioned trial and previous failures, it is likely that nonselective anti-fibrotic therapy may also not be the solution to overcome therapy resistance in PDAC (Erkan 2013b).

Considering the normal function of stromal cells (forming a barrier between a noxious stimuli and the body), we have previously argued that PSC are initially activated around genetically defective cells (i.e., Kras mutated) in a preventive manner. This type of activation is also observed in chronic pancreatitis tissues. However, due to the fibrosis created by PSC, the microenvironment becomes gradually more fibrotic and hypoxic (Erkan 2013b). The ensuing stromal barriers specifically hypoxia, acidosis, and reactive oxygen species are not only highly selective but also able to induce genetic instability in the epithelial cells (Gillies et al. 2012). As a result, malignant cancers evolve through negative selection of the fitter clones under the selection pressure applied by their defensive microenvironment (Gillies et al. 2012). These evolved clones are also resistant to conventional therapies that induce apoptosis (Gillies et al. 2012). As mentioned above, the fibrotic stroma also forms a mechanical barrier preventing effective delivery of chemotherapeutics in advanced cancer. However, at this late stage, where selection of aggressive clones has already taken place, applying anti-fibrotic therapy can be a double-edged sword (Erkan 2013c). Since conventional chemotherapeutics are not powerful enough to eradicate all cancer cells (i.e., tumor-promoting cells) in the tumor, breaking down the stromal wall may also lead to the increased dissemination of cancer cells (Erkan 2013c).

6.7 Conclusions and Further Directions

Pancreatic cancer is the fourth deadly cancer worldwide and has a 5-year survival rate of only 6 %. The cellular mechanisms contributing to pancreatic cancer development and progression are still not completely identified. Inflammation has emerged to be a key mediator of pancreatic cancer development. In a paper by Guerra and colleagues, it could be shown that in adult mice the expression of the mutant Kras is not sufficient to induce pancreatic cancer. However, when additionally inflammation was induced, the mice developed pancreatic cancer stressing the importance of inflammation in the development of pancreatic cancer (Guerra et al. 2007). Furthermore, many studies showed the impact of inflammatory molecules on the development and progression of pancreatic cancer. So far, different approaches have been made to inhibit the main inflammatory signaling pathways in pancreatic cancer. Although, having shown promising results in vitro and in vivo experiments, inhibitors of inflammation have not been successful in cancer prevention or cancer progression in clinical trials. Therefore, further research is needed to elucidate the mechanisms through which inflammation contributes to tumor initiation and progression. It is very likely that that there are several altered mechanisms on various levels contributing to the aggressiveness of PDAC. Therefore, effective therapy of PDAC should aim at overcoming various obstacles at several levels.

References

Alberts SR et al (2005) PS-341 and gemcitabine in patients with metastatic pancreatic adenocarcinoma: a North Central Cancer Treatment Group (NCCTG) randomized phase II study. Ann Oncol 16(10):1654–1661

Apte RN et al (2006) The involvement of IL-1 in tumorigenesis, tumor invasiveness, metastasis and tumor-host interactions. Cancer Metastasis Rev 25(3):387–408

Baldwin AS Jr (1996) The NF-kappaB and I kappaB proteins: new discoveries and insights. Annu Rev Immunol 14:649–683

Balkwill F, Mantovani A (2001) Inflammation and cancer: back to Virchow? Lancet 357(9255):539–545

Beg AA, Baldwin AS Jr (1993) The I kappaB proteins: multifunctional regulators of Rel/NF-kappaB transcription factors. Genes Dev 7(11):2064–2070

Bromberg J, Darnell JE Jr (2000) The role of STATs in transcriptional control and their impact on cellular function. Oncogene 19(21):2468–2473

Cantero D et al (1997) Enhanced expression of urokinase plasminogen activator and its receptor in pancreatic carcinoma. Br J Cancer 75(3):388–395

Cao X et al (1996) Activation and association of Stat3 with Src in v-Src-transformed cell lines. Mol Cell Biol 16(4):1595–1603

Chen Z et al (1995) Signal-induced site-specific phosphorylation targets I kappaB alpha to the ubiquitin-proteasome pathway. Genes Dev 9(13):1586–1597

Chow JY et al (2010) TGF-beta downregulates PTEN via activation of NF-kappaB in pancreatic cancer cells. Am J Physiol Gastrointest Liver Physiol 298(2):G275–G282

Chu J et al (2003) Potential involvement of the cyclooxygenase-2 pathway in the regulation of tumor-associated angiogenesis and growth in pancreatic cancer. Mol Cancer Ther 2(1):1–7

Chu GC et al (2007) Stromal biology of pancreatic cancer. J Cell Biochem 101(4):887–907

Conroy T et al (2011) FOLFIRINOX versus gemcitabine for metastatic pancreatic cancer. New Engl J Med 364(19):1817–1825

Corcoran RB et al (2011) STAT3 plays a critical role in KRAS-induced pancreatic tumorigenesis. Cancer Res 71(14):5020–5029

Daroqui MC et al (2012) TGF-beta autocrine pathway and MAPK signaling promote cell invasiveness and in vivo mammary adenocarcinoma tumor progression. Oncol Rep 28(2):567–575

DiDonato JA, Mercurio F, Karin M (2012) NF-kappaB and the link between inflammation and cancer. Immunol Rev 246(1):379–400

Ding XZ, Tong WG, Adrian TE (2001) Cyclooxygenases and lipoxygenases as potential targets for treatment of pancreatic cancer. Pancreatology 1(4):291–299

Dragovich T et al (2008) Gemcitabine plus celecoxib in patients with advanced or metastatic pancreatic adenocarcinoma: results of a phase II trial. Am J Clin Oncol 31(2):157–162

Dvorak HF (1986) Tumors: wounds that do not heal. Similarities between tumor stroma generation and wound healing. New Engl J Med 315(26):1650–1659

Eibl G et al (2003) PGE(2) is generated by specific COX-2 activity and increases VEGF production in COX-2-expressing human pancreatic cancer cells. Biochem Biophys Res Commun 306(4):887–897

Eibl G et al (2005) Growth stimulation of COX-2-negative pancreatic cancer by a selective COX-2 inhibitor. Cancer Res 65(3):982–990

Ellenrieder V et al (2001) TGF-beta-induced invasiveness of pancreatic cancer cells is mediated by matrix metalloproteinase-2 and the urokinase plasminogen activator system. Int J Cancer 93(2):204–211

El-Rayes BF et al (2004) Cyclooxygenase-2-dependent and -independent effects of celecoxib in pancreatic cancer cell lines. Mol Cancer Ther 3(11):1421–1426

Erkan M (2013a) The role of pancreatic stellate cells in pancreatic cancer. Pancreatology 13(2):106–109

Erkan M (2013b) Understanding the stroma of pancreatic cancer: coevolution of the microenvironment with the epithelial carcinogenesis. J Pathol 231(1):4–7

Erkan M (2013c) The role of pancreatic stellate cells in pancreatic cancer. Pancreatol official J. Int. Assoc Pancreatol 13(2):106–109

Erkan M et al (2009) Cancer-stellate cell interactions perpetuate the hypoxia-fibrosis cycle in pancreatic ductal adenocarcinoma. Neoplasia 11(5):497–508

Erkan M et al (2012) The role of stroma in pancreatic cancer: diagnostic and therapeutic implications. Nat Rev Gastroenterol Hepatol 9(8):454–467

Esposito I et al (2002) The stem cell factor-c-kit system and mast cells in human pancreatic cancer. Lab Invest 82(11):1481–1492

Esposito I et al (2004) Inflammatory cells contribute to the generation of an angiogenic phenotype in pancreatic ductal adenocarcinoma. J Clin Pathol 57(6):630–636

Farrow B et al (2004) Inflammatory mechanisms contributing to pancreatic cancer development. Ann Surg 239(6):763–769 (discussion 769-71)

Feurino LW et al (2007) IL-6 stimulates Th2 type cytokine secretion and upregulates VEGF and NRP-1 expression in pancreatic cancer cells. Cancer Biol Ther 6(7):1096–1100

Frank DA (2007) STAT3 as a central mediator of neoplastic cellular transformation. Cancer Lett 251(2):199–210

Friess H et al (1993a) Enhanced expression of the type II transforming growth factor beta receptor in human pancreatic cancer cells without alteration of type III receptor expression. Cancer Res 53(12):2704–2707

Friess H et al (1993b) Enhanced expression of transforming growth factor beta isoforms in pancreatic cancer correlates with decreased survival. Gastroenterology 105(6):1846–1856

Friess H et al (1999) Growth factors and cytokines in pancreatic carcinogenesis. Ann NY Acad Sci 880:110–121

Fukuda A et al (2011) Stat3 and MMP7 contribute to pancreatic ductal adenocarcinoma initiation and progression. Cancer Cell 19(4):441–455

Funahashi H et al (2007) Delayed progression of pancreatic intraepithelial neoplasia in a conditional Kras(G12D) mouse model by a selective cyclooxygenase-2 inhibitor. Cancer Res 67(15):7068–7071

Gaspar NJ et al (2007) Inhibition of transforming growth factor beta signaling reduces pancreatic adenocarcinoma growth and invasiveness. Mol Pharmacol 72(1):152–161

Gillies RJ, Verduzco D, Gatenby RA (2012) Evolutionary dynamics of carcinogenesis and why targeted therapy does not work. Nat Rev Cancer 12(7):487–493

Greco E et al (2005) Pancreatic cancer cells invasiveness is mainly affected by interleukin-1beta not by transforming growth factor-beta1. Int J Biol Markers 20(4):235–241

Greten FR et al (2002) Stat3 and NF-kappaB activation prevents apoptosis in pancreatic carcinogenesis. Gastroenterology 123(6):2052–2063

Guerra C et al (2007) Chronic pancreatitis is essential for induction of pancreatic ductal adenocarcinoma by K-Ras oncogenes in adult mice. Cancer Cell 11(3):291–302

Guerra C et al (2011) Pancreatitis-induced inflammation contributes to pancreatic cancer by inhibiting oncogene-induced senescence. Cancer Cell 19(6):728–739

Gukovsky I et al (1998) Early NF-kappaB activation is associated with hormone-induced pancreatitis. Am J Physiol 275(6 Pt 1):G1402–G1414

Hahm KB et al (2000) Loss of TGF-beta signaling contributes to autoimmune pancreatitis. J Clin Invest 105(8):1057–1065

Han B, Ji B, Logsdon CD (2001) CCK independently activates intracellular trypsinogen and NF-kappaB in rat pancreatic acinar cells. Am J Physiol Cell Physiol 280(3):C465–C472

Hanahan D, Weinberg RA (2000) The hallmarks of cancer. Cell 100(1):57–70

Hayden MS, Ghosh S (2011) NF-kappaB in immunobiology. Cell Res 21(2):223–244

Hennig R et al (2002) 5-Lipoxygenase and leukotriene B(4) receptor are expressed in human pancreatic cancers but not in pancreatic ducts in normal tissue. Am J Pathol 161(2):421–428

Hennig R et al (2005) 5-Lipoxygenase, a marker for early pancreatic intraepithelial neoplastic lesions. Cancer Res 65(14):6011–6016

Hermanova M et al (2008) Expression of COX-2 is associated with accumulation of p53 in pancreatic cancer: analysis of COX-2 and p53 expression in premalignant and malignant ductal pancreatic lesions. Eur J Gastroenterol Hepatol 20(8):732–739

Huang B et al (2008) TLR signaling by tumor and immune cells: a double-edged sword. Oncogene 27(2):218–224

Huang C et al (2010) Effects of IL-6 and AG490 on regulation of Stat3 signaling pathway and invasion of human pancreatic cancer cells in vitro. J Exp Clin Cancer Res 29:51

Huang H et al (2013) Activation of nuclear factor-kappaB in acinar cells increases the severity of pancreatitis in mice. Gastroenterology 144(1):202–210

Ikebe M et al (2009) Lipopolysaccharide (LPS) increases the invasive ability of pancreatic cancer cells through the TLR4/MyD88 signaling pathway. J Surg Oncol 100(8):725–731

Israel A (2010) The IKK complex, a central regulator of NF-kappaB activation. Cold Spring Harb Perspect Biol 2(3):a000158

Ito H et al (2004) Prostaglandin E2 enhances pancreatic cancer invasiveness through an Ets-1-dependent induction of matrix metalloproteinase-2. Cancer Res 64(20):7439–7446

Jacobetz MA et al (2013) Hyaluronan impairs vascular function and drug delivery in a mouse model of pancreatic cancer. Gut 62(1):112–120

Karin M (1998) The NF-kappaB activation pathway: its regulation and role in inflammation and cell survival. Cancer J Sci Am 4(Suppl 1):S92–S99

Karin M et al (2002) NF-kappaB in cancer: from innocent bystander to major culprit. Nat Rev Cancer 2(4):301–310

Kawakami K, Kawakami M, Puri RK (2001) Overexpressed cell surface interleukin-4 receptor molecules can be successfully targeted for antitumor cytotoxin therapy. Crit Rev Immunol 21(1–3):299–310

Kleeff J, Korc M (1998) Up-regulation of transforming growth factor (TGF)-beta receptors by TGF-beta1 in COLO-357 cells. J Biol Chem 273(13):7495–7500

Kleeff J et al (1999a) Smad6 suppresses TGF-beta-induced growth inhibition in COLO-357 pancreatic cancer cells and is overexpressed in pancreatic cancer. Biochem Biophys Res Commun 255(2):268–273

Kleeff J et al (1999b) The TGF-beta signaling inhibitor Smad7 enhances tumorigenicity in pancreatic cancer. Oncogene 18(39):5363–5372

Kong R et al (2010) Downregulation of nuclear factor-kappaB p65 subunit by small interfering RNA synergizes with gemcitabine to inhibit the growth of pancreatic cancer. Cancer Lett 291(1):90–98

Kuwada Y et al (2003) Potential involvement of IL-8 and its receptors in the invasiveness of pancreatic cancer cells. Int J Oncol 22(4):765–771

Lee JY, Hennighausen L (2005) The transcription factor Stat3 is dispensable for pancreatic beta-cell development and function. Biochem Biophys Res Commun 334(3):764–768

Lesina M et al (2011) Stat3/Socs3 activation by IL-6 transsignaling promotes progression of pancreatic intraepithelial neoplasia and development of pancreatic cancer. Cancer Cell 19(4):456–469

Li M et al (2008) Interleukin-8 increases vascular endothelial growth factor and neuropilin expression and stimulates ERK activation in human pancreatic cancer. Cancer Sci 99(4):733–737

Li H et al (2011) STAT3 knockdown reduces pancreatic cancer cell invasiveness and matrix metalloproteinase-7 expression in nude mice. PLoS ONE 6(10):e25941

Ling L, Cao Z, Goeddel DV (1998) NF-kappaB-inducing kinase activates IKK-alpha by phosphorylation of Ser-176. Proc Natl Acad Sci USA 95(7):3792–3797

Liptay S et al (2003) Mitogenic and antiapoptotic role of constitutive NF-kappaB/Rel activity in pancreatic cancer. Int J Cancer 105(6):735–746

Lipton A et al (2010) Phase II trial of gemcitabine, irinotecan, and celecoxib in patients with advanced pancreatic cancer. J Clin Gastroenterol 44(4):286–288

Logsdon CD, Keyes L, Beauchamp RD (1992) Transforming growth factor-beta (TGF-beta 1) inhibits pancreatic acinar cell growth. Am J Physiol 262(2 Pt 1):G364–G368

Lowenfels AB et al (1993) Pancreatitis and the risk of pancreatic cancer. International Pancreatitis Study Group. New Engl J Med 328(20):1433–1437

Lu Z et al (1997) Presence of two signaling TGF-beta receptors in human pancreatic cancer correlates with advanced tumor stage. Dig Dis Sci 42(10):2054–2063

Mace TA et al (2013) Pancreatic cancer-associated stellate cells promote differentiation of myeloid-derived suppressor cells in a STAT3-dependent manner. Cancer Res 73(10):3007–3018

Malka D et al (2002) Risk of pancreatic adenocarcinoma in chronic pancreatitis. Gut 51(6):849–852

Maniati E et al (2011) Crosstalk between the canonical NF-kappaB and Notch signaling pathways inhibits Ppargamma expression and promotes pancreatic cancer progression in mice. J Clin Invest 121(12):4685–4699

Massague J, Blain SW, Lo RS (2000) TGFbeta signaling in growth control, cancer, and heritable disorders. Cell 103(2):295–309

Matsuo Y et al (2004) Enhanced angiogenesis due to inflammatory cytokines from pancreatic cancer cell lines and relation to metastatic potential. Pancreas 28(3):344–352

Means AL et al (2005) Pancreatic epithelial plasticity mediated by acinar cell transdifferentiation and generation of nestin-positive intermediates. Development 132(16):3767–3776

Melisi D et al (2008) LY2109761, a novel transforming growth factor beta receptor type I and type II dual inhibitor, as a therapeutic approach to suppressing pancreatic cancer metastasis. Mol Cancer Ther 7(4):829–840

Melisi D et al (2009) Secreted interleukin-1alpha induces a metastatic phenotype in pancreatic cancer by sustaining a constitutive activation of nuclear factor-kappaB. Mol Cancer Res 7(5):624–633

Michl P, Gress TM (2013) Current concepts and novel targets in advanced pancreatic cancer. Gut 62(2):317–326

Miyamoto M et al (1998) Effect of interleukin-8 on production of tumor-associated substances and autocrine growth of human liver and pancreatic cancer cells. Cancer Immunol Immunother 47(1):47–57

Miyamoto Y et al (2001) Interleukin-6 inhibits radiation induced apoptosis in pancreatic cancer cells. Anticancer Res 21(4A):2449–2456

Miyatsuka T et al (2006) Persistent expression of PDX-1 in the pancreas causes acinar-to-ductal metaplasia through Stat3 activation. Genes Dev 20(11):1435–1440

Moore MJ et al (2007) Erlotinib plus gemcitabine compared with gemcitabine alone in patients with advanced pancreatic cancer: a phase III trial of the National Cancer Institute of Canada Clinical Trials Group. J Clin Oncol 25(15):1960–1966

Morak MJ et al (2011) Phase II trial of Uracil/Tegafur plus leucovorin and celecoxib combined with radiotherapy in locally advanced pancreatic cancer. Radiother Oncol J Eur Soc Ther Radiol Oncol 98(2):261–264

Neoptolemos JP et al (2010) Adjuvant chemotherapy with fluorouracil plus folinic acid vs gemcitabine following pancreatic cancer resection: a randomized controlled trial. JAMA 304(10):1073–1081

Ochi A et al (2012) Toll-like receptor 7 regulates pancreatic carcinogenesis in mice and humans. J Clin Invest 122(11):4118–4129

Okada S et al (1998) Elevated serum interleukin-6 levels in patients with pancreatic cancer. Jpn J Clin Oncol 28(1):12–15

Olive KP et al (2009) Inhibition of Hedgehog signaling enhances delivery of chemotherapy in a mouse model of pancreatic cancer. Science 324(5933):1457–1461

Pahl HL (1999) Activators and target genes of Rel/NF-kappaB transcription factors. Oncogene 18(49):6853–6866

Pan X et al (2008) Nuclear factor-kappaB p65/relA silencing induces apoptosis and increases gemcitabine effectiveness in a subset of pancreatic cancer cells. Clin Cancer Res 14(24):8143–8151

Patterson GI, Padgett RW (2000) TGF beta-related pathways. Roles in *Caenorhabditis* elegans development. Trends Genet 16(1):27–33

Prokopchuk O et al (2005) Interleukin-4 enhances proliferation of human pancreatic cancer cells: evidence for autocrine and paracrine actions. Br J Cancer 92(5):921–928

Provenzano PP et al (2012) Enzymatic targeting of the stroma ablates physical barriers to treatment of pancreatic ductal adenocarcinoma. Cancer Cell 21(3):418–429

Sanford DE et al (2013) Inflammatory monocyte mobilization decreases patient survival in pancreatic cancer: a role for targeting the CCL2/CCR2 axis. Clin Cancer Res 19(13):3404–3415

Sawai H et al (2006) Interleukin-1alpha enhances the aggressive behavior of pancreatic cancer cells by regulating the alpha6beta1-integrin and urokinase plasminogen activator receptor expression. BMC Cell Biol 7:8

Schmiegel W et al (1993) Tumor necrosis factor alpha induces the expression of transforming growth factor alpha and the epidermal growth factor receptor in human pancreatic cancer cells. Proc Natl Acad Sci USA 90(3):863–867

Sclabas GM et al (2003) Restoring apoptosis in pancreatic cancer cells by targeting the nuclear factor-kappaB signaling pathway with the anti-epidermal growth factor antibody IMC-C225. J Gastrointest Surg 7(1):37–43 (discussion 43)

Shuai K et al (1993) A single phosphotyrosine residue of Stat91 required for gene activation by interferon-gamma. Science 261(5129):1744–1746

Shuai K et al (1994) Interferon activation of the transcription factor Stat91 involves dimerization through SH2-phosphotyrosyl peptide interactions. Cell 76(5):821–828

Siegel R, Naishadham D, Jemal A (2013) Cancer statistics, 2013. CA Cancer J Clin 63(1):11–30

Simeone DM, Pham T, Logsdon CD (2000) Disruption of TGFbeta signaling pathways in human pancreatic cancer cells. Ann Surg 232(1):73–80

Steinle AU et al (1999) NF-kappaB/Rel activation in cerulein pancreatitis. Gastroenterology 116(2):420–430

Strieter RM et al (1995) Role of C-X-C chemokines as regulators of angiogenesis in lung cancer. J Leukoc Biol 57(5):752–762

Takamori H et al (2000) Autocrine growth effect of IL-8 and GROalpha on a human pancreatic cancer cell line, Capan-1. Pancreas 21(1):52–56

Talar-Wojnarowska R et al (2009) Clinical significance of interleukin-6 (IL-6) gene polymorphism and IL-6 serum level in pancreatic adenocarcinoma and chronic pancreatitis. Dig Dis Sci 54(3):683–689

Thompson JE et al (1995) I kappaB-beta regulates the persistent response in a biphasic activation of NF-kappaB. Cell 80(4):573–582

Verma IM et al (1995) Rel/NF-kappaB/I kappaB family: intimate tales of association and dissociation. Genes Dev 9(22):2723–2735

Villanueva A et al (1998) Disruption of the antiproliferative TGF-beta signaling pathways in human pancreatic cancer cells. Oncogene 17(15):1969–1978

Von Hoff DD et al (2011) Gemcitabine plus nab-paclitaxel is an active regimen in patients with advanced pancreatic cancer: a phase I/II trial. J Clin Oncol 29(34):4548–4554

Winter JM et al (2012) Survival after resection of pancreatic adenocarcinoma: results from a single institution over three decades. Ann Surg Oncol 19(1):169–175

Wolf JS et al (2001) IL (interleukin)-1alpha promotes nuclear factor-kappaB and AP-1-induced IL-8 expression, cell survival, and proliferation in head and neck squamous cell carcinomas. Clin Cancer Res 7(6):1812–1820

Xiong HQ et al (2004) NF-kappaB activity blockade impairs the angiogenic potential of human pancreatic cancer cells. Int J Cancer 108(2):181–188

Xu D et al (2010) Cancer cell-derived IL-1alpha promotes HGF secretion by stromal cells and enhances metastatic potential in pancreatic cancer cells. J Surg Oncol 102(5):469–477

Yamamoto Y, Gaynor RB (2001) Therapeutic potential of inhibition of the NF-kappaB pathway in the treatment of inflammation and cancer. J Clin Invest 107(2):135–142

Yip-Schneider MT et al (2000) Cyclooxygenase-2 expression in human pancreatic adenocarcinomas. Carcinogenesis 21(2):139–146

Yoshikawa K et al (2012) Impact of tumor-associated macrophages on invasive ductal carcinoma of the pancreas head. Cancer Sci 103(11):2012–2020

Zhong Z, Wen Z, Darnell JE Jr (1994) Stat3: a STAT family member activated by tyrosine phosphorylation in response to epidermal growth factor and interleukin-6. Science 264(5155):95–98

Chapter 7
The Role of Inflammation in Prostate Cancer

Karen S. Sfanos, Heidi A. Hempel and Angelo M. De Marzo

Abstract In the United States and in "Westernized" countries, the prevalence of both prostate cancer and prostate inflammation is very high, indicating that the two pathologies could be causally related. Indeed, chronic inflammation is now regarded as an "enabling" characteristic of human cancer. Prostate cancer incidence is thought to be mediated in part by genetics, but also by environmental exposures, including the same exposures that may contribute to the development of prostatic inflammation. As our understanding of the role of inflammation in cancer deepens, it is increasingly apparent that "inflammation" as a whole is a complex entity that does not always play a negative role in cancer etiology. In fact, inflammation can play potentially dichotomous (both pro and antitumorigenic) roles depending on the nature and the cellular makeup of the immune response. This chapter will focus on reviewing the current state of knowledge on the role of innate and adaptive immune cells within the prostate tumor microenvironment and their seemingly complex role in prostate cancer in preventing versus promoting initiation and progression of the disease.

7.1 Introduction: Inflammation in the Adult Prostate and Prostate Cancer Risk

The prevalence of both prostate cancer and prostatic inflammation is at near-epidemic levels in the USA and in "Westernized" countries (Nelson et al. 2013). Prostate cancer incidence is thought to be mediated in part by genetics, but also by environmental exposures, including the same exposures that may contribute to the

K. S. Sfanos · H. A. Hempel · A. M. De Marzo (✉)
Department of Pathology, The Johns Hopkins University School of Medicine, Baltimore, MD, USA
e-mail: ademarz@jhmi.edu

B. B. Aggarwal et al. (eds.), *Inflammation and Cancer*, Advances in Experimental Medicine and Biology 816, DOI: 10.1007/978-3-0348-0837-8_7, © Springer Basel 2014

development of prostatic inflammation. Inflammation of the prostate, e.g., prostatitis, is a heterogeneous disease entity that is categorized by the National Institutes of Health (NIH) consensus classification as chronic prostatitis/chronic pelvic pain syndrome (CPPS). CPPS is divided into four categories, the first three of which relate to men with symptoms of disease: (1) acute bacterial prostatitis; (2) chronic bacterial prostatitis; (3) chronic prostatitis/CPPS; and (4) asymptomatic inflammatory prostatitis (Krieger et al. 1999). Whereas there is some epidemiological evidence associating symptomatic prostatitis with prostate cancer risk (Palapattu et al. 2005), a comprehensive analysis of the influence of prostatic inflammation on prostate cancer initiation and/or progression is difficult to perform due to the very high prevalence of prostatic inflammation that occurs in the absence of symptoms. Asymptomatic prostatic inflammation (i.e., "histological prostatitis") is a very common finding in the prostate of the adult male, as indicated by histological analysis of biopsies from men tested for prostate cancer due to elevated prostate-specific antigen (PSA) levels, radical prostatectomy specimens from men being treated for prostate cancer, transurethral resection of the prostate (TURP) specimens from men treated for benign prostatic hyperplasia (BPH), and autopsy specimens (Stimac et al. 2009; Gui-zhong et al. 2011; Ugurlu et al. 2010; Fujita et al. 2011; Delongchamps et al. 2008; Nickel et al. 1999; De Marzo et al. 2007). Accordingly, prostatic inflammation has been linked to all major diseases of the human prostate including BPH, prostatitis syndromes, and prostate cancer. Although the stimulus for this near-universal phenomenon of asymptomatic prostatic inflammation in the adult male remains elusive, multiple different sources are proposed to contribute, as shown in Fig. 7.1, including infectious agents, hormonal alterations (Ellem et al. 2009), physical trauma due to the formation of corpora amylacea, urine reflux, dietary factors, and prostate cancer (i.e., tumor-elicited immune responses) (De Marzo et al. 2007; Sfanos and De Marzo 2012; Sfanos et al. 2009b).

Of particular note, there is a significant amount of literature that supports an early role for prostatic inflammation in the development of a putative risk factor/precursor lesion to prostate cancer development, namely proliferative inflammatory atrophy (PIA). PIA is a term given to regions of prostatic atrophy associated with inflammatory cell infiltrates that develop at a high frequency in older men and can involve very large regions of the prostate. The proliferating atrophic epithelial cells of PIA appear to be regenerating in response to cellular damage, show signs of oxidative stress, and are hypothesized to serve at times as the direct precursor cells to prostatic intraepithelial neoplasia (PIN) and/or prostate cancer (Putzi and De Marzo 2000; Nelson et al. 2003). Indeed, morphological transitions between PIA, PIN, and prostate cancer have been described (Putzi and De Marzo 2000; Wang et al. 2009). Furthermore, PIA contains some of the hallmark changes found in PIN and prostate cancer, including downregulation of the tumor suppressors *NKX*3.1 and p27, and a fraction of PIA lesions exhibit methylation of deoxycytidine residues within the cytosine–guanine–dinucleotide (CpG) island near the glutathione S-transferase-π (*GSTP1*) promoter region (which occurs at a high frequency in prostate cancer and PIN lesions), leading to silencing of *GSTP1* (De Marzo et al. 1999; Bethel et al. 2006; Nakayama et al. 2003) (Fig. 7.2). The role

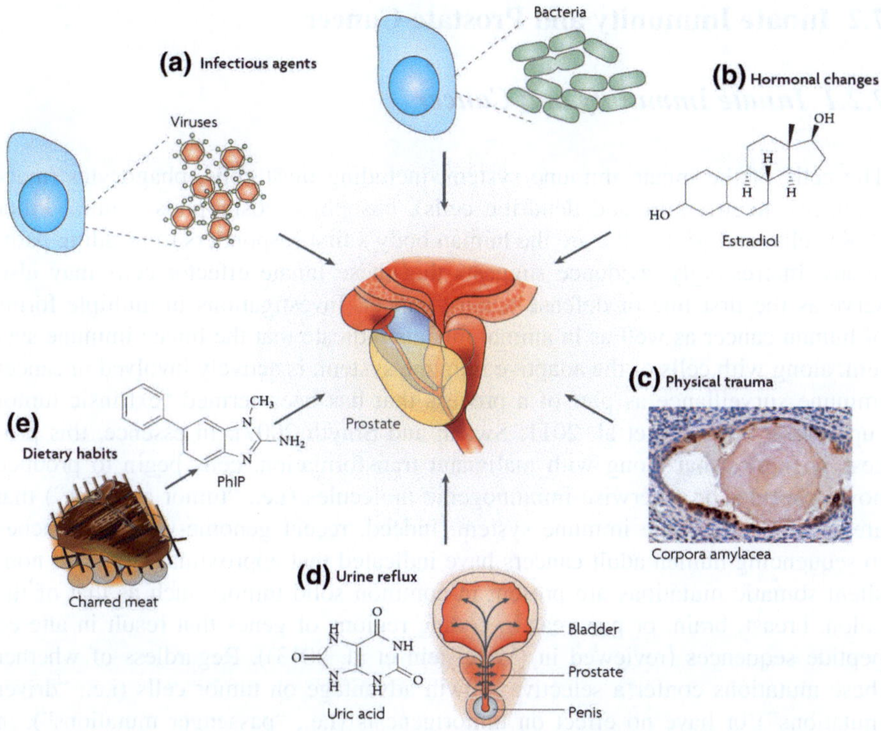

Fig. 7.1 Potential sources of prostatic inflammation. Reprinted from De Marzo et al. (2007)

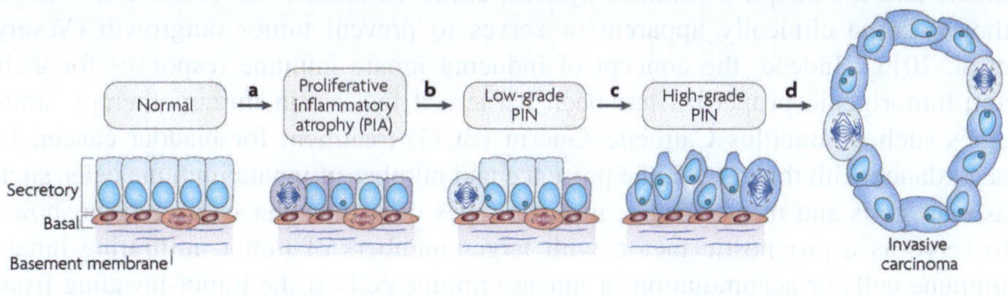

Fig. 7.2 Proposed progression model for prostate cancer development. Adapted from De Marzo et al. (2007)

of prostatic inflammation in the development of prostate cancer precursor lesions remains a topic of keen significance, and this issue has been widely covered by recent reviews and book chapters (Sfanos and De Marzo 2012; Nelson et al. 2013; De Marzo et al. 2007; De Marzo 2007; Lucia et al. 2010). This chapter, therefore, will focus on reviewing the current state of knowledge on the role of innate and adaptive immune cells within the prostate tumor microenvironment and their potentially dichotomous role in preventing versus promoting progression of the disease.

7.2 Innate Immunity and Prostate Cancer

7.2.1 Innate Immunity and Cancer

The cells of the innate immune system, including mast cells, phagocytes (macrophages, neutrophils, and dendritic cells), basophils, eosinophils, natural killer (NK) cells, and γδ T cells, are the human body's first responders to invading pathogens. Interestingly, evidence suggests that these innate effector cells may also serve as the first line of defense against cancer. Investigations in multiple forms of human cancer as well as in animal models indicate that the innate immune system, along with cells of the adaptive immune system, is actively involved in cancer immune surveillance as part of a process that has been termed "extrinsic tumor suppression" (Vesely et al. 2011; Swann and Smyth 2007). In essence, this process presumes that along with malignant transformation, cells begin to produce novel peptides or otherwise immunogenic molecules (i.e., "tumor antigens") that are recognized by the immune system. Indeed, recent genome-wide approaches to sequencing human adult cancers have indicated that approximately 30–70 non-silent somatic mutations are present in common solid tumors such as that of the colon, breast, brain, or pancreas in coding regions of genes that result in altered peptide sequences (reviewed in (Vogelstein et al. 2013)). Regardless of whether these mutations confer a selective growth advantage on tumor cells (i.e., "driver mutations") or have no effect on tumorigenesis (i.e., "passenger mutations"), in principle, these altered peptide sequences can serve as tumor-specific antigens (Vogelstein et al. 2013). The elicited response, mediated by cells of both the innate and the adaptive immune system, either eliminates the tumor cells before they become clinically apparent or serves to prevent tumor outgrowth (Vesely et al. 2011). Indeed, the concept of inducing innate immune responses for their anti-tumorigenic properties has been harnessed by certain immunotherapy strategies such as Bacillus Calmette–Guérin (BCG) treatment for bladder cancer. In accordance with this model, the presence and number of innate immune cells, such as mast cells and macrophages, in some types of human cancer have been shown to serve as a prognostic factor, with larger numbers of tumor-infiltrating innate immune cells or accumulation of innate immune cells at the tumor-invading front conferring a better prognosis (Welsh et al. 2005; Fleischmann et al. 2009; Rajput et al. 2008; Forssell et al. 2007; Zhou et al. 2010; Li et al. 2009a). However, as inflammation in cancer is truly a "double-edged sword," there are many important exceptions to this rule (Hagemann et al. 2007). One notable exception is the innate immune cells involved in dampening and/or regulating immune responses such as the myeloid-derived suppressor cell (MDSC) lineage of human myeloid progenitors (Ostrand-Rosenberg and Sinha 2009). Furthermore, innate immune cells can produce pro-inflammatory cytokines, such as IL-6 and IL-1β, and factors that enhance cell migration and invasiveness, such as matrix metalloproteinases (MMPs) and CC family chemokines, which have been shown to promote tumor initiation and/or progression (Kang et al. 2010; Li et al. 2009b; Allavena et al.

2008; Kaler et al. 2009; Loberg et al. 2006; Mizutani et al. 2009). Therefore, the influence of innate immune cells on cancer prevention versus cancer progression is often very difficult to discern (Disis 2010; Zhang et al. 2012), and whether these various cells provoke pro-growth versus growth-suppressive effects may relate to the specific tissue type in question, the disease temporal state (e.g., initiation, promotion, local extension/progression, metastasis), host genetic factors, and/or environmental cofactors such as local (or systemic) coinfection and dietary exposures.

In regard to prostate cancer, a number of studies have been carried out to determine the prognostic significance of tumor-infiltrating innate immune cells. Herein, although this research is still relatively early overall in terms of the scope of what can be done, we will summarize these efforts and specifically focus on the prognostic significance of prostate-infiltrating innate immune cells.

7.2.2 Mast Cells in Prostate Cancer

Mast cells are best known for their role in allergic reactions, where IgE–antigen complex (IgE–Ag) binding to the mast cell receptor FceRI stimulates degranulation, releasing effector molecules such as histamine, serotonin, leukotrienes, and proteoglycans (Galinsky and Nechushtan 2008; Galli 2000). However, mast cells have also been shown to play a significant role in defense against parasites, to be key players in controlling bacterial infection, and to be very important producers of immunoregulatory cytokines (Galinsky and Nechushtan 2008; Krishnaswamy et al. 2001; Arock et al. 1998; Gordon and Galli 1990; Gordon et al. 1990). What makes mast cells particularly interesting in cancer biology, however, lies in the dynamic way in which these cells reside in and interact with the microenvironment in their target tissues. Mast cell functions can have very potent effects on their environment, effects that can be powerfully pro- or anti-tumorigenic, depending on the circumstances (Fig. 7.3). These functions are very dynamic and are subject to manipulation by outside forces, possibly even by the surrounding cancer cells (Galinsky and Nechushtan 2008; Theoharides and Conti 2004). As such it is likely that mast cells play different roles in different cancers and different cancer stages (Pittoni and Colombo 2012). This possibility is, in fact, reflected in the literature. There have been a number of studies in many different cancers attempting to correlate mast cell density in or around the tumor, with the results varying from associating mast cell density with good prognosis, poor prognosis, and having no association with prognosis at all, even between studies in the same cancer (Galinsky and Nechushtan 2008; Pittoni and Colombo 2012; Fisher et al. 1989; Ribatti et al. 2003; Iamaroon et al. 2003; Ribatti et al. 1999; Molin et al. 2002; Molin 2004; Ribatti et al. 2005; Tuna et al. 2006; Fisher et al. 1985; Aaltomaa et al. 1993; Dabiri et al. 2004; Welsh et al. 2005; Chan et al. 2005; Johansson et al. 2010; Sari et al. 1999; Fleischmann et al. 2009). In prostate cancer specifically, higher numbers of "intratumoral" mast cells have been shown to be correlated with lower Gleason grade and better prognosis (Johansson et al. 2010;

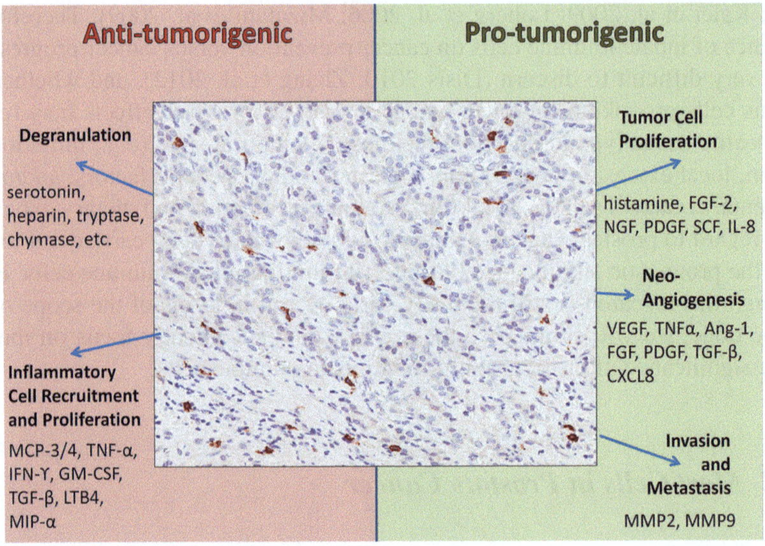

Fig. 7.3 Potential biological roles for mast cells in prostate cancer. Figure shows a photomicrograph from a region of human prostatic adenocarcinoma stained for mast cells (*brown* staining cells) by immunohistochemistry (H.A. Hempel, A.M. De Marzo, K.S. Sfanos, unpublished observations). Original magnification, ×100

Fleischmann et al. 2009; Sari et al. 1999); however, the opposite finding has also been reported (Nonomura et al. 2007). These and other studies on mast cells in human cancers were performed using a variety of techniques and without a standardized definition of "intratumoral" versus "peritumoral" mast cells. Nevertheless, the notion of mast cells having different effects in different circumstances is an attractive one and is consistent with what is known about mast cell biology.

Mast cells, such as most immune cells, originate in the bone marrow. However, mast cells travel to their targets before their final stages of development, and their final differentiation into different subtypes is dictated in large part by the microenvironment of their resident tissues (Galinsky and Nechushtan 2008; Theoharides and Conti 2004). The two main subtypes of mast cells are commonly known as MC_{TC}, which express chymase, tryptase, carboxypeptidase, and cathepsin G and are usually found in mucosa, and MC_T, which express mainly tryptase and are usually localized to connective tissues (Krishnaswamy et al. 2001; Irani et al. 1986; Khazaie et al. 2011). These two subtypes also differ in number, type, and content of secretory granules, as well as which stimuli to which they will respond (Theoharides and Conti 2004). These subtypes are not exhaustive, however, as mast cells have been discovered with phenotypes outside of these. In addition, there is significant evidence to suggest that mast cell differentiation is not final, and phenotype and mast cell protease profile can be changed based on different conditions in their microenvironment, including exposure to different cytokines, the presence of fibroblasts, and different host organ tissues (Galinsky and Nechushtan 2008; Lee et al. 1998; Gurish et al. 1995). As such, it is reasonable to suggest that mast cell phenotype will be very different depending on differing conditions, such as in vitro versus in vivo, and on different cancers and cancer stages. The best known method of mast cell effector function is via degranulation, which is the release of the previously synthesized contents of intracellular granules in response to IgE–Ag binding to the mast cell receptor. These contents include effector molecules such as serotonin, histamine, heparin, tryptase, and chymase, among others, many of which with pro-inflammatory, anti-tumorigenic properties. However, there is also significant evidence for a method for "piecemeal degranulation" of mast cells, allowing for the selective release of cytokines without the release of the entire secretory granule (Crivellato et al. 2003). This alternative activation model helps to fuel the mechanistic side of the argument for the pro-tumorigenic potential of mast cells, as it provides the potential for the selective release of pro-tumorigenic cytokines such as IL-1 and IL-6 (Lacy and Stow 2011) and effector molecules such as MMP9 in the absence of anti-tumorigenic mast cell granule components. The mast cell subtype also comes into play here, as different subtypes will have different effector molecules available to them and thus can have different effects on the tumor upon degranulation, piecemeal or otherwise. In addition to these, mast cells are also potent producers of immune modulating cytokines, chemokines, angiogenic factors, and proteases, all of which can cause significant changes in the tumor microenvironment (Khazaie et al. 2011).

Mast cells are known to produce many different angiogenic molecules, including VEGF, histamine, TNF-α, and Ang-1, and thus have been suspected for some time to play a significant role in tumor angiogenesis and possibly even in the angiogenic switch (Maltby et al. 2009). There have been several studies supporting this idea, including a transplantation multiple myeloma mouse model, in which it was found that transplanting mast cells with plasmacytoma tumors resulted in significantly higher vascularization (Nakayama et al. 2004). In addition, one study in a squamous carcinoma mouse model demonstrated a significant decrease in premalignant angiogenesis in mast cell-deficient mice (Coussens et al. 1999). Evidence in humans for a role for mast cells in tumor angiogenesis is also mounting, such as in one study correlating melanoma progression with mast cell density and simultaneously increased vascular density (Ribatti et al. 2005). However, some have also suggested a role for mast cells in suppressing angiogenesis by providing receptors that can "soak up" angiogenic factors (Theoharides and Conti 2004). In addition, there are studies correlating mast cell density with cancer progression without finding a correlation with angiogenesis, suggesting that mast cells may also have a role in tumor promotion aside from blood vessel development (Molin 2004; Molin et al. 2002). In human prostate cancer, mast cell densities have not been correlated with neovascularization; however, in an orthotopic rat model, implantation of AT-1 tumor cells resulted in peritumoral recruitment of mast cells and an increase in peritumoral vascular density (Johansson et al. 2010). Furthermore, castration was found to result in mast cell recruitment to the prostate both in men and in the AT-1 tumor model and the Dunning rat model, and this correlated with an increase in vascular density in the Dunning model (Johansson et al. 2010).

In addition to the possible roles for mast cells in angiogenesis, the role of mast cells in tissue remodeling is of particular interest in tumor promotion and includes a possible connection in prostate cancer. The idea that the extracellular matrix (ECM) plays a significant role in tumor promotion has gained importance in recent years (Bissell and Hines 2011; LaBarge et al. 2009; van Dijk et al. 2013). Mast cells produce potent proteases, including chymase, tryptase, collagenases, MMP9, and other gelatinases, and cysteinyl cathepsins. As such, research into the role of mast cells in ECM modulation and tumor invasion is also gaining ground (Khazaie et al. 2011). One study in prostate cancer explored the role of mast cell MMP9 in early prostate tumor progression in transgenic adenocarcinoma of the mouse prostate (TRAMP) mice, arguing that lower-grade prostate tumors would need mast cell-derived MMP9 for invasion, since well-differentiated prostate tumor cells do not produce MMP9 (Pittoni et al. 2011). The results did in fact suggest that mast cell MMP9 was necessary for early tumor invasion in mice. Immunohistochemistry (IHC) studies in human prostate cancer tissues showed a positive correlation between increased mast cell density, MMP9 production confined almost entirely to tumor-infiltrating mast cells, and well-differentiated tumors—supporting the observations in the TRAMP mouse studies (Pittoni et al. 2011). Whether mast cell-derived MMP9 plays a role in driving early invasion of human prostate cancer is yet to be elucidated.

In addition to the direct effects mast cells might have on cancer cells and their microenvironment, mast cells may also affect cancer through their roles as potent immune modulators. Mast cells are capable of both suppressing and promoting inflammatory responses, depending on the circumstances (Galinsky and Nechushtan 2008). In fact, mast cells are known to produce a number of cytokines and chemokines capable of recruiting, activating, suppressing, and driving the differentiation of both innate and adaptive immune cells, including neutrophils, basophils, macrophages, lymphocytes (such as B cells, T_H2 T cells, and T_{reg} cells), and NK cells. As such, mast cells are also capable of anti- or pro-tumorigenic effects through the suppression or activation of the inflammatory response and could also have a significant effect on other inflammatory cells in different cancers.

Studies both in vivo in mice and in vitro in mouse and human cells have demonstrated mast cell influences on cancer cells, with one in vivo study showing decreased mitotic index and increased apoptosis in intestinal polyps and two in vitro studies showing increased proliferation and invasion upon treatment with mast cell-conditioned medium (Khazaie et al. 2011; Gounaris et al. 2007; Cheon et al. 2011; Strouch et al. 2010). This activity of mast cells has been theorized to be due to the production of tryptase, which is reported to promote proliferation of colon cancer cells, fibroblasts, and other cell types (Yoshii et al. 2005; Cairns and Walls 1996; Berger et al. 2001; Gruber et al. 1997; Levi-Schaffer and Piliponsky 2003; Frungieri et al. 2002). Mast cell histamine has also been suggested to play a role in tumor cell proliferation; however, the literature is not in agreement with whether it promotes or suppresses proliferation (Theoharides and Conti 2004). In contrast, mast cell effector molecules such as IL-4 and TNF-α could result in tumor cell death (Gooch et al. 1998; Gordon and Galli 1990).

As mast cells and cancer cells evolve in the same microenvironment, the interactions between the two could change significantly. With the myriad of mast cell effector molecules, there is a delicate balance between the anti- and pro-tumorigenic capabilities of mast cells that can conceivably change very dramatically with time, even within the same tumor. It is possible that even if mast cells cannot serve as an independent prognostic factor for all cancers, they might be an indicator of cancer aggressiveness and invasiveness (Galinsky and Nechushtan 2008). In addition, it is very important that this ever-evolving relationship with cancer be better understood before any mast cell-targeted therapies are attempted. Since mast cells may have the potential to be pro-tumorigenic or anti-tumorigenic depending on the microenvironment, even in the same cancer, certain therapies may be beneficial at certain stages of cancer and detrimental in others (Pittoni and Colombo 2012; Pittoni et al. 2011). As such, mast cells have great potential in cancer research, and many possible roles of mast cells in prostate cancer continue to be an important area of study.

7.2.3 Macrophages in Prostate Cancer

The current understanding of tumor-associated macrophages (TAMs) is that they are a heterogeneous group of cells that can be further classified into subsets based on both phenotypic and functional characteristics. Analogous to the T_H1 and T_H2 classification of T-cell lineages, activated macrophages are generally classified into "M1" or "M2" macrophage subsets. M1 macrophages are "classically" activated, acute-phase macrophages that produce a number of pro-inflammatory cytokines such as IL-1β, IL-6, IL-12, IL-23, and TNF. In contrast, M2 or "alternatively" activated macrophages have been described as immune regulators and produce the anti-inflammatory cytokines IL-10 and TGF-β1 (Edin et al. 2012). In most cases, macrophages that infiltrate the tumor microenvironment are considered to be M2 macrophages, and as such, these cells may play a role in dampening anticancer immune responses, leading to tumor immune escape (Hao et al. 2012) (Fig. 7.4).

In prostate cancer, several studies have aimed to correlate TAM numbers with disease prognosis. Studies in prostate cancer have almost exclusively used IHC for the pan-macrophage-specific cell surface marker, CD68, to quantify the number of TAMs in benign and cancerous regions of the prostate. In one of the earliest studies on macrophage numbers in prostate cancer, macrophage density was found to be significantly lower in benign areas adjacent to prostate tumors than within the tumor itself (Shimura et al. 2000). Furthermore, the majority of TAMs (84 %) were found to be distributed within the tumor-associated stroma as opposed to within direct contact with cancer cells or within the lumen of cancerous glands. Interestingly, although TAM density within prostate tumors was positively associated with Gleason score (i.e., higher numbers of TAMs in higher Gleason score tumors), lower numbers of TAMs were shown to be significantly associated with higher clinical stage and the presence of positive lymph nodes. Furthermore,

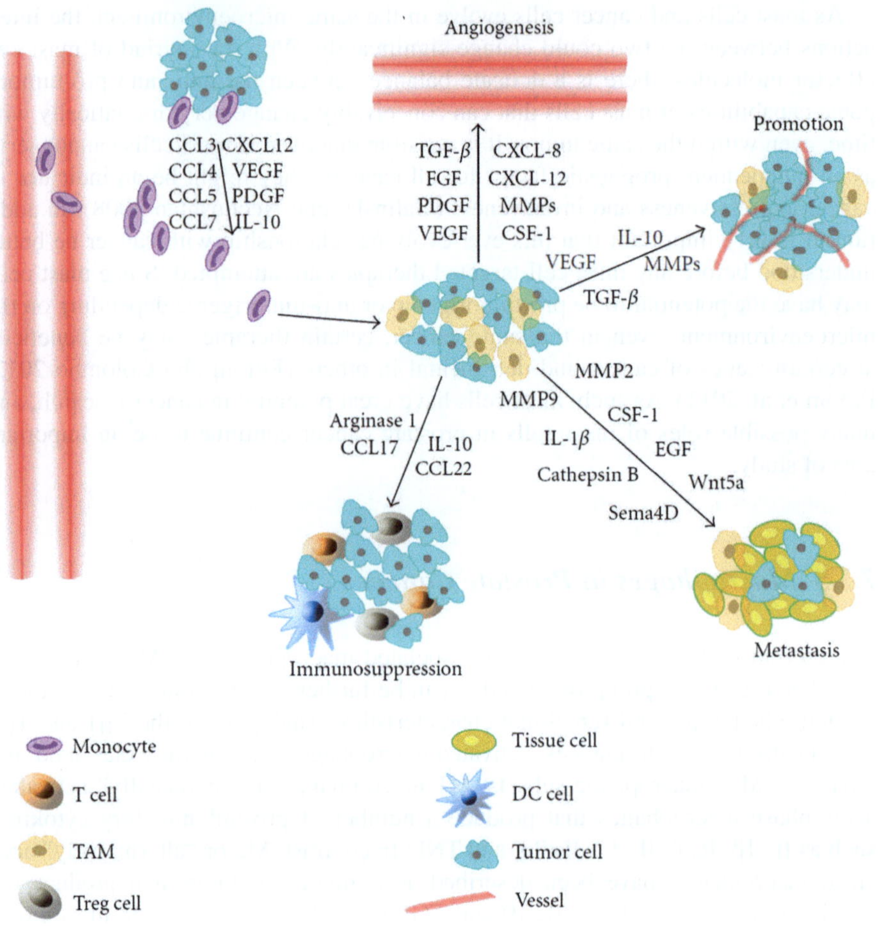

Fig. 7.4 Inflammatory cells within tumor microenvironment and their potential biological roles. Differentiation of monocytes into tumor-associated macrophages (TAM) with differing biological roles may be mediated by secretion of cytokines and growth factors by tumor cells and stromal cells within the tumor microenvironment. Reprinted from Hao et al. (2012)

reduced TAM numbers were found to be an independent predictor for time to PSA-detected disease progression (Shimura et al. 2000). This same group later reported that lower numbers of prostate-infiltrating class A macrophage scavenger receptor (SR-A)-expressing cells (dendritic cells and macrophages) were similarly associated with higher clinical stage and positive lymph nodes and predictive of shorter time to PSA progression (Yang et al. 2004). Although the intriguing positive association of macrophage numbers with Gleason score has held up in multiple additional studies, TAM quantification as an independent prognostic factor for time to PSA progression has varied (Lissbrant et al. 2000; Wang et al. 2005; Nonomura et al. 2011). In a study on disease progression after hormone therapy for prostate cancer, TAM densities as assayed by IHC for CD68 on patient's prostate biopsy specimens prior to treatment were found to be positively correlated with Gleason score and clinical stage (Nonomura et al. 2011). Furthermore, in contrast to the studies by Shimura et al. (2000) and Yang et al. (2004), Nonomura et al. reported that increased numbers of TAMs were significantly associated with PSA progression and serve as a prognostic indicator for decreased time to progression-free survival (Nonomura et al. 2011).

Richardsen et al. (2008) also reported that the production of macrophage colony-stimulating factor (M-CSF) and colony-stimulating factor-1 receptor (CSF-1R) is significantly greater in tumor cells and in stromal areas in the primary tumors of patients with metastatic prostate cancer compared to those without metastatic disease. The mechanism by which macrophages may promote prostate cancer invasion may be mediated in part by secretion of proteases that act on the ECM. Of interest is the serine protease urokinase plasminogen activator (uPA) that stimulates the plasminogen activation system upon binding to urokinase receptor (uPAR). Cleavage of the $\alpha6\beta1$ integrin by uPA has been shown in in vivo studies to increase tumor cell motility, invasion, and prostate cancer metastasis (Ports et al. 2009). Further in vitro studies indicated that this process may be mediated by TAMs (Sroka et al. 2011). Likewise, the cathepsin proteases, and specifically cathepsin K and cathepsin S, are also of interest in this regard. Cathepsins K and S are both lysosomal cysteine proteases. Whereas cysteine cathepsins are generally thought to serve in intracellular lysosomal protein degradation and turnover, these two cathepsins (K and S) can be secreted by macrophages (Punturieri et al. 2000) and may potentially play an important role in ECM remodeling to promote tumor invasion and progression. Macrophage-secreted cathepsin-mediated tumor invasion has been previously demonstrated in multiple forms of cancer (Vasiljeva et al. 2006; Gocheva et al. 2010). In prostate cancer specifically, macrophage-secreted cathepsin S was found in the TRAMP mouse model as a protein of interest in advanced disease as assessed by differential protein-profiling studies of normal prostate, primary tumors of differing histological grades, and metastatic tumors (Lindahl et al. 2009). IHC for CD68 costained with cathepsin S demonstrated that both in TRAMP tumors and in human prostate tumors, cathepsin S is produced primarily by TAMs. Furthermore, the number of cathepsin S-secreting macrophages was found to be significantly higher in castration-resistant prostate cancer as opposed to hormone naïve prostate cancer in patients with high-grade prostate tumors (Lindahl et al. 2009). Another recent study in prostate cancer demonstrated that cathepsin K-deficient mice had a significant reduction in tumor growth and bone resorption when PC3 cells were injected into the tibia compared to wild-type mice (Herroon et al. 2013). This phenomenon was specific to bone, as PC3 cells implanted subcutaneously had similar growth in both wild-type and cathepsin K knockout animals. By IHC, cathepsin K was found to be restricted to osteoclasts and macrophages in this model (Herroon et al. 2013). The role of macrophage-secreted cathepsins remains an area of active interest in prostate cancer invasion, progression, and potentially metastasis.

Further illustrations of the potential role of macrophages in prostate cancer progression involve the large body of work studying macrophage inhibitory cytokine-1 (MIC-1) and its potential prognostic value. MIC-1, also known as prostate-derived factor (PDF), GDF15, PLAB, NAG-1, or PTGFB, is a member of the transforming growth factor beta (TGF-β) superfamily that was initially discovered during cDNA library screens for genes associated with macrophage activation (Bootcov et al. 1997). Although little is known to date regarding the cellular receptor for MIC-1 or its signaling pathways, studies both in vitro and in vivo indicate a generalized anti-inflammatory role for this molecule (Breit et al. 2011). MIC-1 is up-regulated in inflammatory conditions, and this molecule is also produced by cancer cells in multiple types of human cancer. Systemic levels of MIC-1 are indicative of poor prognosis in cancer, cardiovascular disease, chronic renal and heart failure, and pulmonary embolism, and recent studies suggest that serum MIC-1 levels may even serve as a novel predictor of all-cause mortality (Wiklund et al. 2010). In prostate cancer, high serum levels of MIC-1 have been consistently shown to be correlated with poor prognosis (Brown et al. 2009; Selander et al. 2007; Welsh et al. 2003). Furthermore, serum MIC-1 levels have been shown to increase the specificity of PSA testing for prostate cancer (Brown et al. 2006). MIC-1 has been previously shown to be overexpressed in prostate cancer tissues versus benign tissues in gene expression microarray studies, with a magnitude of differential expression between tumor and matched normal tissue that is similar to other well-known genes that are differentially expressed in prostate cancer such as alpha-methylacyl-CoA racemase (AMACR) and hepsin (Welsh et al. 2001). MIC-1 protein levels are also increased in prostate tumor tissues versus benign, and this finding has been demonstrated in multiple studies utilizing protein-profiling analyses (Cheung et al. 2004; Hood et al. 2005). By IHC, MIC-1 levels are low in normal prostate epithelium and progressively higher in the suspected prostate cancer precursor lesion, high-grade prostatic intraepithelial neoplasia (HGPIN), and prostate cancer (Rasiah et al. 2006). Similar to the studies in serum, high levels of MIC-1 protein or mRNA in prostate cancer tissues has been shown to act as an indicator of poor prognosis (Rasiah et al. 2006; Nakamura et al. 2003; Bauskin et al. 2005).

The mechanism by which MIC-1 serves as a prognostic indicator in prostate cancer may involve multiple potential processes. Immunohistochemical studies of MIC-1 production in the prostate have not addressed the potential production of MIC-1 by prostate-infiltrating inflammatory cells (e.g., macrophages). However, as prostate cancer is known to develop in an organ that contains a great deal of unexplained acute and chronic inflammation in adulthood, it is likely that MIC-1 may serve as a "bridge" molecule linking inflammation to cancer development (Karan et al. 2009). Furthermore, the production of MIC-1 by prostate cancer cells may serve to inhibit prostate-infiltrating macrophages that are involved in antitumor immune responses. MIC-1 has been shown in in vitro systems to reduce cell adhesion and induce cell detachment of prostate cancer cells in culture (Liu et al.

2003). This finding provides a potential mechanism whereby MIC-1 production may contribute to tumor dissemination and metastasis.

7.2.4 Toll-Like Receptors (TLRs)

TLRs are a class of molecules associated with innate immunity that are expressed on cells such as macrophages and dendritic cells. TLRs recognize structurally conserved pathogen-derived products such as lipopolysaccharide (LPS) contained in Gram-negative bacteria. TLRs are also involved in tissue homeostasis and play a role in tissue repair and regeneration. There are significant data to demonstrate that TLRs may serve a role as negative regulators of cancer, as many anticancer therapeutic agents have been based on administration of TLR agonists (e.g., the historical use of Coley's toxin as a cancer treatment and the currently used strategy of BCG treatment for bladder cancer) (Rakoff-Nahoum and Medzhitov 2009). On the other hand, TLRs have also been implicated in the promotion of tumorigenesis, which may involve recruitment of macrophages to sites of tissue injury in the developing tumor (Rakoff-Nahoum and Medzhitov 2009). In prostate cancer, early evidence of a role for TLRs in prostate cancer development came from genetic studies of TLR polymorphisms associated with prostate cancer risk. Specifically, multiple studies have shown that single nucleotide polymorphisms (SNPs) in TLR4 and the TLR1-6-10 gene cluster are associated with prostate cancer risk (Chen et al. 2005; Zheng et al. 2004; Sun et al. 2005; Kim et al. 2012), although results have varied among cohorts (Chen et al. 2007; Shui et al. 2012). At the tissue level, TLRs have been reported to be up-regulated by prostate cancer cells as assessed by IHC. For example, TLR3, TLR4, and TLR9 were shown to be produced by prostate tumor cells as assayed by IHC, and interestingly, high expression of these TLRs as assayed by real-time PCR was found to correlate with biochemical recurrence (Gonzalez-Reyes et al. 2011). The mechanism by which this relationship may arise, however, remains unclear, as, on the contrary, TLR stimulation in cancer cells in prostate cancer models has also been consistently shown to result in the upregulation of inflammatory cytokines and induction of apoptosis and/or anti-tumor immune responses (Paone et al. 2008; Harashima et al. 2012; Chin et al. 2010; Galli et al. 2010; Andreani et al. 2007).

7.2.5 IL-6 in Prostate Cancer

Interleukin-6 (IL-6) is a pleiotropic cytokine that elicits multiple physiological processes including immune responses, hematopoiesis, and cellular proliferation and differentiation. IL-6 has also been implicated in a number of pathophysiologic processes and may also play an important role in carcinogenesis, including promotion of tumor cell adhesion, invasion, proliferation, and neoangiogenesis. Increasing evidence indicates that IL-6 may contribute to the progression of prostate cancer, and a high systemic level of IL-6 is considered to be a sign of a more aggressive clinical course (Smith et al. 2001; Okamoto et al. 1997; Twillie et al. 1995). IL-6 is secreted by a variety of cell types such as T cells, macrophages, endothelial cells, and fibroblasts. In addition, studies have suggested that IL-6 is secreted by prostate adenocarcinoma cells (Hobisch et al. 2000). IL-6 is responsible for skewing cellular differentiation of multiple cell types including B cells, T_H17 cells, and myeloid cells (Kimura and Kishimoto 2010; Cheng et al. 2011; Tanner and Tosato 1992). As such, both systemic and local production of IL-6 may drive accumulation of immune cell subtypes. For example, IL-6, along with CCL2 (CC chemokine ligand 2), can induce the differentiation of $CD11b^+$ monocytes into M2-type macrophages, indicating that systemic and/or local IL-6 production in prostate cancer patients may lead to differentiation and accumulation of this immune-suppressive, pro-tumorigenic subset of macrophages (Roca et al. 2009). There is additional evidence that CCL2 may assist in recruitment of macrophages to the tumor site and promote tumor cell metastasis to bone (Loberg et al. 2006; Mizutani et al. 2009). Furthermore, in experiments using the TRAMP murine model, high circulating levels of IL-6 were associated with recruitment of MDSCs (Wu et al. 2012); abrogation of IL-6 in this model inhibited the recruitment of MDSCs, slowed tumor growth, and attenuated angiogenesis (Wu et al. 2012).

A number of studies have been conducted to gain understanding of how IL-6 might act locally on tumor cells to contribute to prostate cancer development and progression. One line of investigation has aimed to identify a role for IL-6 in progression of prostate cancer to androgen independence via direct regulation of androgen receptor transactivation and/or androgen synthesis in prostate cancer cells (Lee et al. 2003; Malinowska et al. 2009; Chun et al. 2009). Finally, it has also been suggested that a positive feedback loop between IL-6 activation, STAT3 activation, and NF-κB activation in cancer maintains cells in an "epigenetic transformed" state that might transform "non-stem cancer cells" into "cancer stem-like cells" (Iliopoulos et al. 2011).

7.2.6 Additional Innate Immune Cells in Prostate Cancer

There are additional innate immune cells that potentially play a role in prostate cancer as indicated by studies in animal and/or in vitro models, but do not as of yet have significant data in human prostate cancer tissues. One notable example of this is the MDSC lineage of myeloid progenitors. MDSCs accumulate in the tumor microenvironment as well as the blood, lymph nodes, and bone marrow in association with several forms of human cancer and may contribute to tumor immune escape due to their general functional role in immune suppression (Ostrand-Rosenberg and Sinha 2009). In regard to prostate cancer, multiple murine models of prostate cancer demonstrate accumulation of MDSCs in tumors along with a potential contribution to tumor progression (Wu et al. 2012; Svensson et al. 2011; Rigamonti et al. 2011).

Finally, whereas we have reviewed different subsets of innate immune cells as separate entities in this chapter, it is entirely possible that multiple different innate immune cells contribute to prostate cancer etiology in concert. In support of this, when 320 SNPs in 46 genes involved in the innate immunity pathway were examined in a large cohort of advanced prostate cancer cases and non-diseased controls, the whole pathway was found to be significantly associated with prostate cancer risk (Kazma et al. 2012). The authors of this particular study conclude that the innate immunity pathway may play a "modest role" in advanced prostate cancer through "multiple small effects" (Kazma et al. 2012). Relatedly, reports from the Glasgow Inflammation Outcome Study, a previously described cohort of cancer patients in north Glasgow, UK (Proctor et al. 2010), describe the use of markers of "systemic inflammation" to predict disease outcome in prostate cancer patients (Shafique et al. 2012). Results from this study indicated that prostate cancer patients with elevated modified Glasgow Prognostic Score (mGPS—a combination of assays for serum levels of C-reactive protein and albumin) predicted poorer 5-year overall and relative survival, excess risk of death, and high-grade (Gleason grade 8–10) disease (Shafique et al. 2012). C-reactive protein is an acute-phase protein and a measure of systemic inflammation. Interestingly, prediagnostic levels of C-reactive protein do not appear to be associated with the development of prostate cancer (Platz et al. 2004). Similar findings to the Glasgow studies are apparent in studies aiming to determine why men of African American (AA) race are two to three times more likely to die from prostate cancer that European Americans (EA) (Horner et al. 2009). Gene expression microarray studies of prostate cancer tissues from AA and EA men have consistently shown overexpression of gene sets involving inflammation pathways in AA samples (Powell et al. 2013; Reams et al. 2009; Wallace et al. 2008). This includes differentially expressed gene clustering in pathways involved in immune response, interleukins, and cytokine signaling and overexpression of specific genes such as IL-6, IL-8, and IL-1β (Powell et al. 2013; Reams et al. 2009; Wallace et al. 2008).

7.3 Adaptive Immunity and Prostate Cancer

7.3.1 Adaptive Immunity and Cancer

The cells of the adaptive immune system (also known as the "acquired" immune system) are more generally considered to be the "second-line" response against invading pathogens, as they typically require costimulation from innate immune cells (i.e., in the form of antigen presentation to cellular receptors) to drive cellular proliferation and a pathogen antigen-specific response. Cells of the adaptive immune system include T lymphocytes (i.e., CD4+ and CD8+ T cells) and B lymphocytes (B cells). Like the cells of the innate immune system, cells involved in adaptive immunity are known to play paradoxical roles in cancer development. For example, whereas CD8+ T cells are thought to be major effector cells in anti-tumor immune responses, it is now well known that chronic inflammation, which is characteristically mediated by the cells of the adaptive immune system, plays a significant role in cancer initiation and progression. Indeed, chronic inflammation is now regarded as one of the "hallmarks" of human cancer (Hanahan and Weinberg 2011). This is especially apparent in types of cancer that are known to be associated with infectious agents and where chronic inflammation-associated lesions are known risk factors for cancer development (Sfanos and De Marzo 2012). One well-known example of this is *Helicobacter pylori* (*H. pylori*)-induced gastritis, gastric ulcers, and gastric atrophy as risk factor lesions for the development of gastric cancer.

7.3.2 Tumor-Infiltrating Lymphocytes (TIL) and Prostate Cancer

The presence of intratumoral T cells, or TIL, is generally indicative of good prognosis in cancer and thought to be indicative of local reaction to the tumor and the initiation of an anti-tumor immune response (Zhang et al. 2003; Clemente et al. 1996; Rao et al. 2010). CD8+ T cells (e.g., cytotoxic T cells or "killer" T cells) are of particular interest in this regard, as they may serve as the primary effector cells in cancer cell elimination (Pardoll 2002). Along these lines, multiple studies also show that the presence of tumor-infiltrating CD8+ T cells in particular is indicative of good prognosis (Naito et al. 1998; Liu et al. 2012; Schumacher et al. 2001). In prostate cancer, a limited number of studies have attempted to identify and quantify prostate TIL and correlate the presence of TIL with prostate cancer prognosis. One study in particular that quantified TIL in 325 prostatic adenocarcinomas with clinical follow-up data found that absent or "weak" TIL within the tumor was significantly associated with tumor progression and death from prostate cancer (Vesalainen et al. 1994). In contrast, a study analyzing CD3+ T cells on tissue microarrays (TMAs) containing tissue from 2,144 prostate cancer samples found no significant correlation between the number of CD3+ TIL and tumor stage, Gleason grade, preoperative PSA level, or lymph node involvement (Flammiger et al. 2012). Intriguingly, this study found that either very low or very high numbers of CD3+ TIL (as opposed to intermediate levels) were significantly associated with shortened PSA recurrence-free survival (Flammiger et al. 2012). A study by Richardsen et al. (2008) reported that CD3+ cells in tumor areas and stromal areas were significantly higher in the primary tumors of patients with metastatic prostate cancer versus those without metastatic disease. Another study quantifying TIL in 188 radical prostatectomy specimens on TMAs found that high numbers of TIL was an independent predictor of short PSA recurrence-free survival together with high Gleason score (Karja et al. 2005). Likewise, a study that quantified inflammation as a whole in 161 radical prostatectomies found a significant correlation between "high-grade" inflammation in and surrounding malignant glands and postoperative biochemical recurrence (Irani et al. 1999). McArdle et al. (2004) reported on a series of 80 cases that increased CD4+ TIL was associated with poor outcome in prostate cancer patients. One potential explanation for the difference in results between studies may involve the heterogeneous nature of prostate cancer (and prostate tumor-associated inflammation) that may not be adequately represented on TMAs as opposed to whole tissue sections. Another potential explanation may involve the fact that many of these studies aimed to quantify TIL as a whole and did not attempt to quantify different T-cell subtypes, such as the different T_{HELPER} subsets of T cells (T_H1, T_H2, T_H17) or regulatory T cells (T_{reg}), and it is known that the different subtypes can play varying and opposing roles in the tumor microenvironment (Kennedy and Celis 2008). T_{reg}, for example, which are characterized by high expression of CD25 and FoxP3 and play a suppressive role in immune responses, are known to actively suppress anti-tumor immune responses (Mougiakakos et al. 2010).

The analysis and quantification of T-cell subsets in prostate tissue samples is challenging, as these cells are typically differentiated by the different cytokines that they secrete. IHC is often not a reliable assay for secreted cytokines, and the isolation of immune cells from prostate tumor or tissue samples for use in flow cytometry can be technically challenging. Nevertheless, one study did isolate TIL from radical prostatectomy specimens using a fine-needle aspiration technique and quantitatively assayed for separate CD4+ T-cell subsets (T_H1, T_H2, T_H17, T_{reg}) using flow cytometry (Sfanos et al. 2008). The results of this study indicated that T_H1 cells are quantitatively most abundant in the prostate of cancer patients and that T_H2 cells are almost completely absent. Furthermore, prostate-infiltrating T_H1, T_H17, and T_{reg} cells are significantly elevated when compared to levels in the peripheral blood of the cancer patients, with the most significant skewing toward the CD4+ T_H17 and T_{reg} phenotype (Sfanos et al. 2008). Finally, although the sample size was limited ($n = 20$), greater numbers of CD4+ T_H17 TIL were significantly associated with lower pathologic Gleason score (Sfanos et al. 2008). Of interest, this finding of higher numbers of T_H17 cells in lower-grade tumors is inconsistent with literature in other types of cancer (Zhang et al. 2008; Grivennikov et al. 2012); however, there does not appear to be a consensus as to whether T_H17 cells are pro- or anti-tumorigenic (Wilke et al. 2011; Martin et al. 2012; Zou and Restifo 2010), and they can possibly be both depending on the inflammatory microenvironment and the stage of the tumor. One potential limitation to the Sfanos et al. study was that the entire peripheral zone of the prostate (where prostate cancer typically arises) was sampled and likely sampled areas that contained both cancerous and benign regions. Therefore, localization of T-cell subsets in prostate tumor versus benign prostate tissues was not conducted. This type of analysis would likely need to be performed in frozen or formalin-fixed paraffin-embedded (FFPE) tissues using in situ hybridization-based assays.

One study of note did utilize IHC for IL-17 to determine that IL-17-producing macrophages accumulate in areas of PIA (Vykhovanets et al. 2011). T_{reg} cells have been examined in additional studies in prostate cancer patients and have consistently been found to be elevated in tumor tissues (Miller et al. 2006; Kiniwa et al. 2007); however, levels in peripheral blood vary (Miller et al. 2006; Yokokawa et al. 2008). These studies also demonstrate the suppressive activity of CD4+ T_{reg} (Miller et al.

2006; Yokokawa et al. 2008; Kiniwa et al. 2007), as well as CD8+ T_{reg} (Kiniwa et al. 2007), isolated from peripheral blood and tumor tissues of prostate cancer patients. CD8+ T_{reg} cells are the newest class of T cells shown to exert suppressive effects on CD4+ T cells (Leavy 2010). Another molecule of interest with respect to its general suppressive function in regard to human prostate cancer is programmed death 1 or PD-1. PD-1 is an inhibitory marker on T cells and is associated with a non-functional or "exhausted" phenotype (Barber et al. 2006; Chen 2004; Freeman et al. 2000). This molecule along with its ligand, PD-L1, may serve as a method of immune escape in human tumors. As such, the PD-1 pathway has been targeted in multiple immunotherapy strategies for different cancers, and preliminary studies in human trials remain promising (Dotti 2009; Turnis et al. 2012). At least two studies have assayed for the presence of PD-1 in prostate tumors. One study identified very high levels of PD-1 expression (close to 90 % of prostate-infiltrating CD8+ T cells in some patients) on prostate-infiltrating CD8+ lymphocytes isolated from prostatectomy tissues and assayed by flow cytometry (Sfanos et al. 2009a). PD-1 was likewise found to be elevated in CD8+ T cells in the peripheral blood of prostate cancer patients compared to controls (Sfanos et al. 2009a). In a separate study that assayed for the presence of PD-1^+ lymphocytes in prostate tissues via IHC, clusters of PD-1^+ T cells were found to surround most prostate tumors (Ebelt et al. 2009). Furthermore, overexpression of PD-1 in cancer patients may be associated with poor disease outcome, and this pathway remains of interest in prostate cancer immunotherapy strategies (Barach et al. 2011; Dulos et al. 2012).

7.3.3 B Cells and Prostate Cancer

Very few studies have assessed a potential contribution of B lymphocytes to prostate cancer etiology, although these cells are present in the prostate tumor microenvironment (Flammiger et al. 2012). One study of note, however, indicated a potential role for B cell-derived lymphotoxin in the development of hormone-refractory prostate cancer (Ammirante et al. 2010). Here, IKK-β (inhibitor of nuclear factor kappa-B kinase subunit beta) ablation in bone marrow-derived cells in mice allografted with MYC-CaP cells delayed the development of castration-resistant cancer after castration. IKK-β ablation in bone marrow-derived cells was found to have abolished lymphotoxin production by B cells, and this property was found to be specifically responsible for delayed growth of castration-independent cancer (Ammirante et al. 2010).

7.4 Concluding Remarks

Herein, we have attempted to comprehensively review the field to date regarding the role of both innate and adaptive immunity in the prostate cancer microenvironment. There are clear indications that prostate tumor-infiltrating immune cells contribute to prostate cancer initiation and/or progression; however, these cells may play a dichotomous role, acting in the context of both pro-tumorigenic and anti-tumorigenic depending on the stage of disease, type of inflammation, and/or the tumor microenvironment. Further research in human specimens as well as animal models of prostate cancer will assist in the elucidation of these roles, which may prove to be imperative in the rational design of prostate cancer prevention and treatment strategies.

References

Aaltomaa S, Lipponen P, Papinaho S, Kosma V (1993) Mast cells in breast cancer. Anticancer Res 13(3):785–788

Allavena P, Sica A, Garlanda C, Mantovani A (2008) The Yin-Yang of tumor-associated macrophages in neoplastic progression and immune surveillance. Immunol Rev 222(1):155–161. doi:10.1111/j.1600-065X.2008.00607.x

Ammirante M, Luo J-L, Grivennikov S, Nedospasov S, Karin M (2010) B-cell-derived lymphotoxin promotes castration-resistant prostate cancer. Nature 464:302–305. doi:10.1038/nature08782

Andreani V, Gatti G, Simonella L, Rivero V, Maccioni M (2007) Activation of toll-like receptor 4 on tumor cells in vitro inhibits subsequent tumor growth in vivo. Cancer Res 67(21):10519–10527. doi:10.1158/0008-5472.can-07-0079

Arock M, Ross E, Lai-Kuen R, Averlant G, Gao Z, Abraham SN (1998) Phagocytic and tumor necrosis factor alpha response of human mast cells following exposure to gram-negative and gram-positive bacteria. Infect Immun 66(12):6030–6034

Barach YS, Lee JS, Zang X (2011) T cell coinhibition in prostate cancer: new immune evasion pathways and emerging therapeutics. Trends Mol Med 17(1):47–55. doi:http://dx.doi.org/10.1016/j.molmed.2010.09.006

Barber DL, Wherry EJ, Masopust D, Zhu B, Allison JP, Sharpe AH, Freeman GJ, Ahmed R (2006) Restoring function in exhausted CD8 T cells during chronic viral infection. Nature 439(7077):682–687. doi:http://www.nature.com/nature/journal/v439/n7077/suppinfo/nature04444_S1.html

Bauskin AR, Brown DA, Junankar S, Rasiah KK, Eggleton S, Hunter M, Liu T, Smith D, Kuffner T, Pankhurst GJ, Johnen H, Russell PJ, Barret W, Stricker PD, Grygiel JJ, Kench JG, Henshall SM, Sutherland RL, Breit SN (2005) The propeptide mediates formation of stromal stores of PROMIC-1: role in determining prostate cancer outcome. Cancer Res 65(6):2330–2336. doi:10.1158/0008-5472.can-04-3827

Berger P, Perng D-W, Thabrew H, Compton SJ, Cairns JA, McEuen AR, Marthan R, Tunon De Lara J-M, Walls AF (2001) Tryptase and agonists of PAR-2 induce the proliferation of human airway smooth muscle cells. J Appl Physiol 91(3):1372–1379

Bethel CR, Faith D, Li X, Guan B, Hicks JL, Lan F, Jenkins RB, Bieberich CJ, De Marzo AM (2006) Decreased NKX3.1 protein expression in focal prostatic atrophy, prostatic intraepithelial neoplasia, and adenocarcinoma: association with Gleason score and chromosome 8p deletion. Cancer Res 66(22):10683–10690. doi:10.1158/0008-5472.can-06-0963

Bissell MJ, Hines WC (2011) Why don't we get more cancer? A proposed role of the microenvironment in restraining cancer progression. Nat Med 17(3):320–329. doi:http://www.nature.com/nm/journal/v17/n3/abs/nm.2328.html#supplementary-information

Bootcov MR, Bauskin AR, Valenzuela SM, Moore AG, Bansal M, He XY, Zhang HP, Donnellan M, Mahler S, Pryor K, Walsh BJ, Nicholson RC, Fairlie WD, Por SB, Robbins JM, Breit SN (1997) MIC-1, a novel macrophage inhibitory cytokine, is a divergent member of the TGF-β superfamily. Proc Natl Acad Sci 94(21):11514–11519

Breit SN, Johnen H, Cook AD, Tsai VWW, Mohammad MG, Kuffner T, Zhang HP, Marquis CP, Jiang L, Lockwood G, Lee-Ng M, Husaini Y, Wu L, Hamilton JA, Brown DA (2011) The TGF-β superfamily cytokine, MIC-1/GDF15: a pleotrophic cytokine with roles in inflammation, cancer and metabolism. Growth Factors 29(5):187–195. doi:10.3109/08977194.2011.607137

Brown DA, Stephan C, Ward RL, Law M, Hunter M, Bauskin AR, Amin J, Jung K, Diamandis EP, Hampton GM, Russell PJ, Giles GG, Breit SN (2006) Measurement of serum levels of macrophage inhibitory cytokine 1 combined with prostate-specific antigen improves prostate cancer diagnosis. Clin Cancer Res 12(1):89–96. doi:10.1158/1078-0432.ccr-05-1331

Brown DA, Lindmark F, Stattin P, Bälter K, Adami H-O, Zheng SL, Xu J, Isaacs WB, Grönberg H, Breit SN, Wiklund FE (2009) Macrophage inhibitory cytokine 1: a new prognostic marker in prostate cancer. Clin Cancer Res 15(21):6658–6664. doi:10.1158/1078-0432.ccr-08-3126

Cairns JA, Walls AF (1996) Mast cell tryptase is a mitogen for epithelial cells. Stimulation of IL-8 production and intercellular adhesion molecule-1 expression. J Immunol 156(1):275–283

Chan JK, Magistris A, Loizzi V, Lin F, Rutgers J, Osann K, DiSaia PJ, Samoszuk M (2005) Mast cell density, angiogenesis, blood clotting, and prognosis in women with advanced ovarian cancer. Gynecol Oncol 99(1):20–25. doi:http://dx.doi.org/10.1016/j.ygyno.2005.05.042

Chen L (2004) Co-inhibitory molecules of the B7-CD28 family in the control of T-cell immunity. Nat Rev Immunol 4(5):336–347

Chen Y-C, Giovannucci E, Lazarus R, Kraft P, Ketkar S, Hunter DJ (2005) Sequence variants of toll-like receptor 4 and susceptibility to prostate cancer. Cancer Res 65(24):11771–11778. doi:10.1158/0008-5472.can-05-2078

Chen Y-C, Giovannucci E, Kraft P, Lazarus R, Hunter DJ (2007) Association between toll-like receptor gene cluster (TLR6, TLR1, and TLR10) and prostate cancer. Cancer Epidemiol Biomark Prev 16(10):1982–1989. doi:10.1158/1055-9965.epi-07-0325

Cheng L, Wang J, Li X, Xing Q, Du P, Su L, Wang S (2011) Interleukin-6 induces Gr-1+CD11b+ myeloid cells to suppress CD8+ T cell-mediated liver injury in mice. PLoS ONE 6(3):e17631. doi:10.1371/journal.pone.0017631

Cheon EC, Khazaie K, Khan MW, Strouch MJ, Krantz SB, Phillips J, Blatner NR, Hix LM, Zhang M, Dennis KL, Salabat MR, Heiferman M, Grippo PJ, Munshi HG, Gounaris E, Bentrem DJ (2011) Mast cell 5-lipoxygenase activity promotes intestinal polyposis in APCΔ468 mice. Cancer Res 71(5):1627–1636. doi:10.1158/0008-5472.can-10-1923

Cheung PK, Woolcock B, Adomat H, Sutcliffe M, Bainbridge TC, Jones EC, Webber D, Kinahan T, Sadar M, Gleave ME, Vielkind J (2004) Protein profiling of microdissected prostate tissue links growth differentiation factor 15 to prostate carcinogenesis. Cancer Res 64(17):5929–5933. doi:10.1158/0008-5472.can-04-1216

Chin AI, Miyahira AK, Covarrubias A, Teague J, Guo B, Dempsey PW, Cheng G (2010) Toll-like receptor 3–mediated suppression of TRAMP prostate cancer shows the critical role of type I interferons in tumor immune surveillance. Cancer Res 70(7):2595–2603. doi:10.1158/0008-5472.can-09-1162

Chun JY, Nadiminty N, Dutt S, Lou W, Yang JC, Kung H-J, Evans CP, Gao AC (2009) Interleukin-6 regulates androgen synthesis in prostate cancer cells. Clin Cancer Res 15(15):4815–4822. doi:10.1158/1078-0432.ccr-09-0640

Clemente CG, Mihm MC, Bufalino R, Zurrida S, Collini P, Cascinelli N (1996) Prognostic value of tumor infiltrating lymphocytes in the vertical growth phase of primary cutaneous melanoma. Cancer 77(7):1303–1310. doi:10.1002/(sici)1097-0142(19960401)77:7<1303:aid-cncr12>3.3.co;2-0

Coussens LM, Raymond WW, Bergers G, Laig-Webster M, Behrendtsen O, Werb Z, Caughey GH, Hanahan D (1999) Inflammatory mast cells up-regulate angiogenesis during squamous epithelial carcinogenesis. Genes Dev 13(11):1382–1397

Crivellato E, Nico B, Mallardi F, Beltrami CA, Ribatti D (2003) Piecemeal degranulation as a general secretory mechanism? Anat Rec Part A Discov Mol Cell Evol Biol 274A(1):778–784. doi:10.1002/ar.a.10095

Dabiri S, Huntsman D, Makretsov N, Cheang M, Gilks B, Bajdik C, Gelmon K, Chia S, Hayes M (2004) The presence of stromal mast cells identifies a subset of invasive breast cancers with a favorable prognosis. Mod Pathol 17(8):1025

De Marzo AM (2007) The pathology of human prostatic atrophy and inflammation. In: Chung LK, Isaacs W, Simons J (eds) Prostate cancer. Contemporary Cancer Research. Humana Press, pp 33–48. doi:10.1007/978-1-59745-224-3_2

De Marzo AM, Marchi VL, Epstein JI, Nelson WG (1999) Proliferative inflammatory atrophy of the prostate: implications for prostatic carcinogenesis. Am J Pathol 155(6):1985–1992. doi:http://dx.doi.org/10.1016/S0002-9440(10)65517-4

De Marzo AM, Platz EA, Sutcliffe S, Xu J, Gronberg H, Drake CG, Nakai Y, Isaacs WB, Nelson WG (2007) Inflammation in prostate carcinogenesis. Nat Rev Cancer 7(4):256–269

Delongchamps NB, de la Roza G, Chandan V, Jones R, Sunheimer R, Threatte G, Jumbelic M, Haas GP (2008) Evaluation of prostatitis in autopsied prostates—is chronic inflammation more associated with benign prostatic hyperplasia or cancer? J Urol 179(5):1736–1740. doi:http://dx.doi.org/10.1016/j.juro.2008.01.034

Disis ML (2010) Immune regulation of cancer. J Clin Oncol 28(29):4531–4538. doi:10.1200/jco.2009.27.2146

Dotti G (2009) Blocking PD-1 in cancer immunotherapy. Blood 114(8):1457–1458. doi:10.1182/blood-2009-05-223412

Dulos J, Carven GJ, van Boxtel SJ, Evers S, Driessen-Engels LJA, Hobo W, Gorecka MA, de Haan AFJ, Mulders P, Punt CJA, Jacobs JFM, Schalken JA, Oosterwijk E, van Eenennaam H, Boots AM (2012) PD-1 blockade augments Th1 and Th17 and suppresses Th2 responses in peripheral blood from patients with prostate and advanced melanoma cancer. J Immunother 35(2):169–178 110.1097/CJI.1090b1013e318247a318244e318247

Ebelt K, Babaryka G, Frankenberger B, Stief CG, Eisenmenger W, Kirchner T, Schendel DJ, Noessner E (2009) Prostate cancer lesions are surrounded by FOXP3+, PD-1+ and B7-H1+ lymphocyte clusters. Eur J Cancer 45(9):1664–1672. doi:http://dx.doi.org/10.1016/j.ejca.2009.02.015

Edin S, Wikberg ML, Dahlin AM, Rutegård J, Öberg Å, Oldenborg P-A, Palmqvist R (2012) The distribution of macrophages with a M1 or M2 phenotype in relation to prognosis and the molecular characteristics of colorectal cancer. PLoS ONE 7(10):e47045. doi:10.1371/journal.pone.0047045

Ellem SJ, Wang H, Poutanen M, Risbridger GP (2009) Increased endogenous estrogen synthesis leads to the sequential induction of prostatic inflammation (prostatitis) and prostatic pre-malignancy. Am J Pathol 175(3):1187–1199. doi:http://dx.doi.org/10.2353/ajpath.2009.081107

Fisher E, Sass R, Watkins G, Johal J, Fisher B (1985) Tissue mast cells in breast cancer. Breast Cancer Res Treat 5(3):285–291. doi:10.1007/bf01806023

Fisher ER, Paik SM, Rockette H, Jones J, Caplan R, Fisher B (1989) Prognostic significance of eosinophils and mast cells in rectal cancer: findings from the National Surgical Adjuvant Breast and Bowel Project (protocol R-01). Human Pathol 20(2):159–163. doi:http://dx.doi.org/10.1016/0046-8177(89)90180-9

Flammiger A, Bayer F, Cirugeda-Kühnert A, Huland H, Tennstedt P, Simon R, Minner S, Bokemeyer C, Sauter G, Schlomm T, Trepel M (2012) Intratumoral T but not B lymphocytes are related to clinical outcome in prostate cancer. APMIS 120(11):901–908. doi:10.1111/j.1600-0463.2012.02924.x

Fleischmann A, Schlomm T, Köllermann J, Sekulic N, Huland H, Mirlacher M, Sauter G, Simon R, Erbersdobler A (2009) Immunological microenvironment in prostate cancer: high mast cell densities are associated with favorable tumor characteristics and good prognosis. Prostate 69(9):976–981. doi:10.1002/pros.20948

Forssell J, Öberg Å, Henriksson ML, Stenling R, Jung A, Palmqvist R (2007) High macrophage infiltration along the tumor front correlates with improved survival in colon cancer. Clin Cancer Res 13(5):1472–1479. doi:10.1158/1078-0432.ccr-06-2073

Freeman GJ, Long AJ, Iwai Y, Bourque K, Chernova T, Nishimura H, Fitz LJ, Malenkovich N, Okazaki T, Byrne MC, Horton HF, Fouser L, Carter L, Ling V, Bowman MR, Carreno BM, Collins M, Wood CR, Honjo T (2000) Engagement of the PD-1 immunoinhibitory receptor by a novel B7 family member leads to negative regulation of lymphocyte activation. J Exp Med 192(7):1027–1034. doi:10.1084/jem.192.7.1027

Frungieri MB, Weidinger S, Meineke V, Köhn FM, Mayerhofer A (2002) Proliferative action of mast-cell tryptase is mediated by PAR2, COX2, prostaglandins, and PPARγ: possible relevance to human fibrotic disorders. Proc Natl Acad Sci 99(23):15072–15077. doi:10.1073/pnas.232422999

Fujita K, Hosomi M, Tanigawa G, Okumi M, Fushimi H, Yamaguchi S (2011) Prostatic inflammation detected in initial biopsy specimens and urinary pyuria are predictors of negative repeat prostate biopsy. J Urol 185(5):1722–1727. doi:http://dx.doi.org/10.1016/j.juro.2010.12.058

Galinsky DST, Nechushtan H (2008) Mast cells and cancer—no longer just basic science. Crit Rev Oncol/Hematol 68(2):115–130. doi:http://dx.doi.org/10.1016/j.critrevonc.2008.06.001

Galli SJ (2000) Mast cells and basophils. Curr Opin Hematol 7(1):32–39

Galli R, Starace D, Busà R, Angelini DF, Paone A, De Cesaris P, Filippini A, Sette C, Battistini L, Ziparo E, Riccioli A (2010) TLR stimulation of prostate tumor cells induces chemokine-mediated recruitment of specific immune cell types. J Immunol 184(12):6658–6669. doi:10.4049/jimmunol.0902401

Gocheva V, Wang H-W, Gadea BB, Shree T, Hunter KE, Garfall AL, Berman T, Joyce JA (2010) IL-4 induces cathepsin protease activity in tumor-associated macrophages to promote cancer growth and invasion. Genes Dev 24(3):241–255. doi:10.1101/gad.1874010

Gonzalez-Reyes S, Fernandez J, Gonzalez L, Aguirre A, Suarez A, Gonzalez J, Escaff S, Vizoso F (2011) Study of TLR3, TLR4, and TLR9 in prostate carcinomas and their association with biochemical recurrence. Cancer Immunol Immunother 60(2):217–226

Gooch JL, Lee AV, Yee D (1998) Interleukin 4 inhibits growth and induces apoptosis in human breast cancer cells. Cancer Res 58(18):4199–4205

Gordon JR, Galli SJ (1990) Mast cells as a source of both preformed and immunologically inducible TNF-[alpha]/cachectin. Nature 346(6281):274–276

Gordon J, Burd P, Galli S (1990) Mast cells as a source of multifunctional cytokines. Immunol Today 11(12):458–464

Gounaris E, Erdman SE, Restaino C, Gurish MF, Friend DS, Gounari F, Lee DM, Zhang G, Glickman JN, Shin K, Rao VP, Poutahidis T, Weissleder R, McNagny KM, Khazaie K (2007) Mast cells are an essential hematopoietic component for polyp development. Proc Natl Acad Sci 104(50):19977–19982. doi:10.1073/pnas.0704620104

Grivennikov SI, Wang K, Mucida D, Stewart CA, Schnabl B, Jauch D, Taniguchi K, Yu G-Y, Osterreicher CH, Hung KE, Datz C, Feng Y, Fearon ER, Oukka M, Tessarollo L, Coppola V, Yarovinsky F, Cheroutre H, Eckmann L, Trinchieri G, Karin M (2012) Adenoma-linked barrier defects and microbial products drive IL-23/IL-17-mediated tumour growth. Nature 491(7423):254–258. doi:http://www.nature.com/nature/journal/v491/n7423/abs/nature11465.html#supplementary-information

Gruber BL, Kew RR, Jelaska A, Marchese MJ, Garlick J, Ren S, Schwartz LB, Korn JH (1997) Human mast cells activate fibroblasts: tryptase is a fibrogenic factor stimulating collagen messenger ribonucleic acid synthesis and fibroblast chemotaxis. J Immunol 158(5):2310–2317

Gui-zhong LI, Libo M, Guanglin H, Jianwei W (2011) The correlation of extent and grade of inflammation with serum PSA levels in patients with IV prostatitis. Int Urol Nephrol 43(2):295–301. doi:10.1007/s11255-010-9825-5

Gurish MF, Pear WS, Stevens RL, Scott ML, Sokol K, Ghildyal N, Webster MJ, Hu X, Austen KF, Baltimore D, Friend DS (1995) Tissue-regulated differentiation and maturation of a v-abl-immortalized mast cell-committed progenitor. Immunity 3(2):175–186

Hagemann T, Balkwill F, Lawrence T (2007) Inflammation and cancer: a double-edged sword. Cancer Cell 12(4):300–301. doi:http://dx.doi.org/10.1016/j.ccr.2007.10.005

Hanahan D, Weinberg Robert A (2011) Hallmarks of cancer: the next generation. Cell 144(5):646–674. doi:http://dx.doi.org/10.1016/j.cell.2011.02.013

Hao N-B, Lü M-H, Fan Y-H, Cao Y-L, Zhang Z-R, Yang S-M (2012) Macrophages in tumor microenvironments and the progression of tumors. Clin Dev Immunol 2012:11. doi:10.1155/2012/948098

Harashima N, Inao T, Imamura R, Okano S, Suda T, Harada M (2012) Roles of the PI3K/Akt pathway and autophagy in TLR3 signaling-induced apoptosis and growth arrest of human prostate cancer cells. Cancer Immunol Immunother 61(5):667–676. doi:10.1007/s00262-011-1132-1

Herroon MK, Rajagurubandara E, Rudy DL, Chalasani A, Hardaway AL, Podgorski I (2013) Macrophage cathepsin K promotes prostate tumor progression in bone. Oncogene 32(12):1580–1593. doi:http://www.nature.com/onc/journal/v32/n12/suppinfo/onc2012166s1.html

Hobisch A, Rogatsch H, Hittmair A, Fuchs D, Bartsch G, Klocker H, Culig Z (2000) Immunohistochemical localization of interleukin-6 and its receptor in benign, premalignant and malignant prostate tissue. J Pathol 191(3):239–244. doi:10.1002/1096-9896(2000)9999:9999<:aid-path633>3.0.co;2-x

Hood BL, Darfler MM, Guiel TG, Furusato B, Lucas DA, Ringeisen BR, Sesterhenn IA, Conrads TP, Veenstra TD, Krizman DB (2005) Proteomic analysis of formalin-fixed prostate cancer tissue. Mol Cell Proteomics 4(11):1741–1753. doi:10.1074/mcp.M500102-MCP200

Horner M, Ries L, Krapcho M, Neyman N, Aminou R, Howlader N, Altekruse SF, Feuer EJ, Huang L, Mariotto A, Miller BA, Lewis DR, Eisner MP, Stinchcomb DG, E BK (2009) SEER Cancer Statistics Review, 1975–2006. National Cancer Institute, Bethesda, MD

Iamaroon A, Pongsiriwet S, Jittidecharaks S, Pattanaporn K, Prapayasatok S, Wanachantararak S (2003) Increase of mast cells and tumor angiogenesis in oral squamous cell carcinoma. J Oral Pathol Med 32(4):195–199. doi:10.1034/j.1600-0714.2003.00128.x

Iliopoulos D, Hirsch HA, Wang G, Struhl K (2011) Inducible formation of breast cancer stem cells and their dynamic equilibrium with non-stem cancer cells via IL6 secretion. Proc Natl Acad Sci 108(4):1397–1402. doi:10.1073/pnas.1018898108

Irani AA, Schechter NM, Craig SS, DeBlois G, Schwartz LB (1986) Two types of human mast cells that have distinct neutral protease compositions. Proc Natl Acad Sci 83(12):4464–4468

Irani J, Goujon J-M, Ragni E, Peyrat L, Hubert J, Saint F, Mottet N (1999) High-grade inflammation in prostate cancer as a prognostic factor for biochemical recurrence after radical prostatectomy. Urology 54(3):467–472. doi:http://dx.doi.org/10.1016/S0090-4295(99)00152-1

Johansson A, Rudolfsson S, Hammarsten P, Halin S, Pietras K, Jones J, Stattin P, Egevad L, Granfors T, Wikström P, Bergh A (2010) Mast cells are novel independent prognostic markers in prostate cancer and represent a target for therapy. Am J Pathol 177(2):1031–1041. doi:http://dx.doi.org/10.2353/ajpath.2010.100070

Kaler P, Godasi B, Augenlicht L, Klampfer L (2009) The NF-kappaB/AKT-dependent Induction of Wnt signaling in colon cancer cells by macrophages and IL-1beta. Cancer Microenviron

Kang J-C, Chen J-S, Lee C-H, Chang J-J, Shieh Y-S (2010) Intratumoral macrophage counts correlate with tumor progression in colorectal cancer. J Surg Oncol 102(3):242–248. doi:10.1002/jso.21617

Karan D, Holzbeierlein J, Thrasher JB (2009) Macrophage inhibitory cytokine-1: possible bridge molecule of inflammation and prostate cancer. Cancer Res 69(1):2–5. doi:10.1158/0008-5472.can-08-1230

Karja V, Aaltomaa S, Lipponen P, Isotalo T, Talja M, Mokka R (2005) Tumour-infiltrating lymphocytes: a prognostic factor of PSA-free survival in patients with local prostate carcinoma treated by radical prostatectomy. Anticancer Res 25(6C):4435–4438

Kazma R, Mefford JA, Cheng I, Plummer SJ, Levin AM, Rybicki BA, Casey G, Witte JS (2012) Association of the innate immunity and inflammation pathway with advanced prostate cancer risk. PLoS ONE 7(12):e51680. doi:10.1371/journal.pone.0051680

Kennedy R, Celis E (2008) Multiple roles for CD4+ T cells in anti-tumor immune responses. Immunol Rev 222(1):129–144. doi:10.1111/j.1600-065X.2008.00616.x

Khazaie K, Blatner N, Khan M, Gounari F, Gounaris E, Dennis K, Bonertz A, Tsai F, Strouch M, Cheon E, Phillips J, Beckhove P, Bentrem D (2011) The significant role of mast cells in cancer. Cancer Metastasis Rev 30(1):45–60

Kim H, Bae J, Chang I, Kim K, Lee J, Shin H, Lee J, Kim W-J, Kim W, Myung S (2012) Sequence variants of toll-like receptor 4 (TLR4) and the risk of prostate cancer in Korean men. World J Urol 30(2):225–232. doi:10.1007/s00345-011-0690-3

Kimura A, Kishimoto T (2010) IL-6: regulator of Treg/Th17 balance. Eur J Immunol 40(7):1830–1835. doi:10.1002/eji.201040391

Kiniwa Y, Miyahara Y, Wang HY, Peng W, Peng G, Wheeler TM, Thompson TC, Old LJ, Wang R-F (2007) CD8+ Foxp3+ regulatory T cells mediate immunosuppression in prostate cancer. Clin Cancer Res 13(23):6947–6958. doi:10.1158/1078-0432.ccr-07-0842

Krieger J, Nyberg L, Nickel J (1999) NIH consensus definition and classification of prostatitis. JAMA 282(3):236–237. doi:10-1001/pubs.JAMA-ISSN-0098-7484-282-3-jac90006

Krishnaswamy G, Kelley J, Johnson D, Youngberg G, Stone W, Huang S, Bieber J, Chi D (2001) The human mast cell: functions in physiology and disease. Front Biosci 6:D1109–D1127

LaBarge MA, Nelson CM, Villadsen R, Fridriksdottir A, Ruth JR, Stampfer MR, Petersen OW, Bissell MJ (2009) Human mammary progenitor cell fate decisions are products of interactions with combinatorial microenvironments. Integr Biol 1(1):70–79

Lacy P, Stow JL (2011) Cytokine release from innate immune cells: association with diverse membrane trafficking pathways. Blood 118(1):9–18. doi:10.1182/blood-2010-08-265892

Leavy O (2010) Regulatory T cells: CD8+ TReg cells join the fold. Nat Rev Immunol 10(10):680–681

Lee Y-M, Jippo T, Kim D-K, Katsu Y, Tsujino K, Morii E, Kim H-M, Adachi S, Nawa Y, Kitamura Y (1998) Alteration of protease expression phenotype of mouse peritoneal mast cells by changing the microenvironment as demonstrated by in situ hybridization histochemistry. Am J Pathol 153(3):931–936. doi:http://dx.doi.org/10.1016/S0002-9440(10)65634-9

Lee SO, Lou W, Hou M, de Miguel F, Gerber L, Gao AC (2003) Interleukin-6 promotes androgen-independent growth in LNCaP human prostate cancer cells. Clin Cancer Res 9(1):370–376

Levi-Schaffer F, Piliponsky AM (2003) Tryptase, a novel link between allergic inflammation and fibrosis. Trends Immunol 24(4):158–161. doi:http://dx.doi.org/10.1016/S1471-4906(03)00058-9

Li Y-W, Qiu S-J, Fan J, Gao Q, Zhou J, Xiao Y-S, Xu Y, Wang X-Y, Sun J, Huang X-W (2009a) Tumor-infiltrating macrophages can predict favorable prognosis in hepatocellular carcinoma after resection. J Cancer Res Clin Oncol 135(3):439–449. doi:10.1007/s00432-008-0469-0

Li Y-Y, Hsieh L-L, Tang R-P, Liao S-K, Yeh K-Y (2009b) Interleukin-6 (IL-6) released by macrophages induces IL-6 secretion in the human colon cancer HT-29 cell line. Hum Immunol 70(3):151–158. doi:http://dx.doi.org/10.1016/j.humimm.2009.01.004

Lindahl C, Simonsson M, Bergh A, Thysell E, Antti H, Sund M, Wikstrom P (2009) Increased levels of macrophage-secreted cathepsin S during prostate cancer progression in TRAMP mice and patients. Cancer Genomics Proteomics 6(3):149–159

Lissbrant I, Stattin P, Wikstrom P, Damber J, Egevad L, Bergh A (2000) Tumor associated macrophages in human prostate cancer: relation to clinicopathological variables and survival. Int J Oncol 17(3):445–451

Liu T, Bauskin AR, Zaunders J, Brown DA, Pankurst S, Russell PJ, Breit SN (2003) Macrophage inhibitory cytokine 1 reduces cell adhesion and induces apoptosis in prostate cancer cells. Cancer Res 63(16):5034–5040

Liu S, Lachapelle J, Leung S, Gao D, Foulkes W, Nielsen T (2012) CD8+ lymphocyte infiltration is an independent favorable prognostic indicator in basal-like breast cancer. Breast Cancer Res 14(2):R48

Loberg RD, Day LL, Harwood J, Ying C, St John LN, Giles R, Neeley CK, Pienta KJ (2006) CCL2 (Monocyte chemoattractant protein-1) is a potent regulator of prostate cancer cell migration and proliferation. Neoplasia 8(7):578–586

Lucia M, Lambert J, Platz EA, De Marzo AM (2010) Inflammation as a target in prostate cancer. In: Figg WD, Chau CH, Small EJ (eds) Drug management of prostate cancer. Springer, New York, NY, pp 375–386

Malinowska K, Neuwirt H, Cavarretta IT, Bektic J, Steiner H, Dietrich H, Moser PL, Fuchs D, Hobisch A, Culig Z (2009) Interleukin-6 stimulation of growth of prostate cancer in vitro and in vivo through activation of the androgen receptor. Endocr Relat Cancer 16(1):155–169. doi:10.1677/erc-08-0174

Maltby S, Khazaie K, McNagny KM (2009) Mast cells in tumor growth: angiogenesis, tissue remodelling and immune-modulation. Biochimica et Biophysica Acta (BBA) Rev Cancer 1796(1):19–26. doi:http://dx.doi.org/10.1016/j.bbcan.2009.02.001

Martin F, Apetoh L, Ghiringhelli F (2012) Controversies on the role of Th17 in cancer: a TGF-β-dependent immunosuppressive activity? Trends Mol Med 18(12):742–749

McArdle PA, Canna K, McMillan DC, McNicol AM, Campbell R, Underwood MA (2004) The relationship between T-lymphocyte subset infiltration and survival in patients with prostate cancer. Br J Cancer 91(3):541–543

Miller AM, Lundberg K, Özenci V, Banham AH, Hellström M, Egevad L, Pisa P (2006) CD4+CD25high T cells are enriched in the tumor and peripheral blood of prostate cancer patients. J Immunol 177(10):7398–7405

Mizutani K, Sud S, McGregor N, Martinovski G, Rice B, Craig M, Varsos Z, Roca H, Pienta K (2009) The chemokine CCL2 increases prostate tumor growth and bone metastasis through macrophage and osteoclast recruitment. Neoplasia 11(11):1235–1242

Molin D (2004) Bystander cells and prognosis in Hodgkin lymphoma. Review based on a doctoral thesis. Ups J Med Sci 109(3):179–228

Molin D, Edström A, Glimelius I, Glimelius B, Nilsson G, Sundström C, Enblad G (2002) Mast cell infiltration correlates with poor prognosis in Hodgkin's lymphoma. Br J Haematol 119(1):122–124. doi:10.1046/j.1365-2141.2002.03768.x

Mougiakakos D, Choudhury A, Lladser A, Kiessling R, Johansson CC (2010) Regulatory T cells in cancer. In: George FVW, George K (eds) Advances in cancer research, vol 107. Academic Press, pp 57–117. doi:http://dx.doi.org/10.1016/S0065-230X(10)07003-X

Naito Y, Saito K, Shiiba K, Ohuchi A, Saigenji K, Nagura H, Ohtani H (1998) CD8+ T cells infiltrated within cancer cell nests as a prognostic factor in human colorectal cancer. Cancer Res 58(16):3491–3494

Nakamura T, Scorilas A, Stephan C, Yousef GM, Kristiansen G, Jung K, Diamandis EP (2003) Quantitative analysis of macrophage inhibitory cytokine-1 (MIC-1) gene expression in human prostatic tissues. Br J Cancer 88(7):1101–1104

Nakayama M, Bennett CJ, Hicks JL, Epstein JI, Platz EA, Nelson WG, De Marzo AM (2003) Hypermethylation of the human glutathione S-transferase-π gene (GSTP1) CpG island is present in a subset of proliferative inflammatory atrophy lesions but not in normal or hyperplastic epithelium of the prostate: a detailed study using laser-capture microdissection. Am J Pathol 163(3):923–933. doi:http://dx.doi.org/10.1016/S0002-9440(10)63452-9

Nakayama T, Yao L, Tosato G (2004) Mast cell-derived angiopoietin-1 plays a critical role in the growth of plasma cell tumors. J Clin Investig 114(9):1317–1325. doi:10.1172/jci22089

Nelson WG, De Marzo AM, Isaacs WB (2003) Prostate cancer. N Engl J Med 349(4):366–381. doi:10.1056/NEJMra021562

Nelson W, Sfanos K, DeMarzo A, Yegnasubramanian S (2013) Prostate inflammation and prostate cancer. In: Klein EA, Jones JS (eds) Management of prostate cancer, current clinical urology. Humana Press, New York, NY, pp 103–115

Nickel JC, Downey J, Young I, Boag S (1999) Asymptomatic inflammation and/ or infection in benign prostatic hyperplasia. BJU International 84(9):976–981. doi:10.1046/j.1464-410x.1999.00352.x

Nonomura N, Takayama H, Nishimura K, Oka D, Nakai Y, Shiba M, Tsujimura A, Nakayama M, Aozasa K, Okuyama A (2007) Decreased number of mast cells infiltrating into needle biopsy specimens leads to a better prognosis of prostate cancer. Br J Cancer 97(7):952–956

Nonomura N, Takayama H, Nakayama M, Nakai Y, Kawashima A, Mukai M, Nagahara A, Aozasa K, Tsujimura A (2011) Infiltration of tumour-associated macrophages in prostate biopsy specimens is predictive of disease progression after hormonal therapy for prostate cancer. BJU Int 107(12):1918–1922. doi:10.1111/j.1464-410X.2010.09804.x

Okamoto M, Lee C, Oyasu R (1997) Interleukin-6 as a paracrine and autocrine growth factor in human prostatic carcinoma cells in vitro. Cancer Res 57(1):141–146

Ostrand-Rosenberg S, Sinha P (2009) Myeloid-derived suppressor cells: linking inflammation and cancer. J Immunol 182(8):4499–4506. doi:10.4049/jimmunol.0802740

Palapattu GS, Sutcliffe S, Bastian PJ, Platz EA, De Marzo AM, Isaacs WB, Nelson WG (2005) Prostate carcinogenesis and inflammation: emerging insights. Carcinogenesis 26(7):1170–1181. doi:10.1093/carcin/bgh317

Paone A, Starace D, Galli R, Padula F, De Cesaris P, Filippini A, Ziparo E, Riccioli A (2008) Toll-like receptor 3 triggers apoptosis of human prostate cancer cells through a PKC-α-dependent mechanism. Carcinogenesis 29(7):1334–1342. doi:10.1093/carcin/bgn149

Pardoll D (2002) T cells take aim at cancer. Proc Natl Acad Sci 99(25):15840–15842. doi:10.1073/pnas.262669499

Pittoni P, Colombo MP (2012) The dark side of mast cell-targeted therapy in prostate cancer. Cancer Res 72(4):831–835. doi:10.1158/0008-5472.can-11-3110

Pittoni P, Tripodo C, Piconese S, Mauri G, Parenza M, Rigoni A, Sangaletti S, Colombo MP (2011) Mast cell targeting hampers prostate adenocarcinoma development but promotes the occurrence of highly malignant neuroendocrine cancers. Cancer Res. doi:10.1158/0008-5472.can-11-1637

Platz EA, De Marzo AM, Erlinger TP, Rifai N, Visvanathan K, Hoffman SC, Helzlsouer KJ (2004) No association between pre-diagnostic plasma C-reactive protein concentration and subsequent prostate cancer. Prostate 59(4):393–400. doi:10.1002/pros.10368

Ports MO, Nagle RB, Pond GD, Cress AE (2009) Extracellular engagement of α6 integrin inhibited urokinase-type plasminogen activator-mediated cleavage and delayed human prostate bone metastasis. Cancer Res 69(12):5007–5014. doi:10.1158/0008-5472.can-09-0354

Powell IJ, Dyson G, Land S, Ruterbusch J, Bock CH, Lenk S, Herawi M, Everson RB, Giroux CN, Schwartz AG, Bollig-Fischer A (2013) Genes associated with prostate cancer are differentially expressed in African American and European American men. Cancer Epidemiol Biomark Prev. doi:10.1158/1055-9965.epi-12-1238

Proctor MJ, Talwar D, Balmar SM, O'Reilly DSJ, Foulis AK, Horgan PG, Morrison DS, McMillan DC (2010) The relationship between the presence and site of cancer, an inflammation-based prognostic score and biochemical parameters. Initial results of the Glasgow inflammation outcome study. Br J Cancer 103(6):870–876

Punturieri A, Filippov S, Allen E, Caras I, Murray R, Reddy V, Weiss SJ (2000) Regulation of elastinolytic cysteine proteinase activity in normal and cathepsin K–deficient human macrophages. J Exp Med 192(6):789–800. doi:10.1084/jem.192.6.789

Putzi MJ, De Marzo AM (2000) Morphologic transitions between proliferative inflammatory atrophy and high-grade prostatic intraepithelial neoplasia. Urology 56(5):828–832. doi:http://dx.doi.org/10.1016/S0090-4295(00)00776-7

Rajput A, Turbin D, Cheang M, Voduc D, Leung S, Gelmon K, Gilks CB, Huntsman D (2008) Stromal mast cells in invasive breast cancer are a marker of favourable prognosis: a study of 4,444 cases. Breast Cancer Res Treat 107(2):249–257. doi:10.1007/s10549-007-9546-3

Rakoff-Nahoum S, Medzhitov R (2009) Toll-like receptors and cancer. Nat Rev Cancer 9(1):57–63

Rao UNM, Lee SJ, Luo W, Mihm MC, Kirkwood JM (2010) Presence of tumor-infiltrating lymphocytes and a dominant nodule within primary melanoma are prognostic factors for relapse-free survival of patients with thick (T4) primary melanoma: pathologic analysis of the E1690 and E1694 intergroup trials. Am J Clin Pathol 133(4):646–653. doi:10.1309/ajcptxmefovywda6

Rasiah KK, Kench JG, Gardiner-Garden M, Biankin AV, Golovsky D, Brenner PC, Kooner R, O'Neill GF, Turner JJ, Delprado W, Lee CS, Brown DA, Breit SN, Grygiel JJ, Horvath LG, Stricker PD, Sutherland RL, Henshall SM (2006) Aberrant neuropeptide Y and macrophage inhibitory cytokine-1 expression are early events in prostate cancer development and are associated with poor prognosis. Cancer Epidemiol Biomark Prev 15(4):711–716. doi:10.1158/1055-9965.epi-05-0752

Reams RR, Agrawal D, Davis M, Yoder S, Odedina F, Kumar N, Higginbotham J, Akinremi T, Suther S, Soliman K (2009) Microarray comparison of prostate tumor gene expression in African-American and Caucasian American males: a pilot project study. Infect Agents Cancer 4(Suppl 1):S3

Ribatti D, Vacca A, Nico B, Quondamatteo F, Ria R, Minischetti M, Marzullo A, Herken R, Roncali L, Dammacco F (1999) Bone marrow angiogenesis and mast cell density increase simultaneously with progression of human multiple myeloma. Br J Cancer 79(3–4):451–455

Ribatti D, Vacca A, Ria R, Marzullo A, Nico B, Filotico R, Roncali L, Dammacco F (2003) Neovascularisation, expression of fibroblast growth factor-2, and mast cells with tryptase activity increase simultaneously with pathological progression in human malignant melanoma. Eur J Cancer 39(5):666–674. doi:http://dx.doi.org/10.1016/S0959-8049(02)00150-8

Ribatti D, Finato N, Crivellato E, Marzullo A, Mangieri D, Nico B, Vacca A, Beltrami CA (2005) Neovascularization and mast cells with tryptase activity increase simultaneously with pathologic progression in human endometrial cancer. Am J Obstet Gynecol 193(6):1961–1965. doi:http://dx.doi.org/10.1016/j.ajog.2005.04.055

Richardsen E, Uglehus RD, Due J, Busch C, Busund LTR (2008) The prognostic impact of M-CSF, CSF-1 receptor, CD68 and CD3 in prostatic carcinoma. Histopathology 53(1):30–38. doi:10.1111/j.1365-2559.2008.03058.x

Rigamonti N, Capuano G, Ricupito A, Jachetti E, Grioni M, Generoso L, Freschi M, Bellone M (2011) Modulators of arginine metabolism do not impact on peripheral T-cell tolerance and disease progression in a model of spontaneous prostate cancer. Clin Cancer Res 17(5):1012–1023. doi:10.1158/1078-0432.ccr-10-2547

Roca H, Varsos ZS, Sud S, Craig MJ, Ying C, Pienta KJ (2009) CCL2 and interleukin-6 promote survival of human CD11b+ peripheral blood mononuclear cells and induce M2-type macrophage polarization. J Biol Chem 284(49):34342–34354. doi:10.1074/jbc.M109.042671

Sari S, Çandir Ö, Öztürk K (1999) Mast cell variations in tumour tissue and with histopathological grading in specimens of prostatic adenocarcinoma. BJU Int 84(7):851–853. doi:10.1046/j.1464-410x.1999.00245.x

Schumacher K, Haensch W, Röefzaad C, Schlag PM (2001) Prognostic significance of activated CD8+ T cell infiltrations within esophageal carcinomas. Cancer Res 61(10):3932–3936

Selander KS, Brown DA, Sequeiros GB, Hunter M, Desmond R, Parpala T, Risteli J, Breit SN, Jukkola-Vuorinen A (2007) Serum macrophage inhibitory cytokine-1 concentrations correlate with the presence of prostate cancer bone metastases. Cancer Epidemiol Biomark Prev 16(3):532–537. doi:10.1158/1055-9965.epi-06-0841

Sfanos KS, De Marzo AM (2012) Prostate cancer and inflammation: the evidence. Histopathology 60(1):199–215. doi:10.1111/j.1365-2559.2011.04033.x

Sfanos KS, Bruno TC, Maris CH, Xu L, Thoburn CJ, DeMarzo AM, Meeker AK, Isaacs WB, Drake CG (2008) Phenotypic analysis of prostate-infiltrating lymphocytes reveals TH17 and Treg skewing. Clin Cancer Res 14(11):3254–3261. doi:10.1158/1078-0432.ccr-07-5164

Sfanos KS, Bruno TC, Meeker AK, De Marzo AM, Isaacs WB, Drake CG (2009a) Human prostate-infiltrating CD8+ T lymphocytes are oligoclonal and PD-1+. Prostate 69(15):1694–1703. doi:10.1002/pros.21020

Sfanos KS, Wilson BA, De Marzo AM, Isaacs WB (2009b) Acute inflammatory proteins constitute the organic matrix of prostatic corpora amylacea and calculi in men with prostate cancer. Proc Natl Acad Sci 106(9):3443–3448. doi:10.1073/pnas.0810473106

Shafique K, Proctor MJ, McMillan DC, Qureshi K, Leung H, Morrison DS (2012) Systemic inflammation and survival of patients with prostate cancer: evidence from the Glasgow inflammation outcome study. Prostate Cancer Prostatic Dis 15(2):195–201

Shimura S, Yang G, Ebara S, Wheeler TM, Frolov A, Thompson TC (2000) Reduced infiltration of tumor-associated macrophages in human prostate cancer: association with cancer progression. Cancer Res 60(20):5857–5861

Shui IM, Stark JR, Penney KL, Schumacher FR, Epstein MM, Pitt MJ, Stampfer MJ, Tamimi RM, Lindstrom S, Sesso HD, Fall K, Ma J, Kraft P, Giovannucci E, Mucci LA (2012) Genetic variation in the toll-like receptor 4 and prostate cancer incidence and mortality. Prostate 72(2):209–216. doi:10.1002/pros.21423

Smith PC, Hobisch A, Lin D-L, Culig Z, Keller ET (2001) Interleukin-6 and prostate cancer progression. Cytokine Growth Factor Rev 12(1):33–40. doi:http://dx.doi.org/10.1016/S1359-6101(00)00021-6

Sroka IC, Sandoval CP, Chopra H, Gard JMC, Pawar SC, Cress AE (2011) Macrophage-dependent cleavage of the laminin receptor α6β1 in prostate cancer. Mol Cancer Res 9(10):1319–1328. doi:10.1158/1541-7786.mcr-11-0080

Stimac G, Reljic A, Spajic B, Dimanovski J, Ruzic B, Ulamec M, Sonicki Z, Kraus O (2009) Aggressiveness of inflammation in histological prostatitis-correlation with total and free prostate specific antigen levels in men with biochemical criteria for prostate biopsy. Scott Med J 54(3):8–12. doi:10.1258/rsmsmj.54.3.8

Strouch MJ, Cheon EC, Salabat MR, Krantz SB, Gounaris E, Melstrom LG, Dangi-Garimella S, Wang E, Munshi HG, Khazaie K, Bentrem DJ (2010) Crosstalk between mast cells and pancreatic cancer cells contributes to pancreatic tumor progression. Clin Cancer Res 16(8):2257–2265. doi:10.1158/1078-0432.ccr-09-1230

Sun J, Wiklund F, Zheng SL, Chang B, Bälter K, Li L, Johansson J-E, Li G, Adami H-O, Liu W, Tolin A, Turner AR, Meyers DA, Isaacs WB, Xu J, Grönberg H (2005) Sequence variants in toll-like receptor gene cluster (TLR6-TLR1-TLR10) and prostate cancer risk. J Natl Cancer Inst 97(7):525–532. doi:10.1093/jnci/dji070

Svensson RU, Haverkamp JM, Thedens DR, Cohen MB, Ratliff TL, Henry MD (2011) Slow disease progression in a C57BL/6 Pten-deficient mouse model of prostate cancer. Am J Pathol 179(1):502–512. doi:http://dx.doi.org/10.1016/j.ajpath.2011.03.014

Swann JB, Smyth MJ (2007) Immune surveillance of tumors. J Clin Investig 117(5):1137–1146. doi:10.1172/jci31405

Tanner J, Tosato G (1992) Regulation of B-cell growth and immunoglobulin gene transcription by interleukin-6. Blood 79(2):452–459

Theoharides TC, Conti P (2004) Mast cells: the JEKYLL and HYDE of tumor growth. Trends Immunol 25(5):235–241. doi:http://dx.doi.org/10.1016/j.it.2004.02.013

Tuna B, Yorukoglu K, Unlu M, Mungan MU, Kirkali Z (2006) Association of mast cells with microvessel density in renal cell carcinomas. European Urol 50(3):530–534. doi:http://dx.doi.org/10.1016/j.eururo.2005.12.040

Turnis ME, Korman AJ, Drake CG, Vignali DAA (2012) Combinatorial immunotherapy: PD-1 may not be LAG-ing behind any more. OncoImmunology 1(7):1172–1174

Twillie DA, Eisenberger MA, Carducci MA, Hseih W-S, Kim WY, Simons JW (1995) Interleukin-6: a candidate mediator of human prostate cancer morbidity. Urology 45(3):542–549. doi:http://dx.doi.org/10.1016/S0090-4295(99)80034-X

Ugurlu O, Yaris M, Oztekin CV, Kosan TM, Adsan O, Cetinkaya M (2010) Impacts of antibiotic and anti-inflammatory therapies on serum prostate-specific antigen levels in the presence of prostatic inflammation: a prospective randomized controlled trial. Urol Int 84(2):185–190. doi:10.1159/000277596

van Dijk M, Göransson SA, Strömblad S (2013) Cell to extracellular matrix interactions and their reciprocal nature in cancer. Exp Cell Res (0). doi:http://dx.doi.org/10.1016/j.yexcr.2013.02.006

Vasiljeva O, Papazoglou A, Krüger A, Brodoefel H, Korovin M, Deussing J, Augustin N, Nielsen BS, Almholt K, Bogyo M, Peters C, Reinheckel T (2006) Tumor cell-derived and macrophage-derived cathepsin B promotes progression and lung metastasis of mammary cancer. Cancer Res 66(10):5242–5250. doi:10.1158/0008-5472.can-05-4463

Vesalainen S, Lipponen P, Talja M, Syrjänen K (1994) Histological grade, perineural infiltration, tumour-infiltrating lymphocytes and apoptosis as determinants of long-term prognosis in prostatic adenocarcinoma. European J Cancer 30(12):1797–1803. doi:http://dx.doi.org/10.1016/0959-8049(94)E0159-2

Vesely MD, Kershaw MH, Schreiber RD, Smyth MJ (2011) Natural innate and adaptive immunity to cancer. Annu Rev Immunol 29(1):235–271. doi:10.1146/annurev-immunol- 031210-101324

Vogelstein B, Papadopoulos N, Velculescu VE, Zhou S, Diaz LA, Kinzler KW (2013) Cancer genome landscapes. Science 339(6127):1546–1558. doi:10.1126/science.1235122

Vykhovanets E, Maclennan G, Vykhovanets O, Gupta S (2011) IL-17 Expression by macrophages is associated with proliferative inflammatory atrophy lesions in prostate cancer patients. Int J Clin Exp Pathol 4(6):552–565

Wallace TA, Prueitt RL, Yi M, Howe TM, Gillespie JW, Yfantis HG, Stephens RM, Caporaso NE, Loffredo CA, Ambs S (2008) Tumor immunobiological differences in prostate cancer between African–American and European–American men. Cancer Res 68(3):927–936. doi:10.1158/0008-5472.can-07-2608

Wang W, Bergh A, Damber J-E (2005) Cyclooxygenase-2 expression correlates with local chronic inflammation and tumor neovascularization in human prostate cancer. Clin Cancer Res 11(9):3250–3256. doi:10.1158/1078-0432.ccr-04-2405

Wang W, Bergh A, Damber J-E (2009) Morphological transition of proliferative inflammatory atrophy to high-grade intraepithelial neoplasia and cancer in human prostate. Prostate 69(13):1378–1386. doi:10.1002/pros.20992

Welsh JB, Sapinoso LM, Su AI, Kern SG, Wang-Rodriguez J, Moskaluk CA, Frierson HF, Hampton GM (2001) Analysis of gene expression identifies candidate markers and pharmacological targets in prostate cancer. Cancer Res 61(16):5974–5978

Welsh JB, Sapinoso LM, Kern SG, Brown DA, Liu T, Bauskin AR, Ward RL, Hawkins NJ, Quinn DI, Russell PJ, Sutherland RL, Breit SN, Moskaluk CA, Frierson HF, Hampton GM (2003) Large-scale delineation of secreted protein biomarkers overexpressed in cancer tissue and serum. Proc Natl Acad Sci 100(6):3410–3415. doi:10.1073/pnas.0530278100

Welsh TJ, Green RH, Richardson D, Waller DA, O'Byrne KJ, Bradding P (2005) Macrophage and mast-cell invasion of tumor cell islets confers a marked survival advantage in non-small-cell lung cancer. J Clin Oncol 23(35):8959–8967. doi:10.1200/jco.2005.01.4910

Wiklund FE, Bennet AM, Magnusson PKE, Eriksson UK, Lindmark F, Wu L, Yaghoutyfam N, Marquis CP, Stattin P, Pedersen NL, Adami H-O, Grönberg H, Breit SN, Brown DA (2010) Macrophage inhibitory cytokine-1 (MIC-1/GDF15): a new marker of all-cause mortality. Aging Cell 9(6):1057–1064. doi:10.1111/j.1474-9726.2010.00629.x

Wilke CM, Kryczek I, Wei S, Zhao E, Wu K, Wang G, Zou W (2011) Th17 cells in cancer: help or hindrance? Carcinogenesis 32(5):643–649. doi:10.1093/carcin/bgr019

Wu C-T, Hsieh C-C, Lin C-C, Chen W-C, Hong J-H, Chen M-F (2012) Significance of IL-6 in the transition of hormone-resistant prostate cancer and the induction of myeloid-derived suppressor cells. J Mol Med 90(11):1343–1355. doi:10.1007/s00109-012-0916-x

Yang G, Addai J, W-h Tian, Frolov A, Wheeler TM, Thompson TC (2004) Reduced infiltration of class A scavenger receptor positive antigen-presenting cells is associated with prostate cancer progression. Cancer Res 64(6):2076–2082. doi:10.1158/0008-5472.can-03-4072

Yokokawa J, Cereda V, Remondo C, Gulley JL, Arlen PM, Schlom J, Tsang KY (2008) Enhanced functionality of CD4+CD25highFoxP3+ regulatory T cells in the peripheral blood of patients with prostate cancer. Clin Cancer Res 14(4):1032–1040. doi:10.1158/1078-0432.ccr-07-2056

Yoshii M, Jikuhara A, Mori S, Iwagaki H, Takahashi HK, Nishibori M, Tanaka N (2005) Mast cell tryptase stimulates DLD-1 carcinoma through prostaglandin- and MAP kinase-dependent manners. J Pharmacol Sci 98(4):450–458

Zhang L, Conejo-Garcia JR, Katsaros D, Gimotty PA, Massobrio M, Regnani G, Makrigiannakis A, Gray H, Schlienger K, Liebman MN, Rubin SC, Coukos G (2003) Intratumoral T cells, recurrence, and survival in epithelial ovarian cancer. N Engl J Med 348(3):203–213. doi:10.1056/NEJMoa020177

Zhang B, Rong G, Wei H, Zhang M, Bi J, Ma L, Xue X, Wei G, Liu X, Fang G (2008) The prevalence of Th17 cells in patients with gastric cancer. Biochem Biophys Res Commun 374(3):533–537. doi:http://dx.doi.org/10.1016/j.bbrc.2008.07.060

Zhang Q-w, Liu L, Gong C-Y, Shi H-S, Zeng Y-H, Wang X-Z, Zhao Y-W, Wei Y-Q (2012) Prognostic significance of tumor-associated macrophages in solid tumor: a meta-analysis of the literature. PLoS ONE 7(12):e50946. doi:10.1371/journal.pone.0050946

Zheng SL, Augustsson-Bälter K, Chang B, Hedelin M, Li L, Adami H-O, Bensen J, Li G, Johnasson J-E, Turner AR, Adams TS, Meyers DA, Isaacs WB, Xu J, Grönberg H (2004) Sequence variants of toll-like receptor 4 are associated with prostate cancer risk: results from the cancer prostate in Sweden Study. Cancer Res 64(8):2918–2922. doi:10.1158/0008-5472.can-03-3280

Zhou Q, Peng R-Q, Wu X-J, Xia Q, Hou J-H, Ding Y, Zhou Q-M, Zhang X, Pang Z-Z, Wan D-S, Zeng Y-X, Zhang X-S (2010) The density of macrophages in the invasive front is inversely correlated to liver metastasis in colon cancer. J Transl Med 8(1):13

Zou W, Restifo NP (2010) TH17 cells in tumour immunity and immunotherapy. Nat Rev Immunol 10(4):248–256

Chapter 8
The Role of Inflammation in Bladder Cancer

Georgios Gakis

Abstract The aim of this book chapter is to present the latest basic research developments on the role of inflammation in bladder cancer and provide insights into their future clinical significance in preventing bladder carcinogenesis and progression. Bladder cancer is a highly immunogenic malignancy. Urothelial cancer cells aim to manipulate the immune system by inhibiting its cytotoxic function while stimulating the secretion of growth promoting factors. Cytokine-induced imbalances in the distribution and differentiation of tumor-infiltrating cytotoxic cells can boost bladder cancer cell proliferation. Tumor-induced release of excessive amount of cytokines causes an "inflammatory storm" which drives metastasis formation via degradation of extracellular matrix proteins. Tumor-related selective cyclooxygenase-2 (COX-2) upregulation suppresses the cell-mediated immune response via aberrant prostaglandin metabolism resulting in failure of differentiation of myeloid cell progenitors into mature antigen-presenting cells. T cells are capable of increasing the oxidative stress on bladder cancer cells via induction of COX-2 and STEAP expression. Some evidence also suggests that COX-2 activation may be also involved in inflammation-mediated cancer stem cell proliferation. Antibodies against the VEGF-co-receptor neuropilin decrease the angiogenetic potential of bladder cancer cells. Inflammation-based predictive bladder cancer models have demonstrated to accurately predict response to treatment both in the curative and palliative setting. While randomized trials do not support a clinical benefit for the use of anti-inflammatory drugs (i.e., celecoxib, atorvastatin) in preventing recurrence of low-grade bladder cancer, further investigations are warranted in the setting of high-grade tumors since the immune response to cancer stimuli is most probably more pronounced in advanced stages.

G. Gakis (✉)
Department of Urology, University Hospital Tübingen, Eberhard-Karls University, Hoppe-Seyler-Strasse 3, 72076 Tübingen, Germany
e-mail: georgios.gakis@googlemail.com; georgios.gakis@med.uni-tuebingen.de

B. B. Aggarwal et al. (eds.), *Inflammation and Cancer*, Advances in Experimental Medicine and Biology 816, DOI: 10.1007/978-3-0348-0837-8_8,

8.1 Introduction

In Western countries, bladder cancer is the sixth most common cause of cancer death in men and the eight most common cause in women. In the United States, the incidence rate of bladder cancer has increased between the years 1973 and 2009 from 21 to 26/100,000 person-years. Stage-specific analyses have confirmed an increase in the incidence of localized and distant tumor stages. Meanwhile, improved 5-year survival rates were noted for all stages, except for distant disease (Abdollah et al. 2013). Similarly, in Germany, a pronounced increase in the incidence of approximately 35 % in men and 75 % in women has been noted between the years 1980 and 2004, which is the second highest bladder cancer incidence worldwide after Denmark. Despite this sharp increase in the incidence, the age-standardized mortality has dropped around 20 % in men and 40 % in men (Robert-Koch-Institut 2010).

Approximately 70–75 % of all bladder malignancies are diagnosed in superficial tumor stages (Stenzl et al. 2011). Superficial bladder cancer is characterized by a high recurrence rate and a relatively low progression rate (Babjuk et al. 2011). Due to this, lifelong surveillance regimens are necessary to detect recurrences at the earliest possible stage. This is the reason why bladder cancer causes the highest costs of all cancer entities in health care systems (Stenzl et al. 2008). Despite the use of recently introduced sophisticated treatment methods based on the combination of urine-based markers, fluorescence-guided cystoscopy, and intravesical instillations (Gakis et al. 2010), 25–30 % of all primary cases demonstrate histologically muscle invasion which is associated with concurrent distant metastatic lesions in 20 % of the patients (Stenzl et al. 2011).

Effective bladder cancer control requires an intact immune system (Balkwill and Mantovani 2001). When bladder cancer cells invade into the subepithelial tissue, further invasion can be arrested by intravesical instillations of Bacille-Calmette-Guerin (BCG), which provides long-term recurrence-free survival in about two-thirds of the patients (Kawai et al. 2013). However, the mechanisms that mediate the antiproliferative effects of BCG on cancer cells are poorly understood (Kawai et al. 2013). The clinical benefits seen in BCG patients suggest that the immune system itself plays an important role in arresting bladder cancer progression (Kawai et al. 2013). However, when tumor cells infiltrate into the muscle layer of the bladder, the risk of micrometastatic disease increases significantly. Therefore, at this stage, the chance of cure can be increased by radical surgical treatment in conjunction with neoadjuvant cisplatinum-based chemotherapy which, has shown to especially in patients with advanced tumor stages (Gakis et al. 2013). In the last years, there is an increasing awareness in the uro-oncological community that the immune system plays a critical role in bladder cancer progression (Gakis et al. 2011). The aim of this review is to provide molecular and clinical evidence for the role of inflammation in bladder cancer development and progression.

8.2 Evidence Acquisition

This review aims to describe the latest basic research developments on the role of inflammation in bladder cancer and provide clinical insights into their future role in preventing bladder carcinogenesis and progression. For this, a systematic Medline literature search was performed along with a free-text protocol, using one or several combinations of the following terms: *angiogenesis, bladder cancer, cytotoxic, immune system, inflammation, invasion, in vitro, in vivo, macrophage, metastasis, molecule, pathway, proliferation, T-cell, urothelial carcinoma.*

8.3 Inflammatory Cells and Pathways in Bladder Cancer

Systemic inflammation is a common host response to any tumorigenic process (Trikha et al. 2003). The microenvironment in tumor tissues resembles a status of chronic inflammation (Balkwill and Mantovani 2001). The immune response to cancer is ensured by macrophages, granulocytes, and lymphocytes (Balkwill and Mantovani 2001). The exact mechanism through which the invasive potential of bladder cancer cells is regulated by the immune system remains elusive. Recent evidence suggests that macrophages play a key role in regulating the metastatic potential of bladder cancer cells. Immunohistochemical studies of patients with high-grade or early-invasive bladder cancer treated with BCG have revealed that the number of macrophages infiltrating into the cancer area in relation to the number of macrophages in the tumor-surrounding lamina propria is of prognostic value (Ajili et al. 2013). A lower cancer area-to-lamina propria ratio has been associated with an improved recurrence-free survival. These data suggest that effective bladder cancer elimination requires the ability of macrophages to migrate largely into peritumoral area. However, this migration potential is differentially expressed as there are distinct subtypes of macrophages which exert pro- and anti-inflammatory effects (Edin et al. 2012). For this reason, a recent in vitro study investigated the cytotoxic effects of pro-inflammatory type-1 macrophages and anti-inflammatory type-2 macrophages on the human urothelial cancer cell line T24. The number of viable T24 cells was considerably higher in T24 cell/macrophage-2 co-cultures than in T24 cell/macrophage-1 co-cultures. In the latter co-cultures, an increase in tumor necrosis factor (TNF)-α gene expression and phosphoinositide 3-kinase (PI3K)/Akt signaling pathway activity was observed which was also associated with enhanced cellular invasiveness. Conversely, macrophage-2-derived factors suppressed the inhibitory effect of macrophage-1-derived factors on T24-cell growth, while exogenous interleukin (IL)-10 administration reversed the effects of macrophage-1-mediated arrest of cell growth on T24 cell/macrophage-1 co-cultures. Of note, while the invasive potential of T24 cells decreased after inhibition of PI3K pathway or TNF-α receptor blockade, it did not affect cell viability (Dufresne et al. 2011). This suggests that, besides activation of macrophages, cancer cell elimination requires further action of the immune system. These two macrophage subtypes show opposite effects in terms of their invasive potential.

Further molecular characterization of these subtypes helps to understand the divergent effects on cancer cells. A recent study analyzed myeloid cells from peripheral blood and tumor tissue collected from patients with urothelial carcinomas. Both blood and tissue analyses showed that two major CD11b(+) myeloid cell subsets were present: granulocyte-type CD15(high) CD33(low) cells and monocyte-type CD15(low) CD33(high) cells. Interestingly, the number of circulating granulocytic but not monocytic myeloid cells was markedly increased in cancer patients compared to healthy individuals. Both myeloid cell subsets produced substantial amounts of proinflammatory chemokines. Granulocytic myeloid cells were able to inhibit in vitro T-cell proliferation via induction of CD4(+) T regulatory cells. Further analysis revealed that tumor tissues were infiltrated with both monocyte–macrophage CD11b(+)-HLA-DR(+) and granulocytic CD11b(+)-CD15(+)-HLA-DR(−) myeloid cells (Eruslanov et al. 2012). Collectively, these studies suggest that different subtypes of activated inflammatory myeloid cells not only interfere with cancer cells but also with the T-cell system, thereby regulating the invasive potential of cancer cells and the functional efficiency of the local immune response.

To effectively eliminate cancer cells, natural killer (NK) cells, CD4(+), and CD8(+) T cells are of fundamental importance. In this respect, in vitro BCG models are ideally suited to elucidate the interactions between the immune and bladder cancer cells. Human interferon-alpha 2B-secreting recombinant BCG augments interferon-γ (IFN-γ) and interleukin-2 (IL-2) production by T helper cells (Liu et al. 2009). This, in turn, potentiates cytotoxic effects of peripheral blood mononuclear cells (PBMCs) on bladder cancer cells. Blockage of IFN-α, IFN-γ, or IL-2 by neutralizing antibodies after rBCG-IFN-α stimulation of cancer cells reduced the ability of PBMC to induce T-cell cytotoxicity. Conversely, NK and CD8(+) T cells are also able to enhance PBMC cytotoxicity after exposure to BCG-IFN-α (Liu et al. 2009).

An imbalance in the distribution of tumor-infiltrating T_h17 cells and regulatory T cells in the tumor area and peripheral blood seems to contribute to the development or progression of bladder carcinoma. Upon interleukin stimulation, T helper cells differentiate into T_h17 cells which are capable of producing large amounts of cytokines. Using flow cytometric analyses, patients with bladder cancer exhibited enriched T_h17 cells in the bladder tumor and a higher proportion of regulatory T cells in peripheral blood compared with healthy controls. Exposure to IL-2 converted T regulatory cells into T_h17 cells (Chi et al. 2010). Taken together, cytokine-induced imbalances in the distribution and differentiation of tumor-infiltrating cytotoxic cells and macrophages provoke a dysregulation of the immune system, thereby promoting bladder cancer cell growth.

8.4 Role of Inflammatory Molecules in the Development of Bladder Cancer: Evidence from In Vitro Studies

8.4.1 Role of Inflammatory Molecules in the Transformation of Bladder Cancer Cells

Chronic inflammation may not only be the host's response to bladder cancer development but also actually elicit bladder carcinogenesis. Secreted protein acidic and rich in cysteine (SPARC), a glycoprotein located in the extracellular matrix which is increasingly expressed during tissue remodeling, has been recently implicated with bladder carcinogenesis. SPARC-deficient mice and their wild-type littermates were exposed to chemical bladder carcinogens. Loss of SPARC accelerated the development of urothelial preneoplastic (such as atypia and dysplasia) and neoplastic conditions. SPARC-deficient animals showed a stronger accumulation of reactive oxygen species, increased urothelial cell proliferation, and carcinogen-induced inflammation. Interestingly, loss of SPARC was associated with an increased activation of pro-inflammatory macrophages and NF-κB overexpression. In experimental and spontaneous metastatic models, tumor- and stroma-derived SPARCs reduced tumor cell growth and metastasis formation via inhibition of cancer-related inflammation and lung colonization. These data indicate that SPARCs are produced both in cancer- and non-cancer-related compartments of bladder carcinomas, where they suppress bladder carcinogenesis and progression via modulation of the inflammatory response to cancer cells (Said et al. 2013).

The two isoforms of the enzyme cyclooxygenase catalyze the initial step in the formation of prostaglandins (PGs). PGs are involved in various inflammatory cell processes, i.e., inflammation, immune response, and carcinogenesis. Urothelial cells predominantly express high levels of COX-1, while bladder cancer cells show COX-2 overexpression (Boström et al. 2001). Therefore, the mechanisms that modify the expression of COX isoforms may possibly contribute to the transformation of normal urothelial cells to cancer cells. In in vitro studies, exposure to IFN-α decreased significantly the expression of COX-1 in 5637 and T24 bladder cancer cells, while an increased COX-2 expression was found in both cell lines (Boström et al. 2001). These findings suggest that IFN-α plays a role in COX-2 upregulation in urothelial cancer cells.

Bacterial lipopolysaccharides have been found to exert tumorigenic influence on the non-tumorigenic rat urothelial cell line MYP3 via cytokine-mediated increase in oxidative stress (i.e., hydrogen oxide) (Okamoto et al. 1996). Hydrogen oxide is a potent transforming agent which is released during inflammatory conditions of the bladder mucosa. Besides IFN-α, an increase in TNF-α release during inflammation has been causally related to the transformation of normal urothelial cells to malignant cells. In a prior study, it was demonstrated that number of colonies of MYP3 cells, which had been exposed to hydrogen oxide and subsequently to TNF-α, markedly increased as compared to untreated controls. Conversely, exposure to TNF-α alone was associated with a strong increase in intracellular hydrogen oxide concentration. Importantly, the use of antioxidants, i.e., α-tocopherol, resulted in a significant reduction in the number of colonies induced by TNF-α exposure. These data reveal that inflammation is able to induce malignant transformation of normal urothelial cells via induction of TNF-α-dependent release of hydrogen oxide (Okamoto et al. 1996; Okamoto and Oyasu 1997).

8.4.2 Role of Inflammatory Molecules in the Survival of Bladder Cancer Cells

Activation of distinct inflammatory pathways may also be important for improved survival of bladder cancer cells. Non-steroidal anti-inflammatory drugs (NSAIDs) are known to be potent inhibitors of COX-2 and capable of inducing apoptosis of bladder cancer cells. In bladder cancer cell lines, exposure to NSAIDs (i.e., ibuprofen) induces the expression of the proximate cell membrane glycoprotein, p75 neurotrophin receptor (p75NTR). A high expression of p75NTR correlates negatively with cancer cell viability. Transfection of bladder cancer cells prior to NSAID exposure with vectors carrying domain-deleted p75NTR products known to be strong antagonists of the intact p75NTR protein decreased cancer cell viability (Khwaja et al. 2004). These observations suggest that p75NTR modulates the antineoplastic effects of NSAIDs in cancer cells, while inhibition of p75NTR protein diminishes their viability.

Another recently discovered group of cell surface proteins, the human six-transmembrane epithelial antigen of the prostate (STEAP) protein family, consists of at least five homologous members that are frequently overexpressed in urological cancers. Basically, these proteins are oxidoreductases involved in the regulation of various physiological cell functions, including iron uptake and turnover, reaction to inflammatory stress, and acid and glucose metabolism (Grunewald et al. 2012). Isolation of specific STEAP-derived epitopes and in vitro vaccination with T helper cells from bladder cancer patients and healthy individuals has shown to stimulate T helper cells. In fact, STEAP peptides behave as promiscuous T-cell epitopes by stimulating T cells in the context of multiple major histocompatibility complex class II alleles (Azumi et al. 2010). Collectively, T cells are able to increase the oxidative stress on bladder cancer cells via induction of STEAP expression. Due to their membrane-linked location and high expression levels, STEAPs represent promising targets for future cell- and antibody-based immunotherapy in bladder cancer (Grunewald et al. 2012).

8.4.3 Role of Inflammatory Molecules in the Proliferation of Bladder Cancer Cells

In contrast to traditional immunological theories signifying that only B lymphocytes are capable of expressing immunoglobulins on their cell surface, a recent study reported that the expression of immunoglobulin G (IgG) messenger RNA (mRNA) and protein was also present on the bladder cancer cell surface. In two human urothelial cancer cell lines, T24 and BIU-87, and in tissues of 56 patients with urothelial carcinoma, IgG mRNA and IgG proteins were detectable. Increased cell apoptosis and inhibited cell growth via activation of the caspase pathway was observed after blockade of tumor-derived IgG by either antihuman IgG antibody or antisense oligonucleotides. Furthermore, in xenotransplant models, antihuman IgG antibody was able to suppress tumor growth. Moreover, adding either antihuman IgG antibody or antisense oligonucleotides to the bladder cancer cell line T24 enhanced its sensitivity to mitomycin C (Liang et al. 2013). Besides immunoglobulines, tumor-derived exosomes exert antiproliferative effects on bladder cancer cells. Exosomes are multi-protein complexes which are capable of degrading RNA. Tumor-specific exosomes are promising tumor vaccines antigens but show low antiproliferative activity. To enhance their immunogenicity, melanoma-antigen-1 (MAGE-1)-expressing T24 cells were transfected with a plasmid encoding the glycosyl-phosphatidylinositol-anchored interleukin 2 (GPI-IL-2) gene. Hereafter, IL-2 was found on the cell surface in the GPI-anchored form. The tumor-derived GPI-IL-2 exosome contained bioactive GPI-IL-2 and tumor-associated antigen MAGE-1. The proliferation of T cells and the antigen-specific cytotoxic T lymphocyte response was found to be more pronounced in exosomes expressing GPI-IL-2-pulsed dendritic cells. In future, these observations may pave the way for exosome-based tumor immunotherapeutic strategies as an alternative approach to traditional immunoglobulin-based immunotherapy.

8.4.4 Role of Inflammatory Molecules in the Invasion, Metastasis, and Angiogenesis of Bladder Cancer Cells

Inflammatory processes are not only necessary for carcinogenesis but also necessary for metastasis formation. The Rho-GDP dissociation inhibitor (RhoGDI2) suppresses the metastatic potential of various human bladder cancer cell lines (Gildea et al. 2002). In patients with muscle-invasive bladder cancer, increased RhoGDI2 expression has been associated with inferior survival (Theodorescu et al. 2004). Versican, a complex and versatile extracellular matrix protein, is a key regulatory molecule in cancer-related inflammation and is also associated with invasive and metastatic cancer stages (Wight 2002). It acts as a substrate to be depleted during invasion by cancer cells in order to facilitate metastasis formation. This metastasis-promoting effect depends on the recruitment of macrophages. Thus, versican is an integral component in order to establish a highly inflammatory microenvironment (Said and Theodorescu 2012). The excessive "crosstalks" between the immune system and cancer cells cause an "inflammatory cytokine storm" that drives cancer cell colonization. Targeting versican or the associated excessive release of cytokines represents a promising strategy to delay the evolution of metastases (Said et al. 2012).

Colonization of distant organs by cancer cells requires first their adhesion to the vascular endothelium. Selectin ligands are transmembrane glycoproteins on cancer cells that bind to selectins on the endothelial surface, thereby enabling the adhesion and migration of cancer cells and leukocytes through the endothelium. Functioning selectin ligands require Sialyl-Lewis tetrasaccharides which are cofactors that facilitate metastasis formation (St Hill 2011).

Following extravasation, cancer cells induce local neovascularization in order to supply with oxygen and nutrients. Therefore, the question arises whether the degree of inflammatory response may also trigger angiogenesis. VEGF receptors and their co-receptors, neuropilins (NRPs) are constituently expressed on normal urothelial cells. In animal models of BCG-induced chronic inflammation, the two VEGF receptor types (VEGFR1 and VEGFR2) and their associated co-receptors (NRP1 and NRP2) were markedly upregulated indicating neovascularization (Saban et al. 2010). In BCG-treated mice, after systemic application of neutralizing NRP antibodies (against their binding site on VEGFs) and following periodic BCG exposure, a depletion of a fluorescent internalizable tracer, called scVEGF/Cy5.5, was found both in cancer cells and in the urothelium which was histologically associated with a decrease in BCG-induced blood vessel density. Treatment with NRP1-neutralizing antibodies also diminished tumor infiltration by PMNCs and dendritic cells. These data suggest that NRPs can regulate the cancer-induced vascular and inflammatory responses (Saban et al. 2010).

8.4.5 Role of Inflammatory Molecules in the Development of Bladder Cancer: Evidence from In Vivo Studies

An established method of inducing bladder cancer in animal models is exposure to *N*-butyl-*N*-(4-hydroxybutyl)nitrosamine (BBN). Targeting COX-2 by pharmacological inhibition has been shown to reduce the incidence of preneoplastic and neoplastic lesions in the BBN-pretreated bladder mucosa and reduce serum transforming growth factor-β1 and C-reactive protein (CRP) levels (Parada et al. 2009). As the cyclooxygenase pathway regulates prostaglandin metabolism and cancer cells are able to deregulate the immune system, it seems prudent to investigate whether potential aberrations in prostaglandin metabolism may enhance tumor cell growth. Fast-growing SW780-bladder tumor mice xenografts were transfected with heterogeneous CD11b myeloid cell subsets including tumor-associated macrophages and myeloid-derived suppressor cells. It was demonstrated that bladder tumors secreted substantial amounts of prostaglandin E_2 (PGE_2). Moreover, when normal bone marrow myeloid cell progenitor cells were cultured in the presence of a bladder tumor-conditioned medium enriched for PGE_2, they did not only fail to differentiate into mature antigen-presenting cells (APCs) but acquired the phenotype of myeloid-derived suppressor cells (Eruslanov et al. 2011).

Another interesting pathway of attenuation of bladder tumor growth is the adenosine pathway. Accumulation of adenosine in tumors leads to an inactivation of immune cells and limits their ability to eliminate cancer cells. Conversely, blockade of adenosine A2 receptors activates cytotoxic T cells and stimulates dendritic cells. Basically, there are two adenosine receptor subtypes [A(2A) and A(2B)] which can be blocked in a selective and non-selective manner. Receptor analyses have shown that the antitumoral effects of adenosine blockers are mainly mediated by the selective adenosine A(2B) receptor. ATL801 is a selective A(2B) receptor antagonist which induces the secretion of IFN-γ and IFN-inducible chemokine CXCL10. CXCL10 is a ligand for CXCR3 expressed on tumor-infiltrating cytotoxic T cells. Accordingly, administration of ATL801 in CXCR3-deficient bladder tumor mice did not show to decelerate tumor growth (Cekic et al. 2012). Taken together, these data suggest that selective adenosine (2B) receptor blockers activate dendritic cells and enhance CXCR3-mediated cytotoxic response to bladder cancer growth. Whether a combined approach by a concurrent blockade of A(2B) and COX-2 receptors might result in superior tumor growth inhibition awaits further investigation.

8.5 Evidence from Patients for the Role of Inflammation in Bladder Cancer

Migration of macrophages into tumor tissues is essential for effective tumor cell elimination. Increasing evidence suggests that the pro-inflammatory cytokine macrophage migration inhibitory factor (MIF) serves as a link between inflammation and carcinogenesis. Anti-thrombin III, an endogenous serine protease inhibitor, which is known to inactivate several enzymes of the blood coagulation cascade, also acts as an inhibitory binding protein for MIF. In the serum, an increased MIF concentration was found in bladder cancer patients compared to healthy individuals, while the concentration of ATIII-MIF complexes was decreased in cancer patients. These data suggest that increased circulating levels of bioactive MIF are present in the sera of bladder cancer patients (Meyer-Siegler et al. 2010).

In recent years, besides increasing evidence for the role of inflammation in bladder cancer, the presence of cancer stem cells has been suggested to be causative for the high risk of recurrence and progression (van der Horst et al. 2012). Therefore, the question arises whether inflammation is capable of activating cancer stem cells. Data from immunohistochemical analyses show that the immunoreactivity of distinct stemness markers (Oct3/4 and CD44v6) and COX-2 is significantly higher in cystitis and cancer patients compared to healthy controls. Interestingly, the nuclear localization of COX-2 was significantly associated with upregulation of Oct3/4 and CD44v6 in bladder cancer tissues irrespective of the degree of inflammation. Therefore, COX-2 activation may be also involved in inflammation-mediated cancer stem cell proliferation during bladder carcinogenesis (Thanan et al. 2012).

From a clinical point of view, as the degree of inflammation potentially reflects tumor aggressiveness (Siemes et al. 2006), the use of serum markers for measuring the degree of systemic inflammation may be useful in counseling patients for neoadjuvant and adjuvant treatment. Candidate markers which can be easily assessed in daily clinical practice include interleukin-6, leukocyte levels, and serum CRP (Siemes et al. 2006). In this respect, CRP is a highly sensitive marker of acute and chronic inflammation (Ledue et al. 1998). After interleukin-6 mediated release by hepatocytes, CRP acts an opsonizing agent for cancer cell detection and elimination. However, interleukin-6 can also be released by tumor cells themselves, facilitating cancer cell survival by pleiotrophic effects (Trikha et al. 2003). Consequently, elevated serum CRP levels are not only an epiphenomenon of the tumor microenvironment but also a critical component of the host's response to the tumor.

A recent screening study among healthy individuals showed that elevated CRP indicates a higher risk of developing bladder cancer (Trichopoulos et al. 2006). In patients undergoing radical surgery for bladder cancer, preoperative serum CRP levels have been shown to predict local tumor stage and prognosis. A novel prediction model for cancer-specific survival after radical cystectomy, termed TNR-C Score (Gakis et al. 2011), which accounts for critical determinants for survival (**T**umor-stage lymph **N**ode density, **R**esection margin status, and **C**RP level), yielded a considerably high predictive accuracy of 79 %. In the following, further investigations have confirmed the clinical significance of pretreatment CRP levels and kinetics in predicting response to first-line and second-line chemotherapy in metastatic bladder cancer (Saito et al. 2012; Ishioka et al. 2012).

8.6 Inhibitors of Inflammation for the Prevention and Treatment of Bladder Cancer

In the last years, anticarcinogenic properties have been attributed to 3-hydroxy-3-methylglutaryl-coenzyme A (HMGCoA) reductase inhibitors which are effective pharmacological substances for lowering serum LDL cholesterol levels. The anticarcinogenic effects of atorvastatin on bladder carcinogenesis were also recently investigated in a BBN-treated rodent model. The incidence of bladder carcinomas was significantly lower in the atorvastatin/BBN group compared to BBN alone. Nevertheless, recent large meta-analyses have not demonstrated a significant benefit of statins in decreasing cancer incidence and mortality (Cholesterol Treatment Trialists' Collaboration 2012). Similarly, a randomized, double-blind, placebo-controlled trial was set up to determine whether celecoxib, a potent COX-2 inhibitor, could reduce the time to recurrence in patients with non-muscle-invasive bladder at high risk for recurrence. A total of 146 patients were randomized to receive either 200 mg celecoxib or placebo administered orally twice daily for at least 12 months. While celecoxib was well tolerated, the intention-to-treat analysis revealed no statistically significant increase in the time to recurrence in the celecoxib group compared with placebo. However, celecoxib had a marginally significant effect on reducing metachronous recurrences (Sabichi et al. 2011). While these results do not support a clinical benefit for the long-term use of celecoxib in preventing recurrence of low-grade bladder cancer, further investigations are warranted as the immune response to cancer stimuli may probably be more pronounced in advanced tumor stages.

8.7 Conclusions and Future Directions

In conclusion, bladder cancer is a highly immunogenic malignancy. Yet, the exact mechanisms through which bladder cancer cells silence the immune system during tumor progression remain largely elusive. Current evidence suggests that bladder cancer cells aim to trigger an "inflammatory cytokine storm" that stimulates the secretion of tumor growth promoting factors while attenuating the cytotoxic function of immune cells. The degree of inflammatory response also triggers the formation of distant metastatic clones. One of the key regulatory events in bladder cancer progression seems to be COX-2 upregulation which leads to an aberrant prostaglandin metabolism and suppresses the cytotoxic function of immune cells. Additionally, COX-2 activation may be also involved in inflammation-mediated cancer stem cell proliferation. Immune cells can attenuate the angiogenetic potential of bladder cancer cells by inhibiting endothelial adhesion and the VEGF receptor signaling pathway. Taken together, the identification of novel target molecules involved in dysregulation of the immune system provides a rationale for a variety of novel targeted approaches in bladder cancer. In light of results from randomized studies on the chemopreventive effects of NSAIDs in bladder cancer, we must acknowledge that optimal selection of appropriate candidates based on established predictive marker models is of paramount importance in order to maximize the clinical benefit of inflammation-based therapeutic strategies.

References

Abdollah F, Gandaglia G, Thuret R, Schmitges J, Tian Z, Jeldres C, Passoni NM, Briganti A, Shariat SF, Perrotte P, Montorsi F, Karakiewicz PI, Sun M (2013) Incidence, survival and mortality rates of stage-specific bladder cancer in United States: a trend analysis. Cancer Epidemiol. doi:10.1016/j.canep.2013.02.002

Ajili F, Kourda N, Darouiche A, Chebil M, Boubaker S (2013) Prognostic value of tumor-associated macrophages count in human non-muscle-invasive bladder cancer treated by BCG immunotherapy. Ultrastruct Pathol 37(1):56–61

Azumi M, Kobayashi H, Aoki N, Sato K, Kimura S, Kakizaki H, Tateno M (2010) Six-transmembrane epithelial antigen of the prostate as an immunotherapeutic target for renal cell and bladder cancer. J Urol 183(5):2036–2044

Babjuk M, Oosterlinck W, Sylvester R, Kaasinen E, Böhle A, Palou-Redorta J, Rouprêt M (2011) EAU guidelines on non-muscle-invasive urothelial carcinoma of the bladder, the 2011 update. Eur Urol 59(6):997–1008

Balkwill F, Mantovani A (2001) Inflammation and cancer: back to Virchow? Lancet 357(9255):539–545

Boström PJ, Aaltonen V, Söderström KO, Uotila P, Laato M (2001a) Expression of cyclooxygenase-1 and -2 in urinary bladder carcinomas in vivo and in vitro and prostaglandin E2 synthesis in cultured bladder cancer cells. Pathology 33(4):469–474

Boström PJ, Uotila P, Rajala P, Nurmi M, Huhtaniemi I, Laato M (2001b) Interferon-alpha inhibits cyclooxygenase-1 and stimulates cyclooxygenase-2 expression in bladder cancer cells in vitro. Urol Res 29(1):20–24

Cekic C, Sag D, Li Y, Theodorescu D, Strieter RM, Linden J (2012) Adenosine A2B receptor blockade slows growth of bladder and breast tumors. J Immunol 188(1):198–205

Chi LJ, Lu HT, Li GL, Wang XM, Su Y, Xu WH, Shen BZ (2010) Involvement of T helper type 17 and regulatory T cell activity in tumour immunology of bladder carcinoma. Clin Exp Immunol 161(3):480–489

Cholesterol Treatment Trialists' (CTT) Collaboration (2012) Lack of effect of lowering LDL cholesterol on cancer: meta-analysis of individual data from 175,000 people in 27 randomised trials of statin therapy. PLoS One 7(1):e29849

Dufresne M, Dumas G, Asselin E, Carrier C, Pouliot M, Reyes-Moreno C (2011) Pro-inflammatory type-1 and anti-inflammatory type-2 macrophages differentially modulate cell survival and invasion of human bladder carcinoma T24 cells. Mol Immunol 48(12–13):1556–1567

Edin S, Wikberg M, Dahlin AM, Rutegård J, Öberg Å, Oldenborg PA, Palmqvist R (2012) The distribution of macrophages with a M1 or M2 phenotype in relation to prognosis and the molecular characteristics of colorectal cancer. PLoS ONE 7(10):e47045

Eruslanov E, Daurkin I, Vieweg J, Daaka Y, Kusmartsev S (2011) Aberrant PGE2 metabolism in bladder tumor microenvironment promotes immunosuppressive phenotype of tumor-infiltrating myeloid cells. Int Immunopharmacol 11(7):848–855

Eruslanov E, Neuberger M, Daurkin I, Perrin GQ, Algood C, Dahm P, Rosser C, Vieweg J, Gilbert SM, Kusmartsev S (2012) Circulating and tumor-infiltrating myeloid cell subsets in patients with bladder cancer. Int J Cancer 130(5):1109–1119

Gakis G, Kruck S, Stenzl A (2010) Can the burden of follow-up in low-grade noninvasive bladder cancer be reduced by photodynamic diagnosis, perioperative instillations, imaging, and urine markers? Curr Opin Urol 20(5):388–392

Gakis G, Todenhöfer T, Stenzl A (2011a) The prognostic value of hematological and systemic inflammatory disorders in invasive bladder cancer. Curr Opin Urol 21(5):428–433

Gakis G, Todenhöfer T, Renninger M, Schilling D, Sievert KD, Schwentner C, Stenzl A (2011b) Development of a new outcome prediction model in carcinoma invading the bladder based on preoperative serum C-reactive protein and standard pathological risk factors: the TNR-C score. BJU Int 108(11):1800–1805

Gakis G, Efstathiou JA, Lerner SP, Cookson MS, Keegan KA, Guru KA, Shipley WU, Heidenreich A, Schoenberg MP, Sagaloswky AI, Soloway MS, Stenzl A (2013) ICUD-EAU International Consultation on bladder cancer 2012: radical cystectomy and bladder preservation for muscle-invasive urothelial carcinoma of the bladder. Eur Urol 63(1):45–57

Gildea JJ, Seraj MJ, Oxford G, Harding MA, Hampton GM, Moskaluk CA, Frierson HF, Conaway MR, Theodorescu D (2002) RhoGDI2 is an invasion and metastasis suppressor gene in human cancer. Cancer Res 62(22):6418–6423

Grunewald TG, Bach H, Cossarizza A, Matsumoto I (2012) The STEAP protein family: versatile oxidoreductases and targets for cancer immunotherapy with overlapping and distinct cellular functions. Biol Cell 104(11):641–657

Ishioka J, Saito K, Sakura M, Yokoyama M, Matsuoka Y, Numao N, Koga F, Masuda H, Fujii Y, Kawakami S, Kihara K (2012) Development of a nomogram incorporating serum C-reactive protein level to predict overall survival of patients with advanced urothelial carcinoma and its evaluation by decision curve analysis. Br J Cancer 107(7):1031–1036

Kawai K, Miyazaki J, Joraku A, Nishiyama H, Akaza H (2013) Bacillus Calmette-Guerin (BCG) immunotherapy for bladder cancer: current understanding and perspectives on engineered BCG vaccine. Cancer Sci 104(1):22–27

Khwaja F, Allen J, Lynch J, Andrews P, Djakiew D (2004) Ibuprofen inhibits survival of bladder cancer cells by induced expression of the p75NTR tumor suppressor protein. Cancer Res 64(17):6207–6213

Ledue TB, Weiner DL, Sipe JD, Poulin SE, Collins MF, Rifai N (1998) Analytical evaluation of particle-enhanced immunonephelometric assays for C-reactive protein, serum amyloid A and mannose-binding protein in human serum. Ann Clin Biochem 35(Pt 6):745–753

Liang PY, Li HY, Zhou ZY, Jin YX, Wang SX, Peng XH, Ou SJ (2013) Overexpression of immunoglobulin G prompts cell proliferation and inhibits cell apoptosis in human urothelial carcinoma. Tumour Biol. doi:10.1007/s13277-013-0717-z

Liu W, O'Donnell MA, Chen X, Han R, Luo Y (2009) Recombinant bacillus Calmette-Guérin (BCG) expressing interferon-alpha 2B enhances human mononuclear cell cytotoxicity against bladder cancer cell lines in vitro. Cancer Immunol Immunother 58(10):1647–1655

Meyer-Siegler KL, Cox J, Leng L, Bucala R, Vera PL (2010) Macrophage migration inhibitory factor anti-thrombin III complexes are decreased in bladder cancer patient serum: complex formation as a mechanism of inactivation. Cancer Lett 290(1):49–57

Okamoto M, Oyasu R (1997) Transformation in vitro of a nontumorigenic rat urothelial cell line by tumor necrosis factor-alpha. Lab Invest 77(2):139–144

Okamoto M, Kawai K, Reznikoff CA, Oyasu R (1996) Transformation in vitro of a nontumorigenic rat urothelial cell line by hydrogen peroxide. Cancer Res 56(20):4649–4653

Parada B, Sereno J, Reis F, Teixeira-Lemos E, Garrido P, Pinto AF, Cunha MF, Pinto R, Mota A, Figueiredo A, Teixeira F (2009) Anti-inflammatory, anti-proliferative and antioxidant profiles of selective cyclooxygenase-2 inhibition as chemoprevention for rat bladder carcinogenesis. Cancer Biol Ther 8(17):1615–1622

Robert-Koch-Institut (2010) Krebs in Deutschland. Berlin, pp 84–88

Saban MR, Sferra TJ, Davis CA, Simpson C, Allen A, Maier J, Fowler B, Knowlton N, Birder L, Wu XR, Saban R (2010) Neuropilin-VEGF signaling pathway acts as a key modulator of vascular, lymphatic, and inflammatory cell responses of the bladder to intravesical BCG treatment. Am J Physiol Renal Physiol 299(6):F1245–F1256

Sabichi AL, Lee JJ, Grossman HB, Liu S, Richmond E, Czerniak BA, De la Cerda J, Eagle C, Viner JL, Palmer JL, Lerner SP (2011) A randomized controlled trial of celecoxib to prevent recurrence of nonmuscle-invasive bladder cancer. Cancer Prev Res (Phila) 4(10):1580–1589

Said N, Theodorescu D (2012) RhoGDI2 suppresses bladder cancer metastasis via reduction of inflammation in the tumor microenvironment. Oncoimmunology 1(7):1175–1177

Said N, Sanchez-Carbayo M, Smith SC, Theodorescu D (2012) RhoGDI2 suppresses lung metastasis in mice by reducing tumor versican expression and macrophage infiltration. J Clin Invest 122(4):1503–1518

Said N, Frierson HF, Sanchez-Carbayo M, Brekken RA, Theodorescu D (2013) Loss of SPARC in bladder cancer enhances carcinogenesis and progression. J Clin Invest. doi:10.1172/JCI64782

Saito K, Urakami S, Komai Y, Yasuda Y, Kubo Y, Kitsukawa S, Okubo Y, Yamamoto S, Yonese J, Fukui I (2012) Impact of C-reactive protein kinetics on survival of patients with advanced urothelial carcinoma treated by second-line chemotherapy with gemcitabine, etoposide and cisplatin. BJU Int 110(10):1478–1484

Siemes C, Vissser LE, Coebergh JW, Splinter TA, Witteman JC, Uitterlinden AG, Hofman A, Pols HA, Stricker BH (2006) C-reactive protein levels, variation in the C-reactive protein gene, and cancer risk: the Rotterdam study. J Clin Oncol 24(33):5216–5222

St Hill CA (2011) Interactions between endothelial selectins and cancer cells regulate metastasis. Front Biosci 16:3233–3251

Stenzl A, Hennenlotter J, Schilling D (2008) Can we still afford bladder cancer? Curr Opin Urol 18(5):488–492

Stenzl A, Cowan NC, De Santis M, Kuczyk MA, Merseburger AS, Ribal MJ, Sherif A, Witjes JA (2011) Treatment of muscle-invasive and metastatic bladder cancer: update of the EAU guidelines. Eur Urol 59(6):1009–1018

Thanan R, Murata M, Ma N, Hammam O, Wishahi M, El Leithy T, Hiraku Y, Oikawa S, Kawanishi S (2012) Nuclear localization of COX-2 in relation to the expression of stemness markers in urinary bladder cancer. Mediators Inflamm 2012:165879. doi:10.1155/2012/165879

Theodorescu D, Sapisono LM, Conaway MR, Oxford G, Hampton GM, Frierson HF Jr (2004) Reduced expression of metastasis suppressor RhoGDI2 is associated with decreased survival for patients with bladder cancer. Clin Cancer Res 10(11):3800–3806

Trichopoulos D, Psaltopoulou T, Orfanos P, Trichopoulou A, Boffetta P (2006) Plasma C-reactive protein and risk of cancer: a prospective study from Greece. Cancer Epidemiol Biomarkers Prev 15(2):381–384

Trikha M, Corringham R, Klein B, Rossi JF (2003) Targeted anti-interleukin-6 monoclonal antibody therapy for cancer: a review of the rationale and clinical evidence. Clin Cancer Res 9(13):4653–4665

van der Horst G, Bost L, van der Pluijm G (2012) Epithelial plasticity, cancer stem cells, and the tumor-supportive stroma in bladder carcinoma. Mol Cancer Res 10(8):995–1009

Wight TN (2002) Versican: a versatile extracellular matrix proteoglycan in cell biology. Curr Opin Cell Biol 14(5):617–623

Chapter 9
The Role of Inflammation in Kidney Cancer

Antonio Roma de Vivar Chevez, James Finke and Ronald Bukowski

Abstract Renal cell carcinoma (RCC) constitutes more than 90 % of primary kidney tumors with the development of metastatic disease in the lung, bone, liver, and brain. Clear-cell RCC (CCRCC) is the most common histologic form of sporadic kidney cancer where the majority of tumors have inactivation of the von Hippel–Lindau (VHL) tumor-suppressor gene resulting in the accumulation of hypoxia-inducible factor (HIF) leading to dysregulation of cell growth and angiogenesis. Understanding of the genetic changes in RCC and the downstream events have led to the development of tyrosine kinase inhibitors (TKI) that target HIF-regulated proteins which currently represents front-line therapy for metastatic disease although resistance develops in most patients overtime. Despite the fact that RCC is an immunogenic tumor, there is mounting evidence that immune cells and inflammatory pathways can enhance tumor growth and immune escape. However, recent studies are beginning to uncover the mechanisms of immune escape in RCC, and the role inflammatory immune cells and cytokines play is this process. These new findings have led to renewed interest in the use of immunotherapy for the treatment of this disease that includes strategies to regulate inflammatory responses. Here, we will discuss the different inflammatory signaling pathways (e.g., VHL, hypoxia, TNF-α, STAT, and TGF-β) and the downstream transcription factors, cytokines, and chemokines involved in tumor development, and disease progression. This will include assessment of the role inflammatory molecules (e.g., pVHL, TGFb, IL6, select chemokines/chemokine receptors) play in promoting cell transformation, survival, proliferation of tumor cells, and metastasis derived from in vitro and in vivo studies. Included is a section on how select inflammatory cells (TAM, MDSC, and neutrophils) promote tumor evasion of immune cells. We also provide examples of molecules/cells that correlate

A. R. de Vivar Chevez · J. Finke · R. Bukowski (✉)
Cleveland Clinic Lerner College of Medicine, Case Western Reserve University, Cleveland, OH, USA
e-mail: bukow464@sbcglobal.net

B. B. Aggarwal et al. (eds.), *Inflammation and Cancer*, Advances in Experimental Medicine and Biology 816, DOI: 10.1007/978-3-0348-0837-8_9, © Springer Basel 2014

negatively (CXCL12, CXCR4, and MMP, neutrophils, and MDSC) and positively (TH1 cells, IP-10, and MIG) with tumor progression and survival. Finally, there is a discussion of different inhibitors of inflammation that may be useful in the treatment of RCC.

9.1 Introduction

An estimated 65,150 new cases of kidney cancer will be diagnosed in the USA in 2013 resulting in 13,680 deaths. Kidney cancer incidence has increased by 3.1 % per year from 2005 to 2009 while death rates have decreased by 5 % in the same time period. The increased incidence is mainly explained by an increase in early-stage diagnosis incidentally during abdominal imaging for unrelated issues; there are, however, no current recommendations for a screening test for the general population. Incidence appears to be reaching a plateau for the first time in several decades. Renal cell carcinoma (RCC) are tumors arising from the renal tubular epithelial cells and account for more than 90 % of primary kidney tumors. RCC represents the eighth most common malignancy in adults in the USA and more than 50 % of individuals present with metastatic disease (American Cancer Society 2008).

Clear-cell RCC (CCRCC) represents the most common histological type of RCC, accounting for up to 75 % of all renal cancer cases, followed by papillary (15 %), oncocytoma (5 %), and chromophobe (5 %) (Devita et al. 2011). CCRCC can affect all patient age groups but is most commonly found in their 60s or 70s, predominantly in men (male-to-female ratio of 2:1) (Cheville et al. 2003).

The extent of the disease determines the treatment of RCC, and it greatly influences survival. Due to its location in the retroperitoneum, RCC tumors can frequently grow unnoticed for many years until the development of metastasis. Historically, less than 50 % of patients have localized disease at presentation, 20 % have local invasion, and 30–40 % of patients have metastatic disease at the time of diagnosis (Golimbu et al. 1986; Zisman et al. 2002). However, recent data (2003–2009) from the surveillance, epidemiology, and end results (SEER) program reflect a pronounced increase in RCC with localized tumors at the time of diagnosis, which brings the percentage of localized disease to a range of 61–71 % depending on the demographic group.

Survival

The overall 5-year relative survival for kidney cancer has increased from 51 % in the early 1980s to over 73 % in the past decade (Howlader et al. 2013). Tumors of the renal pelvis carry a worse prognosis than RCC tumors (5-year survival of 50 vs. 72 %, respectively). Early diagnosis (i.e., at a local stage) increases the 5-year survival rate to 91 %. Unfortunately, this percentage drops to 10 % in patients presenting with metastatic disease (Cohen and McGovern 2005).

Major gene products associated with kidney cancer

Von Hippel–Lindau is a tumor-suppressor gene located on chromosome 3p that encodes a protein with the same name (pVHL). This gene has been associated with predisposition to various types of cancer including pheochromocytomas, hemangioblastomas, and CCRCC. VHL disease is a dominantly inherited familial cancer syndrome initiated by mutations in the VHL tumor-suppressor gene (Ong et al. 2007). The genetic studies from families with this genetic predisposition have been extensive, and this has led to a better understanding of the development of RCC. VHL inactivation is also a common feature of sporadic CCRCC the most abundant histological form of kidney cancer. Although inactivation of VHL is a critical event in the pathogenesis of most CCRCC, it is not sufficient to cause this disease (Li and Kaelin 2011). The gene product pVHL interacts with other proteins to form the complex called E3-ubiquitin. This complex targets specific proteins to undergo proteosomal degradation. pVHL provides target specificity to this complex, and one of its major functions is to bind to the HIFs HIF-1α and HIF-2α to promote their proteosomal degradation. It is now known that pVHL plays a critical role in the cell's response to hypoxic changes (Maher et al. 2011). HIF proteins are hydroxylated under normoxic conditions; pVHL binds to this hydroxylated form of the HIF molecule, tagging it for degradation and keeping it in a relatively low level within the cells. When hypoxic conditions ensue, however, HIF proteins are not hydroxylated and cannot be recognized by pVHL and its concentrations begin to rise. In RCC patients, VHL gene mutations produce non-functional pVHL which are not able to target HIF proteins for degradation, and therefore, they accumulate regardless of the cells redox state. HIF-1 and HIF-2 are transcription factors that regulate a group of genes important to tumor survival and hypoxic gene response. These genes (including VEGF, PDGFβ, TGFα, Cyclin D1) are implicated in several biologic responses including angiogenesis, proliferation, apoptosis, and metabolism (see Fig. 9.1).

Current Therapies for Kidney Cancer Surgery

Surgery is the most effective treatment for localized RCC. Radical nephrectomy is the most common operation for T1a tumors (i.e., less than 4 cm in diameter). It consists of the complete removal of Gerota's fascia and its contents. Adrenal sparing surgery is recommended for T1a tumors of the inferior pole (Golimbu et al. 1986). Patients with a small (<4 cm), usually incidentally found mass, have a survival rate of 90 % or greater when partial or radical nephrectomy is performed. The role of surgery in metastatic disease, however, is only limited to symptom palliation, and nephrectomy alone has no survival benefits in this group of patients (Dekernion et al. 1978). There have been reports of spontaneous regression of metastatic renal cancer following removal of the primary tumor. This rare occurrence (~1 %), however, is not an indication for surgery in metastatic disease as a single modality treatment (Middleton 1980). Advanced RCC can be treated surgically as part of a multimodal therapy such as immunotherapy (Flanigan et al. 2001).

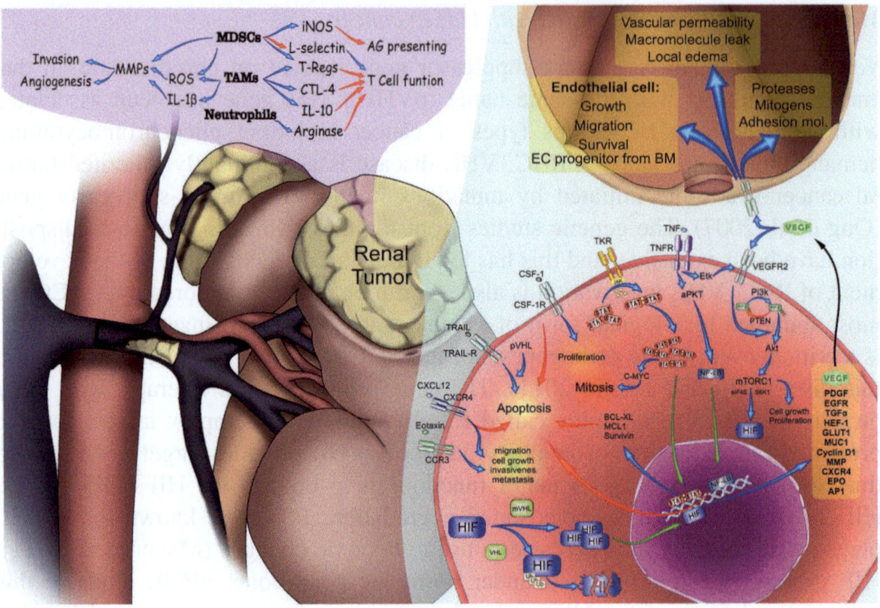

Fig. 9.1 This figure provides a summary of the changes in the infiltrating immune cells that promote immune suppression and angiogenesis resulting in tumor evasion (*top left*, *purple*). Also detailed are the different signaling pathways associated with RCC development, growth, and survival (*lower right*, *pink*). Included is a depiction of the central role VHL silencing has on the constitutive activation of HIF transcription leading to gene expression of different molecules involved in tumor growth. The impact of proangiogenic protein production has on promotion of the tumor vasculature is depicted (*upper right*). This figure also highlights the importance of inflammatory proteins and their receptors in regulating RCC development and growth. *Red arrows* represent inhibition or downregulation, while *blue* represents stimulation or upregulation; *green arrows* indicate nuclear translocation of transcription factors

Chemotherapy

Chemotherapy has shown poor efficacy for advanced stage RCC in numerous clinical trials. Single-agent regimens have shown response rates of 5–6 % in trials involving over 4,000 cases and more than 30 individual agents (Motzer et al. 2000; Yagoda et al. 1995). 5-fluorouracil and gemcitabine combinations have yielded slightly better response rates (10–15 %) (Rini et al. 2005; Stadler et al. 2006).

Immunotherapy

Clear-cell RCCs are considered an immunogenic tumor based on several observations that include rare but documented cases of spontaneous regression sometimes associated with cytoreductive nephrectomy, significant immune infiltrate in some tumors, identification of tumor-associated antigens expressed by RCC, and their sensitivity to immunotherapy.

Cytokine therapy

Cytokines represent an active, non-specific immunotherapy for the treatment of metastatic kidney cancer, and the most studied include interleukin-2 (IL-2) and interferon-alpha.

IL-2

IL-2 was approved by the FDA for the treatment of advanced RCC, and melanoma over two decades ago and for years was the first-line agent for metastatic RCC. Administration of recombinant IL-2 is associated with a 20–25 % objective response rate in patients with kidney cancer. In different clinical trials, the 5-year survival rate for these patients was almost 20 % of the responders (Clement and McDermott 2009; Halama et al. 2010; Escudier 2010; Dillman et al. 2011). High-dose IL-2, however, has profound side effects, in particular, one characterized as a "cytokine storm" or capillary leak syndrome, but the mechanism behind it is not clearly understood. Clinically, this results in hypotension, cardiac, renal, pulmonary, gastrointestinal, cerebral, and hepatic toxicity (Finkelstein et al. 2010). Strategies to improve efficacy and/or reduce the side effect profile have been unsuccessful; agent combination such as TNF, iNOS, or VEGF inhibition, IFN-α administration did not significantly improve outcome (Halama et al. 2010; Escudier 2010). Efforts to identify which patients are more likely to respond to IL-2 have identified possible biomarkers. Complete responders to IL-2 therapy have unique protein and gene expression patterns, but clinical trials have failed to identify markers that can be use prospectively (Clement and McDermott 2009). The cloning and production of recombinant IL-2 allowed for the in vitro expansion of lymphokine-activated killer cells (LAK). These cells were administered to patients as a form of adoptive immunotherapy. The majority of LAK cells are derived from precursor cells with the immunological marker spectrum CD3(−), CD11(+), CD14(−), CD16(+), CD56(+). Following activation with IL-2, cells express the markers CD2(+), CD3(−), CD56(+) and typically represent activated NK cells (Fortis et al. 1991). However, IL2 combined with LAK cell infusion did not improve the therapeutic activity of IL2 (Law et al. 1995).

IFN-α

IFN-α is a glycoprotein that has antitumor effects along with immunomodulative, antiproliferative, and differentiation-inducing activities (Neidhart 1986; McDermott and Rini 2007). Overall response rates range between 10 and 15 % with different dose regimens and preparations. A meta-analysis involving 6,117 patients with metastatic RCC between 1995 and 2004 showed a median improvement in survival of 3.8 months (Coppin et al. 2005). This small but significant improved survival and a lower treatment-related toxicity (and cost) resulted in a wide spread use of IFN-α in metastatic RCC. IFN-α has been tested in clinical trials with multiple other agents including IL-2 at different doses, chemotherapeutic drugs (5-fluorouracil, vinblastine, cis-retinoic acid), targeted therapy agents (sorafenib, sunitinib, bevacizumab), and even combination of these three classes of drugs, and although modest synergy has been observed in phase II clinical trials, strong phase III clinical trial data to support the use of any of this combinations over IFN-α alone are still lacking (Rini and Campbell 2009). However, there are clinical variables that can stratify patients into favorable, intermediate, or poor risk with median survival of 30, 14, and 5 months, respectively. These data were gathered from six prospective clinical trials, and the clinical variables were: low Karnofsky performance status, high lactate dehydrogenase, low serum hemoglobin, high corrected serum calcium and time from diagnosis (of RCC) to IFN-α therapy of less than one year.

Checkpoint inhibitors as immunotherapy

Tumors, including RCC, escape immune destruction by multiple mechanisms. This includes using the body's own protective pathways that normally prevent autoimmunity such as immune checkpoints leading to termination of immune responses after T cell activation (Pardoll 2012; Tang and Heng 2013). Current therapies include the use of antibodies directed toward select checkpoint molecules such as CTLA-4 (cytotoxic T lymphocyte-associated antigen 4). CTLA-4 is known to be an inhibitory regulator of T cell expansion which counter acts the CD28-mediated co-stimulation initiated by B7-1 and B7-2 ligands (Peggs et al. 2009). Genetic disruption of CTLA-4 expression results in a T-cell-dominated lymphoproliferative syndrome leading to significant autoimmune disease. However, the use of blocking antibodies to CTLA-4 in mouse and humans can enhance immunological responses to cancer (Shrikant et al. 1999). Indeed, clinical studies in patients with metastatic RCC and melanoma demonstrated that treatment with anti-CTLA4 antibody (ipilimumab) has significant clinical activity. Interestingly, there was a significant association between autoimmune events noted in these patients and tumor regression (Yang et al. 2007; Tang and Heng 2013). However, autoimmunity mediated by anti-CTLA4 antibody treatment is a significant complication in some patients.

The other T cell co-inhibitory receptor that has been shown to suppress T cell function is PD-1 (Programmed death 1). PD-1 is expressed after T cell activation, and when PD-1 receptors binds to its ligands PD-L1 (B7-H1) or PD-L2, T cell function is blocked (Tang and Heng 2013; Freeman et al. 2000); approximately 56 % of RCC tumors have infiltration of PD-1^+ T cells, and patients with PD-1^+ immune cells were at significant risk of cancer-specific death when compared to PD-1-negative patients (Thompson et al. 2007). Additionally, the ligand PD-L1 is known to be expressed on a portion of renal tumors (30 %), and expression of this ligand is associated with poor prognosis (Thompson et al. 2004, 2006). Anti-PD1 antibodies have shown significant efficacy in several tumor types (25 %) including RCC, melanoma, and non-small-cell lung cancer (Topalian et al. 2012; Lipson et al. 2013). Although less studied anti-PD-L1 antibody has also demonstrated antitumor activity in RCC patients (Brahmer et al. 2012), these studies and others suggest that blocking PD-1 interaction with its ligands is a new and viable approach to the treatment of metastatic RCC and will likely to lead to interesting combinational studies.

Targeted therapy drugs

Discovery of the VHL gene as a landmark mutation for both familial as well as sporadic cases of RCC resulted in an extensive characterization of the downstream pathway of this gene product functions. This eventually led to identification of specific molecules involved in RCC development and subsequently the identification of drugs that specifically act on these pathways.

VEGF receptor inhibitors

VEGF is typically produced by fibroblast and stromal cells; however, RCC cells are able to produce this protein in large amounts as a consequence of silencing of the VHL gene (Edgren et al. 1999). Binding of this protein to its receptor ultimately results in blood vessel formation. Sunitinib maleate is a multitargeted tyrosine kinase inhibitor that is available in oral form. It has antitumor and antiangiogenic activity in part through inhibition of VEGF receptors, whether its activity is also related to other receptors it binds to remains unclear (PDGF receptors as well as Flt-3, c-Kit, and CSF1R) (Mendel et al. 2003). Two Phase II clinical trials involving 63 and 106 patients with advanced RCC, response rates were 40 and 39 %, respectively, and a median progression-free survival of 8.7 and 8.3 months, respectively. No complete responses were observed in these studies (Motzer et al. 2006a, b). A phase III international trial compared sunitinib to IFN-α as first-line treatment for advanced RCC (Motzer et al. 2007). The median progression-free survival and objective response rate were 47.3 weeks and 37 % for sunitinib and 24.9 weeks and 9 % for IFN-α. This led to the use of sunitinib as one of the standard first-line therapies for advanced RCC. Additional TKI have been developed and have demonstrated clinical efficacy in mRCC, and this includes axitinib, pazopanib, and sorafenib. Current studies are comparing these different TKI in terms of their antitumor activity as well as toxicity. Although these TKI have significant clinical activity, RCC patients eventually become resistant to the drug possibly by different mechanisms. Another interesting feature of select TKI such as sunitinib is that they can moderate immune suppression and improve T cell function in the tumor bearing host. Sunitinib has been reported to reduce the number of myeloid-derived suppressor cells and T-regulatory cells in RCC patients and enhance T cell production of IFNγ (van Cruijsen et al. 2008; Ko et al. 2009; Finke et al. 2008). Subsequent studies in multiple mouse models have shown that sunitinib can enhance the efficacy of immunotherapy including vaccines (Bose et al. 2011; Farsaci et al. 2012), IL-12 plus 4-1BB activation (Farsaci et al. 2012) and adoptive T cell therapy (Kujawski et al. 2010).

mTOR inhibitors

Another important cellular pathway in the biology of RCC involves the mammalian target of rapamycin (mTOR). This serine–threonine protein kinase is critical for cell proliferation, metabolism, protein synthesis, and angiogenesis, and its activation was found in around 60 % of primary CCRCC (Robb et al. 2007); furthermore, its activation worsens the prognosis of localized and metastatic kidney cancer patients (Pantuck et al. 2007). Three analogs of rapamycin with mTOR inhibition properties have been tested clinically: temsirolimus, everolimus, and deforolimus. The first two have been extensively tested in RCC as second-line agents in metastatic RCC that progressed after treatment with a TKI as first-line drug treatment. Compared to IFNγ, IV infusion of temsirolimus improved the overall survival of poor prognosis population with RCC (Hudes et al. 2007). Everolimus can be taken orally as a second-line agent after progressive disease following TKI treatment; its efficacy and safety in this patient population have been established in a phase III clinical trial involving 416 patients. PFS was 4.9 and 1.9 months for the everolimus and placebo groups, respectively (Motzer et al. 2008).

Combination therapy

There are a number of combinational studies that are being developed, and some are underway. This includes combining anti-CTLA-4 antibodies with either anti-PD1 or anti-PDL-1 antibodies as a strategy that will block two checkpoint pathways of T cell suppression. Other studies are combining checkpoint blockade inhibitory antibodies with TKI since the latter are known to reduce angiogenesis but can also reduce immune suppression by targeting myeloid-derived suppressor cells and Treg cells (Ko et al. 2009; Ozao-Choy et al. 2009). Another focus is to combine agents that reduce immune suppression mediated by different mechanisms along with different immunotherapy approaches that are designed to stimulate the immune system. Clinical trials are underway testing whether sunitinib will synergize with two different vaccine strategies to promote an antitumor immune response and improve overall survival. This includes vaccination of RCC patients with DCs expressing tumor-associated antigens following their transfection with autologous tumor RNA (Argos Inc) or with a cocktail of peptides constituting multiple proteins that are overexpressed on RCC (Immatics Biotechnology). It also seems likely that additional studies will include combining these and other vaccines with checkpoint blockade antibodies.

9.2 Inflammatory Signaling Pathways Associated with Kidney Cancer

VHL pathway

Inflammation is mediated by certain environmental and pathogenic factors which include upregulation of HIF-1α and the production of proinflammatory proteins leading to the concept that hypoxia plays a role in inflammatory processes in

RCC (Reuter et al. 2010; Fitzgerald et al. 2012). As mentioned earlier, the transcription factors, HIF-1 and HIF-2, initiate transcription of a large set of genes important in several biologic responses including angiogenesis, proliferation, apoptosis, and metabolism (Fig. 9.1) (Kaelin 2009). The proteins produced as a consequence of VHL silencing include those involved in angiogenesis [vascular endothelial growth factor (VEGF), glycolysis (phosphoglycerate kinase), glucose transport (Glut-1), and erythropoiesis (erythropoietin)]; the chemokine receptor CXCR4 has also been identified as an HIF target (Staller et al. 2003), suggesting that HIF activation may contribute to the metastatic potential of cancer cells.

Hypoxia

A recent study (Fitzgerald et al. 2012) suggests that the inflammatory cytokines interleukin-6 and interleukin-8 (IL-6 and IL-8) are secreted from RCC cells after exposure to hypoxia (VHL deficient RCC cells). Furthermore, the NADPH oxidase isoform, Nox4, plays an important role in hypoxia-induced IL-6 and IL-8 production in RCC. Additionally, the AMP-activated protein kinase (AMPK) is a key regulator of NOX oxidase protein expression. AMPK is a sensor of cellular sensor status that has been shown to play a role in the regulation of cell inflammatory processes. Ex vivo studies by Fitzgerald et al. showed that enhanced levels of IL-6 and IL-8 result in RCC cell invasion and that activation of AMPK reduces Nox4 expression, IL-6 and IL-8 production, and RCC cell invasion. These findings shed light on a possible mechanism by which AMPK and Nox4 are linked to inflammation-induced RCC metastasis and that activation of AMPK may represent a relevant therapeutic strategy to reduce IL-6- and IL-8-induced inflammation and cell invasion in RCC.

VEGF

Binding of VEGF to its receptor initiates a complex of signaling cascades that promotes various cellular processes essential for new vessel formation including; increased vascular permeability, endothelial cell growth, migration, and survival of preexisting vasculature. VEGF also mobilizes endothelial progenitor cells from the bone marrow to sites of neovascularization.

The exact mechanism by which VEGF changes vascular permeability is not clearly understood but this change leads to macromolecule leak to the extravascular space and followed by edema formation. This change in the extravascular microenvironment makes it more proangiogenic compared to the stromal baseline conditions (Dvorak 2002). Additionally, VEGF promotes antiapoptotic proteins like bcl-2 and A1 which inactivates upstream caspases. This is mediated by activation of the PI3K-Akt pathway and promotes survival of endothelial cells. VEGF signaling increases the expression of several genes in endothelial cells, including several proteases, mitogens, and adhesion molecules that ultimately promote endothelial cell changes in cytoskeleton, cell morphology, and migration and invasion (Zachary 2001).

mTOR pathways

Protein kinase B (Akt) and mTOR are key players in processes involved in oncogenic transformation including cell survival, angiogenesis, and proliferation. mTOR is part of two major signaling complexes, mTORC1 and mTORC2, with two different functional roles. mTORC1 promotes cell proliferation and growth; mTORC2 modulates cell polarity and cytoskeleton rearrangement. Signaling of the mTORC1 pathway is initiated by growth factors binding PI3K on the cell membrane, this in turn phosphorylates PIP2 to PIP3, and this step is negatively regulated by PTEN. However, PIP3 activates Akt, which inhibits TSC (tuberous sclerosis complex) results in an overall upregulation of mTORC1 (Lieberthal and Levine 2009). In addition to its effects in cell growth and proliferation, mTOR activation leads to HIF accumulation; this is mediated through downstream proteins S6K1 and eIF-4E. PTEN is inactive in 20–30 % of RCC tumors (Brenner et al. 2002); furthermore, these mTOR-related proteins measured by tissue microarray from 375 patients with RCC were found more active in tissue samples from higher grade tumor and poor prognostic features (Pantuck et al. 2007), and some of these biomarkers (pAkt and p-S6K1) could be predictive of response with mTOR inhibition therapy (temsirolimus) (Cho et al. 2007).

TNF pathway

TNF has many different effects on tumor cells mostly dependent on ligation of each of its receptors (TNFR1 and TNFR2). Ligation of TNFR1 activates apoptotic signaling kinase and NF-κB promoting apoptosis. TNFR2 ligation leads to activation of EtK and VEGFR2, stimulates the transcription of antiapoptotic proteins, and promotes entry into the cell cycle acting as an autocrine growth factor in ccRCC (Al-Lamki et al. 2010). Thus, strategies to reduce TNFR2 expression or to selectively block signaling through TNFR2 may be more effective than global TNF blockade to reduce tumor progression. Malignant transformation of tubuloendothelial cells changes the profile of TNFR2 expression, in fact at both tissue level and plasma levels of TNFR2 have been shown to be elevated in RCC, and this elevation correlates with malignant grade of ccRCC (Elsasser-Beile et al. 2000; Al-Lamki et al. 2010). Furthermore, TNF-α may play a role in tumorigenesis in RCC, TNF-α-induced epithelial–mesenchymal transition and promotes tumor invasion by repressing E-cadherin, upregulating vimentin, activating matrix metalloproteinase 9 (Ho et al. 2012; Chuang et al. 2008).

STAT signaling pathways

The signal transducers and activators of transcription (STAT) factors represent downstream effectors of cytokine and growth factor receptor signaling. STATs are dual role proteins with both cytoplasmic signaling function and nuclear transcription factors capability. Cytokines and growth factors associated with tyrosine kinase receptors, cytoplasmic tyrosine kinases or molecules with intrinsic kinase activity use STAT to transmit cytoplasmic signals (van Boxel-Dezaire et al. 2006).

The persistent cytokine and growth factor signaling observed in cancer and chronic inflammation leads to accumulation of activated STAT proteins, and this persistent STAT activation has been observed in several types of cancer including RCC (Buettner et al. 2002; Horiguchi et al. 2002). In the setting of constant STAT activation, resulting in persistence of STAT in the nucleus and dysregulated gene expression eventually will alter the genotype of the cell. Constitutive expression of STAT3 induces expression of BCL-XL, MCL1, and survivin, which have antiapoptotic functions. Blocking STAT3 signaling can block the expression of these proteins and makes cells more susceptible to apoptosis (Catlett-Falcone et al. 1999; Aoki et al. 2003). STAT3 also induces C-MYC expression which prevents cells from reaching terminal differentiation and maintains mitotic cell capabilities (Bowman et al. 2001).

9.3 Role of Inflammatory Molecules in the Development of Kidney Cancer: In Vitro Studies

The development and transformation of cancer cells, as well as invasion and metastasis is influenced by a complex interaction of inflammatory mediators including cytokines, chemokines, their receptors, and downstream signaling pathways. This inflammatory signaling profile promotes proliferation of tumor cells as well as a microenvironment rich in growth factors, activated inflammatory cells and factors that support angiogenesis, migration and invasion (Balkwill 2004). An increasing number of cytokines and chemokines are been found to be related to RCC, and they often correlate with bad prognosis or high malignant grade. This includes CXCR4, CCR3, IL-6, IL-1β, and TNF-α which are among the inflammatory markers found upregulated in RCC (Johrer et al. 2005; Yoshida et al. 2002; Dosquet et al. 1994).

9.3.1 Role of Inflammatory Molecules in the Transformation of Kidney Cancer Cells

Early in the formation of primary epithelial tumors, cells show excessive proliferation, angiogenesis, and invasiveness. This is thought to be initially characterized by the invasion of the basement membrane which is the first step for tumor cells to eventually disseminate and metastasize. The ability to advance through the basement membrane is not exclusive of tumor cells, normal cells can do this as part of the epithelial to mesenchymal transition (EMT) which is tightly regulated genetically and biochemically. Activation of this phenotype is postulated as a key step in malignant transformation of epithelial cells and is characterized by altered morphology, adhesion, migration, and cellular architecture (Thiery 2002). Expression of vimentin and nuclear translocation of β-catenin are some of the molecular markers of EMT; cells also show resistance to apoptosis and increased migration capacity. An invasion assay using CCRCC lines with mutated VHL showed that tumor-derived IL-6, TNF-α, IL-1, and matrix metalloproteinase-2 (MMP2) promoted tumor invasion. The most invasive cell lines showed higher levels of mRNA of these proinflammatory cytokines and MMP2 and produced more TNF-α, which was correlated with stronger invasive ability (Chuang et al. 2008). TNF-α has shown to enhance migration of RCC cell lines via activation of PI3K/Akt pathway which in turn inactivates GSK-3β pathway (Sourbier et al. 2006) which has been reported to be involved in the regulation of EMT (Luo 2009). Moreover, inhibition of PI3K/AKT reactivated the GSK-3β suppression of EMT in TNF-α-conditioned RCC cells (Ho et al. 2012).

pVHL can play an HIF-independent role in tumor transformation. VHL mutation results in dysregulation of HIF-1α which in turn activates a cascade of events that favor tumor growth and proliferation. However, the mechanism by which a normal kidney cell undergoes oncogenic transformation is poorly understood. Some in vitro studies have shown that VHL has HIF-1α-independent effect on RCC cells, and such effect could play an important role in tumor initiation. In fact, overexpression of non-degradable HIF proteins in the absence of VHL mutation leads to proliferation of normal-appearing blood vessels but no oncogenic transformation (Elson et al. 2001). pVHL directly binds to fibronectin which interacts with integrin to bridge cells to the extracellular matrix in vitro, and this assembly is defective in mutant pVHL cells (Ohh et al. 1998). pVHL stabilizes tumor-suppressor gene p53 which mediates cell cycle arrest and apoptosis. Additionally, pVHL also suppresses the expression of the mitogen cyclin D1 which is required for cells to exit the cell cycle upon serum starvation in vitro (Roe et al. 2006; Zatyka et al. 2002; Pause et al. 1998). Functional VHL seems also to be required for the formation of the primary cilium, which occurs in cells reaching quiescence, and its dysfunction is associated with the formation of renal cyst which often precedes tumor formation (Esteban et al. 2006; Lutz and Burk 2006). Together, these experiments suggest that there are independent functions of VHL separable from its interactions with HIF-1α that likely play an important role in the oncogenic transformation of kidney cells in RCC.

Transforming growth factor (TGF) β1 is a member of the TGF-β superfamily. This cytokine plays a role in wound healing, fibrinogenesis, and tissue remodeling and can strongly influence the growth and phenotype of several types of cells (Massague et al. 1992). Overexpression has been observed in different kinds of cancer, including RCC. Primary RCC cells as well as different RCC cell lines express TGF-β1, and a majority of cell lines are resistant to growth-suppressive effect of exogenous TGF-β1 (Ramp et al. 1997). This suggests that transformation and/or progression of human RCC could be related to TGF-β1 resistance to growth inhibition. Transfection of wild-type VHL gene into the human RCC line 786-O lacking WT pVHL suppressed TGF-β message mainly at the posttranscriptional level showing that TGF-β is a target for pVHL. However, this line was unresponsive to TGF-β because it lacked the TGF-β type II receptor. While VHL mutations appear early in RCC development, a second genetic event resulting in loss of TGF-β type II receptor expression and resistant to the antiproliferative effect of TGF-β can occur. Additionally, the biological significance of increased TGF-β levels in RCC appears to be the stimulation of angiogenesis, and therefore, blocking the angiogenic effect of TGF-β could be a strategy to reducing RCC growth (Ananth et al. 1999).

9.3.2 Role of Inflammatory Molecules in the Survival of Kidney Cancer Cells

The production of IL-6, a proinflammatory cytokine, is associated with poor prognosis in patients with metastatic RCC. IL-6 causes upregulation of the suppressor of cytokine signaling-3 (SOCS3) which plays a role in IFN-α resistance in RCC by inactivating cytokine-induced janus kinase/signal transducer and activator of transcription (JAK/STAT) pathway (Tomita et al. 2011). IFN-α stimulation induced IL-6 secretion and both IL-6 and SOCS3 mRNA expression in RCC cell lines. Adding an antihuman IL-6 receptor blocking antibody, tocilizumab, to IFN-α-treated RCC cell lines significantly suppressed cell proliferation compared to IFN-α stimulation alone. Tocilizumab also inhibited the IFN-α-induced mRNA expression of SOCS3. Treatment with tocilizumab in IFN-α-stimulated RCC cells enhanced phosphorylation of STAT1 and inhibited SOCS3 expression and the phosphorylation of both STAT3 and ERK (Oguro et al. 2013). This experiment suggests that autocrine IL-6 secretion after IFN-α treatment can promote tumor cell survival possibly through upregulation of SOCS3 and STAT3 activation. IL-6 decreases the antitumor effects of IFN-α treatment. This inhibition can be reversed when an IL-6 receptor blocking antibody is utilized.

TNF-α plays a major role in several inflammatory pathways; it regulates cytotoxicity, survival, and apoptotic responses (Wajant et al. 2003). RCC cell lines with a non-functional VHL protein were shown to be resistant to TNF-α-induced cytotoxicity. Insertion of a wild-type pVHL plasmid into the RCC cells reconstituted the sensitivity to TNF-α compared to empty plasmid insertion as measured by an Annexin-V assay going from 2 and 12 % to 32 and 61 % after 48–72-h treatment with TNF-α (Qi and Ohh 2003). TNF-α can both induce cell survival and cell death depending on expression of receptors and regulation of downstream signaling. FADD recruitment to the TNFR1 starts the caspase cascade, which results in apoptosis. In contrast, TNF-α also activates aPKC, which results in translocation of NF-κB into the nucleus and subsequently suppression of apoptosis.

Another member of the TNF family, TNF-related apoptosis-inducing ligand (TRAIL) is produced by most normal tissue cells. Binding of TRAIL to its receptor results in apoptosis, primarily in tumor cells. Most RCC cell lines express TRAIL-R1 and TRAIL-R2 receptors; however, the majority of RCC cell lines are resistant to TRAIL-mediated apoptosis (Ramp et al. 2003). Constitutively activated NF-κB correlates with resistance to TRAIL-induced apoptosis in RCC cell lines (Oya et al. 2001). VHL protein has been shown to bind several aPKC isoforms and targets them for ubiquitination and degradation (Okuda et al. 2001). The nuclear fraction of RCC cell lines was analyzed by electrophoretic mobility shift assay and showed higher basal level of NF-κB capable of binding its DNA motifs compared with wild-type VHL reconstituted cells. Furthermore, treatment with TNF-α showed a significant rise in NF-κB in the nucleus of WT VHL reconstituted cells compared to a lower response in non-reconstituted cells (Qi and Ohh 2003). This suggests that in addition to downregulation of HIF proteins and their target genes, VHL is a positive regulator of apoptosis and RCC cells with a mutated VHL display resistant to NF-κB-mediated apoptosis. Functional VHL protein may be required for TNF-α and TRAIL-induced apoptotic cell death.

CSF-1 is highly regulated in the kidney and plays an important role in renal tubular injury by promoting repair and inhibiting apoptosis (Menke et al. 2009). It also participates in progression of several epithelial tumors (Morandi et al. 2011). RCC cell lines were found to co-express CSF-1, and its receptor CSF-1R stimulation with TNF-α significantly upregulates this expression at the RNA and protein level. Moreover, expression of CSF-1 and CSF-1R is induced in tubular epithelial cells when treated with supernatant from an RCC cell culture in a concentration dependent fashion and with greater response when the supernatant was from stimulated RCC cells. Treatment of RCC and TEC cell lines with CSF-1 showed increased cell proliferation in a dose-dependent manner, and this response was inhibited with a blocking antibody. RCC cell lines stimulated with TNF-α/LPS showed an increased rate of apoptosis, and adding a blocking anti-CSF-1R Ab further increased the response (Menke et al. 2012). CSF-1 may have an autocrine and paracrine role in RCC promoting tumor cell proliferation, and decreasing apoptosis.

9.3.3 Role of Inflammatory Molecules in the Proliferation of Kidney Cancer Cells

Chemokine role in proliferation and trafficking

Chemokines are proinflammatory cytokines involved in several immune reactions including inflammation, infection, tissue repair, and many others, and have been shown to have an important role in tumor growth and metastasis (Wang et al. 1998). CXCL12 is a chemokine whose expression has been found decreased in rapidly dividing cells such as fibroblast and liver cells (Jiang et al. 1994) and in several kinds of solid tumors, it binds to a G protein coupled receptor CXCR4 and its expression is commonly elevated in cancer cells including RCC (Begum et al. 1999; Shibuta et al. 1997; Rempel et al. 2000; Sehgal et al. 1998).

The expression of CXCL12 and its receptor was measured by RT-PCR in 4 primary human kidney cancer cell lines (Schrader et al. 2002). CXCR4 was elevated in all 4 cell lines analyzed in particular in A-498 cells. This elevation of CXCR4 in RCC cells is likely due to a loss of inhibition by the pVHL. CXCR4 was shown to be one of the target genes of HIF and reconstitution of pVHL in an

RCC cell line resulted in significant downregulation of CXCR4 gene (Staller et al. 2003). Treatment with a recombinant ligand (rhCXCL12 alpha) induced changes in intracellular calcium levels in A-498 RCC cells, proving functionality of this receptor. Furthermore, a cDNA expression array showed increased stimulation of cell cycle and apoptosis-related genes compared to unstimulated A-498 cells. Upon binding of CXCL12 to CXCR4, a signaling cascade is initiated, the complex is internalized and localizes into the nucleus (Wang et al. 2009). Silencing of the CXCR4 receptor by RNA interference in A-498 cells induced apoptosis and inhibited cell growth, migration, and invasiveness compared to control cells (Wang et al. 2012b). Previous studies have shown that CXCR4-expressing cancer cells commonly metastasize to organs that express abundant CXCL12 (Muller et al. 2001), and this chemotactic property could also play an important role in RCC tumor migration. Moreover, while this HIF-dependent expression of CXCR4 takes place in other solid tumors in response to hypoxia, RCC cells could manifest this CXCR4 activation much earlier in the tumor progression. Thus, CXCR4 expression could provide kidney cancer cells with an increased ability to regulate the cell cycle, invade tissue barriers, migrate to other organs, and inhibit apoptosis.

A-498 cells also express CCR3, CCR6, CXCR2, CXCR3, and CXCR4 on both mRNA and protein levels (Johrer et al. 2005). CCR3 is a receptor for eotaxin-1 which has been characterized as a potent eosinophil chemoattractant but may also play an important role in the proliferation of RCC cells. CCR3 and eotaxin-1 mRNA expression is high in a wide range of organs including small intestine, colon, heart, kidney, and pancreas (Levina et al. 2009). Proinflammatory cytokines including TNF-α, IL-1, IFN-α, and IL-4 induce eotaxin-1 expression in vitro in a variety of tissues (Garcia-Zepeda et al. 1996a, b; Schrader et al. 2002; Mochizuki et al. 1998). Binding of eotaxin-1 to its receptors leads to activation of G proteins, increased intracellular calcium, cytoskeletal rearrangements, activation of mitogen-activated protein kinase pathway, and receptor internalization (Zimmermann et al. 1999). When A-498 kidney cancer cells were treated with eotaxin-1, there was upregulation of intracellular Ca^{2+}, internalization of the receptor-ligand complex that coincided with increased cell proliferation compared to control (Johrer et al. 2005).

9.3.4 Role of Inflammatory Molecules in the Invasion, Metastasis, and Angiogenesis of Kidney Cancer Cells

Invasion and metastasis

Metastasis represents the worst prognostic feature of several kinds of cancer. Kidney cancer in particular presents a dramatic drop in the 5-year survival rate from over 90 % to a mere 10 % when metastasis is present at diagnosis (Cohen and McGovern 2005). For a tumor to become invasive a complex series, chemical interactions must take place between tumor cells, extracellular matrix, adhesion molecules, and blood vessels to allow the tumor cells to escape from the primary tumor site. Inflammatory molecules play an important role in RCC that allows these interactions to occur.

MMPs are metalloendopeptidases that have the ability to disrupt the extracellular matrix continuity, thereby playing an important role in the inflammatory response and in promoting histological processes such as tissue remodeling and angiogenesis. MMPs also participate in pathological processes like cirrhosis, arthritis, and metastasis (Yoon et al. 2003). The loss of VHL function has been linked with upregulation of gene and protein MMP expression through HIF up-regulation (Petrella et al. 2005). Specifically, MT1-MMP gene is a target of HIF-2α, and MT1-MMP is thought to be a key mediator of invasion and angiogenesis (Seiki and Yana 2003). An experiment using RCC cells either wild-type (WT8) and null (pRc-9) for VHL looked at their invasive characteristics. The pRc-9 cells had increased capacity to degrade and invade in a type I collagen matrix transwell assay compared to WT8 cells. Expression of HIF-2α or MT1-MMP in the WT8 cells, via transfection, promoted collagen degradation and invasion of these cells comparable to levels seen in pRc-9 cells (Petrella and Brinckerhoff 2006).

Tissue inhibitors of metalloproteinases (TIMPs) are endogenous inhibitors of MMPs that protect tissues by regulating their function, and a high MMP to TIMP ratio in a particular tumor has been found to correlate with malignant grade. MMP-2 and MMP-9 are increased in RCC tissue (Kallakury et al. 2001; Kugler et al. 1998) and overexpressed in RCC cell lines analyzed after oxidative stress. However, the levels of their inhibitors TIMP-1 and TIMP-2 remained unchanged compared to unstressed cells. Silencing MMP-9 reduced the expression of MMP-9 in a RCC cell line (Caki-2) as well as their invasiveness, but cell proliferation was not affected (Ueno et al. 2009). The increase in MMP to TIMP ratio may represent a mechanism by which RCC cells acquire invasive capabilities in the presence of oxidative stress inducers such as tumor-associated macrophages (TAMs) (Hemmerlein et al. 2004).

In addition to ROS, TAMs from RCC specimens have been shown to secrete high amounts of IL1-β (Ikemoto et al. 2003). Treatment of serum starved human 786-0 VHL null RCC cell line with IL-1β resulted in induction of tumor cell invasion in a type I collagen-coated transwell assay. Furthermore, pretreatment of RCC cells with a pan-MMP inhibitor, blocked IL-1β-induced invasion thereby demonstrating a MMP-dependent effect of IL-1β in promoting cell invasion. Moreover, IL-1β potently induced the expression of MMP-1, MMP-3, and MMP-10 (which have collagen I degradation activity) at the mRNA and protein levels in a dose-dependent fashion (Ikemoto et al. 2003).

Urokinase-type plasminogen activator (uPA) has been known to mediate invasion and metastasis of various tumor cells, its expression has been found elevated in kidney tumors, and it possibly correlates with aggressive phenotype (Andreasen et al. 2000; Swiercz et al. 1998). The protein C inhibitor (PCI) is an endogenous inhibitor of several protease enzymes including protein C and uPA. In humans, PCI is mainly produced by the liver and other tissues including the reproductive track, and the kidney also produces it in lesser amounts (Laurell et al. 1992;

Francis and Thomas 1984). PCI is found in tissues in complex with uPA, which inhibits it suggesting a role of PCI in protecting tissues from unopposed uPA; in fact, PCI knockout mice have been reported to grow normally but are infertile, this is thought to be due to disruption of the blood–testis barrier (Uhrin et al. 2000). uPA has been known to mediate invasion and metastasis of various tumor cells. An experiment using purified PCI to treat Caki-1, a kidney cancer cell line that expresses uPA (but not PCI) showed that PCI inhibited cell invasion in a dose-dependent fashion in gel matrix assay, heat inactivation of PCI, or addition of a PCI antibody blocked this inhibition and treatment with an uPA antibody also inhibited cell migration (Wakita et al. 2004).

RCC, especially the clear-cell type, develops a densely vascular architecture. The VHL gene plays a crucial role in the cellular response to oxygen, and its ability regulates critical regulators of angiogenesis through the HIF transcription factors (Iliopoulos et al. 1996). In the renal tumor setting, HIF-2α is responsible for activation of cyclin-D1, TGF-α, and VEGF pathways (Raval et al. 2005). VEGF angiogenic activity is mediated through interaction with other proangiogenic factors many of which are also gene targets of HIF, some of these molecules, like angioprotein-1, provide antiapoptotic properties and vessel stability; erythropoietin, also a target of HIF, promotes endothelial cell growth and migration (Heeschen et al. 2003; Yamakawa et al. 2004).

MMPs can disrupt the extracellular matrix and promote tumor cell migration; this disruption of the tissue also allows for pericyte invasion and activation through release of growth factors bound to the extracellular matrix; this step is necessary for new vessel formation and is also facilitated by platelet-derived growth factor receptor (PDGFR) activation on the pericyte (Yamakawa et al. 2004). PDGF-B and TGF-β1 participate in smooth muscle cell recruitment and stabilization (Carmeliet and Jain 2000).

9.4 Role of Inflammatory Molecules in the Development of Kidney Cancer: In Vivo Studies

Animal models

The most widely used murine tumor model is the RENCA cell line that arose spontaneously in Balb/c mice (Wigginton et al. 1996). More recently, streptozotocin-induced renal cell tumor lines including SIRCC-1.15 (designated RCC#15) have been developed and characterized. The Streptozotocin tumor develops spontaneous metastases to lung and mesenteric lymph nodes following into kidneys (Gruys et al. 2001). Both of these tumor models are sensitive to different forms of immunotherapy; however, neither have the molecular and cellular features of human CCRCC as they lack the loss of the VHL gene function and the constitutive expression of HIF and its targets. Conditional models of VHL inactivation and VHL knockout mice have been produced but they do not develop spontaneous RCC (Kleymenova et al. 2004; Rankin et al. 2006; Haase et al. 2001). A mouse model that specifically express a mutated, constitutively active HIF-1α in kidney cells was recently developed and shows characteristics of VHL disease including spontaneous kidney tumors (Fu et al. 2011); this model could be a closer step to better explore the biology of RCC in an in vivo model. Clearly, additional studies are needed to develop tumor models that come closer to mimicking human RCC. The implantation of human clear-cell tumors into *nu/nu* mice is currently being used to study the signaling pathways of RCC and metabolism of this tumor along with TKI resistance (Gameiro et al. 2013; Huang et al. 2010; Karam et al. 2011). Another model uses tissue slices from freshly collected RCC specimens to be implanted under the renal capsule in nu/nu mice (Thong et al. 2014). The major drawback to the use of xenograft models in nude mice or NOD-skid is that the role of immune cells in either promoting tumor growth (infiltrating macrophages) or eradication of tumor via immunotherapy cannot be examined.

9.5 Evidence from Patients for the Role of Inflammation in Kidney Cancer

The production of different inflammatory cytokines, chemokines, and growth factors by RCC cells and tumor stromal cells stimulates the activation, expansion, and trafficking of various immune cells into the tumor where they can promote tumor progression by enhancing angiogenesis and initiating T cell immune suppression (Fig 9.1) (Gabrilovich et al. 2012).

9.5.1 Immune Inflammatory cells

TAMs

Tumor-associated macrophages or TAMs are cells that originate from recruited myeloid cells such as monocytes and MDSC. These myeloid cells are highly plastic and tumor-derived factors recruit and sustain them to support angiogenesis, tissue remodeling, and immune suppression (Sica and Bronte 2007). TAMs can constitute a significant component of solid tumors, and depending on the microenvironment, they can present different phenotypes (Sica and Bronte 2007; Biswas and Mantovani 2010). In RCC microenvironment, there is an increased metabolism of arachidonic acid partly due to the enzyme 15-lypoxygenase (LOX) highly expressed in RCC TAMs. This, in turn, increases production of hydroxyeicosatetraenoic acids (HETE). An upregulated LOX-HETE pathway in RCCs tumor microenvironment affects the immune phenotype of TAMs. For example, RCC TAMs secrete immunosuppressive Interleukin-10 and the proinflammatory chemokine CCL2. IL-10-producing macrophages are considered “regulatory macrophages” in a recently proposed classification, and their presence could negatively affect prognosis as well as efficacy of tumor vaccines and other kinds of immunotherapy (Mosser and Edwards 2008). RCC TAMs also induce upregulation of CTLA-4, IL-10-secreting TILs, and FoxP3+ T cells, a tolerogenic subset of tumor infiltrating lymphocytes called Tregs (Daurkin et al. 2011). And, as discussed above, their ability to induce oxidative stress and produce IL1-β could favor a more invasive and proangiogenic phenotype in RCC cells. RCC tumors with high-infiltration TAMs were significantly associated with poor prognosis, and inflammatory cytokines TAMs produce, including IL-1β, TNF-α, and IL-6, are also independent factors of poor prognosis in RCC (Yoshida et al. 2002; Komohara et al. 2011).

MDSC

Myeloid-derived suppressor cells constitute a heterogenous cell population with immunosuppressive and angiogenic properties that originate from the bone marrow under pathologic conditions such as cancer. These cells have the morphology of immature granulocytes, monocytes, and dendritic cells (DCs) (Gabrilovich 2004). These cells are functionally defined by their capacity to suppress T cell immunity via different mechanisms (Gabrilovich 2004; Peranzoni et al. 2010). MDSC express enzymes (e.g., arginase 1) that can deplete select amino acids in the tumor microenvironment (L-arginine and L-cysteine), thereby limiting the availability of these amino acid which are necessary for lymphocyte activation (13) (Srivastava et al. 2010). Some MDSC produce reactive oxygen species (ROS) and/or inducible nitric oxide synthase, resulting in reduced CTL activity and IFN-γ production (Corzo et al. 2009; Kusmartsev et al. 2008; Cohen et al. 2012; Ko et al. 2010). MDSC indirectly inhibit T cell immunity by stimulating expansion of regulatory T cells (Treg) (Huang et al. 2006; Pan et al. 2010). MDSC can also reduce L-selectin expression of naïve T cells, reducing their ability to enter peripheral lymph nodes where DC presents antigen (Hanson et al. 2009). Besides mediating immunosuppression, MDSC can stimulate angiogenesis. Injecting nude mice with MDSC plus tumor cells compared to tumor alone increased vascular density and maturation within the tumor that was dependent metallomatrix protein 9 (MMP9) production. Interestingly, a subset of MDSC can associate with tumor endothelium followed by their differentiation into endothelial cells (Yang et al. 2004). Furthermore, the production of VEGF and bFGF by MDSC is STAT3 dependent since MDSC- mediated angiogenesis can be blocked by STAT3 inhibitors (Kujawski et al. 2008). Similar to mouse models, granulocytic (G) MDSC (CD33+HLADR−CD15+CD14−) dominate in the blood of patients with different types of cancer including RCC, GBM, lung, and pancreatic cancer (Rodriguez et al. 2009; Zea et al. 2005; Peggs et al. 2009; Ko et al. 2010; Youn et al. 2012; Sippel et al. 2011). Monocytic (CD33+HLADR−CD15−CD14+) are also present in modest numbers in RCC patients while a population of MDSC not typically seen in mouse models are prevalent in RCC, the linage negative subset (CD33+HLADR−CD15−CD14−) (11, 23, 25). The granulocytic MDSC are known to be suppressive. The impact-increased MDSC numbers in the blood has on tumor progression were recently assessed in RCC patients. High pretreatment levels of M-MDSC and G-MDSC in mRCC patients correlated with reduced overall survival (Walter et al. 2012).

The abnormal expansion of MDSC is attributable to the heightened production of several growth factors such as G-CSF, GM-CSF, IL6, VEGF, S100, and SCF (Gabrilovich 2004). Additional molecules expressed in the tumor microenvironment stimulate MDSC activation, and this includes prostaglandins, and select cytokines IFN-γ, IL-4, IL-13, and TGF-β.

Neutrophils

Increased neutrophil numbers in the peripheral blood have been identified as a predictor for shorter overall survival in metastatic RCC patients (Choueiri et al. 2007; Donskov and von der Maase 2006; Donskov 2013; Lopez-Lago et al. 2013; Negrier et al. 2002). More recently it was reported that the presence of intratumoral CD66b+ neutrophils in RCC patients with localized disease was linked to higher tumor size, lower recurrence-free survival, and reduced overall survival (Jensen et al. 2009). It may be that the negative impact of neutrophils on RCC patient outcome is linked to the evidence that neutrophils from RCC patients are immunosuppressive. Peripheral blood from RCC patients contain already mature, activated neutrophils with suppressive activity resulting from their expression of arginase. Because of their similarities to granulocytic MDSC, they were identified as G-MDSC (Rodriguez et al. 2009; Zea et al. 2005). These findings were similar to the work of Schmielau and Finn who earlier showed that the presence of granulocytes from pancreatic, colon, and breast cancer patients had T cell suppressive activity and their presence correlated with reduced T cell zeta-chain expression and decreased cytokine production. They also showed that healthy donor resting granulocytes could be converted to suppressive cells by exposure to the chemotactic peptide N-formyl-L-methionyl–L-leucyl–L-phenylanine (fmlp) (Schmielau and Finn 2001). However, other studies suggest that human G-MDSC constitute immature neutrophils (CD16−CD33+HLADR−CD66b+) because they display low to absent expression of the neutrophil maturation marker CD16 (FcRγ1) (Brandau et al. 2011). Additional functional and gene array studies are clearly needed to define the interrelationship between G-MDSC, patient neutrophils, and activated neutrophils from healthy donors.

9.5.2 *Chemokines Receptors (CXCR4, CXCR3 enoxin) and Ligands, Cytokines (IL-6, IFNγ, IL-4,) that Correlates with Prognosis*

Angiogenesis, invasion, and metastasis

As cancer progresses, the phenotype of cells, microenvironment, and the immune responses exhibit changes (often orchestrated by tumor cells) that allow this progression to take place. Real-time PCR and immunohistochemistry staining of specimens from RCC patients with localized or metastatic RCC showed that primary human RCC tumors are immunogenic and expresses high levels of HLA class I mRNA and proinflammatory cytokines and chemokines. In contrast, metastatic RCC is characterized by an immunosuppressive microenvironment, decreased expression of HLA class I, reduced level of IFN-γ and suppression of IP-10, VEGF and SDF-1 at both mRNA and protein level (Romero et al. 2006). This may indicate that a switch in the tumor cells, its microenvironment, or both may provide an escape for tumor cells from the cytotoxic response and favor tumor invasion and metastasis.

The macrophage migration inhibitory factor (MIF) is a cytokine with roles in autoimmunity diseases, obesity, and cancer; it promotes inflammation and can prolong immune responses. This cytokine is regulated by hypoxia and is one of the HIF target genes (Bernhagen et al. 1993; Welford et al. 2006). MIF is expressed and correlated with poor prognosis in a number of solid tumors (Du et al. 2013). In RCC, MIF was found in most tumor specimens, and it correlated with the presence of circulating MIF in RCC patients. shRNA inhibition of MIF expression in RCC cell lines or the use of a direct antagonist reduced their proliferation rate. Similarly, inhibition of MIF receptors CD74 or CD44 resulted in inhibition of cell proliferation. Western blot analysis showed MIF signaling through CD74 and CD44 increases Src expression and degradation of p27 which could represent a mechanism for promotion of cell growth (Du et al. 2013).

Inflammatory molecules as prognostic tools

Inflammation-associated molecules have been increasingly studied as prognostic factors or predictors of response. CRP is an acute phase reactant discovered almost a century ago and is used in the clinic as a non-specific early marker of inflammation. CRP is mainly synthesized in the liver under different stimuli, mainly by IL-6 and IL-1β. Cancer patients often have elevated plasma levels of CRP, and it correlates with survival in many solid tumors (Roxburgh and McMillan 2010; Trichopoulos et al. 2006). In RCC, CRP is too used as a prognostic factor for patients undergoing surgery as well as receiving systemic therapy (Saito and Kihara 2013; Saito et al. 2009). IL-6 levels are elevated in patients with RCC, they correlate with CRP levels and correlate with, poor prognosis, survival, and response to treatment, both immunotherapy and targeted systemic therapy (Michaelson and Stadler 2013; Kallio et al. 2001; Blay et al. 1992).

As discussed earlier, CXCL12 and its receptors, CXCR4 and CXCR7, play an important role in kidney cancer cells' survival and proliferation; CXCR4 has been found unregulated in RCC tumors while CXCL12 is decreased compared to surrounding tissues (Schrader et al. 2002; D'Alterio et al. 2010a). The presence of this cytokines and receptors in tumor specimens has been correlated with poor prognosis. A total of 560 RCC patients' specimens from three different studies were evaluated for CXCR4 and CXCR7 through immunohistochemistry. High CXCR4 and high CXCR7 expression predicted poor disease-free survival (DFS). Both CXCR4 and CXCR7 were found to have a significant negative correlation with survival independently in multivariate analysis. A total of 97 specimens evaluated showed CXCL12 expression which was correlated with poor overall survival and DFS. Furthermore, RT-PCR analysis of 49 tumor samples showed that the presence of CXCR4 and CXCR7 correlated with symptoms at the time of diagnosis and lymph nodes status (D'Alterio et al. 2010b; Wang et al. 2012a; D'Alterio et al. 2010a). Screening for the chemokine receptor CXCR3 (receptor for eotaxin-1 discussed above) in 219 tumor specimens found this expression in almost a third of the samples, and its expression was found to correlate with high tumor grade (Johrer et al. 2005). Two ligands for this receptor are CXC chemokines, I-TAC and Mig, and they have antiangiogenic activities; however, RCC samples showed high levels of both in vascular smooth muscle, pericytes of tumor tissues compared to corresponding normal tissue. This paradoxical expression suggests a stronger opposing angiogenic stimuli or a possible dual role of these chemokines generally considered angiostatic (Suyama et al. 2005).

In contrast with the above markers, Th1-associated cytokines could indicate favorable prognosis. A total of 67 tumor specimens from sporadic RCC cases were analyzed by rt-PCR for Th1- (IP-10, ITAC, MIG, MIP-1β, and RANTES) and Th2- (MDC and eotaxin) associated genes. TH1 genes were higher compared to normal kidney tissue, and it correlated with IFNγ expression. More importantly, out of 59 patients who underwent curative surgery, 9 patients had recurrence, and none of them presented high TH1-related cytokines IP-10, ITAC, MIP-1β, and RANTES, and 1 patient with high MIG had recurrence after surgery (mean follow up of 45.7 ± 29.3 months). Similarly, patients with high eotaxin expression had no tumor recurrence after surgery (Kondo et al. 2006).

Matrix metalloproteinases (MMPs) and their regulators, TIMPs, are implicated in RCCs invasive potential (see in vitro section). A total of 153 RCC sections were analyzed for MMP2, MMP9, TIMP1, and TIMP2 by immune staining, and it was found that their increased expression (including TIMPs) correlated with poor prognostic characteristics including survival, and high tumor grade (Kallakury et al. 2001). The paradoxical correlation of TIMPs expression with poor prognostic features suggest a more complex biology of these inhibitors, in fact, when the ratio of MMPs to TIMPs in RCC tumors was compared to normal kidney tissue, it was found that tumors cells had a ratio of 2.4 MMP:TIMP (based on a ratio of 1 for normal kidney) for localized tumors and 4.86 for advanced disease suggesting that a balance of these molecules has probably more prognostic value than the absolute number (Kugler et al. 1998).

9.6 Inhibitors of Inflammation for the Prevention and Treatment of Kidney Cancer

NSAIDs

Studies on the use of anti-inflammatory drugs and kidney cancer have been inconsistent. The overall risk of cancer in patients who use NSAIDs is reduced compared to patients not taking this drugs (Bardia et al. 2007); this is thought to be due to COX-2 inhibition, reduced inflammation, and effects on cell proliferation and apoptosis (Leahy et al. 2002). Cho et al. (2011) used prospective data of two different cohorts with 126,000 women and men followed for 16 and 20 years, respectively. Lifestyle questionnaires every 2 years enquiring about NSAIDs use and illnesses including RCC were done. Aspirin and acetaminophen, which are among the most used analgesics, use were not associated with RCC risk, consistent with previous reports (Tavani et al. 2010). In contrast, increased risk of RCC was associated with non-aspirin NSAIDs; the absolute risk differences for users vs. nonusers of non-aspirin NSAIDs were 9.15 per 100,000 person years in women and 10.92 per 100,000 person years in men and a pooled multivariate relative risk of 1.51 suggesting an increased risk of RCC with longer use of non-aspirin NSAIDs (Cho et al. 2011). Although the absolute risk for NSAIDs users compared to nonusers is relatively small, the ubiquitous use of NSAIDs worldwide should emphasize the significance of these results.

COX-2 inhibitors

Cyclooxygenase-2 (COX-2) is an important enzyme involved in the synthesis of prostaglandins. In cancer, COX-2 has been linked to several stages of development of tumors including cell growth, antiapoptosis, and angiogenesis (Koga et al. 2004; Sawaoka et al. 1999; Masferrer et al. 2000). COX-2 inhibitors have been used in preclinical and clinical studies to inhibit tumor growth and angiogenesis and as a chemopreventive drug in different solid tumors (Rao et al. 2002; Wang et al. 2013; Fujimura et al. 2007). RCC cell lines overexpress COX-2, and it has a role in cell invasion capabilities (Chen et al. 2004a, b). Although in vivo studies showed COX-2 enhanced tumorigenesis and angiogenesis in a human RCC xenograft, and human RCC specimens showed expression of COX-2, human clinical trials using a selective COX-2 inhibitor in combination with IFN-α resulted in no added clinical activity compared to IFN-α alone. Furthermore, selective treatment of patients whose tumors showed high immunostaining for COX-2 did not benefited from COX-2 inhibition when treated with IFN-α. Selecting high COX-2 expressing tumors could also represent a selection of highly immunosuppressive tumors which could explain this lack of additional response. (Rini et al. 2006; Schwandt et al. 2011).

Statins as an anti-inflammatory drug in kidney cancer

Statins are a group of drugs that inhibit HMG-CoA reductase enzyme and lower blood cholesterol levels. Although not traditionally considered anti-inflammatory drugs, statins have been found to have effects on inflammation and immunomodulation (Schonbeck and Libby 2004). Moreover, statins can reduce cell growth and proliferation of several types of cancer cells, and recent studies are looking at statins as potential anticancer agents (Sassano and Platanias 2008; Gauthaman et al. 2009). Clinically, studies looking at the overall risk of cancer in patients taking statins have had variable results from reduced overall risk, neutral effect, and one study found higher cancer incidence correlated with lower LDL-cholesterol levels (Farwell et al. 2008; Dale et al. 2006; Alsheikh-Ali et al. 2007). Khurana et al. (2008) looked nearly 500,000 records of veterans who visited the VA Health Care System over a period of 5.6 years, multivariate analysis adjusting for age, race, sex, body mass index (BMI), and smoking showed an overall 44 % RCC risk reduction in patients taking statins. Mechanistically, the effect of statins on renal cancer cells has been shown to inhibit cell growth, proliferation, invasion, and pro-apoptotic effects in vitro, it also leads to cell cycle arrest with upregulation of p21 and p53 (Fang et al. 2013; Horiguchi et al. 2004). Protein analysis showed elevated Bax and decreased Bcl-2; the balance of these two apoptosis-related proteins favors apoptosis when it favors Bax. Looking downstream, cleaved caspase-3 (an effector caspase) and cleaved PARP (a caspase-3 target) levels were also elevated; furthermore, a statin (simvastatin) mediated these effects by targeting the AKT/mTOR pathway which is commonly activated in RCC as discussed in the beginning of this chapter. Similarly, phosphorylation of ERK and IL-6 induced JAK2/STAT3 pathway that results in increased proliferation, migration, and invasion of RCC cells was also inhibited by statin pretreatment. In vivo models showed that statins inhibited tumor growth, metastasis, and induced apoptosis in the tumors and, consistent with in vitro experiments; AKT, ERK, and STAT3 phosphorylation were decreased (Fang et al. 2013; Horiguchi et al. 2004).

Reduction in number and function of suppressive MDSC

Because MDSC are immunosuppressive, and angiogenic multiple strategies are being examined to reduce the number and/or function in tumor bearing mice and humans (Gabrilovich 2004; Najjar and Finke 2013). Strategies tested in RCC patients and mouse models includes the use of all-trans retinoic acid (ATRA) to drive the differentiation of immature myeloid cells into mature cells without suppressive activity (Kusmartsev et al. 2008). In RCC patients treated with ATRA, the number of MDSC in the blood was significantly reduced, and this reduction was associated with an increase in tetanus-toxoid-specific T cell responses (Mirza et al. 2006). Others are testing whether MDSC can be converted into tumoricidal macrophages by the use of CD40 ligand, TLR agonists, and/or T1-type cytokines (Beatty et al. 2011; Shirota et al. 2012; Liscovsky et al. (2011); Zembala et al. 1994). Additional studies using a different approach demonstrated that blocking reactive oxygen species production in MDSC with synthetic triterpenoid (CDDO, Me) reduced the suppressive activity of MDSC isolated from patients with RCC (Nagaraj et al. 2010). In a mouse model, this approach did not alter the number of MDSC in the spleens but did reduce their suppressive activity and decreased tumor growth. Select TKI that are used to treat metastatic RCC patients can reduce the number of MDSC by promoting cell death. Sunitinib (front-line therapy) significantly reduces the number of MDSC in the peripheral blood (Ko et al. 2009; van Cruijsen et al. 2008) along with restoring Type-1 T cell IFN-γ responses (Ko et al. 2009; Finke et al. 2008). Additionally, select chemotherapy agents can also reduce MDSC levels in cancer patients (Gabrilovich 2004; Najjar and Finke 2013). In select mouse tumor models, sunitinib therapy when combined with vaccines and/or adoptive therapy can enhance tumor regression, improve survival, and increase development of antitumor T cell responses compared to either treatment alone (Bose et al. 2011; Farsaci et al. 2012; Kujawski et al. 2010; Ozao-Choy et al. 2009).

Reduction in tumor-promoting TAM

IL-10 and CCL2 production by RCC TAM is likely mediated by overexpression of the enzyme 15-lipoxygenase-2 (15-LOX2), resulting in production of the biologically active lipid 15 (S) HETE. Inhibition of the lipoxygenase pathway by the inhibitor NDGA significantly reduced expression of the chemokine CCL2 by TAM, and in vitro reduced the ability of TAMs to produce IL-10 (Daurkin et al. 2011).

9.7 Conclusions and Future Directions

The last couple of decades have seen exponentially growing evidence linking cancer and inflammation, and with this a shift to our approach to cancer from strictly a disorder of cells with damaged or mutated genes that grow unregulated to one that includes the interaction between tumor cells and the immune system where tumor cells use host's immune mediators to foster their growth and survival, in turn, inflammation becomes chronic and tumors thrive and progress, a view that Rudolph Virchow had over 150 years ago. RCC represents 90 % of primary kidney tumors and is a prototypical tumor that interacts profoundly with the immune system. The gene mutations that result in a loss of function of the VHL gene are a common feature of sporadic and familial cases of RCC. Most solid tumors eventually outgrow their blood supply and enter a constant state of hypoxia; this activates hypoxia-inducible genes via the HIF; in RCC, however, the loss of VHL function results in a constant HIF expression and function early in the tumor formation even in normoxic conditions. Early on there is upregulation of many pathways that promote tumor growth, proliferation, invasion, angiogenesis, antiapoptosis, and evasion of the immune system. These pathways are mediated by targets of HIF which include VEGF, MMPs, chemokines, and chemokine receptors, cyclin-D1, TGF-alpha, angioprotein-1, erythropoietin among others. The VHL protein itself has HIF-independent functions that may favor malignant transformation and tumor progression; it mediates cell–extracellular matrix interactions and assembly, stabilizes p53, suppresses cycling D1, and helps cells reach quiescence.

Surgery remains the most effective treatment for RCC but is limited to localized disease. Surgery for advanced RCC does not improve survival but anecdotal cases of metastatic disease regression after nephrectomy has hints on the control RCC has over immune-tumor interactions. Advanced RCC responds poorly to chemotherapy and/or radiation although it is considered an immunogenic tumor and is modestly responsive non-specific immunotherapy for RCC (IL-2 and IFN-α). While a small percentage of patients achieved cures with this approach, significant toxicity to high-dose IL-2 made way to more specific therapies. HIF target genes and their pathways are now the main focus of the current and developing treatments of RCC (e.g., TKI targeting VEGF and mTOR inhibitors), termed "targeted therapy," and have proven to have greater survival benefit than IL-2 and IFN-α treatment. Therapies targeting checkpoints of the immune system such as CTLA-4 and PD-1 pathways have shown significant activity in some cancer types such as RCC and providing renewed interest in immunotherapy approaches. Additionally, growing evidence is emerging on inflammatory profiles on the patient side that can help predict not only prognosis and survival but also predict response to specific treatment. Inflammatory cytokines usually correlate poor prognosis or advance disease, and immune infiltrating cell profiles can also predict patient outcomes; even xenograft tumor model using fresh tissue tumor samples implanted in nude mice are used in an attempt to predict best response to treatment. Clearly, efforts are been made to characterize both patients and their tumor inflammatory profiles and treatments that target a more specific biology. There are many unanswered questions in the interactions of RCC with the immune system, a better understanding of this bilateral dialog is vital to achieve clinical improvements in patients with RCC.

References

Al-Lamki RS, Sadler TJ, Wang J, Reid MJ, Warren AY, Movassagh M, Lu W, Mills IG, Neal DE, Burge J, Vandenebeele P, Pober JS, Bradley JR (2010) Tumor necrosis factor receptor expression and signaling in renal cell carcinoma. Am J Pathol 177:943–954

Alsheikh-Ali AA, Maddukuri PV, Han H, Karas RH (2007) Effect of the magnitude of lipid lowering on risk of elevated liver enzymes, rhabdomyolysis, and cancer: insights from large randomized statin trials. J Am Coll Cardiol 50:409–418

American Cancer Society (2008) Cancer facts and figures. American Cancer Society, New York

Ananth S, Knebelmann B, Gruning W, Dhanabal M, Walz G, Stillman IE, Sukhatme VP (1999) Transforming growth factor beta1 is a target for the von Hippel-Lindau tumor suppressor and a critical growth factor for clear cell renal carcinoma. Cancer Res 59:2210–2216

Andreasen PA, Egelund R, Petersen HH (2000) The plasminogen activation system in tumor growth, invasion, and metastasis. Cell Mol Life Sci 57:25–40

Aoki Y, Feldman GM, Tosato G (2003) Inhibition of STAT3 signaling induces apoptosis and decreases survivin expression in primary effusion lymphoma. Blood 101:1535–1542

Balkwill F (2004) Cancer and the chemokine network. Nat Rev Cancer 4:540–550

Bardia A, Ebbert JO, Vierkant RA, Limburg PJ, Anderson K, Wang AH, Olson JE, Vachon CM, Cerhan JR (2007) Association of aspirin and nonaspirin nonsteroidal anti-inflammatory drugs with cancer incidence and mortality. J Natl Cancer Inst 99:881–889

Beatty GL, Chiorean EG, Fishman MP, Saboury B, Teitelbaum UR, Sun W, Huhn RD, Song W, Li D, Sharp LL, Torigian DA, O'Dwyer PJ, Vonderheide RH (2011) CD40 agonists alter tumor stroma and show efficacy against pancreatic carcinoma in mice and humans. Science 331:1612–1616

Begum NA, Shibuta K, Mori M, Barnard GF (1999) Reduced expression of the CXCR4 receptor mRNA in hepatocellular carcinoma and lack of inducibility of its ligand alpha-chemokine hIRH/SDF1alpha/PBSF in vitro. Int J Oncol 14:927–934

Bernhagen J, Calandra T, Mitchell RA, Martin SB, Tracey KJ, Voelter W, Manogue KR, Cerami A, Bucala R (1993) MIF is a pituitary-derived cytokine that potentiates lethal endotoxaemia. Nature 365:756–759

Biswas SK, Mantovani A (2010) Macrophage plasticity and interaction with lymphocyte subsets: cancer as a paradigm. Nat Immunol 11:889–896

Blay JY, Negrier S, Combaret V, Attali S, Goillot E, Merrouche Y, Mercatello A, Ravault A, Tourani JM, Moskovtchenko JF et al (1992) Serum level of interleukin 6 as a prognosis factor in metastatic renal cell carcinoma. Cancer Res 52:3317–3322

Bose A, Taylor JL, Alber S, Watkins SC, Garcia JA, Rini BI, Ko JS, Cohen PA, Finke JH, Storkus WJ (2011) Sunitinib facilitates the activation and recruitment of therapeutic anti-tumor immunity in concert with specific vaccination. Int J Cancer 129:2158–2170

Bowman T, Broome MA, Sinibaldi D, Wharton W, Pledger WJ, Sedivy JM, Irby R, Yeatman T, Courtneidge SA, Jove R (2001) Stat3-mediated Myc expression is required for Src transformation and PDGF-induced mitogenesis. Proc Natl Acad Sci USA 98:7319–7324

Brahmer JR, Tykodi SS, Chow LQ, Hwu WJ, Topalian SL, Hwu P, Drake CG, Camacho LH, Kauh J, Odunsi K, Pitot HC, Hamid O, Bhatia S, Martins R, Eaton K, Chen S, Salay TM, Alaparthy S, Grosso JF, Korman AJ, Parker SM, Agrawal S, Goldberg SM, Pardoll DM, Gupta A, Wigginton JM (2012) Safety and activity of anti-PD-L1 antibody in patients with advanced cancer. N Engl J Med 366:2455–2465

Brandau S, Trellakis S, Bruderek K, Schmaltz D, Steller G, Elian M, Suttmann H, Schenck M, Welling J, Zabel P, Lang S (2011) Myeloid-derived suppressor cells in the peripheral blood of cancer patients contain a subset of immature neutrophils with impaired migratory properties. J Leukoc Biol 89:311–317

Brenner W, Farber G, Herget T, Lehr HA, Hengstler JG, Thuroff JW (2002) Loss of tumor suppressor protein PTEN during renal carcinogenesis. Int J Cancer 99:53–57

Buettner R, Mora LB, Jove R (2002) Activated STAT signaling in human tumors provides novel molecular targets for therapeutic intervention. Clin Cancer Res 8:945–954

Carmeliet P, Jain RK (2000) Angiogenesis in cancer and other diseases. Nature 407:249–257

Catlett-Falcone R, Landowski TH, Oshiro MM, Turkson J, Levitzki A, Savino R, Ciliberto G, Moscinski L, Fernandez-Luna JL, Nunez G, Dalton WS, Jove R (1999) Constitutive activation of Stat3 signaling confers resistance to apoptosis in human U266 myeloma cells. Immunity 10:105–115

Chen Q, Shinohara N, Abe T, Harabayashi T, Nonomura K (2004a) Impact of cyclooxygenase-2 gene expression on tumor invasiveness in a human renal cell carcinoma cell line. J Urol 172:2153–2157

Chen Q, Shinohara N, Abe T, Watanabe T, Nonomura K, Koyanagi T (2004b) Significance of COX-2 expression in human renal cell carcinoma cell lines. Int J Cancer 108:825–832

Cheville JC, Lohse CM, Zincke H, Weaver AL, Blute ML (2003) Comparisons of outcome and prognostic features among histologic subtypes of renal cell carcinoma. Am J Surg Pathol 27:612–624

Cho D, Signoretti S, Dabora S, Regan M, Seeley A, Mariotti M, Youmans A, Polivy A, Mandato L, McDermott D, Stanbridge E, Atkins M (2007) Potential histologic and molecular predictors of response to temsirolimus in patients with advanced renal cell carcinoma. Clin Genitourin Cancer 5:379–385

Cho E, Curhan G, Hankinson SE, Kantoff P, Atkins MB, Stampfer M, Choueiri TK (2011) Prospective evaluation of analgesic use and risk of renal cell cancer. Arch Intern Med 171:1487–1493

Choueiri TK, Garcia JA, Elson P, Khasawneh M, Usman S, Golshayan AR, Baz RC, Wood L, Rini BI, Bukowski RM (2007) Clinical factors associated with outcome in patients with metastatic clear-cell renal cell carcinoma treated with vascular endothelial growth factor-targeted therapy. Cancer 110:543–550

Chuang MJ, Sun KH, Tang SJ, Deng MW, Wu YH, Sung JS, Cha TL, Sun GH (2008) Tumor-derived tumor necrosis factor-alpha promotes progression and epithelial-mesenchymal transition in renal cell carcinoma cells. Cancer Sci 99:905–913

Clement JM, McDermott DF (2009) The high-dose aldesleukin (IL-2) "select" trial: a trial designed to prospectively validate predictive models of response to high-dose IL-2 treatment in patients with metastatic renal cell carcinoma. Clin Genitourin Cancer 7:E7–E9

Cohen HT, McGovern FJ (2005) Renal-cell carcinoma. N Engl J Med 353:2477–2490

Cohen PA, Ko JS, Storkus WJ, Spencer CD, Bradley JM, Gorman JE, McCurry DB, Zorro-Manrique S, Dominguez AL, Pathangey LB, Rayman PA, Rini BI, Gendler SJ, Finke

JH (2012) Myeloid-derived suppressor cells adhere to physiologic STAT3- vs STAT5-dependent hematopoietic programming, establishing diverse tumor-mediated mechanisms of immunologic escape. Immunol Invest 41:680–710

Coppin C, Porzsolt F, Awa A, Kumpf J, Coldman A, Wilt T (2005) Immunotherapy for advanced renal cell cancer. Cochrane Database Syst Rev CD001425 1–87

Corzo CA, Cotter MJ, Cheng P, Cheng F, Kusmartsev S, Sotomayor E, Padhya T, McCaffrey TV, McCaffrey JC, Gabrilovich DI (2009) Mechanism regulating reactive oxygen species in tumor-induced myeloid-derived suppressor cells. J Immunol 182:5693–5701

D'Alterio C, Cindolo L, Portella L, Polimeno M, Consales C, Riccio A, Cioffi M, Franco R, Chiodini P, Carteni G, Mirone V, Longo N, Marra L, Perdona S, Claudio L, Mascolo M, Staibano S, Falsaperla M, Puglisi M, Martignoni G, Ficarra V, Castello G, Scala S (2010a) Differential role of CD133 and CXCR4 in renal cell carcinoma. Cell Cycle 9:4492–4500

D'Alterio C, Consales C, Polimeno M, Franco R, Cindolo L, Portella L, Cioffi M, Calemma R, Marra L, Claudio L, Perdona S, Pignata S, Facchini G, Carteni G, Longo N, Pucci L, Ottaiano A, Costantini S, Castello G, Scala S (2010b) Concomitant CXCR4 and CXCR7 expression predicts poor prognosis in renal cancer. Curr Cancer Drug Targets 10:772–781

Dale KM, Coleman CI, Henyan NN, Kluger J, White CM (2006) Statins and cancer risk: a meta-analysis. JAMA 295:74–80

Daurkin I, Eruslanov E, Stoffs T, Perrin GQ, Algood C, Gilbert SM, Rosser CJ, Su LM, Vieweg J, Kusmartsev S (2011) Tumor-associated macrophages mediate immunosuppression in the renal cancer microenvironment by activating the 15-lipoxygenase-2 pathway. Cancer Res 71:6400–6409

Dekernion JB, Ramming KP, Smith RB (1978) The natural history of metastatic renal cell carcinoma: a computer analysis. J Urol 120:148–152

Devita VT, Lawrence TS, Rosenberg SA (2011) DeVita, Hellman, and Rosenberg's cancer: principles & practice of oncology. Wolters Kluwer Health/Lippincott Williams & Wilkins, Philadelphia

Dillman RO, Barth NM, Vandermolen LA, Fong WH, Mahdavi KK, McClure SE (2011) Should high-dose interleukin-2 still be the preferred treatment for patients with metastatic renal cell cancer? Cancer Biother Radiopharm 26:273–277

Donskov F (2013) Immunomonitoring and prognostic relevance of neutrophils in clinical trials. Semin Cancer Biol 23:200–207

Donskov F, von der Maase H (2006) Impact of immune parameters on long-term survival in metastatic renal cell carcinoma. J Clin Oncol 24:1997–2005

Dosquet C, Schaetz A, Faucher C, Lepage E, Wautier JL, Richard F, Cabane J (1994) Tumour necrosis factor-alpha, interleukin-1 beta and interleukin-6 in patients with renal cell carcinoma. Eur J Cancer 30A:162–167

Du W, Wright BM, Li X, Finke J, Rini BI, Zhou M, He H, Lal P, Welford SM (2013) Tumor-derived macrophage migration inhibitory factor promotes an autocrine loop that enhances renal cell carcinoma. Oncogene 32:1469–1474

Dvorak HF (2002) Vascular permeability factor/vascular endothelial growth factor: a critical cytokine in tumor angiogenesis and a potential target for diagnosis and therapy. J Clin Oncol 20:4368–4380

Edgren M, Lennernas B, Larsson A, Nilsson S (1999) Serum concentrations of VEGF and b-FGF in renal cell, prostate and urinary bladder carcinomas. Anticancer Res 19:869–873

Elsasser-Beile U, Rindsfuser M, Grussenmeyer T, Schultze-Seemann W, Wetterauer U (2000) Enhanced expression of IFN-gamma mRNA in CD4(+)or CD8(+)tumour-infiltrating lymphocytes compared to peripheral lymphocytes in patients with renal cell cancer. Br J Cancer 83:637–641

Elson DA, Thurston G, Huang LE, Ginzinger DG, McDonald DM, Johnson RS, Arbeit JM (2001) Induction of hypervascularity without leakage or inflammation in transgenic mice overexpressing hypoxia-inducible factor-1alpha. Genes Dev 15:2520–2532

Escudier B (2010) Chemo-immunotherapy in RCC: the end of a story. Lancet 375:613–614

Esteban MA, Harten SK, Tran MG, Maxwell PH (2006) Formation of primary cilia in the renal epithelium is regulated by the von Hippel-Lindau tumor suppressor protein. J Am Soc Nephrol 17:1801–1806

Fang Z, Tang Y, Fang J, Zhou Z, Xing Z, Guo Z, Guo X, Wang W, Jiao W, Xu Z, Liu Z (2013) Simvastatin inhibits renal cancer cell growth and metastasis via AKT/mTOR, ERK and JAK2/STAT3 pathway. PLoS ONE 8:e62823

Farsaci B, Higgins JP, Hodge JW (2012) Consequence of dose scheduling of sunitinib on host immune response elements and vaccine combination therapy. Int J Cancer 130:1948–1959

Farwell WR, Scranton RE, Lawler EV, Lew RA, Brophy MT, Fiore LD, Gaziano JM (2008) The association between statins and cancer incidence in a veterans population. J Natl Cancer Inst 100:134–139

Finke JH, Rini B, Ireland J, Rayman P, Richmond A, Golshayan A, Wood L, Elson P, Garcia J, Dreicer R, Bukowski R (2008) Sunitinib reverses type-1 immune suppression and decreases T-regulatory cells in renal cell carcinoma patients. Clin Cancer Res 14:6674–6682

Finkelstein SE, Carey T, Fricke I, Yu D, Goetz D, Gratz M, Dunn M, Urbas P, Daud A, Deconti R, Antonia S, Gabrilovich D, Fishman M (2010) Changes in dendritic cell phenotype after a new high-dose weekly schedule of interleukin-2 therapy for kidney cancer and melanoma. J Immunother 33:817–827

Fitzgerald JP, Nayak B, Shanmugasundaram K, Friedrichs W, Sudarshan S, Eid AA, Denapoli T, Parekh DJ, Gorin Y, Block K (2012) Nox4 mediates renal cell carcinoma cell invasion through hypoxia-induced interleukin 6- and 8-production. PLoS ONE 7:e30712

Flanigan RC, Salmon SE, Blumenstein BA, Bearman SI, Roy V, McGrath PC, Caton JR Jr, Munshi N, Crawford ED (2001) Nephrectomy followed by interferon alfa-2b compared with interferon alfa-2b alone for metastatic renal-cell cancer. N Engl J Med 345:1655–1659

Fortis C, Ferrero E, Biffi M, Heltai S, Besana C, Bucci E, Tresoldi M, Rugarli C (1991) Recombinant interleukin-2 and lymphokine-activated killer cells in renal cancer patients: II. Characterization of cells cultured ex vivo and their contribution to the in vivo immunomodulation. Cancer Immunol Immunother 33:128–132

Francis RB Jr, Thomas W (1984) Behaviour of protein C inhibitor in intravascular coagulation and liver disease. Thromb Haemost 52:71–74

Freeman GJ, Long AJ, Iwai Y, Bourque K, Chernova T, Nishimura H, Fitz LJ, Malenkovich N, Okazaki T, Byrne MC, Horton HF, Fouser L, Carter L, Ling V, Bowman MR, Carreno BM, Collins M, Wood CR, Honjo T (2000) Engagement of the PD-1 immunoinhibitory receptor by a novel B7 family member leads to negative regulation of lymphocyte activation. J Exp Med 192:1027–1034

Fu L, Wang G, Shevchuk MM, Nanus DM, Gudas LJ (2011) Generation of a mouse model of von Hippel-Lindau kidney disease leading to renal cancers by expression of a constitutively active mutant of HIF1alpha. Cancer Res 71:6848–6856

Fujimura T, Ohta T, Oyama K, Miyashita T, Miwa K (2007) Cyclooxygenase-2 (COX-2) in carcinogenesis and selective COX-2 inhibitors for chemoprevention in gastrointestinal cancers. J Gastrointest Cancer 38:78–82

Gabrilovich D (2004) Mechanisms and functional significance of tumour-induced dendritic-cell defects. Nat Rev Immunol 4:941–952

Gabrilovich DI, Ostrand-Rosenberg S, Bronte V (2012) Coordinated regulation of myeloid cells by tumours. Nat Rev Immunol 12:253–268

Gameiro PA, Yang J, Metelo AM, Perez-Carro R, Baker R, Wang Z, Arreola A, Rathmell WK, Olumi A, Lopez-Larrubia P, Stephanopoulos G, Iliopoulos O (2013) In vivo HIF-mediated reductive carboxylation is regulated by citrate levels and sensitizes VHL-deficient cells to glutamine deprivation. Cell Metab 17:372–385

Garcia-Zepeda EA, Combadiere C, Rothenberg ME, Sarafi MN, Lavigne F, Hamid Q, Murphy PM, Luster AD (1996a) Human monocyte chemoattractant protein (MCP)-4 is a novel CC chemokine with activities on monocytes, eosinophils, and basophils induced in allergic and nonallergic inflammation that signals through the CC chemokine receptors (CCR)-2 and -3. J Immunol 157:5613–5626

Garcia-Zepeda EA, Rothenberg ME, Ownbey RT, Celestin J, Leder P, Luster AD (1996b) Human eotaxin is a specific chemoattractant for eosinophil cells and provides a new mechanism to explain tissue eosinophilia. Nat Med 2:449–456

Gauthaman K, Fong CY, Bongso A (2009) Statins, stem cells, and cancer. J Cell Biochem 106:975–983

Golimbu M, Joshi P, Sperber A, Tessler A, Al-Askari S, Morales P (1986) Renal cell carcinoma: survival and prognostic factors. Urology 27:291–301

Gruys ME, Back TC, Subleski J, Wiltrout TA, Lee JK, Schmidt L, Watanabe M, Stanyon R, Ward JM, Wigginton JM, Wiltrout RH (2001) Induction of transplantable mouse renal cell cancers by streptozotocin: in vivo growth, metastases, and angiogenic phenotype. Cancer Res 61:6255–6263

Haase VH, Glickman JN, Socolovsky M, Jaenisch R (2001) Vascular tumors in livers with targeted inactivation of the von Hippel-Lindau tumor suppressor. Proc Natl Acad Sci USA 98:1583–1588

Halama N, Zoernig I, Jaeger D (2010) Advanced malignant melanoma: immunologic and multimodal therapeutic strategies. J Oncol 2010:689893

Hanson EM, Clements VK, Sinha P, Ilkovitch D, Ostrand-Rosenberg S (2009) Myeloid-derived suppressor cells down-regulate L-selectin expression on CD4+ and CD8+ T cells. J Immunol 183:937–944

Heeschen C, Aicher A, Lehmann R, Fichtlscherer S, Vasa M, Urbich C, Mildner-Rihm C, Martin H, Zeiher AM, Dimmeler S (2003) Erythropoietin is a potent physiologic stimulus for endothelial progenitor cell mobilization. Blood 102:1340–1346

Hemmerlein B, Johanns U, Halbfass J, Bottcher T, Heuser M, Radzun HJ, Thelen P (2004) The balance between MMP-2/-9 and TIMP-1/-2 is shifted towards MMP in renal cell carcinomas and can be further disturbed by hydrogen peroxide. Int J Oncol 24:1069–1076

Ho MY, Tang SJ, Chuang MJ, Cha TL, Li JY, Sun GH, Sun KH (2012) TNF-alpha induces epithelial-mesenchymal transition of renal cell carcinoma cells via a GSK3beta-dependent mechanism. Mol Cancer Res 10:1109–1119

Horiguchi A, Oya M, Shimada T, Uchida A, Marumo K, Murai M (2002) Activation of signal transducer and activator of transcription 3 in renal cell carcinoma: a study of incidence and its association with pathological features and clinical outcome. J Urol 168:762–765

Horiguchi A, Sumitomo M, Asakuma J, Asano T, Asano T, Hayakawa M (2004) 3-hydroxy-3-methylglutaryl-coenzyme a reductase inhibitor, fluvastatin, as a novel agent for prophylaxis of renal cancer metastasis. Clin Cancer Res 10:8648–8655

Howlader NNA, Krapcho M, Garshell J, Neyman N, Altekruse SF, Kosary CL, Yu M, Ruhl J, Tatalovich Z, Cho H, Mariotto A, Lewis DR, Chen HS, Feuer EJ, Cronin KA (2013) SEER cancer statistics review, 1975–2010. National Cancer Institute (Posted to the SEER web site)

Huang B, Pan PY, Li Q, Sato AI, Levy DE, Bromberg J, Divino CM, Chen SH (2006) Gr-1+CD115+ immature myeloid suppressor cells mediate the development of tumor-induced T regulatory cells and T-cell anergy in tumor-bearing host. Cancer Res 66:1123–1131

Huang D, Ding Y, Zhou M, Rini BI, Petillo D, Qian CN, Kahnoski R, Futreal PA, Furge KA, Teh BT (2010) Interleukin-8 mediates resistance to antiangiogenic agent sunitinib in renal cell carcinoma. Cancer Res 70:1063–1071

Hudes G, Carducci M, Tomczak P, Dutcher J, Figlin R, Kapoor A, Staroslawska E, Sosman J, McDermott D, Bodrogi I, Kovacevic Z, Lesovoy V, Schmidt-Wolf IG, Barbarash O, Gokmen E, O'Toole T, Lustgarten S, Moore L, Motzer RJ, Global AT (2007) Temsirolimus, interferon alfa, or both for advanced renal-cell carcinoma. N Engl J Med 356:2271–2281

Ikemoto S, Yoshida N, Narita K, Wada S, Kishimoto T, Sugimura K, Nakatani T (2003) Role of tumor-associated macrophages in renal cell carcinoma. Oncol Rep 10:1843–1849

Iliopoulos O, Levy AP, Jiang C, Kaelin WG Jr, Goldberg MA (1996) Negative regulation of hypoxia-inducible genes by the von Hippel-Lindau protein. Proc Natl Acad Sci USA 93:10595–10599

Jensen HK, Donskov F, Marcussen N, Nordsmark M, Lundbeck F, von der Maase H (2009) Presence of intratumoral neutrophils is an independent prognostic factor in localized renal cell carcinoma. J Clin Oncol 27:4709–4717

Jiang W, Zhou P, Kahn SM, Tomita N, Johnson MD, Weinstein IB (1994) Molecular cloning of TPAR1, a gene whose expression is repressed by the tumor promoter 12-O-tetradecanoylphorbol 13-acetate (TPA). Exp Cell Res 215:284–293

Johrer K, Zelle-Rieser C, Perathoner A, Moser P, Hager M, Ramoner R, Gander H, Holtl L, Bartsch G, Greil R, Thurnher M (2005) Up-regulation of functional chemokine receptor CCR3 in human renal cell carcinoma. Clin Cancer Res 11:2459–2465

Kaelin WG Jr (2009) Treatment of kidney cancer: insights provided by the VHL tumor-suppressor protein. Cancer 115:2262–2272

Kallakury BV, Karikehalli S, Haholu A, Sheehan CE, Azumi N, Ross JS (2001) Increased expression of matrix metalloproteinases 2 and 9 and tissue inhibitors of metalloproteinases 1 and 2 correlate with poor prognostic variables in renal cell carcinoma. Clin Cancer Res 7:3113–3119

Kallio JP, Tammela TL, Marttinen AT, Kellokumpu-Lehtinen PL (2001) Soluble immunological parameters and early prognosis of renal cell cancer patients. J Exp Clin Cancer Res 20:523–528

Karam JA, Zhang XY, Tamboli P, Margulis V, Wang H, Abel EJ, Culp SH, Wood CG (2011) Development and characterization of clinically relevant tumor models from patients with renal cell carcinoma. Eur Urol 59:619–628

Khurana V, Caldito G, Ankem M (2008) Statins might reduce risk of renal cell carcinoma in humans: case-control study of 500,000 veterans. Urology 71:118–122

Kleymenova E, Everitt JI, Pluta L, Portis M, Gnarra JR, Walker CL (2004) Susceptibility to vascular neoplasms but no increased susceptibility to renal carcinogenesis in Vhl knockout mice. Carcinogenesis 25:309–315

Ko JS, Zea AH, Rini BI, Ireland JL, Elson P, Cohen P, Golshayan A, Rayman PA, Wood L, Garcia J, Dreicer R, Bukowski R, Finke JH (2009) Sunitinib mediates reversal of myeloid-derived suppressor cell accumulation in renal cell carcinoma patients. Clin Cancer Res 15:2148–2157

Ko JS, Rayman P, Ireland J, Swaidani S, Li G, Bunting KD, Rini B, Finke JH, Cohen PA (2010) Direct and differential suppression of myeloid-derived suppressor cell subsets by sunitinib is compartmentally constrained. Cancer Res 70:3526–3536

Koga T, Shibahara K, Kabashima A, Sumiyoshi Y, Kimura Y, Takahashi I, Kakeji Y, Maehara Y (2004) Overexpression of cyclooxygenase-2 and tumor angiogenesis in human gastric cancer. Hepatogastroenterology 51:1626–1630

Komohara Y, Hasita H, Ohnishi K, Fujiwara Y, Suzu S, Eto M, Takeya M (2011) Macrophage infiltration and its prognostic relevance in clear cell renal cell carcinoma. Cancer Sci 102:1424–1431

Kondo T, Nakazawa H, Ito F, Hashimoto Y, Osaka Y, Futatsuyama K, Toma H, Tanabe K (2006) Favorable prognosis of renal cell carcinoma with increased expression of chemokines associated with a Th1-type immune response. Cancer Sci 97:780–786

Kugler A, Hemmerlein B, Thelen P, Kallerhoff M, Radzun HJ, Ringert RH (1998) Expression of metalloproteinase 2 and 9 and their inhibitors in renal cell carcinoma. J Urol 160:1914–1918

Kujawski M, Kortylewski M, Lee H, Herrmann A, Kay H, Yu H (2008) Stat3 mediates myeloid cell-dependent tumor angiogenesis in mice. J Clin Invest 118:3367–3377

Kujawski M, Zhang C, Herrmann A, Reckamp K, Scuto A, Jensen M, Deng J, Forman S, Figlin R, Yu H (2010) Targeting STAT3 in adoptively transferred T cells promotes their in vivo expansion and antitumor effects. Cancer Res 70:9599–9610

Kusmartsev S, Su Z, Heiser A, Dannull J, Eruslanov E, Kubler H, Yancey D, Dahm P, Vieweg J (2008) Reversal of myeloid cell-mediated immunosuppression in patients with metastatic renal cell carcinoma. Clin Cancer Res 14:8270–8278

Laurell M, Christensson A, Abrahamsson PA, Stenflo J, Lilja H (1992) Protein C inhibitor in human body fluids. Seminal plasma is rich in inhibitor antigen deriving from cells throughout the male reproductive system. J Clin Invest 89:1094–1101

Law TM, Motzer RJ, Mazumdar M, Sell KW, Walther PJ, O'Connell M, Khan A, Vlamis V, Vogelzang NJ, Bajorin DF (1995) Phase III randomized trial of interleukin-2 with or without lymphokine-activated killer cells in the treatment of patients with advanced renal cell carcinoma. Cancer 76:824–832

Leahy KM, Ornberg RL, Wang Y, Zweifel BS, Koki AT, Masferrer JL (2002) Cyclooxygenase-2 inhibition by celecoxib reduces proliferation and induces apoptosis in angiogenic endothelial cells in vivo. Cancer Res 62:625–631

Levina V, Nolen BM, Marrangoni AM, Cheng P, Marks JR, Szczepanski MJ, Szajnik ME, Gorelik E, Lokshin AE (2009) Role of eotaxin-1 signaling in ovarian cancer. Clin Cancer Res 15:2647–2656

Li L, Kaelin WG Jr (2011) New insights into the biology of renal cell carcinoma. Hematol Oncol Clin North Am 25:667–686

Lieberthal W, Levine JS (2009) The role of the mammalian target of rapamycin (mTOR) in renal disease. J Am Soc Nephrol 20:2493–2502

Lipson EJ, Sharfman WH, Drake CG, Wollner I, Taube JM, Anders RA, Xu H, Yao S, Pons A, Chen L, Pardoll DM, Brahmer JR, Topalian SL (2013) Durable cancer regression off-treatment and effective reinduction therapy with an anti-PD-1 antibody. Clin Cancer Res 19:462–468

Liscovsky MV, Ranocchia RP, Alignani DO, Gorlino CV, Moron G, Maletto BA, Pistoresi-Palencia MC (2011) CpG-ODN+IFN-gamma confer pro- and anti-inflammatory properties to peritoneal macrophages in aged mice. Exp Gerontol 46:462–467

Lopez-Lago MA, Posner S, Thodima VJ, Molina AM, Motzer RJ, Chaganti RS (2013) Neutrophil chemokines secreted by tumor cells mount a lung antimetastatic response during renal cell carcinoma progression. Oncogene 32:1752–1760

Luo J (2009) Glycogen synthase kinase 3beta (GSK3beta) in tumorigenesis and cancer chemotherapy. Cancer Lett 273:194–200

Lutz MS, Burk RD (2006) Primary cilium formation requires von hippel-lindau gene function in renal-derived cells. Cancer Res 66:6903–6907

Maher ER, Neumann HP, Richard S (2011) von Hippel-Lindau disease: a clinical and scientific review. Eur J Hum Genet 19:617–623

Masferrer JL, Leahy KM, Koki AT, Zweifel BS, Settle SL, Woerner BM, Edwards DA, Flickinger AG, Moore RJ, Seibert K (2000) Antiangiogenic and antitumor activities of cyclooxygenase-2 inhibitors. Cancer Res 60:1306–1311

Massague J, Cheifetz S, Laiho M, Ralph DA, Weis FM, Zentella A (1992) Transforming growth factor-beta. Cancer Surv 12:81–103

McDermott DF, Rini BI (2007) Immunotherapy for metastatic renal cell carcinoma. BJU Int 99:1282–1288

Mendel DB, Laird AD, Xin X, Louie SG, Christensen JG, Li G, Schreck RE, Abrams TJ, Ngai TJ, Lee LB, Murray LJ, Carver J, Chan E, Moss KG, Haznedar JO, Sukbuntherng J, Blake RA, Sun L, Tang C, Miller T, Shirazian S, McMahon G, Cherrington JM (2003) In vivo antitumor activity of SU11248, a novel tyrosine kinase inhibitor targeting vascular endothelial growth factor and platelet-derived growth factor receptors: determination of a pharmacokinetic/pharmacodynamic relationship. Clin Cancer Res 9:327–337

Menke J, Iwata Y, Rabacal WA, Basu R, Yeung YG, Humphreys BD, Wada T, Schwarting A, Stanley ER, Kelley VR (2009) CSF-1 signals directly to renal tubular epithelial cells to mediate repair in mice. J Clin Invest 119:2330–2342

Menke J, Kriegsmann J, Schimanski CC, Schwartz MM, Schwarting A, Kelley VR (2012) Autocrine CSF-1 and CSF-1 receptor coexpression promotes renal cell carcinoma growth. Cancer Res 72:187–200

Michaelson MD, Stadler WM (2013) Predictive markers in advanced renal cell carcinoma. Semin Oncol 40:459–464

Middleton AW Jr (1980) Indications for and results of nephrectomy for metastatic renal cell carcinoma. Urol Clin North Am 7:711–717

Mirza N, Fishman M, Fricke I, Dunn M, Neuger AM, Frost TJ, Lush RM, Antonia S, Gabrilovich DI (2006) All-trans-retinoic acid improves differentiation of myeloid cells and immune response in cancer patients. Cancer Res 66:9299–9307

Mochizuki M, Bartels J, Mallet AI, Christophers E, Schroder JM (1998) IL-4 induces eotaxin: a possible mechanism of selective eosinophil recruitment in helminth infection and atopy. J Immunol 160:60–68

Morandi A, Barbetti V, Riverso M, Sbarba PD, Rovida E (2011) The colony-stimulating factor-1 (CSF-1) receptor sustains ERK1/2 activation and proliferation in breast cancer cell lines. PLoS ONE 6:e27450

Mosser DM, Edwards JP (2008) Exploring the full spectrum of macrophage activation. Nat Rev Immunol 8:958–969

Motzer RJ, Hutson TE, Tomczak P, Michaelson MD, Bukowski RM, Rixe O, Oudard S, Negrier S, Szczylik C, Kim ST, Chen I, Bycott PW, Baum CM, Figlin RA (2007) Sunitinib versus interferon alfa in metastatic renal-cell carcinoma. N Engl J Med 356:115–124

Motzer RJ, Escudier B, Oudard S, Hutson TE, Porta C, Bracarda S, Grunwald V, Thompson JA, Figlin RA, Hollaender N, Urbanowitz G, Berg WJ, Kay A, Lebwohl D, Ravaud A, Group R-S (2008) Efficacy of everolimus in advanced renal cell carcinoma: a double-blind, randomised, placebo-controlled phase III trial. Lancet 372:449–456

Motzer RJ, Murphy BA, Bacik J, Schwartz LH, Nanus DM, Mariani T, Loehrer P, Wilding G, Fairclough DL, Cella D, Mazumdar M (2000) Phase III trial of interferon alfa-2a with or without 13-cis-retinoic acid for patients with advanced renal cell carcinoma. J Clin Oncol 18:2972–2980

Motzer RJ, Michaelson MD, Redman BG, Hudes GR, Wilding G, Figlin RA, Ginsberg MS, Kim ST, Baum CM, Deprimo SE, Li JZ, Bello CL, Theuer CP, George DJ, Rini BI (2006a) Activity of SU11248, a multitargeted inhibitor of vascular endothelial growth factor receptor and platelet-derived growth factor receptor, in patients with metastatic renal cell carcinoma. J Clin Oncol 24:16–24

Motzer RJ, Rini BI, Bukowski RM, Curti BD, George DJ, Hudes GR, Redman BG, Margolin KA, Merchan JR, Wilding G, Ginsberg MS, Bacik J, Kim ST, Baum CM, Michaelson MD (2006b) Sunitinib in patients with metastatic renal cell carcinoma. JAMA 295:2516–2524

Muller A, Homey B, Soto H, Ge N, Catron D, Buchanan ME, McClanahan T, Murphy E, Yuan W, Wagner SN, Barrera JL, Mohar A, Verastegui E, Zlotnik A (2001) Involvement of chemokine receptors in breast cancer metastasis. Nature 410:50–56

Nagaraj S, Youn JI, Weber H, Iclozan C, Lu L, Cotter MJ, Meyer C, Becerra CR, Fishman M, Antonia S, Sporn MB, Liby KT, Rawal B, Lee JH, Gabrilovich DI (2010) Anti-inflammatory triterpenoid blocks immune suppressive function of MDSCs and improves immune response in cancer. Clin Cancer Res 16:1812–1823

Najjar YG, Finke JH (2013) Clinical perspectives on targeting of myeloid derived suppressor cells in the treatment of cancer. Front Oncol 3:49

Negrier S, Escudier B, Gomez F, Douillard JY, Ravaud A, Chevreau C, Buclon M, Perol D, Lasset C (2002) Prognostic factors of survival and rapid progression in 782 patients with metastatic renal carcinomas treated by cytokines: a report from the Groupe Francais d'Immunotherapie. Ann Oncol 13:1460–1468

Neidhart JA (1986) Interferon therapy for the treatment of renal cancer. Cancer 57:1696–1699

Oguro T, Ishibashi K, Sugino T, Hashimoto K, Tomita S, Takahashi N, Yanagida T, Haga N, Aikawa K, Suzutani T, Yamaguchi O, Kojima Y (2013) Humanised antihuman IL-6R antibody with interferon inhibits renal cell carcinoma cell growth in vitro and in vivo through suppressed SOCS3 expression. Eur J Cancer 49:1715–1724

Ohh M, Yauch RL, Lonergan KM, Whaley JM, Stemmer-Rachamimov AO, Louis DN, Gavin BJ, Kley N, Kaelin WG Jr, Iliopoulos O (1998) The von Hippel-Lindau tumor suppressor protein is required for proper assembly of an extracellular fibronectin matrix. Mol Cell 1:959–968

Okuda H, Saitoh K, Hirai S, Iwai K, Takaki Y, Baba M, Minato N, Ohno S, Shuin T (2001) The von Hippel-Lindau tumor suppressor protein mediates ubiquitination of activated atypical protein kinase C. J Biol Chem 276:43611–43617

Ong KR, Woodward ER, Killick P, Lim C, Macdonald F, Maher ER (2007) Genotype-phenotype correlations in von Hippel-Lindau disease. Hum Mutat 28:143–149

Oya M, Ohtsubo M, Takayanagi A, Tachibana M, Shimizu N, Murai M (2001) Constitutive activation of nuclear factor-kappaB prevents TRAIL-induced apoptosis in renal cancer cells. Oncogene 20:3888–3896

Ozao-Choy J, Ma G, Kao J, Wang GX, Meseck M, Sung M, Schwartz M, Divino CM, Pan PY, Chen SH (2009) The novel role of tyrosine kinase inhibitor in the reversal of immune suppression and modulation of tumor microenvironment for immune-based cancer therapies. Cancer Res 69:2514–2522

Pan PY, Ma G, Weber KJ, Ozao-Choy J, Wang G, Yin B, Divino CM, Chen SH (2010) Immune stimulatory receptor CD40 is required for T-cell suppression and T regulatory cell activation mediated by myeloid-derived suppressor cells in cancer. Cancer Res 70:99–108

Pantuck AJ, Seligson DB, Klatte T, Yu H, Leppert JT, Moore L, O'Toole T, Gibbons J, Belldegrun AS, Figlin RA (2007) Prognostic relevance of the mTOR pathway in renal cell carcinoma: implications for molecular patient selection for targeted therapy. Cancer 109:2257–2267

Pardoll DM (2012) The blockade of immune checkpoints in cancer immunotherapy. Nat Rev Cancer 12:252–264

Pause A, Lee S, Lonergan KM, Klausner RD (1998) The von Hippel-Lindau tumor suppressor gene is required for cell cycle exit upon serum withdrawal. Proc Natl Acad Sci USA 95:993–998

Peggs KS, Quezada SA, Chambers CA, Korman AJ, Allison JP (2009) Blockade of CTLA-4 on both effector and regulatory T cell compartments contributes to the antitumor activity of anti-CTLA-4 antibodies. J Exp Med 206:1717–1725

Peranzoni E, Zilio S, Marigo I, Dolcetti L, Zanovello P, Mandruzzato S, Bronte V (2010) Myeloid-derived suppressor cell heterogeneity and subset definition. Curr Opin Immunol 22:238–244

Petrella BL, Brinckerhoff CE (2006) Tumor cell invasion of von Hippel Lindau renal cell carcinoma cells is mediated by membrane type-1 matrix metalloproteinase. Mol Cancer 5:66

Petrella BL, Lohi J, Brinckerhoff CE (2005) Identification of membrane type-1 matrix metalloproteinase as a target of hypoxia-inducible factor-2 alpha in von Hippel-Lindau renal cell carcinoma. Oncogene 24:1043–1052

Qi H, Ohh M (2003) The von Hippel-Lindau tumor suppressor protein sensitizes renal cell carcinoma cells to tumor necrosis factor-induced cytotoxicity by suppressing the nuclear factor-kappaB-dependent antiapoptotic pathway. Cancer Res 63:7076–7080

Ramp U, Caliskan E, Mahotka C, Krieg A, Heikaus S, Gabbert HE, Gerharz CD (2003) Apoptosis induction in renal cell carcinoma by TRAIL and gamma-radiation is impaired by deficient caspase-9 cleavage. Br J Cancer 88:1800–1807

Ramp U, Jaquet K, Reinecke P, Nitsch T, Gabbert HE, Gerharz CD (1997) Acquisition of TGF-beta 1 resistance: an important progression factor in human renal cell carcinoma. Lab Invest 76:739–749

Rankin EB, Tomaszewski JE, Haase VH (2006) Renal cyst development in mice with conditional inactivation of the von Hippel-Lindau tumor suppressor. Cancer Res 66:2576–2583

Rao CV, Indranie C, Simi B, Manning PT, Connor JR, Reddy BS (2002) Chemopreventive properties of a selective inducible nitric oxide synthase inhibitor in colon carcinogenesis, administered alone or in combination with celecoxib, a selective cyclooxygenase-2 inhibitor. Cancer Res 62:165–170

Raval RR, Lau KW, Tran MG, Sowter HM, Mandriota SJ, Li JL, Pugh CW, Maxwell PH, Harris AL, Ratcliffe PJ (2005) Contrasting properties of hypoxia-inducible factor 1 (HIF-1) and HIF-2 in von Hippel-Lindau-associated renal cell carcinoma. Mol Cell Biol 25:5675–5686

Rempel SA, Dudas S, Ge S, Gutierrez JA (2000) Identification and localization of the cytokine SDF1 and its receptor, CXC chemokine receptor 4, to regions of necrosis and angiogenesis in human glioblastoma. Clin Cancer Res 6:102–111

Reuter S, Gupta SC, Chaturvedi MM, Aggarwal BB (2010) Oxidative stress, inflammation, and cancer: how are they linked? Free Radic Biol Med 49:1603–1616

Rini BI, Campbell SC (2009) Renal cell carcinoma. People's Medical Pub. House, McGraw Hill Education, Shelton, Maidenhead

Rini BI, Weinberg V, Small EJ (2005) A phase I trial of fixed dose rate gemcitabine and capecitabine in metastatic renal cell carcinoma. Cancer 103:553–558

Rini BI, Weinberg V, Dunlap S, Elchinoff A, Yu N, Bok R, Simko J, Small EJ (2006) Maximal COX-2 immunostaining and clinical response to celecoxib and interferon alpha therapy in metastatic renal cell carcinoma. Cancer 106:566–575

Robb VA, Karbowniczek M, Klein-Szanto AJ, Henske EP (2007) Activation of the mTOR signaling pathway in renal clear cell carcinoma. J Urol 177:346–352

Rodriguez PC, Ernstoff MS, Hernandez C, Atkins M, Zabaleta J, Sierra R, Ochoa AC (2009) Arginase I-producing myeloid-derived suppressor cells in renal cell carcinoma are a subpopulation of activated granulocytes. Cancer Res 69:1553–1560

Roe JS, Kim H, Lee SM, Kim ST, Cho EJ, Youn HD (2006) p53 stabilization and transactivation by a von Hippel-Lindau protein. Mol Cell 22:395–405

Romero JM, Aptsiauri N, Vazquez F, Cozar JM, Canton J, Cabrera T, Tallada M, Garrido F, Ruiz-Cabello F (2006) Analysis of the expression of HLA class I, proinflammatory cytokines and chemokines in primary tumors from patients with localized and metastatic renal cell carcinoma. Tissue Antigens 68:303–310

Roxburgh CS, McMillan DC (2010) Role of systemic inflammatory response in predicting survival in patients with primary operable cancer. Future Oncol 6:149–163

Saito K, Kihara K (2013) Role of C-reactive protein in urological cancers: a useful biomarker for predicting outcomes. Int J Urol 20:161–171

Saito K, Tatokoro M, Fujii Y, Iimura Y, Koga F, Kawakami S, Kihara K (2009) Impact of C-reactive protein kinetics on survival of patients with metastatic renal cell carcinoma. Eur Urol 55:1145–1153

Sassano A, Platanias LC (2008) Statins in tumor suppression. Cancer Lett 260:11–19

Sawaoka H, Tsuji S, Tsujii M, Gunawan ES, Sasaki Y, Kawano S, Hori M (1999) Cyclooxygenase inhibitors suppress angiogenesis and reduce tumor growth in vivo. Lab Invest 79:1469–1477

Schmielau J, Finn OJ (2001) Activated granulocytes and granulocyte-derived hydrogen peroxide are the underlying mechanism of suppression of t-cell function in advanced cancer patients. Cancer Res 61:4756–4760

Schonbeck U, Libby P (2004) Inflammation, immunity, and HMG-CoA reductase inhibitors: statins as antiinflammatory agents? Circulation 109:II18–II26

Schrader AJ, Lechner O, Templin M, Dittmar KE, Machtens S, Mengel M, Probst-Kepper M, Franzke A, Wollensak T, Gatzlaff P, Atzpodien J, Buer J, Lauber J (2002) CXCR4/CXCL12 expression and signalling in kidney cancer. Br J Cancer 86:1250–1256

Schwandt A, Garcia JA, Elson P, Wyckhouse J, Finke JH, Ireland J, Triozzi P, Zhou M, Dreicer R, Rini BI (2011) Clinical and immunomodulatory effects of celecoxib plus interferon-alpha in metastatic renal cell carcinoma patients with COX-2 tumor immunostaining. J Clin Immunol 31:690–698

Sehgal A, Keener C, Boynton AL, Warrick J, Murphy GP (1998) CXCR-4, a chemokine receptor, is overexpressed in and required for proliferation of glioblastoma tumor cells. J Surg Oncol 69:99–104

Seiki M, Yana I (2003) Roles of pericellular proteolysis by membrane type-1 matrix metalloproteinase in cancer invasion and angiogenesis. Cancer Sci 94:569–574

Shibuta K, Begum NA, Mori M, Shimoda K, Akiyoshi T, Barnard GF (1997) Reduced expression of the CXC chemokine hIRH/SDF-1alpha mRNA in hepatoma and digestive tract cancer. Int J Cancer 73:656–662

Shirota Y, Shirota H, Klinman DM (2012) Intratumoral injection of CpG oligonucleotides induces the differentiation and reduces the immunosuppressive activity of myeloid-derived suppressor cells. J Immunol 188:1592–1599

Shrikant P, Khoruts A, Mescher MF (1999) CTLA-4 blockade reverses CD8+ T cell tolerance to tumor by a CD4+ T cell- and IL-2-dependent mechanism. Immunity 11:483–493

Sica A, Bronte V (2007) Altered macrophage differentiation and immune dysfunction in tumor development. J Clin Invest 117:1155–1166

Sippel TR, White J, Nag K, Tsvankin V, Klaassen M, Kleinschmidt-Demasters BK, Waziri A (2011) Neutrophil degranulation and immunosuppression in patients with GBM: restoration of cellular immune function by targeting arginase I. Clin Cancer Res 17:6992–7002

Sourbier C, Lindner V, Lang H, Agouni A, Schordan E, Danilin S, Rothhut S, Jacqmin D, Helwig JJ, Massfelder T (2006) The phosphoinositide 3-kinase/Akt pathway: a new target in human renal cell carcinoma therapy. Cancer Res 66:5130–5142

Srivastava MK, Sinha P, Clements VK, Rodriguez P, Ostrand-Rosenberg S (2010) Myeloid-derived suppressor cells inhibit T-cell activation by depleting cystine and cysteine. Cancer Res 70:68–77

Stadler WM, Halabi S, Rini B, Ernstoff MS, Davila E, Picus J, Barrier R, Small EJ (2006) A phase II study of gemcitabine and capecitabine in metastatic renal cancer: a report of Cancer and Leukemia Group B protocol 90008. Cancer 107:1273–1279

Staller P, Sulitkova J, Lisztwan J, Moch H, Oakeley EJ, Krek W (2003) Chemokine receptor CXCR4 downregulated by von Hippel-Lindau tumour suppressor pVHL. Nature 425:307–311

Suyama T, Furuya M, Nishiyama M, Kasuya Y, Kimura S, Ichikawa T, Ueda T, Nikaido T, Ito H, Ishikura H (2005) Up-regulation of the interferon gamma (IFN-gamma)-inducible chemokines IFN-inducible T-cell alpha chemoattractant and monokine induced by IFN-gamma and of their receptor CXC receptor 3 in human renal cell carcinoma. Cancer 103:258–267

Swiercz R, Wolfe JD, Zaher A, Jankun J (1998) Expression of the plasminogen activation system in kidney cancer correlates with its aggressive phenotype. Clin Cancer Res 4:869–877

Tang PA, Heng DY (2013) Programmed death 1 pathway inhibition in metastatic renal cell cancer and prostate cancer. Curr Oncol Rep 15:98–104

Tavani A, Scotti L, Bosetti C, Dal Maso L, Montella M, Ramazzotti V, Negri E, Franceschi S, La Vecchia C (2010) Aspirin and risk of renal cell cancer in Italy. Eur J Cancer Prev 19:272–274

Thiery JP (2002) Epithelial-mesenchymal transitions in tumour progression. Nat Rev Cancer 2:442–454

Thompson RH, Gillett MD, Cheville JC, Lohse CM, Dong H, Webster WS, Krejci KG, Lobo JR, Sengupta S, Chen L, Zincke H, Blute ML, Strome SE, Leibovich BC, Kwon ED (2004) Costimulatory B7-H1 in renal cell carcinoma patients: indicator of tumor aggressiveness and potential therapeutic target. Proc Natl Acad Sci USA 101:17174–17179

Thompson RH, Kuntz SM, Leibovich BC, Dong H, Lohse CM, Webster WS, Sengupta S, Frank I, Parker AS, Zincke H, Blute ML, Sebo TJ, Cheville JC, Kwon ED (2006) Tumor B7-H1 is associated with poor prognosis in renal cell carcinoma patients with long-term follow-up. Cancer Res 66:3381–3385

Thompson RH, Dong H, Lohse CM, Leibovich BC, Blute ML, Cheville JC, Kwon ED (2007) PD-1 is expressed by tumor-infiltrating immune cells and is associated with poor outcome for patients with renal cell carcinoma. Clin Cancer Res 13:1757–1761

Thong AE, Zhao H, Ingels A, Valta MP, Nolley R, Santos J, Young SR, Peehl DM (2014) Tissue slice grafts of human renal cell carcinoma: An authentic preclinical model with high engraftment rate and metastatic potential. Urol Oncol 32:43.e23–43.e30

Tomita S, Ishibashi K, Hashimoto K, Sugino T, Yanagida T, Kushida N, Shishido K, Aikawa K, Sato Y, Suzutani T, Yamaguchi O (2011) Suppression of SOCS3 increases susceptibility of renal cell carcinoma to interferon-alpha. Cancer Sci 102:57–63

Topalian SL, Hodi FS, Brahmer JR, Gettinger SN, Smith DC, McDermott DF, Powderly JD, Carvajal RD, Sosman JA, Atkins MB, Leming PD, Spigel DR, Antonia SJ, Horn L, Drake CG, Pardoll DM, Chen L, Sharfman WH, Anders RA, Taube JM, McMiller TL, Xu H, Korman AJ, Jure-Kunkel M, Agrawal S, McDonald D, Kollia GD, Gupta A, Wigginton JM, Sznol M (2012) Safety, activity, and immune correlates of anti-PD-1 antibody in cancer. N Engl J Med 366:2443–2454

Trichopoulos D, Psaltopoulou T, Orfanos P, Trichopoulou A, Boffetta P (2006) Plasma C-reactive protein and risk of cancer: a prospective study from Greece. Cancer Epidemiol Biomarkers Prev 15:381–384

Ueno T, Fukuda N, Tsunemi A, Yao EH, Matsuda H, Tahira K, Matsumoto T, Matsumoto K, Matsumoto Y, Nagase H, Sugiyama H, Sawamura T (2009) A novel gene silencer, pyrrole-imidazole polyamide targeting human lectin-like oxidized low-density lipoprotein receptor-1 gene improves endothelial cell function. J Hypertens 27:508–516

Uhrin P, Dewerchin M, Hilpert M, Chrenek P, Schofer C, Zechmeister-Machhart M, Kronke G, Vales A, Carmeliet P, Binder BR, Geiger M (2000) Disruption of the protein C inhibitor gene results in impaired spermatogenesis and male infertility. J Clin Invest 106:1531–1539

Van Boxel-Dezaire AH, Rani MR, Stark GR (2006) Complex modulation of cell type-specific signaling in response to type I interferons. Immunity 25:361–372

van Cruijsen H, van der Veldt AA, Vroling L, Oosterhoff D, Broxterman HJ, Scheper RJ, Giaccone G, Haanen JB, van den Eertwegh AJ, Boven E, Hoekman K, de Gruijl TD (2008) Sunitinib-induced myeloid lineage redistribution in renal cell cancer patients: CD1c+ dendritic cell frequency predicts progression-free survival. Clin Cancer Res 14:5884–5892

Wajant H, Pfizenmaier K, Scheurich P (2003) Tumor necrosis factor signaling. Cell Death Differ 10:45–65

Wakita T, Hayashi T, Nishioka J, Tamaru H, Akita N, Asanuma K, Kamada H, Gabazza EC, Ido M, Kawamura J, Suzuki K (2004) Regulation of carcinoma cell invasion by protein C inhibitor whose expression is decreased in renal cell carcinoma. Int J Cancer 108:516–523

Walter S, Weinschenk T, Stenzl A, Zdrojowy R, Pluzanska A, Szczylik C, Staehler M, Brugger W, Dietrich PY, Mendrzyk R, Hilf N, Schoor O, Fritsche J, Mahr A, Maurer D, Vass V, Trautwein C, Lewandrowski P, Flohr C, Pohla H, Stanczak JJ, Bronte V, Mandruzzato S, Biedermann T, Pawelec G, Derhovanessian E, Yamagishi H, Miki T, Hongo F, Takaha N, Hirakawa K, Tanaka H, Stevanovic S, Frisch J, Mayer-Mokler A, Kirner A, Rammensee HG, Reinhardt C, Singh-Jasuja H (2012) Multipeptide immune response to cancer vaccine IMA901 after single-dose cyclophosphamide associates with longer patient survival. Nat Med 18:1254–1261

Wang JM, Deng X, Gong W, Su S (1998) Chemokines and their role in tumor growth and metastasis. J Immunol Methods 220:1–17

Wang L, Wang Z, Yang B, Yang Q, Wang L, Sun Y (2009) CXCR4 nuclear localization follows binding of its ligand SDF-1 and occurs in metastatic but not primary renal cell carcinoma. Oncol Rep 22:1333–1339

Wang L, Chen W, Gao L, Yang Q, Liu B, Wu Z, Wang Y, Sun Y (2012a) High expression of CXCR4, CXCR7 and SDF-1 predicts poor survival in renal cell carcinoma. World J Surg Oncol 10:212

Wang L, Huang T, Chen W, Gao X, Zhou T, Wu Z, Sun Y (2012b) Silencing of CXCR4 by RNA interference inhibits cell growth and metastasis in human renal cancer cells. Oncol Rep 28:2043–2048

Wang R, Guo L, Wang P, Yang W, Lu Y, Huang Z, Tang C (2013) Chemoprevention of cancers in gastrointestinal tract with cyclooxygenase 2 inhibitors. Curr Pharm Des 19:115–125

Welford SM, Bedogni B, Gradin K, Poellinger L, Broome Powell M, Giaccia AJ (2006) HIF1alpha delays premature senescence through the activation of MIF. Genes Dev 20:3366–3371

Wigginton JM, Komschlies KL, Back TC, Franco JL, Brunda MJ, Wiltrout RH (1996) Administration of interleukin 12 with pulse interleukin 2 and the rapid and complete eradication of murine renal carcinoma. J Natl Cancer Inst 88:38–43

Yagoda A, Abi-Rached B, Petrylak D (1995) Chemotherapy for advanced renal-cell carcinoma: 1983–1993. Semin Oncol 22:42–60

Yamakawa M, Liu LX, Belanger AJ, Date T, Kuriyama T, Goldberg MA, Cheng SH, Gregory RJ, Jiang C (2004) Expression of angioproteins in renal epithelial and clear cell carcinoma cells: regulation by hypoxia and participation in angiogenesis. Am J Physiol Renal Physiol 287:F649–F657

Yang L, Debusk LM, Fukuda K, Fingleton B, Green-Jarvis B, Shyr Y, Matrisian LM, Carbone DP, Lin PC (2004) Expansion of myeloid immune suppressor Gr+CD11b+ cells in tumor-bearing host directly promotes tumor angiogenesis. Cancer Cell 6:409–421

Yang JC, Hughes M, Kammula U, Royal R, Sherry RM, Topalian SL, Suri KB, Levy C, Allen T, Mavroukakis S, Lowy I, White DE, Rosenberg SA (2007) Ipilimumab (anti-CTLA4 antibody) causes regression of metastatic renal cell cancer associated with enteritis and hypophysitis. J Immunother 30:825–830

Yoon SO, Park SJ, Yun CH, Chung AS (2003) Roles of matrix metalloproteinases in tumor metastasis and angiogenesis. J Biochem Mol Biol 36:128–137

Yoshida N, Ikemoto S, Narita K, Sugimura K, Wada S, Yasumoto R, Kishimoto T, Nakatani T (2002) Interleukin-6, tumour necrosis factor alpha and interleukin-1beta in patients with renal cell carcinoma. Br J Cancer 86:1396–1400

Youn JI, Collazo M, Shalova IN, Biswas SK, Gabrilovich DI (2012) Characterization of the nature of granulocytic myeloid-derived suppressor cells in tumor-bearing mice. J Leukoc Biol 91:167–181

Zachary I (2001) Signaling mechanisms mediating vascular protective actions of vascular endothelial growth factor. Am J Physiol Cell Physiol 280:C1375–C1386

Zatyka M, da Silva NF, Clifford SC, Morris MR, Wiesener MS, Eckardt KU, Houlston RS, Richards FM, Latif F, Maher ER (2002) Identification of cyclin D1 and other novel targets for the von Hippel-Lindau tumor suppressor gene by expression array analysis and investigation of cyclin D1 genotype as a modifier in von Hippel-Lindau disease. Cancer Res 62:3803–3811

Zea AH, Rodriguez PC, Atkins MB, Hernandez C, Signoretti S, Zabaleta J, McDermott D, Quiceno D, Youmans A, O'Neill A, Mier J, Ochoa AC (2005) Arginase-producing myeloid suppressor cells in renal cell carcinoma patients: a mechanism of tumor evasion. Cancer Res 65:3044–3048

Zembala M, Siedlar M, Marcinkiewicz J, Pryjma J (1994) Human monocytes are stimulated for nitric oxide release in vitro by some tumor cells but not by cytokines and lipopolysaccharide. Eur J Immunol 24:435–439

Zimmermann N, Conkright JJ, Rothenberg ME (1999) CC chemokine receptor-3 undergoes prolonged ligand-induced internalization. J Biol Chem 274:12611–12618

Zisman A, Pantuck AJ, Wieder J, Chao DH, Dorey F, Said JW, Dekernion JB, Figlin RA, Belldegrun AS (2002) Risk group assessment and clinical outcome algorithm to predict the natural history of patients with surgically resected renal cell carcinoma. J Clin Oncol 20:4559–4566

Chapter 10
The Role of Inflammation in Gastric Cancer

Kazım Şenol, Murat Bulut Özkan, Selahattin Vural and Mesut Tez

Abstract Gastric cancer, despite its declining incidence rate, is still the second cause of cancer-related death worldwide, killing 750,000 people each year and remaining the second common type of cancer. The best examples of inflammation-associated cancer in human beings may be gastric cancer. Understanding the molecular mechanism of the inflammation in gastric carcinogenesis is important for developing new strategies against gastric cancer.

10.1 Introduction

Cancer is a major public health problem. Every year almost 1 million new cases of gastric cancers are presented and there are about 750,000 deaths caused by gastric cancer. It ranks second in terms of cancer-related deaths after lung and bronchus cancer (Hussain and Harris 2007; Jemal et al. 2011). Although chemotherapy improves life expectancy, complete resection of gastric cancer (R0) via gastrectomy remains insufficient and more than 80 % of patients with advanced gastric cancer die of the recurrent disease within 1 year after diagnosis (Group et al. 2010; Gomceli et al. 2012).

The choice of treatment generally depends on the tumor's size, tumor location, stage of disease, and general health status of patient. Treatment of the gastric cancer consists of surgery, chemotherapy, radiotherapy, and also targeted therapy. Surgery is a common treatment of all stages of gastric cancer. The aim of surgery is to remove as completely as possible all grossly visible tumor tissue and to obtain histologically free surgical margins. Total and subtotal gastrectomy are used for R0 resection. If the tumor is blocking the stomach but the cancer

K. Şenol · M. B. Özkan · S. Vural · M. Tez (✉)
Department of General Surgery, Ankara Numune Research and Training Hospital,
Samanpazarı, Ankara, Turkey
e-mail: mtez@hacettepe.edu.tr

B. B. Aggarwal et al. (eds.), *Inflammation and Cancer*, Advances in Experimental Medicine and Biology 816, DOI: 10.1007/978-3-0348-0837-8_10, © Springer Basel 2014

cannot be completely removed by standard surgery, endoluminal stent placement, endoluminal laser therapy, and gastrojejunostomy are used in palliative surgical procedures. Generally, 3 cycles of chemotherapy regimen are used before and after surgery. Each cycle lasts 3 weeks. The most commonly used drug combinations for gastric cancer are ECF and ECX. ECF contains the drugs epirubicin, cisplatin, and fluorouracil, and ECX contains epirubicin, cisplatin, and capecitabine. Targeted therapy is an another type of treatment of gastric cancer. A drug called trastuzumab has led to significant gains in overall survival if the stomach cancer cells have too much HER2 protein (Misleh et al. 2013).

10.2 Inflammatory Signaling Pathways

Cell proliferation, differentiation, and function are principally arranged with a broad signaling network mediated by stimulative/inhibitory hormones, neurotransmitters, various cytokines, and growth factors. The interactions between cells are the most important factors that keep the balance of this network which can influence cell proliferation in positive or negative ways, as well as these interactions induce a series of differentiated responses in appropriate target cells. When these networks are inappropriately regulated, neoplastic cells may occur with its autonomy of unrestrained growth and may harm the organism even the causes are disappeared (Fedi et al. 2000).

Inflammation is one of the predominant manifestations of innate and adaptive immune systems that different and also alternative inflammatory mechanisms play a part in remodeling of tissue and re-establishment of tissue homeostasis in consequence of infection or injury by exogenous or endogenous means. All pro-inflammatory responses are accompanied by anti-inflammatory responses as a non-homogenous result that depend on type of the pathogen or tissue damage, the genotype of the host, and also discrepancies between the tissue involved. Any disturbance in tissue homeostasis activates the innate immune cells that are first line of defense which quickly migrate into the injured tissue after vasodilatation and in response to chemokine gradients, classically described as the inflammatory stage of wound healing (Velnar et al. 2009). The innate immune system cells are composed of macrophages, mast cells, dendritic cells (DC), and natural killer cells (NK), etc., that regulates the inflammatory response by releasing excessive growth hormones, cytokines, chemokines, matrix-remodeling proteases, reactive oxygen, and nitrogen species on behalf of taking control of the inflammatory process (Coussens and Werb 2002; Nathan 2002). These cells also promote healing by releasing cytokines such as tumor necrosis factor (TNF), interleukin (IL)-1, interleukin (IL)-6 that achieves cell survival, activate stem cells and promote epithelial proliferation. Also, the correlation between tumor-associated macrophage abundance and poor prognosis has been shown (Nowicki et al. 1996). Furthermore, macrophage-deficient mice display reduced progression of tumors to a more malignant phenotype (Bromberg and Wang 2009). NK and DC also play a key role in providing a link between adaptive and innate immune response, and both have crucial roles in maintaining the antigen-specific immunity (de Visser et al. 2006). Th1 response and its accompanying mediators interferon (IFN)-γ are not only necessary for *Helicobacter*-induced inflammation but also for the development of atrophy or metaplasia and spasmolytic polypeptide-expressing metaplasia (SPEM); however, a Th2 response and its mediators (i.e., IL-4) appear to be protective. The presence of a Th1, rather than a Th2, immune response is also associated with better survival in gastric cancer patients (Marshall and Warren 1984).The host response to the inflammation is a key factor takes role within inflammation process leading to carcinogenesis which includes the steps of initiation, promotion, and progression (Kinzler and Vogelstein 1996).

In addition, inappropriate and steady regulation of the immune components may be a cause of chronic inflammation by generating an initiative microenvironment that alters normal cellular homeostasis and advances the stepwise accumulation of genetic and epigenetic alterations of various proto-oncogenes and tumor suppressor genes on behalf of cancer development. These genetic and epigenetic changes include point mutations, deletions, duplications, recombinations, methylation of various tumor-related genes through various mechanisms (Chiba et al. 2012) and also include altered microRNAs expression (Zhang et al. 2008). Although, multiple signaling pathways including increased inflammatory cytokine production, abnormal apoptosis, inappropriate cell proliferation/differentiation, and epithelial transformation are triggering causes of these alterations. The fact is that biology of cell division, differentiation, and apoptosis is exceedingly similar in both normal and cancer cells (Ooi et al. 2009).

Some of the earliest observations in cancer biology as well as recent advances in molecular analyses contribute to our knowledge about the multistep process of gastric carcinogenesis (Yokozaki et al. 1997; Balkwill and Mantovani 2001; Gutierrez-Gonzalez and Wright 2008). Ooi et al. (2009) mentioned in a study that among 70 % of GC patients, three oncogenic pathways are deregulated, which are demonstrated as: proliferation/stem cell pathway (40 % of GCs), NF-κB pathway (46 % of GCs), and Wnt/b-catenin pathway (39 % of GCs). Nuclear factor (NF)-κB and STAT3 pathways have emerged as key regulators of the release of these proinflammatory cytokines, and important mediators of both tumor proliferation and persistence of chronic inflammation. The activation of these pathways results in further cytokine release (Yang 2007; Rius et al. 2008; Guilford et al. 1998). Several studies suggest that association between gastric carcinogenesis and cytokine overexpression, especially IL-1, IL-6, TNF which are also regulated by the NF-κB, showed such a clinical correlation with NF-κB signaling pathway upregulation in gastric cancer cells more than benign disorders such as gastritis (Yin et al. 2013). STAT3 drive in gastric cancer initiation and progression through its activation by cytokines, IL-6 family ligands are expressed in the stomach that IL-6 and IL-11 provide a basis in tumorigenesis (Giraud et al. 2012).

The gastrointestinal tract has rapid epithelial turnover and exposure to injury by infections and dietary toxins. These conditions create very high cancer prevalence. Intestinalization of gastric units, which is called "IM"; phenotypic antralization of fundic units, which is called "spasmolytic polypeptide-expressing metaplasia

(SPEM)"; and the development directly from the stem/progenitor cell zone are three pathways that have been described for gastric carcinogenesis (Fox and Wang 2007; Hoffmann 2008; Slack 1986).

Stem cell activation is a remarkable step in obtaining the tissue repair and self-renewal. Despite the main disadvantages of addressing the response of human immune system in the clinical researches remain obscure, these studies implicate that only a subset of cancer stem cells (CSCs) propagate the tumor (Vries et al. 2010), while the frequency of CSCs greatly increases to possibly more than 25 % of all tumor cells (Shmelkov et al. 2008; Quintana et al. 2008; Kelly et al. 2007). Several signaling pathways such as, Wnt/β-catenin pathway, take role in assuring the homeostasis and maintain the balance of gastric epithelia between progenitor and stem cells (Lickert et al. 2001; Katoh 2007). Additionally, Wnt signaling pathway is described as important steps of tissue repair and stem cell self-renewal in chronic tissue injury-related carcinogenesis (Beachy et al. 2004). It has been shown in a study that Wnt pathway in association with other inflammatory signaling pathways initiates the gastric progenitor cells through the metaplasia-carcinoma sequence in rat gastric mucosa (Oshima et al. 2006). In another mouse model, activated macrophages in the inflamed or *Helicobacter pylori*-infected gastric mucosa express TNF-α, which stimulate the surrounding cells to promote Wnt/β-catenin signaling activity in multistep pathogenesis of inflammation leading to gastric cancer (Oguma et al. 2008).

Cyclooxygenases (COX) are the key enzymes that convert and array of fatty acid substrates into pro-inflammatory prostanoids. There are 2 types of COX genes, type 1 is a physiologic gene that constitutively expressed in many tissues and responsible for the synthesis of prostanoids involved in protection of the gastrointestinal mucosa and for production of the pro-aggregatory prostanoid thromboxane by the platelets. In the contrary, type 2 COX gene is usually undetectable in most tissues. COX-2 is an inducible gene and activated by several stimulus like hormones, pro-inflammatory cytokines, growth factors, and tumor promoters. Also COX-2 has been related to inflammation, reproduction, and carcinogenesis (Taketo 1998; Dannenberg et al. 2001).

Although the subsequent pathways are different, chronic inflammation is the first step in both the intestinal and the diffuse type of gastric cancer. While the intestinal type has a sequence of multifocal atrophic gastritis, IM, and dysplasia, which advances to carcinoma, the diffuse type tends to be primarily genetic in origin (Correa 1995; Nardone et al. 2004). The progress from IM to gastric cancer has a wide range of molecular alterations affecting transcription factors, such as CDX1 and CDX2, telomerases, microsatellite instability, mutations of p53 protein, overexpression of COX-2, cyclin D2, and decreased expression of p27 (Muller et al. 2001). The next step is gastric dysplasia. During the progression of normal tissue through the metaplasia-dysplasia sequence, there are mutations in genes including *p53*, also loss of heterozygosity of the adenomatous polyposis coli gene, overexpression of the anti-apoptotic gene *bcl-2,* and a mixture of polyploidy and aneuploidy (Muller et al. 2001).

As described above, several signaling pathways take place in gastric carcinogenesis, and detection of the form and complexity of interactions between these oncogenic pathways may be helpful in the immediate future to taxonomize the individual gastric cancers into biologically and clinically relevant subgroups (Ooi et al. 2009).

Aside cytokines, members of the nuclear hormone receptor superfamily, which are ligand-activated transcription factors and members, peroxisome proliferator-activated receptors (PPARs) are assigned in multiple tasks. PPARγ, in particular, is involved in the control of inflammation and glucose metabolism and participates in the processes of cellular proliferation, differentiation, and apoptosis. It has been clearly demonstrated that gastric cancer cell lines express PPARγ and PPARγ is implicated in *H. pylori*-related gastric carcinogenesis (Morita et al. 2001; Konturek et al. 2003). PPARγ ligands, especially troglitazone, induce growth inhibition of gastric cancer cell lines, and that PPARγ agonists may have potential in a cancer therapeutic role (Sato et al. 2000). In addition, a study suggested that on the effect of PPARγ agonists, PPARγ antagonists also inhibit the gastric cancer cell lines growth which explains that PPARγ may effect gastric carcinogenesis through a PPARγ-independent pathway (Ma et al. 2009).

10.3 Role of Inflammation in Gastric Cancer

About 150 years ago Rudolph Virchow distinguished that inflammatory cells are existed in tumor tissues suggesting that chronic inflammation played a role in carcinogenesis. Since then it has been established that 25 % of all cancer types related with chronic inflammation (Hussain and Harris 2007). After identifying chronic atrophic gastritis and discover of *H. pylori*, gastric carcinoma has taken place in one of the cancers caused by chronic inflammation.

Over 100 years several studies have been conducted on gastric cancer and its relationship with atrophic gastritis and intestinal metaplasia. There has been a significant progress through the understanding of the development of gastric cancers, after in 1937, Magnus concluded that *the presence of intestinal epithelium in the stomach is the result of the faulty regeneration of surface epithelium in a mucosa repeatedly damaged by gastritis and that it is, in fact, an example of metaplasia resulting form chronic irritation*, and in 1955, Morson suggested that gastric carcinoma has arose from the areas of intestinal metaplasia (Morson 1955; Magnus 1937). Interest in *H. pylori* as a cause of cancer began after the pioneering discoveries of Marshall and Warren in 1983. *H. pylori* infection is the most common bacterial infection worldwide, almost 80 % of the population in developing countries are infected with *H. pylori* (Pounder and Ng 1995). *H. pylori* is a gram-negative spiral-shaped rod that usually acquired in infancy. It has four to six flagella that settle beneath the mucus layer of stomach. This is a defensive mechanism which protects bacteria from low gastric pH. Another defensive mechanism is its highly active urease enzyme which is capable of dividing urea into ammonia and bicarbonate, creating a non-acid microenvironment. *H. pylori* has various virulence factors such as its screw-like shape, lipopolysaccharide, vacuolating cytotoxin

A (VacA), cytotoxin-associated gene A (CagA), and its pathogenicity island (cagPAI). In recent years, there have been some studies about cagA and cagPAI and their relationship with gastric adenocarcinomas (Yamaoka 2010).

After the discovery of *H. pylori* in the late 1980s and 1990s, many researches have been achieved on its effects over the gastric mucosa and linkage to multistep pathogenesis of atrophic gastritis, intestinal metaplasia, and finally gastric cancer sequence (Correa 1988). The pattern of gastritis has also been shown to correlate strongly with the risk of gastric adenocarcinoma. The presence of antral-predominant gastritis, the most common form, confers a higher risk of developing peptic ulcers whereas corpus predominant gastritis and multifocal atrophic gastritis lead to a higher risk of developing gastric ulcers and subsequent gastric cancer. Pathogens that insist a long-term infection, such as *H. pylori,* can lead to the chronic production of pro-tumorigenic cytokines (Grivennikov et al. 2010). The response to *H. pylori* infection and the subsequent pattern of gastritis depends on the genotype of the patients and in particular genetic polymorphisms of IL-1 beta which is an inflammatory mediator triggered by *H. pylori* infection (Milne et al. 2009). *H. pylori* is the most important risk factor that causes chronic gastritis, peptic ulcus, non-cardia adenocarcinomas, and mucosa-associated lymphoid tissue (MALT) lymphoma. Although most of the infected individuals are asymptomatic, 10–15 % of them develop peptic ulcus and only 1 % of them develop gastric malignancy (Ernst et al. 2006). *H. pylori* has been classified by the World Health Organization as a class one carcinogen in 1994 (Hoggart et al. 2002). However, gastric cancer is not prevented by *H. pylori* eradication in all patients. This can be speculated that prevention of *H. pylori*-associated carcinogenesis only benefits those in whom the malignant process has not begun. Understanding the mechanism of inflammation and cancer may provide a powerful tool for understanding cancer development and prognosis.

Also other pathogen-associated inflammatory responses leading to gastric cancer has been identified, especially Epstein–Barr virus (EBV) that has been accounted for 10 % of the total GC cases (Ushiku et al. 2007). As well as Shin et al. (2006) revealed a rare agent human papilloma virus called the John Cunningham virus (JCV), and JCV T-Ag (oncogenic transforming antigen) has been isolated in 21 out of 37 GC (57 %) patients. Besides, other studies has already been concluded that JCV T-Ag DNA sequences are even presented in 80–90 % of colorectal cancers (Dyson et al. 1990; Bollag et al. 1989).

In the literature, association between parasitic infections and gastric cancer has also been described. Toxocariasis infestation-related multiple liver and pulmonary metastatic nodules have been documented in the follow-up of three gastric cancer patients which are fully regressed after anti-biotherapy (Park et al. 2012). In another patient diagnosed as gastric cancer showed Microfilaria infestation in a sample of supraclavicular lymphoid tissue aspiration cytology in the background of malignant cells thought as transmigration along with metastatic emboli in an immunosuppressed state (Kumar 2010). Although, underlying mechanisms of existence of these pathogens, associated malignancy has to be clarified.

Other etiologic factors in gastric cancer are shown in Table 10.1 (Gomceli et al. 2012).

Table 10.1 Etiologic factors in gastric cancer

Genetic factors	Environmental factors	Other factors
Sex	*Helicobacter pylori*	Gastric adenomas
Familial adenomatous polyposis	Epstein–Barr virus	Barrett's esophagus
Hereditary non-polyposis colorectal cancer (Lynch 2)	Nitrites	Hamartomas
Genetic diffuse gastric cancer (E-cadherin–CDH 1 mutation)	Excess alcohol ingestion	Menetrier's disease
Genetic polymorphisms for pro- and anti-inflammatory cytokines	High intake of salted, pickled, or smoked foods	Chronic atrophic gastritis
Polymorphisms for cell receptors of innate immune response	Low intake of fiber, fruits, and vegetables	Gastric metaplasia
Peutz–Jeghers syndrome	Antioxidant consumption (especially ascorbic acid, carotenoids, folates, and tocopherols)	Pernicious anemia
	Tobacco smoking (adenocarcinoma of cardia)	Benign gastric ulcers Fundic gland polyps Hyperplastic polyps Gastric biopsy revealing high-grade dysplasia History of subtotal gastrectomy (>20 year)

Adapted from Gomceli et al. (2012)

10.4 Role of Inflammatory Molecules in Gastric Cancer: Evidence from In Vitro Studies

Inflammatory cytokines are the remarkable determinants cell survival and death. IL-1 and IL-6 activate nuclear factor-κB (NF-κB) and STAT3 pro-survival transcription factors to induce cell survival and tumor development, where as other cytokines such as Fas ligand and TNF-related apoptosis-inducing ligand (TRAIL) induce apoptotic cell death (Kuraishy et al. 2011). It is now well accepted that if the host-mediated anti-tumor activity is incapable of forming immune response via several defending mechanisms, tumor cells undergo immune escape and grow rapidly. Dunn et al. (2004) suggested as in "cancer immunosurveillance" theory that cytokines have dual roles, while such cytokines especially TNF, TRAIL, FasL, and TWEAK are inducing the apoptotic cell death, the other cytokines such as type I interferon (IFN) and TGF-β limit the proliferation of epithelial cells. TNF-α, especially in combination with IFN-γ, were originally described for their anti-tumoral activity, a cytotoxic action against tumor cells by regulating the immune response, host defense and gene expression. It is demonstrated in a study that IFN-γ regulates apoptosis by soluble TNF-R released by IFN-gamma in the injured gastric epithelial cell line induced by TNF (Furuta et al. 2002). IL-12 and IL-18 both allow proliferation of T cells and potent production of IFN-γ, which may lead to a direct anti-proliferative and pro-apoptotic effect on the tumor cells as well as anti-tumor activity (Ye et al. 2007). In a study, IL-18 enhance the proliferation of gastric cancer lines via NF-κB signaling pathway in a dose-dependent manner, where as L-18-pretreated gastric cancer cells, which were cultured with cytokine-activated peripheral blood killer lymphocytes, showed less secretion of IFN-γ or perforin, anti-tumor products of killer lymphocytes, resulting in a decreased susceptibility of cancer cells to killer lymphocytes (Majima et al. 2006). Despite cytokines, several in vitro studies have found that PPARγ activation results in cell cycle arrest and/or apoptosis of gastric cancer cells (Takahashi et al. 1999). Cytokines produced in response to injury have enormous effects on cell survival contributing to tumor initiation, growth, progression, and metastasis, which is yet to be elucidated.

Chronic inflammation plays an important role in tumorigenesis and macrophages are a key player in generating the chronic inflammation microenvironment by being activated persistently until leading to continuous tissue damage (Macarthur et al. 2004). In the acute phase of inflammation, the release of endogenous reactive oxygen (ROS) and nitrogen species (NOS) (O_2^-, H_2O_2, NO, OH, $ONOO^-$, HOCl) from such innate immune cells as macrophages together with other leukocytes contributes a fight back to infection and pathogens (Maeda and Akaike 1998; Leach et al. 1987). However, sustained generation of ROS and NOS may alter proliferating cells via forming a tumorigenic microenvironment that generated in several pathways. Continuous deleterious ROS and NOS exposure triggers amplification of inflammatory cytokine production that stimulates signal transductors, angiogenic factors, and oncogene overexpression and post-translational modification of tumor suppressor genes and also causes direct DNA damage by inhibition of DNA repair in proliferating cells (Federico et al. 2007).

ROS and NOS secretion is under control of pro-inflammatory cytokines through the activation of protein kinases signaling that accumulates the production of free radicals such as hydroxyl radical (OH•), superoxide (O_2^-•), nitric oxide (NO•), and peroxynitrite ($ONOO^-$).

TNF-α induces ROS production in neutrophils, tumor cells, and also endothelial cells via a ceramide-dependent signaling pathway (Corda et al. 2001), while TNF-α, IL-1β, interferon-γ (IFN-γ) stimulates the expression of inducible nitric oxide synthase in inflammatory and epithelial cells. In addition, in an increased cellular oxidative stress process, TNF-α induced excessive production of reactive oxygen species, influence its cytotoxic effects on tumor cells, and arrangement of gene expression (Goossens et al. 1995; Schutze et al. 1992).

TNF-α and IL-1β also induce the formation of $ONOO^-$, which formed by a reaction of NO• with superoxide, is a constitutive producer of IL-8. IL-8 is a potent pro-inflammatory chemokine derived from monocytes, macrophages, and endothelial cells that promote adhesion, migration, invasion, and chemoresistance of gastric cancer cells (Zouki et al. 2001; Kuai et al. 2012). When ROS levels are significantly increased, oxidatively altered nucleic acids (Demple and Harrison 1994) cause DNA damage including strand breaks, intrastrand adducts, and DNA protein cross-links (Valko et al. 2005). In addition, ROS mediates the formation of

8-oxo-7,8-dihydro-20-deoxyguanosine (Inoue and Kawanishi 1995), and *8-nitroguanine* (Yermilov et al. 1995; Akaike et al. 2003), which are considered to be potential biomarkers of oxidative stress (Evans et al. 2004), in relation to cancer-associated inflammation (Valko et al. 2006, 2007). 8-hydroxydeoxyguanine basically alters the nucleotide string by leading to guanine(G)/cytosine(C) to thymine(T)/adenine(A) transversions which are also observed in vivo in the ras gene (Bos 1988) and the v-Ki-ras2 Kirsten rat sarcoma viral oncogene homolog (*K-RAS*) and *TP53* tumor suppressor gene in lung and liver cancers (Takahashi et al. 1989; Hsu et al. 1991).

In an another study, chronic gastritis as a precancerous lesion of gastric cancer, is characterized by the accumulation of oxidative DNA damage that *H. pylori* infection is the major determinant for DNA adduct formation (Farinati et al. 1998). *H. pylori*-infected stomach arranges the microenvironment for the activated neutrophils to provide the ROS or NOS production besides that *H. pylori* itself also produces ROS (Handa et al. 2010).

NO• has a crucial role in inflammation and its functional heterogeneity, between preneoplastic and antineoplastic functions is the remarkable status in the field of cancer biology. NO• and nitric oxide synthase (NOS), *especially overexpression of NOS2*, both have an impact on the post-translational modification of tumor suppressor genes such as p53 and Rb during chronic inflammation (Ying et al. 2005; Hofseth et al. 2003). NO• mediated p53 accumulation and post-translational modification promote gastric cancer progression in association with advanced tumors even with metastasis thereby causing cellular growth arrest, inducing apoptosis and oncogenic mutations in the p53 gene (Rajnakova et al. 2001).

However, *c-MYC oncogene* activation generates sufficient ROS to produce DNA strand breaks, activate p53 pathway in the absence of apoptosis, and cause DNA damage before the S phase in association with ROS induction in normal human fibroblasts (Vafa et al. 2002). Thus, activated oncogenes induce genomic instability in consequence of DNA damage in both precancerous lesions and cancers (Halazonetis et al. 2008)

However, a tumorigenic microenvironment, formed by an unresolved inflammation on account of any deleterious effects of unrestrained release of mediators that already exacerbated by such immune cells, mesenchymal cells, and epithelial cells, contributes to tumor initiation and/or initial tumoral progression. Cytokines are the putative regulators of the inflammation with pro- and anti-inflammatory functions, where INF-γ, TNF, IL-1α/β, IL-6, and chemokines are known to be the major cytokines important for inflammation and cancer development (El-Omar et al. 2000; Ben-Neriah and Karin 2011; Kuraishy et al. 2011).

TNF-α has an important role in both anti-tumoral activity and tumorigenesis with a diversity of response in the chronic inflammation, which ranges between tissue recovery and tissue destruction. TNF-α, produced by malignant cells, leukocytes, and other cells in tumor microenvironments, acts primarily through membrane-bound homotrimeric receptors TNRFI and TNRFII in autocrine and paracrine ways (Locksley et al. 2001). Despite locally high dose of TNF-α exposure destroys the tumor vascularate and causes tumor necrosis, sustained production of TNF-α may facilitate tissue remodeling and stromal development linking to tumor growth and spread as an endogenous tumor promoter (Balkwill and Joffroy 2010). TNF-α can also promote the angiogenesis by inducing a range of angiogenic factors, thymidine phosphorylase, and matrix metalloproteinases (MMPs) (Balkwill and Mantovani 2001; Leek et al. 1998; Balkwill and Joffroy 2010; Aggarwal 2003). In addition, TNF-α has a vital role in DNA damage with the help of other inflammatory cytokines, IFN-γ, and IL-1β, by upregulating iNOS and NO• production which causes direct damage of DNA and inhibits the DNA repair (Jaiswal et al. 2000). Besides that, TNF-α implicates other chemokines via regulating a tumorigenic signaling network, in inflammatory processes leading to tumorigenesis (Balkwill and Joffroy 2010).

Thus, TNF-α secures its position as a major mediator of inflammation-associated carcinogenesis, by contributing a tumorigenic microenvironment via inducing several cytokines, angiogenic factors, and MMPs that cause DNA damage and promote tumor growth and tumor metastasis in the survival of tumor cells through a tumorigenic signaling pathway, NF-κB (Balkwill and Joffroy 2010). NF-κB is a transcription factor, and NF-κB-regulated genes provide several products that inhibit apoptosis and enhance cell cycle progression, angiogenesis, and metastasis, in consequence of forming the IKK complexes which pro-inflammatory cytokines and microbial infections are being stimulated (Karin and Greten 2005; Karin 2006; Luo et al. 2005). Soutto et al. (2011) demonstrated that Trefoil factor 1(TFF1, a tumor suppressor gene) knockout mice leads to activation of IKK complex-regulated NF-κB transcription factors, and hence, NF-κB-mediated inflammatory response causes a multistep carcinogenesis cascade in the progression of gastric carcinogenesis with the help of TNF-α-mediated NF-κB activation through the TNF receptor 1 (TNFR1)/IκB kinase (IKK) pathway. In an another study, Mochizuki et al., also showed that by using a green fluorescent protein (GFP)-tagged human gastric cancer cell line, TNF-α-pretreated mice group exhibits an early progression of peritoneal metastasis which is more significant than the non-pretreated group (Mochizuki et al. 2004). It is still a controversial manner that gastric cancer patients show a significant increase in TNF-α levels.

TNF-α and IL-1β are essential in the initiation of chronic inflammation. Recent works have shown that IL-1β overexpression, in the absence of *H. pylori* infection, is sufficient to cause gastric cancer. In addition, IL-1β is one of the essential pro-inflammatory cytokines modulated during *H. pylori* infection that directs the mucosa toward atrophy, metaplasia, and neoplastic transformation (El-Omar et al. 2000; El-Omar 2001; Pollard 2004). Beales (2002) demonstrated in a study that IL-1β stimulates the proliferation of gastric cancer cell lines via tyrosine kinase-dependent signaling pathway and autocrine stimulation of GM-CSF contributes to this stimulation in a dose-dependent manner. Similar to findings for IL-1β, Uefuji et al. (2005) demonstrated that IL-1α mRNA expression levels were relevant to COX-2 positive cancer cell lines, that exogenous supplement of IL-1α enhances both IL-1α and COX-2 mRNA expression levels which indicates IL-1α-COX-2 pathway might be involved in tumor progression by regulating cancer cell proliferation. Several researchers have demonstrated that IL-1α enhances angiogenesis and vascular endothelial cell proliferation in gastric cancer cell lines (Ma et al. 2008; Furuya et al. 2000).

Recently, direct evidence has also linked IL-6 to inflammation-mediated tumor initiation and proliferation in colon cancer (Bromberg and Wang 2009). IL-6 plays an important role in stimulation of tumor growth and tumor metastasis including the steps of tumor cells invasion of the stroma, intravasation of blood vessels and circulation in the blood. In an in vitro study designed with several gastric cancer cell lines demonstrated that such gastric cancer cell lines expressed IL-6 mRNA, which was an indicator of gastric cancer cell growth, even anti-IL-6 antibody inhibited this process (Ito et al. 1997). In cancer cells, IL-6 expression that leads to tumor invasion and metastasis in gastric cancer may act as in autocrine and paracrine ways. IL-6 can be secreted from cancer cells which combines with IL-6 receptors on the surface of cancer cells, directly promote the cancer cell mitogenic activity in an autocrine pathway (Ashizawa et al. 2005). IL-6 also stimulates cancer cells to produce hepatocyte growth factor (HGF), which combines with the HGF receptor (c-met) expressed on cancer cells, through a paracrine pathway that HGF induces cancer cells to move to the metastatic site by promoting and accelerating invasion as well as lymph node and/or hepatic metastasis (Ashizawa et al. 2005). In addition, it is documented that IL-6, is an important effector of TNF-α and IL-1β actions in vivo (Gangopadhyay et al. 1998). IL-6 promotes the adhesion of cancer cells and endothelial cells via overexpressing the intercellular adhesion molecules such as ICAM, VCAM, and E-selectin in association with TNF-α and IL-1β (Gangopadhyay et al. 1998). IL-6 acts on cancer cells directly via the Janus Kinase (JNK)/signal transducer and activator of transcription 3 pathways (Ashizawa et al. 2005) and may also inhibit DC maturation and, together with the NF-κB-activating cytokines IL-1 and TNF may promote tumor progression. IL-6 can regulate VEGF and angiogenesis in gastric cancer, as demonstrated in another study that increasing dose and duration of IL-6-stimulated gastric cancer cell lines produces significant amount of vascular endothelial growth factor (VEGF) in vivo and in vitro (Huang et al. 2004).

IL-10 and transforming growth factor (TGF)-β are known for not only their effects oversuppressing the host anti-tumor immunity and anti-inflammatory actions, but also are central regulator of regulatory T cell (Treg) which can inhibit immune responses mediated by CD4(+) and CD8(+) cells (Tsujimoto et al. 2010). TGF-β1 expression demonstrated as a clinical prognostic marker and putative angiogenic factor in gastric carcinogenesis that has already been suggested in a study that TGF-β1 expression stimulates angiogenesis via promoting indirectly by VEGF upregulation (Saito et al. 1999).

10.5 Role of Inflammatory Molecules in Gastric Cancer: Evidence from In Vivo Studies

IL-1β, IL-6, IL-8, and TNF-α mRNA expression levels were significantly elevated in *H. pylori*-positive mucosa compared with *H. pylori*-negative mucosa. In *H. pylori*-positive gastric mucosa, IL-1β, IL-6, and IL-8 mRNA expression levels correlated significantly with activity and chronic inflammation scores, and TNF-α mRNA expression levels correlated with chronic inflammation scores. There was a negative association between IL-6 and IL-8 mRNA expression and intestinal metaplasia scores IL-6 and TNF-α mRNA expression levels increased with the severity of atrophic gastritis, while pro-inflammatory cytokine mRNA expression levels were lower in the mucosa with intestinal metaplasia compared to mucosa with extended atrophic gastritis (Isomoto et al. 2012).

Individual differences in the intensity of the inflammatory response (which affects the maintenance, severity, and outcome of *H. pylori* infection) may contribute to gastric mucosa transformation. Moreover, the impact of gene polymorphisms on the activity of key inflammatory molecules is relatively well known.

Previous studies on the association between IL-1 genetic polymorphisms and the risk of gastric cancer have produced controversial results. In a meta-analysis, authors observed that the IL-1B–511T carrier, as well as the IL-1RN*2 carriers, are associated with an increased risk of developing of gastric cancer, markedly the intestinal type. IL-1RN*2 carrier increased the risk of developing gastric cancer among Caucasian. However, the IL-1B–31C and +3954T genotypes are not associated with an increased risk of developing gastric cancer (Wang et al. 2007).

In contrast, these polymorphisms are not consistently related to the risks of esophageal or gastric cardia cancers (El-Omar et al. 2003).

A number of studies have shown that cyclooxygenase-2 (COX-2) gene polymorphisms were associated with gastric cancer. However, the results from different research groups have not been consistent. At present, two polymorphisms in COX-2 have been reported. The promoter region polymorphic variant of −1195G>A and −765G>C has been demonstrated to have a functional effect on COX-2 transcription, which may cause gastric cancer (Pereira et al. 2009; Zhang et al. 2005).

Several studies have examined the association of polymorphisms in tumor necrosis factor-A gene (TNF-A) with gastric cancer risk. However, the meta-analysis of these studies have shown that TNF-A-308AA genotype was associated with a increased risk of gastric cancer, whereas other polymorphisms are not (Gorouhi et al. 2008).

Polymorphisms in the 5′-flanking region of IL-10 at positions −1082 A/G, −819T/C, and −592A/C have been suggested to be associated with gastric cancer risk in different populations (El-Omar et al. 2003; de Oliveira et al. 2012). IL-10-592 AA is a factor of protection against the development of this neoplasm in Asians, but not among Caucasians and Latinos, indicating differences in the genetic background of Asians and other ethnicities (Zhu et al. 2011).

IL-17A has a crucial role in the gastric inflammation and carcinogenesis. Genetic polymorphisms of IL-17A may be involved in methylation-related carcinogenesis in the stomach (Tahara et al. 2010). Similarly, it also indicates that IL8, and maybe IL4R, variants may modify the risk for gastric cancer (Crusius et al. 2008).

Few studies have done combined analysis of different polymorphisms in gastric cancer. El-Omar et al. (2003) analyzed 11 polymorphisms of the IL-1B, IL-1RN, IL-4, IL-6, IL-10, and TNF-A cytokine genes and showed that the risk for non-cardia gastric cancer increased progressively with the number of pro-inflammatory genotypes to 27.3 for three or four polymorphisms. This finding is probably due to an additive effect of the pro-inflammatory profiles of these gene polymorphisms, resulting in an exacerbated immune response. Several studies have demonstrated that the Pro12Ala polymorphism is associated with the high risk of gastric adenocarcinoma (Xu et al. 2010; Lee et al. 2012).

TNF-α-857T carrier showed significantly better overall survival than patients with CC genotype. Gastric cancer patients who have both IL-1β-31 CC and IL-1β-511 TT genotypes and have at least one of the protective genotypes (IL-1β-31 CC, IL-1β-511 TT, TNF-α-857 T carrier) were also associated with better survival. IL-1β-31CC, IL-1β-511TT genotype, and TNF-α-857T carrier may have protective effect against gastric cancer progression (Tahara et al. 2011). Percentages of Tc17 cells in gastric tumors are associated with survival times of patients (Zhuang et al. 2012). Overexpression of TNF-α, IL-6, IL-8, IL-10, IL-18, and IL-33 correlates with several poor prognostic factors such as depth of invasion, distant metastasis, and advanced stage (stage III/IV).

Despite the several studies concluded, the correlation between high serum levels of TNF-α is a prognostic marker in advanced gastric cancer (stage III and IV) patients (Forones et al. 2001; Macri et al. 2006), Wu et al. (1998) suggest that TNF-α value was not an independent prognostic indicator and the role of TNF-α in gastric cancer remains obscure. Gastric cancer patients show different biologic behavior in each of the cases depending on host inflammatory immune conditions. For example, TNF-α gene polymorphism, which is located in the promoter of TNFA gene, effects the prognosis and survival of the patients in such protective and progressive ways (Tahara et al. 2011; Hong et al. 2013). Several studies manifest that IL-6 serum level increase is a significant marker in correlation with tumor size, tumor stage, and metastasis in gastric cancer patients as well as indicator of gastric cancer progression (Ikeguchi et al. 2009; Ashizawa et al. 2005).

On the other hand, low serum levels of IL-12 have been associated with more advanced stages of gastric and colorectal carcinomas and tended to be associated with lymph node metastasis and carcinoembryonic antigen (CEA)-positive tumors greater than 5 cm in diameter (Kawabata et al. 2001; Wu et al. 1998; Nakayama et al. 2000; Sun et al. 2011; Szaflarska et al. 2009). IL-18, previously known as interferon-γ-inducing factor, found elevated in patients with gastric carcinoma stage 2 or 3 (Kawabata et al. 2001).

Also, COX-2 expression is associated with intestinal histologic subtype, proximal location, large tumor size, and advanced stage (Thiel et al. 2011).

Although there are several studies about relation between gastric cancer prognosis and inflammation markers, none of these markers are used in clinical practice.

10.6 Inhibitors of Inflammation for the Prevention and Treatment of Gastric Cancer

Chemoprevention of gastric carcinoma may be divided into three titles: eradication of *H. pylori*, cyclooxygenase inhibitors which directly effects inflammation, and dietary supplements.

Eradication of *H. pylori* for prevention from gastric adenocarcinoma still keeps its uncertainty. But there is a truth that eradication reduces the rates of precancerous lesion such as atrophic gastritis and intestinal metaplasia (Mera et al. 2005). Recent studies state that early eradication of *H. pylori* seems to reduce gastric cancer risk (Fuccio et al. 2009). The key point of eradication is "timing." If the malignant process has begun, eradication therapy loses its significance. Recent long-term studies about the patients with high risk of gastric carcinoma or with patients after endoscopic resection of early gastric carcinoma showed that the eradication therapy did not reduce the risk of development of primary or metachronous gastric cancer (Wong et al. 2004; Maehata et al. 2012). A double-blind randomized study in China showed that gastric cancer still occurred after successful eradication of *H. pylori* and that *H. pylori* eradication did not lead to significant decrease in the incidence of gastric cancer. In the high-risk region of China, 1630 healthy carriers of *H. pylori* were followed for 7.5 years. During the follow-up, the development of gastric cancer was observed in 7 subjects from the *H. pylori* eradication therapy group and 11 subjects from the placebo group, with no significant difference between the two groups. In the subgroup analysis without precancerous lesions (atrophy, intestinal metaplasia, and dysplasia), the incidence of gastric cancer was significantly lower in the *H. pylori* eradication therapy group than in the placebo group (Wong et al. 2004). This study suggested that the preventive effect of *H. pylori* eradication for gastric cancer is sufficient only in patients without an atrophic change (Kato and Asaka 2012).

Right after the study which defines miRNA expression patterns in *H. pylori*-infected gastric mucosa before and after eradication (Matsushima et al. 2011), Shiotani made similar study with patients who underwent endoscopic gastric resection with control biopsies before and 1 year after the eradication therapy (Shiotani et al. 2012). In *H. pylori*-infected mucosa, eradication therapy works as a decreasing factor for vast majority of miRNA which expressed during the *H. pylori*-associated gastritis. But on the other hand, Shiotani underlined that eradication therapy did not improve the abnormal expression of many oncogenic miRNAs in intestinal metaplastic glands or in the gastric mucosa of the high-risk group for gastric cancer (Kato and Asaka 2012).

Several epidemiologic studies have suggested that long-term and regular use of NSAIDs, aspirin in particular, reduce mortality from gastrointestinal metaplasias (Ristimaki et al. 1997). As a result, cyclooxygenase enzyme (COX) is to be thought of a potential therapeutic target in cancer prevention and treatment (Thiel et al. 2011). Firstly, COX-2 inhibitors were tried for prevention therapy of colorectal polyps and cancer; then, recent studies showed that NSAIDs and specific COX-2 inhibitors can play role in prevention of gastric cancer.

In a large prospective cohort study in 2009, Abnet et al. found that regular use of aspirin, or non-aspirin NSAIDs, may reduce the risk of non-cardia gastric cancer. In this study, they reached 2078248 person-years of follow-up in total (mean follow-up is 6.7 years). They found that reported use of aspirin or non-aspirin NSAIDs was associated with a significant 36 % reduction in the risk of non-cardia gastric cancer (Abnet et al. 2009).

Except from NSAIDs, there are several published articles about selective COX-2 inhibitors. In animal models, a study with reflux-induced gastric adenocarcinoma in

Wistar rats that underwent gastrojejunostomy stated that celecoxib has an inhibiting effect on reflux-induced gastric carcinogenesis (Rocha et al. 2009).

In a human trial, patients with gastric preneoplastic lesion, who taken *H. pylori* eradication therapy, received either celecoxib or placebo for 3 months, and a significant improvement in precancerous lesions was observed who received celecoxib for placebo (Zhang et al. 2009). In an another study, etodolac was used as a selective COX-2 inhibitor to demonstrate the preventive effects on cancer development in extensive metaplastic gastritis (Yanaoka et al. 2010). These results strongly suggest that chemoprevention of cancer in the metaplastic stomach is possible by controlling COX-2 expression.

In light of these findings, there is a high probability that in near future, gastric cancer will be prevented by COX inhibition.

There are various studies about diet, nutrition, dietary supplements, and their relation with gastric cancer and also its prevention. According to The World Cancer Research Fund and the American Institute for Cancer Research, non-starchy vegetables and fruits probably protect against stomach cancer. Salt and also salt-preserved foods are probably the causes of this cancer (Wiseman 2008). A prospective study with 10-year follow-up of the Japan Public Health Center study cohort suggested that consumption of vegetables and fruits is associated with diminished gastric cancer risk (Kobayashi et al. 2002). Current epidemiologic and human trial evidence generally indicates that antioxidant foods or supplements provide little protection against gastrointestinal cancers (Jayaprakash and Marshall 2011).

10.7 Conclusions and Future Directions

Gastric cancer is a major health problem in worldwide. Understanding of the mechanism inflammation and cancer may provide a powerful tool for understanding cancer development and prognosis. CSC hypothesis has received more and more attention in last 10 years. This hypothesis will change our daily practice in several types of cancer including gastric cancer. An in-depth understanding of the relation between stem cell and inflammation can lead to development of new drugs and markers that can be used in routine practice.

References

Abnet CC, Freedman ND, Kamangar F, Leitzmann MF, Hollenbeck AR, Schatzkin A (2009) Non-steroidal anti-inflammatory drugs and risk of gastric and oesophageal adenocarcinomas: results from a cohort study and a meta-analysis. Br J Cancer 100(3):551–557. doi:10.1038/sj.bjc.6604880

Aggarwal BB (2003) Signalling pathways of the TNF superfamily: a double-edged sword. Nat Rev Immunol 3(9):745–756. doi:10.1038/nri1184

Akaike T, Okamoto S, Sawa T, Yoshitake J, Tamura F, Ichimori K, Miyazaki K, Sasamoto K, Maeda H (2003) 8-nitroguanosine formation in viral pneumonia and its implication for pathogenesis. Proc Nat Acad Sci USA 100(2):685–690. doi:10.1073/pnas.0235623100

Ashizawa T, Okada R, Suzuki Y, Takagi M, Yamazaki T, Sumi T, Aoki T, Ohnuma S, Aoki T (2005) Clinical significance of interleukin-6 (IL-6) in the spread of gastric cancer: role of IL-6 as a prognostic factor. Gastric Cancer (Official Journal of the International Gastric Cancer Association and the Japanese Gastric Cancer Association) 8(2):124–131. doi:10.1007/s10120-005-0315-x

Balkwill F, Joffroy C (2010) TNF: a tumor-suppressing factor or a tumor-promoting factor? Future Oncol 6(12):1833–1836. doi:10.2217/fon.10.155

Balkwill F, Mantovani A (2001) Inflammation and cancer: back to Virchow? Lancet 357(9255):539–545. doi:10.1016/S0140-6736(00)04046-0

Beachy PA, Karhadkar SS, Berman DM (2004) Tissue repair and stem cell renewal in carcinogenesis. Nature 432(7015):324–331. doi:10.1038/nature03100

Beales IL (2002) Effect of interlukin-1beta on proliferation of gastric epithelial cells in culture. BMC Gastroenterol 2:7

Ben-Neriah Y, Karin M (2011) Inflammation meets cancer, with NF-kappaB as the matchmaker. Nat Immunol 12(8):715–723. doi:10.1038/ni.2060

Bollag B, Chuke WF, Frisque RJ (1989) Hybrid genomes of the polyomaviruses JC virus, BK virus, and simian virus 40: identification of sequences important for efficient transformation. J Virol 63(2):863–872

Bos JL (1988) The ras gene family and human carcinogenesis. Mutat Res 195(3):255–271

Bromberg J, Wang TC (2009) Inflammation and cancer: IL-6 and STAT3 complete the link. Cancer Cell 15(2):79–80. doi:10.1016/j.ccr.2009.01.009

Chiba T, Marusawa H, Ushijima T (2012) Inflammation-associated cancer development in digestive organs: mechanisms and roles for genetic and epigenetic modulation. Gastroenterology 143(3):550–563. doi:10.1053/j.gastro.2012.07.009

Corda S, Laplace C, Vicaut E, Duranteau J (2001) Rapid reactive oxygen species production by mitochondria in endothelial cells exposed to tumor necrosis factor-alpha is mediated by ceramide. Am J Respir Cell Mol Biol 24(6):762–768

Correa P (1988) A human model of gastric carcinogenesis. Cancer Res 48(13):3554–3560

Correa P (1995) *Helicobacter pylori* and gastric carcinogenesis. Am J Surg Pathol 19 (Suppl 1):S37–S43

Coussens LM, Werb Z (2002) Inflammation and cancer. Nature 420(6917):860–867. doi:10.1038/nature01322

Crusius JB, Canzian F, Capella G, Pena AS, Pera G, Sala N, Agudo A, Rico F, Del Giudice G, Palli D, Plebani M, Boeing H, Bueno-de-Mesquita HB, Carneiro F, Pala V, Save VE, Vineis P, Tumino R, Panico S, Berglund G, Manjer J, Stenling R, Hallmans G, Martinez C, Dorronsoro M, Barricarte A, Navarro C, Quiros JR, Allen N, Key TJ, Binghan S, Caldas C, Linseisen J, Kaaks R, Overvad K, Tjonneland A, Buchner FC, Peeters PH, Numans ME, Clavel-Chapelon F, Trichopoulou A, Lund E, Jenab M, Rinaldi S, Ferrari P, Riboli E, Gonzalez CA (2008) Cytokine gene polymorphisms and the risk of adenocarcinoma of the stomach in the European prospective investigation into cancer and nutrition (EPIC-EURGAST). Ann Oncol (Official Journal of the European Society for Medical Oncology/ESMO) 19(11):1894–1902. doi:10.1093/annonc/mdn400

Dannenberg AJ, Altorki NK, Boyle JO, Dang C, Howe LR, Weksler BB, Subbaramaiah K (2001) Cyclo-oxygenase 2: a pharmacological target for the prevention of cancer. Lancet Oncol 2(9):544–551. doi:10.1016/S1470-2045(01)00488-0

de Oliveira JG, Rossi AF, Nizato DM, Miyasaki K, Silva AE (2012) Profiles of gene polymorphisms in cytokines and toll-like receptors with higher risk for gastric cancer. Dig Dis Sci. doi:10.1007/s10620-012-2460-5

de Visser KE, Eichten A, Coussens LM (2006) Paradoxical roles of the immune system during cancer development. Nat Rev Cancer 6(1):24–37. doi:10.1038/nrc1782

Demple B, Harrison L (1994) Repair of oxidative damage to DNA: enzymology and biology. Annu Rev Biochem 63:915–948. doi:10.1146/annurev.bi.63.070194.004411

Dunn GP, Old LJ, Schreiber RD (2004) The immunobiology of cancer immunosurveillance and immunoediting. Immunity 21(2):137–148. doi:10.1016/j.immuni.2004.07.017

Dyson N, Bernards R, Friend SH, Gooding LR, Hassell JA, Major EO, Pipas JM, Vandyke T, Harlow E (1990) Large T antigens of many polyomaviruses are able to form complexes with the retinoblastoma protein. J Virol 64(3):1353–1356

El-Omar EM (2001) The importance of interleukin 1beta in *Helicobacter pylori* associated disease. Gut 48(6):743–747

El-Omar EM, Carrington M, Chow WH, McColl KE, Bream JH, Young HA, Herrera J, Lissowska J, Yuan CC, Rothman N, Lanyon G, Martin M, Fraumeni JF Jr, Rabkin CS (2000) Interleukin-1 polymorphisms associated with increased risk of gastric cancer. Nature 404(6776):398–402. doi:10.1038/35006081

El-Omar EM, Rabkin CS, Gammon MD, Vaughan TL, Risch HA, Schoenberg JB, Stanford JL, Mayne ST, Goedert J, Blot WJ, Fraumeni JF Jr, Chow WH (2003) Increased risk of noncardia gastric cancer associated with proinflammatory cytokine gene polymorphisms. Gastroenterology 124(5):1193–1201

Ernst PB, Peura DA, Crowe SE (2006) The translation of *Helicobacter pylori* basic research to patient care. Gastroenterology 130(1):188–206; quiz 212–183. doi:10.1053/j.gastro.2005.06.032

Evans MD, Dizdaroglu M, Cooke MS (2004) Oxidative DNA damage and disease: induction, repair and significance. Mutat Res 567(1):1–61. doi:10.1016/j.mrrev.2003.11.001

Farinati F, Cardin R, Degan P, Rugge M, Mario FD, Bonvicini P, Naccarato R (1998) Oxidative DNA damage accumulation in gastric carcinogenesis. Gut 42(3):351–356

Federico A, Morgillo F, Tuccillo C, Ciardiello F, Loguercio C (2007) Chronic inflammation and oxidative stress in human carcinogenesis. Int J Cancer 121(11):2381–2386. doi:10.1002/ijc.23192

Fedi P, Kimmelman A, Aaronson SA (2000) Growth factor signal transduction in cancer. In: Bast RC Jr, Kufe DW, Pollock RE et al (ed) Holland-Frei cancer medicine, 5th edn. BC Decker, Hamilton (ON). http://www.ncbi.nlm.nih.gov/books/NBK20800

Forones NM, Mandowsky SV, Lourenco LG (2001) Serum levels of interleukin-2 and tumor necrosis factor-alpha correlate to tumor progression in gastric cancer. Hepatogastroenterology 48(40):1199–1201

Fox JG, Wang TC (2007) Inflammation, atrophy, and gastric cancer. J Clin Investig 117(1):60–69. doi:10.1172/JCI30111

Fuccio L, Zagari RM, Eusebi LH, Laterza L, Cennamo V, Ceroni L, Grilli D, Bazzoli F (2009) Meta-analysis: can *Helicobacter pylori* eradication treatment reduce the risk for gastric cancer? Ann Intern Med 151(2):121–128

Furuta S, Goto H, Niwa Y, Ohmiya N, Kamiya K, Oguri A, Hayakawa T, Mori N (2002) Interferon-gamma regulates apoptosis by releasing soluble tumor necrosis factor receptors in a gastric epithelial cell line. J Gastroenterol Hepatol 17(12):1283–1290

Furuya Y, Ichikura T, Mochizuki H, Shinomiya N (2000) Relationship between interleukin-1-alpha concentration in tumors and cell growth in gastric cancer, determined using flow cytometry. Gastric Cancer (Official Journal of the International Gastric Cancer Association and the Japanese Gastric Cancer Association) 3(2):86–90

Gangopadhyay A, Lazure DA, Thomas P (1998) Adhesion of colorectal carcinoma cells to the endothelium is mediated by cytokines from CEA stimulated Kupffer cells. Clin Exp Metastasis 16(8):703–712

Giraud AS, Menheniott TR, Judd LM (2012) Targeting STAT3 in gastric cancer. Expert Opin Ther Targets 16(9):889–901. doi:10.1517/14728222.2012.709238

Gomceli I, Demiriz B, Tez M (2012) Gastric carcinogenesis. World J Gastroenterol 18(37):5164–5170. doi:10.3748/wjg.v18.i37.5164

Goossens V, Grooten J, De Vos K, Fiers W (1995) Direct evidence for tumor necrosis factor-induced mitochondrial reactive oxygen intermediates and their involvement in cytotoxicity. Proc Natl Acad Sci USA 92(18):8115–8119

Gorouhi F, Islami F, Bahrami H, Kamangar F (2008) Tumour-necrosis factor-A polymorphisms and gastric cancer risk: a meta-analysis. Br J Cancer 98(8):1443–1451. doi:10.1038/sj.bjc.6604277

Grivennikov SI, Greten FR, Karin M (2010) Immunity, inflammation, and cancer. Cell 140(6):883–899. doi:10.1016/j.cell.2010.01.025

Group G, Paoletti X, Oba K, Burzykowski T, Michiels S, Ohashi Y, Pignon JP, Rougier P, Sakamoto J, Sargent D, Sasako M, Van Cutsem E, Buyse M (2010) Benefit of adjuvant chemotherapy for resectable gastric cancer: a meta-analysis. JAMA 303(17):1729–1737. doi:10.1001/jama.2010.534

Guilford P, Hopkins J, Harraway J, McLeod M, McLeod N, Harawira P, Taite H, Scoular R, Miller A, Reeve AE (1998) E-cadherin germline mutations in familial gastric cancer. Nature 392(6674):402–405. doi:10.1038/32918

Gutierrez-Gonzalez L, Wright NA (2008) Biology of intestinal metaplasia in 2008: more than a simple phenotypic alteration. Digestive and Liver Disease (Official Journal of the Italian Society of Gastroenterology and the Italian Association for the Study of the Liver) 40(7):510–522. doi:10.1016/j.dld.2008.02.029

Halazonetis TD, Gorgoulis VG, Bartek J (2008) An oncogene-induced DNA damage model for cancer development. Science 319(5868):1352–1355. doi:10.1126/science.1140735

Handa O, Naito Y, Yoshikawa T (2010) *Helicobacter pylori*: a ROS-inducing bacterial species in the stomach. Inflam Res (Official Journal of the European Histamine Research Society [et al]) 59(12):997–1003. doi:10.1007/s00011-010-0245-x

Hoffmann W (2008) Regeneration of the gastric mucosa and its glands from stem cells. Curr Med Chem 15(29):3133–3144

Hofseth LJ, Saito S, Hussain SP, Espey MG, Miranda KM, Araki Y, Jhappan C, Higashimoto Y, He P, Linke SP, Quezado MM, Zurer I, Rotter V, Wink DA, Appella E, Harris CC (2003) Nitric oxide-induced cellular stress and p53 activation in chronic inflammation. Proc Natl Acad Sci USA 100(1):143–148. doi:10.1073/pnas.0237083100

Hoggart K, Lees L, Davies A (2002) Researching human geography. Hodder Arnold

Hong Y, Ge Z, Jing C, Shi J, Dong X, Zhou F, Wang M, Zhang Z, Gong W (2013) Functional promoter −308G>A variant in tumor necrosis factor alpha gene is associated with risk and progression of gastric cancer in a Chinese population. PLoS ONE 8(1):e50856. doi:10.1371/journal.pone.0050856

Hsu IC, Metcalf RA, Sun T, Welsh JA, Wang NJ, Harris CC (1991) Mutational hotspot in the p53 gene in human hepatocellular carcinomas. Nature 350(6317):427–428. doi:10.1038/350427a0

Huang SP, Wu MS, Shun CT, Wang HP, Lin MT, Kuo ML, Lin JT (2004) Interleukin-6 increases vascular endothelial growth factor and angiogenesis in gastric carcinoma. J Biomed Sci 11(4):517–527. doi:10.1159/000077902

Hussain SP, Harris CC (2007) Inflammation and cancer: an ancient link with novel potentials. Int J Cancer 121(11):2373–2380. doi:10.1002/ijc.23173

Ikeguchi M, Hatada T, Yamamoto M, Miyake T, Matsunaga T, Fukumoto Y, Yamada Y, Fukuda K, Saito H, Tatebe S (2009) Serum interleukin-6 and -10 levels in patients with gastric cancer. Gastric Cancer (Official Journal of the International Gastric Cancer Association and the Japanese Gastric Cancer Association) 12(2):95–100. doi:10.1007/s10120-009-0509-8

Inoue S, Kawanishi S (1995) Oxidative DNA damage induced by simultaneous generation of nitric oxide and superoxide. FEBS Lett 371(1):86–88

Isomoto H, Matsushima K, Inoue N, Hayashi T, Nakayama T, Kunizaki M, Hidaka S, Nakayama M, Hisatsune J, Nakashima M, Nagayasu T, Nakao K, Hirayama T (2012) Interweaving microRNAs and proinflammatory cytokines in gastric mucosa with reference to *H. pylori* infection. J Clin Immunol 32(2):290–299. doi:10.1007/s10875-011-9626-3

Ito R, Yasui W, Kuniyasu H, Yokozaki H, Tahara E (1997) Expression of interleukin-6 and its effect on the cell growth of gastric carcinoma cell lines. Jpn J Cancer Res: Gann 88(10):953–958

Jaiswal M, LaRusso NF, Burgart LJ, Gores GJ (2000) Inflammatory cytokines induce DNA damage and inhibit DNA repair in cholangiocarcinoma cells by a nitric oxide-dependent mechanism. Cancer Res 60(1):184–190

Jayaprakash V, Marshall JR (2011) Selenium and other antioxidants for chemoprevention of gastrointestinal cancers. Best Pract Res Clin Gastroenterol 25(4–5):507–518. doi:10.1016/j.bpg.2011.09.006

Jemal A, Bray F, Center MM, Ferlay J, Ward E, Forman D (2011) Global cancer statistics. CA Cancer J Clin 61(2):69–90. doi:10.3322/caac.20107

Karin M (2006) NF-kappaB and cancer: mechanisms and targets. Mol Carcinog 45(6):355–361. doi:10.1002/mc.20217

Karin M, Greten FR (2005) NF-kappaB: linking inflammation and immunity to cancer development and progression. Nat Rev Immunol 5(10):749–759. doi:10.1038/nri1703

Kato M, Asaka M (2012) Recent development of gastric cancer prevention. Jpn J Clin Oncol 42(11):987–994. doi:10.1093/jjco/hys151

Katoh M (2007) Networking of WNT, FGF, Notch, BMP, and Hedgehog signaling pathways during carcinogenesis. Stem Cell Rev 3(1):30–38

Kawabata T, Ichikura T, Majima T, Seki S, Chochi K, Takayama E, Hiraide H, Mochizuki H (2001) Preoperative serum interleukin-18 level as a postoperative prognostic marker in patients with gastric carcinoma. Cancer 92(8):2050–2055

Kelly PN, Dakic A, Adams JM, Nutt SL, Strasser A (2007) Tumor growth need not be driven by rare cancer stem cells. Science 317(5836):337. doi:10.1126/science.1142596

Kinzler KW, Vogelstein B (1996) Lessons from hereditary colorectal cancer. Cell 87(2):159–170

Kobayashi M, Tsubono Y, Sasazuki S, Sasaki S, Tsugane S, Group JS (2002) Vegetables, fruit and risk of gastric cancer in Japan: a 10-year follow-up of the JPHC Study Cohort I. Int J Cancer 102(1):39–44. doi:10.1002/ijc.10659

Konturek PC, Kania J, Konturek JW, Nikiforuk A, Konturek SJ, Hahn EG (2003) *H. pylori* infection, atrophic gastritis, cytokines, gastrin, COX-2, PPAR gamma and impaired apoptosis in gastric carcinogenesis. Med Sci Monit: Int Med J Exp Clin Res 9(7):SR53–SR66

Kuai WX, Wang Q, Yang XZ, Zhao Y, Yu R, Tang XJ (2012) Interleukin-8 associates with adhesion, migration, invasion and chemosensitivity of human gastric cancer cells. World J Gastroenterol 18(9):979–985. doi:10.3748/wjg.v18.i9.979

Kumar R (2010) Microfilariae in lymph node aspirate associated with metastatic gastric carcinoma: a case report. Acta Cytol 54(3):319–320

Kuraishy A, Karin M, Grivennikov SI (2011) Tumor promotion via injury- and death-induced inflammation. Immunity 35(4):467–477. doi:10.1016/j.immuni.2011.09.006

Leach SA, Thompson M, Hill M (1987) Bacterially catalysed N-nitrosation reactions and their relative importance in the human stomach. Carcinogenesis 8(12):1907–1912

Lee JM, Kim SS, Cho YS (2012) The role of PPARgamma in *Helicobacter pylori* infection and gastric carcinogenesis. PPAR Res 2012:687570. doi:10.1155/2012/687570

Leek RD, Landers R, Fox SB, Ng F, Harris AL, Lewis CE (1998) Association of tumour necrosis factor alpha and its receptors with thymidine phosphorylase expression in invasive breast carcinoma. Br J Cancer 77(12):2246–2251

Lickert H, Kispert A, Kutsch S, Kemler R (2001) Expression patterns of Wnt genes in mouse gut development. Mech Dev 105(1–2):181–184

Locksley RM, Killeen N, Lenardo MJ (2001) The TNF and TNF receptor superfamilies: integrating mammalian biology. Cell 104(4):487–501

Luo JL, Kamata H, Karin M (2005) IKK/NF-kappaB signaling: balancing life and death—a new approach to cancer therapy. J Clin Investig 115(10):2625–2632. doi:10.1172/JCI26322

Ma J, Sawai H, Matsuo Y, Ochi N, Yasuda A, Takahashi H, Wakasugi T, Funahashi H, Sato M, Okada Y, Takeyama H, Manabe T (2008) Interleukin-1alpha enhances angiogenesis and is associated with liver metastatic potential in human gastric cancer cell lines. J Surg Res 148(2):197–204. doi:10.1016/j.jss.2007.08.014

Ma XM, Yu H, Huai N (2009) Peroxisome proliferator-activated receptor-gamma is essential in the pathogenesis of gastric carcinoma. World J Gastroenterol 15(31):3874–3883

Macarthur M, Hold GL, El-Omar EM (2004) Inflammation and Cancer II. Role of chronic inflammation and cytokine gene polymorphisms in the pathogenesis of gastrointestinal malignancy. Am J Physiol Gastrointest Liver Physiol 286(4):G515–G520. doi:10.1152/ajpgi.00475.2003

Macri A, Versaci A, Loddo S, Scuderi G, Travagliante M, Trimarchi G, Teti D, Famulari C (2006) Serum levels of interleukin 1beta, interleukin 8 and tumour necrosis factor alpha as markers of gastric cancer. Biomarkers (Biochemical indicators of exposure, response, and susceptibility to chemicals) 11(2):184–193. doi:10.1080/13547500600565677

Maeda H, Akaike T (1998) Nitric oxide and oxygen radicals in infection, inflammation, and cancer. Biochem Biokhim 63(7):854–865

Maehata Y, Nakamura S, Fujisawa K, Esaki M, Moriyama T, Asano K, Fuyuno Y, Yamaguchi K, Egashira I, Kim H, Kanda M, Hirahashi M, Matsumoto T (2012) Long-term effect of *Helicobacter pylori* eradication on the development of metachronous gastric cancer after endoscopic resection of early gastric cancer. Gastrointest Endosc 75(1):39–46. doi:10.1016/j.gie.2011.08.030

Magnus HA (1937) Observations on the presence of intestinal epithelium in the gastric mucosa. J Pathol Bacteriol 44(2):389–398

Majima T, Ichikura T, Chochi K, Kawabata T, Tsujimoto H, Sugasawa H, Kuranaga N, Takayama E, Kinoshita M, Hiraide H, Seki S, Mochizuki H (2006) Exploitation of interleukin-18 by gastric cancers for their growth and evasion of host immunity. Int J Cancer 118(2):388–395. doi:10.1002/ijc.21334

Marshall BJ, Warren JR (1984) Unidentified curved bacilli in the stomach of patients with gastritis and peptic ulceration. Lancet 1(8390):1311–1315

Matsushima K, Isomoto H, Inoue N, Nakayama T, Hayashi T, Nakayama M, Nakao K, Hirayama T, Kohno S (2011) MicroRNA signatures in *Helicobacter pylori*-infected gastric mucosa. Int J Cancer 128(2):361–370. doi:10.1002/ijc.25348

Mera R, Fontham ET, Bravo LE, Bravo JC, Piazuelo MB, Camargo MC, Correa P (2005) Long term follow up of patients treated for *Helicobacter pylori* infection. Gut 54(11):1536–1540. doi:10.1136/gut.2005.072009

Milne AN, Carneiro F, O'Morain C, Offerhaus GJ (2009) Nature meets nurture: molecular genetics of gastric cancer. Hum Genet 126(5):615–628. doi:10.1007/s00439-009-0722-x

Misleh JG, Santoro P, Strasser JF, Bennett JJ (2013) Multidisciplinary management of gastric cancer. Surg Oncol Clin N Am 22(2):247–264. doi:10.1016/j.soc.2012.12.013

Mochizuki Y, Nakanishi H, Kodera Y, Ito S, Yamamura Y, Kato T, Hibi K, Akiyama S, Nakao A, Tatematsu M (2004) TNF-alpha promotes progression of peritoneal metastasis as demonstrated using a green fluorescence protein (GFP)-tagged human gastric cancer cell line. Clin Exp Metastasis 21(1):39–47

Morita D, Ichikura T, Mochizuki H (2001) The expression of PPAR gamma in gastric cancer. Nihon rinsho Jpn J Clin Med 59(Suppl 4):595–597

Morson BC (1955) Intestinal metaplasia of the gastric mucosa. Br J Cancer 9(3):365–376

Muller A, Homey B, Soto H, Ge N, Catron D, Buchanan ME, McClanahan T, Murphy E, Yuan W, Wagner SN, Barrera JL, Mohar A, Verastegui E, Zlotnik A (2001) Involvement of chemokine receptors in breast cancer metastasis. Nature 410(6824):50–56. doi:10.1038/35065016

Nakayama Y, Shibao K, Sako T, Ohta R, Onitsuka K, Hirata K, Nagata N, Itoh H (2000) Serum levels of interleukin-12 in patients with gastrointestinal cancer. Anticancer Res 20(1C):635–640

Nardone G, Rocco A, Malfertheiner P (2004) Review article: *helicobacter pylori* and molecular events in precancerous gastric lesions. Aliment Pharmacol Ther 20(3):261–270. doi:10.1111/j.1365-2036.2004.02075.x

Nathan C (2002) Points of control in inflammation. Nature 420(6917):846–852. doi:10.1038/nature01320

Nowicki A, Szenajch J, Ostrowska G, Wojtowicz A, Wojtowicz K, Kruszewski AA, Maruszynski M, Aukerman SL, Wiktor-Jedrzejczak W (1996) Impaired tumor growth in colony-stimulating factor 1 (CSF-1)-deficient, macrophage-deficient op/op mouse: evidence for a role of CSF-1-dependent macrophages in formation of tumor stroma. Int J Cancer 65(1):112–119. doi:10.1002/(SICI)1097-0215(19960103)65:1<112:AID-IJC19>3.0.CO;2-I

Oguma K, Oshima H, Aoki M, Uchio R, Naka K, Nakamura S, Hirao A, Saya H, Taketo MM, Oshima M (2008) Activated macrophages promote Wnt signalling through tumour necrosis factor-alpha in gastric tumour cells. EMBO J 27(12):1671–1681. doi:10.1038/emboj.2008.105

Ooi CH, Ivanova T, Wu J, Lee M, Tan IB, Tao J, Ward L, Koo JH, Gopalakrishnan V, Zhu Y, Cheng LL, Lee J, Rha SY, Chung HC, Ganesan K, So J, Soo KC, Lim D, Chan WH, Wong WK, Bowtell D, Yeoh KG, Grabsch H, Boussioutas A, Tan P (2009) Oncogenic pathway combinations predict clinical prognosis in gastric cancer. PLoS Genet 5(10):e1000676. doi:10.1371/journal.pgen.1000676

Oshima H, Matsunaga A, Fujimura T, Tsukamoto T, Taketo MM, Oshima M (2006) Carcinogenesis in mouse stomach by simultaneous activation of the Wnt signaling and prostaglandin E2 pathway. Gastroenterology 131(4):1086–1095. doi:10.1053/j.gastro.2006.07.014

Park S, Kim YS, Kim YJ, Kyung SY, Park JW, Jeong SH, Lee SP (2012) Toxocariasis masquerading as liver and lung metastatic nodules in patents with gastrointestinal cancer: clinicopathologic study of five cases. Dig Dis Sci 57(1):155–160. doi:10.1007/s10620-011-1833-5

Pereira C, Medeiros RM, Dinis-Ribeiro MJ (2009) Cyclooxygenase polymorphisms in gastric and colorectal carcinogenesis: are conclusive results available? Eur J Gastroenterol Hepatol 21(1):76–91. doi:10.1097/MEG.0b013e32830ce7ba

Pollard JW (2004) Tumour-educated macrophages promote tumour progression and metastasis. Nat Rev Cancer 4(1):71–78. doi:10.1038/nrc1256

Pounder RE, Ng D (1995) The prevalence of *Helicobacter pylori* infection in different countries. Aliment Pharmacol Ther 9(Suppl 2):33–39

Quintana E, Shackleton M, Sabel MS, Fullen DR, Johnson TM, Morrison SJ (2008) Efficient tumour formation by single human melanoma cells. Nature 456(7222):593–598. doi:10.1038/nature07567

Rajnakova A, Moochhala S, Goh PM, Ngoi S (2001) Expression of nitric oxide synthase, cyclooxygenase, and p53 in different stages of human gastric cancer. Cancer Lett 172(2):177–185

Ristimaki A, Honkanen N, Jankala H, Sipponen P, Harkonen M (1997) Expression of cyclooxygenase-2 in human gastric carcinoma. Cancer Res 57(7):1276–1280

Rius J, Guma M, Schachtrup C, Akassoglou K, Zinkernagel AS, Nizet V, Johnson RS, Haddad GG, Karin M (2008) NF-kappaB links innate immunity to the hypoxic response through transcriptional regulation of HIF-1alpha. Nature 453(7196):807–811. doi:10.1038/nature06905

Rocha FT, Lourenco LG, Juca MJ, Costa V, Leal AT (2009) Chemoprevention by celecoxib in reflux-induced gastric adenocarcinoma in Wistar rats that underwent gastrojejunostomy. Acta Cirurgica Bras/Sociedade Brasileira para Desenvolvimento Pesquisa em Cirurgia 24(3):189–194

Saito H, Tsujitani S, Oka S, Kondo A, Ikeguchi M, Maeta M, Kaibara N (1999) The expression of transforming growth factor-beta1 is significantly correlated with the expression of vascular endothelial growth factor and poor prognosis of patients with advanced gastric carcinoma. Cancer 86(8):1455–1462

Sato H, Ishihara S, Kawashima K, Moriyama N, Suetsugu H, Kazumori H, Okuyama T, Rumi MA, Fukuda R, Nagasue N, Kinoshita Y (2000) Expression of peroxisome proliferator-activated receptor (PPAR) gamma in gastric cancer and inhibitory effects of PPARgamma agonists. Br J Cancer 83(10):1394–1400. doi:10.1054/bjoc.2000.1457

Schutze S, Potthoff K, Machleidt T, Berkovic D, Wiegmann K, Kronke M (1992) TNF activates NF-kappa B by phosphatidylcholine-specific phospholipase C-induced "acidic" sphingomyelin breakdown. Cell 71(5):765–776

Shin SK, Li MS, Fuerst F, Hotchkiss E, Meyer R, Kim IT, Goel A, Boland CR (2006) Oncogenic T-antigen of JC virus is present frequently in human gastric cancers. Cancer 107(3):481–488. doi:10.1002/cncr.22028

Shiotani A, Uedo N, Iishi H, Murao T, Kanzaki T, Kimura Y, Kamada T, Kusunoki H, Inoue K, Haruma K (2012) *H. pylori* eradication did not improve dysregulation of specific oncogenic miRNAs in intestinal metaplastic glands. J Gastroenterol 47(9):988–998. doi:10.1007/s00535-012-0562-7

Shmelkov SV, Butler JM, Hooper AT, Hormigo A, Kushner J, Milde T, St Clair R, Baljevic M, White I, Jin DK, Chadburn A, Murphy AJ, Valenzuela DM, Gale NW, Thurston G, Yancopoulos GD, D'Angelica M, Kemeny N, Lyden D, Rafii S (2008) CD133 expression is not restricted to stem cells, and both CD133+ and CD133− metastatic colon cancer cells initiate tumors. J Clin Investig 118(6):2111–2120. doi:10.1172/JCI34401

Slack JM (1986) Epithelial metaplasia and the second anatomy. Lancet 2(8501):268–271

Soutto M, Belkhiri A, Piazuelo MB, Schneider BG, Peng D, Jiang A, Washington MK, Kokoye Y, Crowe SE, Zaika A, Correa P, Peek RM Jr, El-Rifai W (2011) Loss of TFF1 is associated with activation of NF-kappaB-mediated inflammation and gastric neoplasia in mice and humans. J Clin Investig 121(5):1753–1767. doi:10.1172/JCI43922

Sun P, Ben Q, Tu S, Dong W, Qi X, Wu Y (2011) Serum interleukin-33 levels in patients with gastric cancer. Dig Dis Sci 56(12):3596–3601. doi:10.1007/s10620-011-1760-5

Szaflarska A, Szczepanik A, Siedlar M, Czupryna A, Sierzega M, Popiela T, Zembala M (2009) Preoperative plasma level of IL-10 but not of proinflammatory cytokines is an independent prognostic factor in patients with gastric cancer. Anticancer Res 29(12):5005–5012

Tahara T, Shibata T, Nakamura M, Yamashita H, Yoshioka D, Okubo M, Yonemura J, Maeda Y, Maruyama N, Kamano T, Kamiya Y, Fujita H, Nakagawa Y, Nagasaka M, Iwata M, Hirata I, Arisawa T (2010) Association between IL-17A, -17F and MIF polymorphisms predispose to CpG island hyper-methylation in gastric cancer. Int J Mol Med 25(3):471–477

Tahara T, Shibata T, Nakamura M, Yamashita H, Yoshioka D, Okubo M, Yonemura J, Maeda Y, Maruyama N, Kamano T, Kamiya Y, Fujita H, Nakagawa Y, Nagasaka M, Iwata M, Hirata I, Arisawa T (2011) Effect of IL-1beta and TNF-alpha polymorphisms on the prognosis and survival of gastric cancer patients. Clin Exp Med 11(4):211–217. doi:10.1007/s10238-010-0129-y

Takahashi T, Nau MM, Chiba I, Birrer MJ, Rosenberg RK, Vinocour M, Levitt M, Pass H, Gazdar AF, Minna JD (1989) p53: A frequent target for genetic abnormalities in lung cancer. Science 246(4929):491–494

Takahashi N, Okumura T, Motomura W, Fujimoto Y, Kawabata I, Kohgo Y (1999) Activation of PPARgamma inhibits cell growth and induces apoptosis in human gastric cancer cells. FEBS Lett 455(1–2):135–139

Taketo MM (1998) Cyclooxygenase-2 inhibitors in tumorigenesis (Part II). J Natl Cancer Inst 90(21):1609–1620

Thiel A, Mrena J, Ristimaki A (2011) Cyclooxygenase-2 and gastric cancer. Cancer Metastasis Rev 30(3–4):387–395. doi:10.1007/s10555-011-9312-1

Tsujimoto H, Ono S, Ichikura T, Matsumoto Y, Yamamoto J, Hase K (2010) Roles of inflammatory cytokines in the progression of gastric cancer: friends or foes? Gastric Cancer (Official Journal of the International Gastric Cancer Association and the Japanese Gastric Cancer Association) 13(4):212–221. doi:10.1007/s10120-010-0568-x

Uefuji K, Ichikura T, Mochizuki H (2005) Increased expression of interleukin-1alpha and cyclooxygenase-2 in human gastric cancer: a possible role in tumor progression. Anticancer Res 25(5):3225–3230

Ushiku T, Chong JM, Uozaki H, Hino R, Chang MS, Sudo M, Rani BR, Sakuma K, Nagai H, Fukayama M (2007) p73 gene promoter methylation in Epstein-Barr virus-associated gastric carcinoma. Int J Cancer 120(1):60–66. doi:10.1002/ijc.22275

Vafa O, Wade M, Kern S, Beeche M, Pandita TK, Hampton GM, Wahl GM (2002) c-Myc can induce DNA damage, increase reactive oxygen species, and mitigate p53 function: a mechanism for oncogene-induced genetic instability. Mol Cell 9(5):1031–1044

Valko M, Morris H, Cronin MT (2005) Metals, toxicity and oxidative stress. Curr Med Chem 12(10):1161–1208

Valko M, Rhodes CJ, Moncol J, Izakovic M, Mazur M (2006) Free radicals, metals and antioxidants in oxidative stress-induced cancer. Chem Biol Interact 160(1):1–40. doi:10.1016/j.cbi.2005.12.009

Valko M, Leibfritz D, Moncol J, Cronin MT, Mazur M, Telser J (2007) Free radicals and antioxidants in normal physiological functions and human disease. Int J Biochem Cell Biol 39(1):44–84. doi:10.1016/j.biocel.2006.07.001

Velnar T, Bailey T, Smrkolj V (2009) The wound healing process: an overview of the cellular and molecular mechanisms. J Int M Res 37(5):1528–1542

Vries RG, Huch M, Clevers H (2010) Stem cells and cancer of the stomach and intestine. Mol Oncol 4(5):373–384. doi:10.1016/j.molonc.2010.05.001

Wang P, Xia HH, Zhang JY, Dai LP, Xu XQ, Wang KJ (2007) Association of interleukin-1 gene polymorphisms with gastric cancer: a meta-analysis. Int J Cancer 120(3):552–562. doi:10.1002/ijc.22353

Wiseman M (2008) The second World Cancer Research Fund/American Institute for Cancer Research expert report. Food, nutrition, physical activity, and the prevention of cancer: a global perspective. Proc Nutr Soc 67(3):253–256. doi:10.1017/S002966510800712X

Wong BC, Lam SK, Wong WM, Chen JS, Zheng TT, Feng RE, Lai KC, Hu WH, Yuen ST, Leung SY, Fong DY, Ho J, Ching CK, Chen JS, China Gastric Cancer Study G (2004) Helicobacter pylori eradication to prevent gastric cancer in a high-risk region of China: a randomized controlled trial. JAMA 291(2):187–194. doi:10.1001/jama.291.2.187

Wu CW, Chi CW, Hsieh MC, Chao MF, Lui WY, P'Eng FK (1998) Serum tumor necrosis factor in patients with gastric cancer. Anticancer Res 18(3A):1597–1599

Xu W, Li Y, Wang X, Chen B, Liu S, Wang Y, Zhao W, Wu J (2010) PPARgamma polymorphisms and cancer risk: a meta-analysis involving 32,138 subjects. Oncol Rep 24(2):579–585

Yamaoka Y (2010) Mechanisms of disease: *Helicobacter pylori* virulence factors. Nat Rev Gastroenterol Hepatol 7(11):629–641. doi:10.1038/nrgastro.2010.154

Yanaoka K, Oka M, Yoshimura N, Deguchi H, Mukoubayashi C, Enomoto S, Maekita T, Inoue I, Ueda K, Utsunomiya H, Iguchi M, Tamai H, Fujishiro M, Nakamura Y, Tsukamoto T, Inada K, Takeshita T, Ichinose M (2010) Preventive effects of etodolac, a selective cyclooxygenase-2 inhibitor, on cancer development in extensive metaplastic gastritis, a *Helicobacter pylori*-negative precancerous lesion. Int J Cancer 126(6):1467–1473. doi:10.1002/ijc.24862

Yang XF (2007) Immunology of stem cells and cancer stem cells. Cell Mol Immunol 4(3):161–171

Ye ZB, Ma T, Li H, Jin XL, Xu HM (2007) Expression and significance of intratumoral interleukin-12 and interleukin-18 in human gastric carcinoma. World J Gastroenterol 13(11):1747–1751

Yermilov V, Rubio J, Becchi M, Friesen MD, Pignatelli B, Ohshima H (1995) Formation of 8-nitroguanine by the reaction of guanine with peroxynitrite in vitro. Carcinogenesis 16(9):2045–2050

Yin Y, Si X, Gao Y, Gao L, Wang J (2013) The nuclear factor-kappaB correlates with increased expression of interleukin-6 and promotes progression of gastric carcinoma. Oncol Rep 29(1):34–38. doi:10.3892/or.2012.2089

Ying L, Marino J, Hussain SP, Khan MA, You S, Hofseth AB, Trivers GE, Dixon DA, Harris CC, Hofseth LJ (2005) Chronic inflammation promotes retinoblastoma protein hyperphosphorylation and E2F1 activation. Cancer Res 65(20):9132–9136. doi:10.1158/0008-5472.CAN-05-1358

Yokozaki H, Kuniyasu H, Semba S, Yasui W, Tahara E (1997) Molecular bases of human stomach carcinogenesis. In: Tahara E (ed) Molecular pathology of gastroenterological cancer. Springer, New York/Tokyo, pp 55–70

Zhang X, Miao X, Tan W, Ning B, Liu Z, Hong Y, Song W, Guo Y, Zhang X, Shen Y, Qiang B, Kadlubar FF, Lin D (2005) Identification of functional genetic variants in cyclooxygenase-2 and their association with risk of esophageal cancer. Gastroenterology 129(2):565–576. doi:10.1016/j.gastro.2005.05.003

Zhang Z, Li Z, Gao C, Chen P, Chen J, Liu W, Xiao S, Lu H (2008) miR-21 plays a pivotal role in gastric cancer pathogenesis and progression. Lab Invest (A Journal of Technical Methods and Pathology) 88(12):1358–1366. doi:10.1038/labinvest.2008.94

Zhang LJ, Wang SY, Huo XH, Zhu ZL, Chu JK, Ma JC, Cui DS, Gu P, Zhao ZR, Wang MW, Yu J (2009) Anti-*Helicobacter pylori* therapy followed by celecoxib on progression of gastric precancerous lesions. World J Gastroenterol 15(22):2731–2738

Zhu Y, Wang J, He Q, Zhang JQ (2011) The association between interleukin-10-592 polymorphism and gastric cancer risk: a meta-analysis. Med Oncol 28(1):133–136. doi:10.1007/s12032-010-9417-3

Zhuang Y, Peng LS, Zhao YL, Shi Y, Mao XH, Chen W, Pang KC, Liu XF, Liu T, Zhang JY, Zeng H, Liu KY, Guo G, Tong WD, Shi Y, Tang B, Li N, Yu S, Luo P, Zhang WJ, Lu DS, Yu PW, Zou QM (2012) CD8(+) T cells that produce interleukin-17 regulate myeloid-derived suppressor cells and are associated with survival time of patients with gastric cancer. Gastroenterology 143(4):951–962, e958. doi:10.1053/j.gastro.2012.06.010

Zouki C, Jozsef L, Ouellet S, Paquette Y, Filep JG (2001) Peroxynitrite mediates cytokine-induced IL-8 gene expression and production by human leukocytes. J Leukoc Biol 69(5):815–824

Chapter 11
The Role of Inflammation in Sarcoma

Jürgen Radons

Abstract Sarcomas encompass a heterogenous group of tumors with diverse pathologically and clinically overlapping features. It is a rarely curable disease, and their management requires a multidisciplinary team approach. Chronic inflammation has emerged as one of the hallmarks of tumors including sarcomas. Classical inflammation-associated sarcomas comprise the inflammatory malignant fibrous histiocytoma and Kaposi sarcoma. The identification of specific chromosomal translocations and important intracellular signaling pathways such as Ras/Raf/MAPK, insulin-like growth factor, PI3K/AKT/mTOR, sonic hedgehog and Notch together with the increasing knowledge of angiogenesis has led to development of targeted therapies that aim to interrupt these pathways. Innovative agents like oncolytic viruses opened the way to design new therapeutic options with encouraging findings. Preclinical evidence also highlights the therapeutic potential of anti-inflammatory nutraceuticals as they can inhibit multiple pathways while being less toxic. This chapter gives an overview of actual therapeutic standards, newest evidence-based studies and exciting options for targeted therapies in sarcomas.

Abbreviations

ANG	Angiogenin
AS	Angiosarcoma
BGS	Baller–Gerold syndrome
BLS	Bloom syndrome
BS	Bone sarcoma
CCS	Clear cell sarcoma

J. Radons (✉)
Department of Radiotherapy and Radiation Oncology, Klinikum rechts der Isar, Technische Universität München, Ismaninger Straße 22, 81675 Munich, Germany
e-mail: raj10062@web.de

B. B. Aggarwal et al. (eds.), *Inflammation and Cancer*, Advances in Experimental Medicine and Biology 816, DOI: 10.1007/978-3-0348-0837-8_11, © Springer Basel 2014

CS	Chondrosarcoma
DBA	Diamond–Blackfan anemia
EC	Endometrial cancer
ECS	Endometrial carcinosarcoma
EFT	Ewing's family tumors
ERK	Extracellular signal-regulated kinase
ES	Ewings's sarcoma
FAK	Focal adhesion kinase
FAP	Familial adenomatous polyposis
FS	Fibrosarcoma
GIST	Gastrointestinal stromal sarcoma
HS	Histiocytic sarcoma
HAS	Hemangiosarcoma
Hh	Hedgehog
HLRCC	Hereditary leiomyomatosis and renal cell cancer
IRS	Insulin receptor substrate
JNK	c-Jun N-terminal kinase
KS	Kaposi sarcoma
KSHV	Kaposi sarcoma-associated herpesvirus
STS	Soft tissue sarcoma
LFS	Li–Fraumeni syndrome
LMS	Leiomyosarcoma
LS	Liposarcoma
MAPK	Mitogen-activated protein kinase
MEK	Mitogen-activated protein kinase kinase
MFH	Malignant fibrous histiocytoma
MM	Malignant mesothelioma
MPNST	Malignant peripheral nerve sheath tumor
mTOR	Mammalian target of rapamycin
NF1	Neurofibromatosis type 1
OPN	Osteopontin
OS	Osteosarcoma
PGHS-2	Prostaglandin H_2 synthase 2
PI3K	Phosphatidylinositol 3-kinase
RB	Retinoblastoma
RMS	Rhabdomyosarcoma
RTS	Rothmund–Thomson syndrome
SS	Synovial sarcoma
STAT	Signal transducer and activator of transcription
TK	Tyrosine kinase
WS	Werner syndrome

11.1 Introduction

11.1.1 Epidemiology

Sarcomas represent a heterogenous group of rare malignant neoplasms of the connective tissue arising from mesenchymal cells. Sarcomas account for 21 % of all pediatric solid malignant cancers and less than 1 % of all adult solid malignant cancers (Lahat et al. 2008). They comprise a group of more than 50 different histological subtypes that can occur at any age and are not restricted to a specific anatomic site. Sarcomas are quite lethal tumor entities due to the lack of distinct symptoms at early stage leading to advanced disease and metastasis at presentation (Burningham et al. 2012). Sarcomas can be divided into soft tissue sarcoma (STS), bone sarcoma (BS), and gastrointestinal stromal sarcoma (GIST; Table 11.1). In the "Surveillance of Rare Cancer in Europe" (RARECARE) project, a large population-based series of data were analyzed to characterize the epidemiology of sarcomas in Europe. By analyzing 45,568 incident cases diagnosed between 1995–2002 for rare sarcomas, the crude incidence was found as being 5.6 per 100,000 per year (increasing with age) with 28,000 new cases a year (Stiller et al. 2013). As given in Table 11.1, STS account for approximately 85 % of all sarcomas diagnosed, while the remaining predominantly consist of malignant BS (14 %). Chondrosarcoma (CS) and osteosarcoma (OS) are the most frequent malignant bone tumors, accounting for more than half of all BS diagnoses. Leiomyosarcoma (LMS) has been identified as being the most frequent STS together with liposarcoma (LS) and unspecified sarcomas. LMS represents the most common sarcoma entity of the uterus, peritoneum, head and neck as well as other genitourinary and visceral sites (Stiller et al. 2013). LS has been found as being the most frequent sarcoma of the limbs whereas phyllodes tumor was the most common in breast and peripheral nerve sheath tumors the most common in the peripheral nerves and autonomic nervous system. It is interesting to note that the Ewing's family tumors (EFT) occur with a high percentage at both, bone and extraosseous sites.

Five-year relative survival for the period 2000–2002 was 58 % for STS, 62 % for BS and 68 % for GIST, respectively. Among STS, the highest survival rate of >90 % could be found in the skin while STS of the heart and mediastinum harbored the lowest survival rates ranging between 10 and 15 %. Vascular sarcomas showed the lowest survival rate among all BS tested with 34 % whereas the highest survival rate was found for epithelial tumors such as adamantinoma (Table 11.1).

The epidemiology of sarcoma is similar in the United States. As demonstrated by the Surveillance, Epidemiology, and End Results (SEER) program (www.seer.cancer.gov), STS is the most frequent sarcoma entity (86 %) followed by BS, the latter accounting for 14 % of all sarcomas. OS and CS were identified as being the most common malignant bone tumors in the United States with the same frequency as can be found in Europe. According to SEER, LS (16.5 %), LMS (13.7 %), malignant fibrous histiocytoma (11.9 %), and fibrosarcoma (6.3 %) represent the most common histologic subtypes of STS. As in the RARECARE project, incidence increases with age and <50 % of cases were primarily located at connective tissue (Toro et al. 2006).

Table 11.1 Epidemiology of sarcomas in Europe during 1995–2002 based on the "Surveillance of Rare Cancer in Europe" (RARECARE) project

Sarcoma entity	Cases	Percentage	Incidence[a]	Survival (%)[b]
Soft tissue sarcoma (STS)	38,526	84.6	4.7	57.8
STS of limbs	8,323	18.3	1.0	68.0
STS of viscera	4,169	9.2		45.6
STS of uterus	4,011	8.8	0.5	49.2
STS of superficial trunk	3,748	8.2	0.5	44.1
STS of skin	2,473	5.4		94.0
STS of head and neck	2,338	5.1	0.3	65.1
STS of retroperitoneum and peritoneum	2,322	5.1		42.0
Other STSs of genitourinary tract	1,954	4.3	0.2	53.7
STS of brain and other parts of the nervous system	1,560	3.4	0.2	52.9
STS of breast	1,526	3.4	0.2	80.8
Embryonal rhabdomyosarcoma of soft tissue (RMS)	511	1.1	<0.1	62.4
Ewing's family tumors of soft tissue	433	1.0	0.1	46.5
Alveolar RMS	264	0.6	<0.1	37.5
STS of paratestis	263	0.5	<0.1	90.0
STS of mediastinum	214	0.5	<0.1	15.3
STS of heart	122	0.3	<0.1	10.7
STS of pelvis	116	0.3	<0.1	42.4
STS of paraorbit	54	0.1	<0.1	75.5
Others	4,636	10.2	n.d.	n.d.
Bone sarcoma (BS)	6,494	14.3	0.8	61.6
Chondrogenic sarcomas	1,969	4.3	0.2	76.7
Osteosarcoma (OS)	1,838	4.0	0.2	53.9
Ewing's family tumors (EFT)	1,053	2.3	0.1	52.8
Chordoma	352	0.8	<0.1	76.4
Epithelial tumors (adamantinoma)	70	0.2	<0.1	82.9
Fibrosarcoma (FS), malignant fibrous histiocytoma (MFH)	147	0.3	<0.1	51.4
Vascular sarcomas	26	0.1	<0.1	33.9
Other bone sarcomas	1,039	2.3	n.d.	n.d.
Gastrointestinal stromal sarcoma (GIST)	548	1.2	0.1	67.7
Total cases analyzed	45,568		45,136	15,141

Table adapted from Stiller et al. (2013)
n.d. not determined
[a]Crude incidence rates per 100,000 in Europe per year
[b]Estimated 5-year relative survival based on the period survival analysis 2000–2002

A recent population-based study from the SEER data base with >48,000 STS cases clearly demonstrated that individuals over 50 years of age have an inferior survival than younger patients (Ferrari et al. 2011), thus confirming results of the RARECARE project. A similar pattern was observed for OS (Mirabello et al. 2009) and CS (Giuffrida et al. 2009), demonstrating the lowest survival rates in the oldest age group. The influence of gender on the incidence of sarcoma is controversially discussed in the literature. According to RARECARE, STS overall had a slightly higher incidence

Table 11.2 Inherited disorders obviously predisposing to sarcoma development

Disorder	Gene, protein	Chromosome	Function
Li–Fraumeni syndrome (LFS)	*TP53*, tumor suppressor p53	17p13.1	DNA repair, apoptosis induction
Rothmund–Thomson syndrome (RTS)	*RECQL4*, RecQ protein-like 4	8q24.3	DNA helicase
RAPADILINO syndrome	*RECQL4*, RecQ protein-like 4	8q24.3	DNA helicase
Baller–Gerold syndrome (BGS)	*RECQL4*, RecQ protein-like 4	8q24.3	DNA helicase
Werner syndrome (WS)	*WRN*, RecQ protein-like 2	8p12	DNA helicase
Bloom syndrome (BLS)	*BLM*, RecQ protein-like 3	15q26.1	DNA helicase
Retinoblastoma (RB)	*RB1*, retinoblastoma 1	13q14.2	Tumor suppressor cell cycle control
Neurofibromatosis type 1 (NF1; *syn.* von Recklinghausen's disease)	*NF1*, neurofibromin	17q11.2	Tumor suppressor, stimulation of proto-oncoprotein p53
Familial GIST syndrome	*CKIT*, c-Kit (CD117)	4q12	Stem cell factor receptor, proto-oncoprotein
	PDGFRA, PDGFR-α		Platelet-derived growth factor receptor alpha
Hereditary leiomyomatosis and renal cell cancer (HLRCC) syndrome	*FH*, fumarate hydratase (fumarase)	1q43	Krebs cycle enzyme, tumor suppressor
Diamond–Blackfan anemia (DBA)	*RPS19*, *RPL5*, *RPL11*, *RPL35A*, *RPS7*, *RPS17*, *RPS24*	Multiple	Ribosomal proteins S19, L5, L11, L35a, S7, S17, S24
Familial adenomatous polyposis (FAP)	*APC*, adenomatous polyposis coli protein	5q21	Tumor suppressor, cell migration, cell adhesion, chromosome segregation, spindle assembly, apoptosis, neuronal differentiation
TDP-43 proteinopathies (frontotemporal lobar degeneration, amyotrophic lateral sclerosis)	*TARDBP*, transactivation response DNA-binding protein (TDP-43)	1p36.22	TDP-43 pathology
	EGR2, Egr-2	10q21	Transcriptional regulation

in females than in males (Stiller et al. 2013), whereas SEER data revealed the direct opposite (Toro et al. 2006; Ferrari et al. 2011).

11.1.2 Major Gene Products

Several inherited genetic syndromes predispose to sarcoma development. Inherited cancer predisposition syndromes represent a heterogeneous group of disorders that are summarized in Table 11.2. Most notably, individuals with Li–Fraumeni syndrome (LFS), neurofibromatosis type 1 (NF1; at risk for malignant peripheral nerve sheath tumors and GIST), or those with familial adenomatous polyposis (FAP; at risk for intraabdominal desmoids tumors) are at high risk of developing sarcomas. LFS was about one of the first genetic syndromes found to be strongly associated with sarcoma development (Li and Fraumeni 1969). It is caused by germ line mutations in the tumor suppressor gene *TP53* (Malkin et al. 1990). Its product, the p53 protein, is a transcription factor playing a crucial role in numerous cellular processes including DNA repair, apoptosis, and cell growth. Mutations in *TP53* will consequently lead to the early development of tumors including sarcomas as a result of genetic instability (Multhoff and Radons 2012). Notably, approximately 30 % of patients meeting clinical criteria for LFS do not harbor *TP53* mutations (Das et al. 2007; Savage and Mirabello 2011) whereas somatic *TP53* mutations can be observed in 30–60 % of STS (Das et al. 2007). In addition to sarcomas, these individuals develop a multitude of tumors such as adrenocortical tumors, leukemias as well as tumors of brain and breast. Mdm-2 has been shown to bind to p53, thus abolishing its function as a transcription factor (Momand et al. 1992; Cordon-Cardo et al. 1994). Overexpression of *MDM2* has been demonstrated in a wide variety of sarcomas including LS and OS (Ladanyi et al. 1993; Leach et al. 1993; Shimada et al. 2006), and *MDM2* amplification to correlate with disease recurrence and metastasis (Gisselsson et al. 2002).

Retinoblastoma (RB), a relatively rare pediatric cancer of the eye, results from mutations in the tumor suppressor gene retinoblastoma 1 (*RB1*) located on chromosome 13q14 with very high penetrance and expressivity (Harbour 2001). This gene encodes the cell cycle regulatory retinoblastoma gene protein (pRb), which is critically involved in controlling cell cycle and differentiation processes as well as preserving chromosomal stability (Knudson 1971). Survivors of hereditary RB are of higher risk for developing secondary malignancies (Wong et al. 1997). Loss of pRb functions has been reported in several sporadic tumors including OS representing the most frequent tumor in patients with RB (Hansen et al. 1985). Long-term survivors of hereditary RB show an increased 20-fold risk of developing and dying from a subsequent nonocular cancer, primarily BS and STS, melanoma and brain tumors (Marees et al. 2008). Survivors of nonhereditary RB are at much lower risk of a subsequent primary cancer, similar to the risk in the general population (Fletcher et al. 2004).

Individuals with mutations in DNA helicase genes are predisposed for the development of OS. Known OS predisposition syndromes include Rothmund–Thomson syndrome (RTS), Werner syndrome (WS), Bloom syndrome (BLS), and RAPADILINO syndrome (Calvert et al. 2012). RTS is a rare autosomal recessive disorder caused by mutations in the DNA helicase gene *RECQL4* located on chromosome 8q24.3 (Wang et al. 2003; Kansara and Thomas 2007). Individuals with RTS typically present with a characteristic sun-sensitive rash during infancy followed by poikiloderma through adulthood. RTS patients may have small statue and skeletal dysplasias. As demonstrated by the group of Sharon Plon, the loss of RECQL4 protein function occurred in two-thirds of RTS patients and was associated with high risk of OS (Wang et al. 2003). Studies are currently under way to examine the role of *RECQL4* mutations in sporadic OS in the general population.

Apart from RTS, WS and BLS are rare autosomal recessive cancer predisposition disorders caused by loss of function of the RecQ helicases Wrn or Blm, respectively. BLS and WS are characterized by replication defects, hyperrecombination events and chromosomal aberrations (Muftuoglu et al. 2008; Shen et al. 2012) leading to genetic instability as one of the hallmarks of cancer (Colotta et al. 2009). Genetic instability is associated with an increased predisposition to a great variety of cancers including sarcoma, e.g., OS, CS, and spindle cell sarcoma (Lahat et al. 2008). *RECQL4* mutations can also lead to Baller–Gerold syndrome (BGS), or RAPADILINO syndrome correlating with an increased risk for OS (Suhasini and Brosh 2013). Diamond–Blackfan anemia (DBA) represents a further inherited disorder which has been found as being associated with an enhanced risk of OS (Lipton et al. 2001). DBA patients exhibit abnormal pre-rRNA maturation patterns, and the majority bears mutations in one of several ribosomal protein genes that encode structural components of the ribosome essential for the correct assembly of the ribosomal subunits. Studies on the most frequently mutated gene, *RPS19*, revealed that mutations prevent the assembly of the ribosomal protein into forming preribosomal particles, thus triggering nucleolar stress pathways (Ellis and Gleizes 2011). However, the role of ribosomal proteins in the pathogenesis of OS remains to be elucidated.

Hereditary leiomyomatosis and renal cell cancer (HLRCC) syndrome is a tumor predisposition syndrome caused by heterozygous germ line mutations in the fumarate hydratase (*FH*) gene (Tomlinson et al. 2002). The condition is characterized by predisposition to benign leiomyomas of the skin and the uterus, renal cell carcinoma (RCC), and uterine LMS (Launonen et al. 2001; Lehtonen et al. 2006). As shown by Pollard et al. (2005a, b), HLRCC tumors were found to overexpress hypoxia-inducible factor-1α (HIF-1α) and hypoxia-responsive genes encoding vascular endothelial growth factor (*VEGF*) and Bcl-2/adenovirus E1B 19 kDa interacting protein 3 (*BNIP3*) accompanied by a higher microvessel density in comparison with the sporadic counterparts. From these findings, the authors postulate that failure of the Krebs cycle in HLRCC tumors causes inappropriate signaling followed by a hypoxic cell state which may lead to angiogenesis as well as clonal expansion and tumor growth through some uncharacterized, cell-autonomous effects.

Several heritable mutations in the genes encoding the stem cell factor receptor c-Kit and platelet-derived growth factor receptor alpha (PDGFR-α) have been identified in patients with familial GIST (Maeyama et al. 2001; Heinrich et al. 2003b). While about 70–80 % of GIST harbor mutations in the proto-oncogene *CKIT*, approximately one–third of the remaining have mutations in *PDGFRA* (Wardelmann et al. 2003; Heinrich et al. 2003a). Mutations in these genes result in constitutive activation of the c-Kit and PDGFR-α signaling pathway culminating in blockage of apoptosis and cell proliferation, respectively (Rubin et al. 2007).

On the other hand, genetic syndromes associated with Ewing's sarcoma (ES), a neoplasm of the undifferentiated small round cells generally affecting the bone and deep soft tissues of children and adolescents, are extremely rare. ES is associated with specific chromosomal translocations resulting in oncogenic fusion transcripts and proteins (Ross et al. 2013). The chimeric proteins commonly represent artificial transcription factors dysregulating gene expression (Xia and Barr 2005) and consequently modifying growth and differentiation processes leading to cell transformation due to their oncogenic potential (May et al. 1993; Scheidler et al. 1996). A genome-wide association study of 401 French individuals with ES recently identified candidate risk loci upstream of *TARDBP* and *EGR2* (Postel-Vinay et al. 2012). *TARDBP* encodes the nuclear transactive response DNA-binding protein 43 (TDP-43) representing the dominant disease protein in amyotrophic lateral sclerosis and a subgroup of frontotemporal lobar degeneration. *TARDBP* shares structural similarities with *EWSR1* and *FUS*, that encode RNA-binding proteins, and early growth response gene 2 (*EGR2*) is a target gene of the *EWSR1/ETS* translocation. Erythroblastosis virus E26 transforming sequence (ETS) family of proteins are transcription factors that modulate the expression of genes involved in various biological processes, including cellular proliferation, differentiation, development, transformation, and apoptosis (Bassuk and Leiden 1997). The study by Postel-Vinay et al. (2012) clearly demonstrated that variants at these loci were associated with expression levels of *TARDBP*, *ADO* (encoding cysteamine dioxygenase), and *EGR2*. Since our knowledge of the oncogenic pathways underlying the pathogenesis of sarcoma is steadily increasing, one can assume that fusion genes characteristic for a certain subtype could have the potential to function as critical targets in diagnosis and therapy.

Moreover, specific molecular markers have been shown to impact STS prognosis. In addition to p53 and PDGFR-α that give rise to GIST, upregulated β-catenin levels correlate with increased proliferative activity in high-grade STS (Kuhnen et al. 2000). Apart from its membranous function as an effective molecule for cell adhesion in sarcomas with epithelioid pattern, β-catenin may act as an oncoprotein in sarcomas with intracytoplasmic and nuclear localization by binding to nuclear DNA (Kuhnen et al. 2000). S-phase kinase-associated protein 2 (Skp-2) catalyzes the ubiquitylation of the tumor suppressors $p27^{Kip-1}$ and $p21^{Waf-1}$ (Fasanaro et al. 2010). In myxofibrosarcomas, Skp-2 overexpression was found as being highly representative of the biological aggressiveness, thus playing an important prognostic role (Huang et al. 2006).

An intriguing novel aspect is presented by Savage and Mirabello (2011) who discuss the putative impact of single nucleotide polymorphisms (SNPs) on the risk of OS. SNPs are the most common type of genetic variation in the genome. Although SNPs do not modify gene expression or protein functions, they can influence a wide variety of biological effects such as upregulation of Mdm-2, a direct negative regulator of p53, and inhibition of the p53 signaling pathway, thereby accelerating tumor formation (Bond et al. 2004). SNPs have been found, among others, in the genes encoding estrogen receptor (*ESR1*), collagen 1α1 (*COL1A1*), vitamin D receptor (*VDR*), Mdm-2 (*MDM2*), insulin-like growth factor receptor 2 (*IGFR2*), Fas protein (*FAS*), and *TGFBR1*6A*, a common hypomorphic variant of transforming growth factor beta receptor 1 (*TGFBR1*). In these genes, genetic variations obviously appear to be associated with an increased risk of OS (Savage and Mirabello 2011).

11.1.3 Current Therapies

Sarcomas represent a complex family of diseases necessitating multidisciplinary therapeutic approaches not only including advanced surgical and/or orthopedic techniques, reconstructive surgery as well as radiotherapy and chemotherapy, but also hormonal and physical therapy as well as specialized targeted therapy and psychosocial support. Expert surgical resection with or without radiotherapy remains the first-line therapy for localized sarcoma (Stojadinovic et al. 2002; O'Sullivan et al. 2002). Of note, the role of adjuvant therapy remains controversial. Radiotherapy can be delivered before, during or after surgery. Although preoperative radiation therapy is favored for certain sarcomas, in the United Kingdom most of STS are treated with postoperative radiotherapy although requiring a higher radiation dose (Grimer et al. 2010b). A similar outcome was observed in a reasonably sized randomized trial of preoperative versus postoperative radiation therapy for large sarcomas of the extremity in Canada (Davis et al. 2005).

The benefits of chemotherapy in sarcoma management remain controversial. Preoperative systemic chemotherapy represents the standard therapy for high-grade OS, ES, and certain RMS (Grimer et al. 2010a). BS such as CS (Grimer et al. 2010a) or other STS entities, including LMS (Gupta et al. 2013) and LS (Crago and Singer 2011), obviously do not significantly benefit from systemic chemotherapy. In contrast, Hensley and coworkers reported on a clinical benefit of the fixed-dose rate gemcitabine plus docetaxel treatment as a first- and second-line therapy in metastatic uterine LMS (Hensley et al. 2008a, b). A recent meta-analysis of ifosfamide-based combination chemotherapy in advanced STS revealed that this combinatorial treatment improves response rates by rendering such tumors resectable, but at the cost of a higher toxicity and a failure to improve one-year survival (Verma et al. 2008). Notably, a further meta-analysis with 1,953 STS patients in 18 randomized trials demonstrated that the combined administration of doxorubicin and ifosfamide significantly improved overall survival compared to doxorubicin administered in monotherapy (Pervaiz et al. 2008). From these data, it can be concluded that a combinatorial treatment with ifosfamide and doxorubicin represents the standard of care for completely resected high-risk sarcomas (Purohit et al. 2011).

A growing body of evidence suggests that sarcoma treatment may differ radically depending on the histologic subtype (Verweij and Baker 2010). The best example is GIST, a form of routinely fatal sarcoma that is driven by aberrant tyrosine kinase signaling. GIST is the most common mesenchymal neoplasm of the gastrointestinal tract and is highly resistant to conventional chemotherapy and radiotherapy. Since our understanding of the pathogenesis of GIST has increased, targeted therapies using specific tyrosine kinase (TK) inhibitors such as imatinib mesylate (Gleevec, STI-571, Novartis) and sunitinib mesylate (Sutent, SU11248, Pfizer) are being investigated in GIST. Clinical response to imatinib was found to correlate with the tumor genotype, i.e., patient tumors harboring mutations in exon 11 of *CKIT* showed the best responses (Debiec-Rychter et al. 2004). Patients with *CKIT* mutations in exon 9 obviously benefit from a higher imatinib dosage.

Results from the Meta-GIST meta-analysis showed that patients whose GIST harbors a *CKIT* mutation in exon 9 garner a longer progression-free survival time when treated initially with high-dose imatinib (800 mg daily) compared with those patients harboring *CKIT* mutations in exon 11 or no mutation (Meta-analysis 2010; Gronchi et al. 2010). Moreover, treatment interruption after three years resulted in tumor progression in most patients with metastatic GIST (Le Cesne et al. 2010), demonstrating that GIST patients benefit from an imatinib treatment. Imatinib treatment has been approved by the Food and Drug Administration (FDA) to decrease the risk of disease recurrence after resection of GIST with significant relapse potential. Although this treatment strategy has improved the quality of life and survival of patients with advanced GIST, several patients did not respond to imatinib. Approaches to treat imatinib-resistant GIST include the use of alternative kinase inhibitors such as sunitinib, dasatinib, nilotinib, AMG-706 (Amgen), the mammalian target of rapamycin (mTOR) inhibitor everolimus (Afinitor, RAD001, Novartis), and the Hsp90 inhibitor retaspimycin hydrochloride (IPI-504).

New drugs for the treatment of STS include eribulin (Halaven, Eisai), an analog of the marine sponge natural product halichondrin B, which functions as a mechanistically unique inhibitor of microtubule dynamics. Eribulin has been approved 2010 by the FDA for the treatment of patients with metastatic breast cancer. In a nonrandomized multicenter phase II study, patients were included if they had progressive or high-grade STS and had received no more than one previous combination chemotherapy or up to two single drugs for advanced disease (Schoffski et al. 2011b). This study clearly demonstrated that 32 % of patients with LMS, 47 % of patients with adipocytic sarcoma, 21 % of patients with synovial sarcoma (SS), and 19 % of other sarcomas were progression-free at 12 weeks after eribulin monotherapy.

Targeting the molecular pathways involved in sarcomagenesis represents a promising novel approach in the treatment of sarcomas. Antagonistic antibodies, TK inhibitors, and inhibitors of downstream molecules of the PI3K (phosphatidylinositol 3-kinase)/AKT/mTOR pathway demonstrated encouraging activities. Table 11.3 summarizes selected chemotherapeutics that have been used in clinical settings for the treatment of different subtypes of sarcoma. Among them, monoclonal antibodies against the insulin-like growth factor 1 receptor (IGF1-R) such as figitumumab, cixutumumab, and ganitumab either alone or in combination with other agents are currently under investigation for patients with sarcomas. The IGF signaling pathway is constitutively activated in and drives cellular growth of a great variety of sarcomas including ES, LS, LMS, RMS, and SS. Therefore, anti-IGF therapy represents a promising therapeutic option in the treatment of sarcoma because it also affects mTOR, one of the downstream effector molecules of PI3K. The participation of mTOR in sarcomagenesis is related to the primordial role of the IGF system in these tumors. Therefore, mTOR inhibitors have been consequently tested for their anti-tumor potential in sarcoma. Sirolimus, temsirolimus, everolimus, and ridaforolimus are analogs of rapamycin, so-called rapalogs, and function as specific mTOR inhibitors (Table 11.3). Clinical trials analyzing the clinical efficacy of rapalogs in monotherapy or combination therapy in sarcomas are ongoing.

Table 11.3 Chemotherapeutics used for the treatment of sarcomas

Agents	Sarcoma subtype	References
Cytostatics		
Dacarbazine plus other drugs (doxorubicin, ifosfamide, mesna)	Advanced STS, uterine LMS	Grimer et al. (2010b), Minobe et al. (2011)
Doxoribucin	Localized respectable and metastatic STS	Sarcoma Meta-analysis Collaboration (1997), Grimer et al. (2010b)
Doxorubicin plus ifosfamide	Locally-advanced STS, SS	Spurrell et al. (2005), Verma et al. (2008), Pervaiz et al. (2008), Kasper et al. (2013)
Epirubicin with/without ifosfamide	STS at high risk of relapse	Petrioli et al. (2002)
Ifosfamide	Advanced STS, e.g., myxoid LS, SS	van Oosterom et al. (2002), Sleijfer et al. (2010)
Eribulin mesylate	High-grade STS	Schoffski et al. (2011b)
	Metastatic breast cancer	Cortes et al. (2011), Cortes et al. (2012)
Gemcitabine plus docetaxel	Metastatic STS, metastatic uterine LMS	Bay et al. (2006), Maki et al. (2007), Hensley et al. (2008a, b)
Ixabepilone plus capecitabine	Metastatic breast cancer	Thomas et al. (2007), Valero et al. (2012)
Paclitaxel	Angiosarcoma (AS)	Fata et al. (1999), Skubitz and Haddad (2005)
Trabectedin	SS, LMS, advanced myoxid/round cell LS	Yovine et al. (2004), Garcia-Carbonero et al. (2004), Demetri et al. (2009a), Gronchi et al. (2012)
Tyrosine kinase/ Angiogenesis inhibitors		
Axitinib	STS, AS	Clinical trials currently ongoing
Bevacizumab	Metastatic STS, AS, epitheloid hemangioendothelioma, fibrous tumors, hemangiopericytomas	D'Adamo et al. (2005), Fuller et al. (2010), Rosen et al. (2010), Park et al. (2011), Agulnik et al. (2013)
Brivanib	Advanced STS	Schwartz et al. (2011)
Cediranib	Alveolar soft part sarcoma (ASPS)	Gardner et al. (2009), Kummar et al. (2011)
Imatinib mesylate	Advanced GIST	Demetri et al. (2002), Verweij et al. (2004), Meta-analysis (2010), Le Cesne et al. (2010), Gronchi et al. (2010)
Pazopanib	Advanced STS, e.g., LMS, SS	Sleijfer et al. (2009), van der Graaf et al. (2012)
Sorafenib	Advanced STS, OS, AS	Maki et al. (2009), von Mehren et al. (2012), Ray-Coquard et al. (2012), Grignani et al. (2012)

(continued)

Table 11.3 continued

Agents	Sarcoma subtype	References
Sunitinib mesylate, sunitinib malate	Imatinib-resistant GIST, extraskeletal myxoid CS, solitary fibrous tumor	Heinrich et al. (2008), George et al. (2009), Demetri et al. (2009b), Stacchiotti et al. (2012a, b)
Tivantinib	Clear cell sarcoma (CCS)	Wagner et al. (2012)
mTOR inhibitors		
Everolimus (RAD001)	Advanced sarcoma, retroperitoneal perivascular epithelioid cell tumor (PEComa), SS	Quek et al. (2011), Gennatas et al. (2012), Ho et al. (2012)
Ridaforolimus (AP23573)	Advanced BS and STS	Mita et al. (2013), Chawla et al. (2012)
Sirolimus (rapamycin)	KS, CS, pretreated STS, OS, ES	Yaich et al. (2012), Bernstein-Molho et al. (2012), Schuetze et al. (2012)
Temsirolimus (CCI-779)	BS, STS, Ewing's family tumors (EFT), malignant PEComa	Italiano et al. (2010), Naing et al. (2012), Schwartz et al. (2012)
Insulin-like growth factor receptor inhibitors		6
Cixutumumab	EFT, refractory BS and STS	Schoffski et al. (2011a), Naing et al. (2012), Schwartz et al. (2012), Malempati et al. (2012), Chugh et al. (2012)
Figitumumab	ES, STS	Toretsky and Gorlick (2010), Olmos et al. (2010), Quek et al. (2011), Juergens et al. (2011)
Ganitumab (AMG 479)	EFT, desmoplastic small round cell tumors (DSRCT), advanced or metastatic RMS, LMS, adipocytic sarcoma, SS	Tolcher et al. (2009), Tap et al. (2012)

A variety of drugs targeting angiogenesis are also being tested in sarcomas. Angiogenesis plays a crucial role in growth and dissemination of tumors. It is well accepted that upregulated expression of pro-angiogenic VEGF represents an independent poor prognostic factor in tumorigenesis (Purohit et al. 2011). Despite an upregulated VEGF expression, overexpression of growth-promoting PDGF-β as well as invasiveness- and angiogenesis-promoting matrix metalloproteinase (MMP) 2 and -9 (MMP-9) and uroplasminogen activator (uPA) has been found as correlating with high tumor grade and diminished overall survival (Purohit et al. 2011). There is now a wealth of evidence indicating that monoclonal antibodies such as bevacizumab and TK inhibitors (e.g., axitinib, brivanib, cediranib, imatinib, pazopanib, sorafenib, sunitinib) harbor promising activity and safety in certain subtypes of sarcoma.

11.2 Inflammatory Signaling Pathways Associated with Sarcoma

Rudolf Virchow (1821–1902) established cellular pathology and coined the phrase *Omnis cellula e cellula* that means "each cell stems from another cell," and he distinguished sarcomas from carcinomas (Virchow 1859). In 1863, Virchow noted leukocytes in neoplastic tissues and postulated a connection between chronic inflammation and development of cancer (Virchow 1863). 60 years later, Francis Harbitz (1867–1950) demonstrated the significance of chronic inflammation with the formation of sarcomas (Harbitz 1924). Epidemiological and experimental studies now provide evidence that the development of cancer is indeed attributed to inflammation. Nowadays, it is generally accepted that up to 25 % of human malignancies are related to chronic inflammation and to viral and bacterial as well as parasitic infections (Hussain and Harris 2007). Chronic inflammation increases the risk of cancer, promotes tumor progression, and supports metastatic spread (Multhoff et al. 2012; Kundu and Surh 2012). The connection between tumorigenesis and inflammation is mediated via intrinsic and extrinsic pathways (Mantovani et al. 2008). The intrinsic pathway is activated by various epigenetic alterations causing inflammation and malignant transformation. Epigenetic alterations comprise mutation-driven proto-oncogene activation, chromosomal rearrangement/amplification, and inactivation of tumor suppressor genes. Transformed cells secrete inflammatory mediators and thus generate an inflammatory microenvironment. The extrinsic pathway is driven by inflammation or infections consequently leading to malignant transformation and further increasing the risk for cancer development. Both pathways converge in tumor cells and induce the activation of several transcription factors such as NF-κB, STAT-3, and HIF-1 culminating in the formation of numerous pro-inflammatory molecules that recruit and activate various leukocyte populations into the tumor microenvironment (for a review see Multhoff et al. 2012). These pro-inflammatory factors include proangiogenic mediators (IL-8, VEGF), growth factors (IL-6, GM-CSF, osteopontin), anti-apoptotic mediators (Bcl-x_L, c-Flip, survivin), cell cycle mediators (cyclin D1, c-Myc), adhesion molecules (ELAM-1, ICAM-1, VCAM-1), invasion-promoting factors (MMP-2/-7/-9, uPA), inflammatory enzymes (lipoxygenase, prostaglandin H_2 synthase 2: PGHS-2), prostaglandins, iNOS, as well as chemokines (CCL2/-20, IL-8, osteopontin), and pro-inflammatory cytokines (IL-1, IL-6, IL-23, TNF, TGF-β, EGF), promoting the malignant phenotype. The tumor cell-derived pro-inflammatory molecules now activate the same transcription factors within tumor cells and cells of the microenvironment. This concerted action of tumor and micromilieu results in a more pronounced generation of inflammatory mediators driving the progression of a positive amplification loop which further triggers tumor growth and invasiveness.

Emerging data suggest that genetic destabilization of tumor cells is regarded as a further hallmark of most human cancers contributing to tumor initiation and progression (Colotta et al. 2009). Apart from the production of cytokines, chemokines, proteases, and prostanoids, inflammatory cells are able to produce reactive oxygen (ROS) and nitrogen species (RNS) acting as chemical effectors in inflammation-driven carcinogenesis (Kundu and Surh 2008). ROS and RNS have been identified in tumor cells as inducers of the oxygen-dependent heterodimeric transcription factor HIF-1 (Sandau et al. 2000) which plays a pivotal role in genetic destabilization of these cells (Koshiji et al. 2005). All of these inflammatory mediators act together in perpetuating and amplifying the inflammatory cascade. On the one hand, they suppress DNA repair mechanisms leading to microsatellite instability. On the other hand, they can cause chromosomal instability culminating in abnormal chromosomal segregation and aneuploidy (Multhoff and Radons 2012). Moreover, the inflammatory factors induce DNA double-strand breaks, affect function of mitotic checkpoint molecules, and dysregulate homologous recombination of DNA double-strand break repair leading to random genetic diversification of tumor cells. Cancer cells harboring the optimal combination of activated oncoproteins and inactivated oncosuppressor proteins will develop the malignant phenotype (Colotta et al. 2009).

Inflammatory processes also play a critical role in sarcomagenesis. The classical tumor with inflammatory etiology is the inflammatory malignant fibrous histiocytoma (MFH) predominantly occurring in adults (Sinkovics 2007a, b). The expression of cytokines in inflammatory MFH may account for local inflammatory cell infiltration and the aggressive nature of the malignant cells (Melhem et al. 1993). In this sarcoma subtype, the inflammatory process is driven by HIF-1 (Koga et al. 2005) which not only plays a crucial role in genetic destabilization of tumor cells but also in tumor angiogenesis, invasion, survival, and growth (Multhoff et al. 2012). As demonstrated by the group of Takaaki Akaike, ROS and RNS induce the formation of 8-nitroguanine, a product of nitrative DNA damage (Ohshima et al. 2006). In MFH patients, 8-nitroguanine formation can be detected predominantly in the nuclei of tumor cells and inflammatory cells in tumor tissues, while HIF-1α, the oxygen-regulated subunit of HIF-1, is expressed in the cytoplasm and nuclei of tumor cells (Hoki et al. 2007b). Apart from HIF-1α, iNOS, NF-κB, and PGHS-2 have been found to colocalize with 8-nitroguanine in MFH tissues and to negatively correlate with the survival indicating an NF-κB-driven sarcomagenesis (Hoki et al. 2007a, b).

Human herpesvirus 8 (HHV8) or Kaposi sarcoma-associated herpesvirus (KSHV) is the known causative oncogenic virus for Kaposi sarcoma (KS), which in general portends a poor prognosis (Mesri et al. 2010). KS is a chronic inflammation-associated malignancy that arises from the initial infection of an appropriate endothelial or progenitor cell by KSHV/HHV8. Cellular hallmarks of KS progression include both the hyperproliferation of KSHV-infected cells and the infiltration of immune modulatory cells into KS lesions, which together result in chronic inflammation, the induction of angiogenesis and tumor growth (Douglas et al. 2010). Recent evidence has pointed to the involvement of the NF-κB pathway in the biology of KSHV and in the pathogenesis of KS (Keller et al. 2006).

Many aspects of KS suggest that chronic inflammation associated with the lesion and/or viral infection plays a role in tumor pathogenesis. A crucial role for inflammation in the pathogenesis of KS is exemplified by the association of KS with the Koebner (or isomorphic) phenomenon, a condition where lesions initiate or recur at inflammatory sites of injury or trauma (Rubin and Stiller 2002), and the recrudescent KS (KS flare) seen with the immune constitution inflammatory syndrome (IRIS; Leidner and Aboulafia 2005). The inflammatory response generated is thought to attract infected cells to the site as well as exacerbate the oncogenic properties of the viruses (Rubin and Stiller 2002). Progression of KS likely depends on a complex and incompletely understood interplay between KSHV and the host immune system that allows for the establishment of a tumor-promoting environment (Douglas et al. 2010).

In addition to the classical tumor-promoting molecules such as cytokines, chemokines, ROS/RNS, matrix-degrading enzymes, the matricellular protein osteopontin (OPN) has been identified as playing a crucial role in inflammation and tumor progression. OPN mediates cell migration, adhesion, and survival in many cell types (Lund et al. 2009). As reviewed by Kundu and Surh (2012), OPN signals via the cell surface receptor RAGE and $\alpha v\beta_3$-integrin. On the one hand, OPN/RAGE interaction leads to upregulation of NADPH oxidase (NOX) and a concomitant raise in ROS levels culminating in activation of AKT and MAPK (mitogen-activated protein kinase) as well as NF-κB. On the other hand, OPN/$\alpha v\beta_3$-integrin interactions lead to direct or indirect activation of NF-κB via the mitogen-activated protein kinase kinase / extracellular signal-regulated protein kinase (MEK/ERK) pathway, regulating the expression of several genes involved in cell survival, angiogenesis, and metastasis and thereby promoting tumor growth (Kundu and Surh 2012).

Several signaling pathways have been identified as playing a crucial role in sarcomagenesis required for neoplastic transformation. These pathways include the Ras/Raf/MAPK pathway, the PI3K/AKT/mTOR pathway as well as the receptor tyrosine kinase c-Met and its ligand hepatocyte growth factor (HGF). Normally, c-Met is expressed by epithelial and mesenchymal cells and regulates several cellular responses such as cell proliferation, survival, motility, invasion, and morphogenesis (Birchmeier et al. 2003). Activation via ligand binding and/or receptor overexpression, amplification, and mutation induces multiple downstream effector proteins and cascades including Ras/Raf/MAPK, PI3K/AKT/mTOR, and STAT-3/-5 (for a review see Liu et al. 2010). The c-Met/HGF pathway represents one of the most commonly dysregulated pathways in human cancers with aberrant signaling found in most solid tumors and hematological malignancies (Birchmeier et al. 2003; Liu et al. 2010). Amplification or overexpression of c-Met has been demonstrated in many cancers including OS and unclassified pleomorphic sarcoma/MFH (Lahat et al. 2011).

Induction of the PI3K/AKT/mTOR and Ras/Raf/MAPK cascades can also be achieved via activation of TK receptors by either growth factors (IGF, HGF, VEGF, bFGF) or upregulation/mutation. This triggers a number of mitogenic processes that promote cell survival and proliferation, anti-apoptotic signals and upregulate expression of cell cycle proteins such as cyclin D1 and CDK4 (Takebe et al. 2011). Moreover, activation/upregulation of Ras culminates in the induction of ERK-1/-2 via Raf and MAPK/ERK kinases (MEK-1/-2) which regulate cell proliferation, survival, differentiation, and migration (Takebe et al. 2011). The possible contribution of these pathways to sarcomagenesis is discussed in detail in Sect. 11.3.

One of the major pathways involved in sarcomagenesis is the insulin-like growth factor (IGF) system. Signaling via the IGF receptor (IGF-1R) plays an important role in normal cell growth and differentiation as well as key aspects of neoplasia such as transformation and anti-apoptotic signaling (Zha and Lackner 2010). The ligands IGF-1 and IGF-2 are both capable of binding and stimulating IGF-1R. Bioavailability of IGF-1 is modulated by circulating IGF-binding proteins (IGFBPs), whereas bioavailability of IGF-2 is modulated both by the IGFBPs and by binding to the IGF-2R, resulting in receptor-mediated internalization and degradation of IGF-2 in lysosomes. Receptor ligation creates multiple docking sites for the adaptor proteins insulin receptor substrate 1 (IRS-1), IRS-2, and Shc. IRS-1 and IRS-2 binding results in activation of PI3K followed by recruitment and activation of AKT by PDK-1 and the mTOR-containing complex mTORC-2 (Guertin and Sabatini 2005). AKT activation exerts anti-apoptotic effects through inhibition of pro-apoptotic factors such as Bad and members of the FOXO family of transcription factors, as well as increased expression of anti-apoptotic proteins such as Bcl-2, Bcl-x_L, and NF-κB (Datta et al. 1999). AKT signaling also impacts glucose metabolism and plays a key role in protein synthesis and cell growth by regulating the activity of the mTORC-1 complex (Efeyan and Sabatini 2010). In contrast, Shc binding to activated IGF-1R activates the Ras/Raf/MAPK pathway and induces transduction of mitogenic signals (Pollak 2008).

As described above, the IGF-1 system is considered as playing a general role in neoplastic transformation and metastasis in a number of cancers including sarcomas. An upregulated expression of IGF-1/-2 or IGF-1R has been identified in various sarcomas such as SS, RMS, LMS, OS, and GIST while in ES, a downregulation of IGFBP-3 can be observed (Quesada and Amato 2012). In this context, preliminary clinical data argue for a link between members of the IGF system to increased cancer risk and pathological alterations in certain tumor types, notably sarcomas (Zha and Lackner 2010).

11.3 Role of Inflammatory Molecules in the Development of Sarcoma: Evidence from In Vitro Studies

11.3.1 Role of Inflammatory Molecules in the Transformation of Sarcoma Cells

There is growing evidence that interconnections among molecular pathways governing tissue differentiation are nodal points for malignant transformation. In this scenario, the discovery of microRNA (miRNA) identified this RNA subtype as a crucial player in tumorigenesis. miRNAs are a class of small RNAs that post-transcriptionally regulate gene expression, triggering not only transformation but also differentiation, and proliferation. Global alterations in miRNAs are frequently observed in a number of disease states including cancer. A comprehensive analysis of miRNA expression profiles of 27 sarcomas using microarray technology and/or small RNA cloning approaches identified distinct miRNA expression profiles among the tumor types as demonstrated by an unsupervised hierarchical clustering, and unique miRNA expression signatures in each tumor class (Subramanian et al. 2008). In GIST, the downregulated expression of miR-221 and miR-222 was suggested to allow for increased translation of *CKIT* and to further enhance its oncogenic potential on the cells. Significant overrepresentation of miR-1, miR-133a, and miR-133b was found in LMS playing a major role in myogenesis and myoblast proliferation. In SS, miR-143 was expressed at very low levels relative to GIST and LMS. The only experimentally verified target for miR-143 is *ERK5* (also known as *MAPK7*) whose role in sarcomagenesis is unclear. *SSX1*, a common 3′-fusion partner gene resulting from a t(X;18)(p11.2;q11.2) translocation in SS (Sturgis and Potter 2003), is predicted to be a target for miR-143, suggesting that underrepresentation of miR-143 in SS tumor cells enables the production of the SYT/SSX-1 oncoprotein (Subramanian et al. 2008; Hisaoka et al. 2011). In alveolar RMS, high levels of miR-335 involved in mesoderm or muscle differentiation can be found (Subramanian et al. 2008). From these data, the authors speculate that the clearly distinct miRNA expression signatures among the tumor types studied might implicate their role in tumorigenesis in these tumors and their potential as diagnostic markers or even therapeutic targets. It is interesting to note that the induction of the cancer stem cell (CSC) phenotype in ES is the result of the combined effect of suppression of miR-145 promoter activity and expression of *EWS/FLI1* fusion gene required for transformation (Riggi et al. 2010). *SOX2*, which participates in the development of pluripotent stem cells, was identified as the target gene of miR-145 and *EWS/FLI1*, thus providing insight how a single oncogene *(EWS/FLI1)* can reprogram cells to display the CSC phenotype (Riggi et al. 2010).

Several groups demonstrated a strikingly decreased expression of miR-1 and miR-133a in alveolar and embryonal RMS cell lines (Yan et al. 2009; Rao et al. 2010). Preclinical studies reported that forced re-expression of miR-206 leads to cell cycle arrest and myogenic differentiation of RMS cells, preventing xenograft growth in vivo by targeting the mRNA of the oncogenic c-Met receptor (Yan et al. 2009; Taulli et al. 2009). miR-1 and miR-206 are downregulated in alveolar and embryonal RMS compared to nonneoplastic skeletal muscle tissues and fail to increase in RMS cell lines in response to differentiation-inducing treatment (Taulli et al. 2009). Moreover, re-expression of miR-1 or miR-206 through lentiviral vectors promotes cell differentiation in alveolar cell lines that are resistant to differentiate cues, and blocks anchorage-independent growth and invasiveness in vitro and in vivo (Taulli et al. 2009). Meanwhile, clusters of hundreds of genes up- (muscle lineage) or downregulated (cell cycle) by miR-206 in RMS were identified, among which c-Met was found as being a direct miR-206 target. Thus, the miR-206-dependent post-transcriptional inhibition of c-Met expression markedly contributes to the anti-tumor effects of this miRNA rendering tissue-specific miRNAs as holding great therapeutic potential.

The miR-155 has been shown to be the most overexpressed miRNA in LS cell lines, and functional investigations assigned an important role in the growth of dedifferentiated LS cells (Zhang et al. 2012). Knockdown of miR-155 retarded tumor cell growth, decreased colony formation, and induced G1/S cell cycle arrest in vitro and blocked tumor growth in murine xenografts in vivo. Casein kinase 1α (CK1α) seems to be the direct target of miR-155 augmenting β-catenin signaling and cyclin D1 expression and promoting tumor cell growth (Zhang et al. 2012).

In inflamed tissue, miR-155 inhibits the repair of DNA double-strand breaks or allows mismatch repairs. According to Sinkovics (2012), these cells assume the "mutator phenotype" and upregulate the expression of hypoxanthine phosphoribosyl-transferase as a consequence of the dramatically enhanced number of DNA strand breaks and mutations. Inflammatory mediators such as TNF, IL-1β, IL-6, IL-8, and LPS are able to upregulate miR-155 in cancer cells. miR-155 increases the proliferation of adenocarcinoma cells and downregulates Wee-1, a recently recognized tumor suppressor and the key inhibitor of cyclin-dependent kinase 1 (Cdk-1), enabling unlimited cell divisions to occur (Enders 2010). Apart from being a regulator of mitotic entry, Wee-1 has been described to affect other cellular processes, including regulation of mitotic spindle formation, positioning and integrity, microtubule stabilization, and heat-shock protein 90 (Hsp90) phosphorylation (Hashimoto et al. 2006; Garcia et al. 2009; Mollapour et al. 2010). Inactivation of Wee-1 by miR-155 represents one of the hallmarks of inflammatory carcinogenesis (Enders 2010; Butz et al. 2010; Tili et al. 2011). Whether downregulation of Wee-1 as can be observed in human sporadic pituitary cancer cells (Butz et al. 2010) also occurs in sarcoma remains to be addressed.

Epithelial–mesenchymal transition (EMT) is the key process driving cancer metastasis characterized by the loss of the epithelial marker E-cadherin, an increase in the mesenchymal markers vimentin and N-cadherin, and an increase in the migratory and invasive behavior (Kraljevic Pavelic et al. 2011). Oncogene/self-renewal factor Bmi-1 has been shown to induce EMT in cancer cells (Yang et al. 2010b). Bmi-1 upregulation is associated with malignant transformation in hepatocellular carcinoma (Sasaki et al. 2008). Recent studies suggest that miRNAs function as crucial modulators for EMT. The group of Noriaki Sakuragi identified Bmi-1 as an essential factor in EMT and in the development of an invasive phenotype in endometrial cancer (EC) cells (Dong et al. 2011). Furthermore, the expression of Bmi-1 could be suppressed by miR-194 via direct binding to the *BMI1* 3′-untranslated region. Ectopic expression of miR-194 in EC cells induced a mesenchymal to epithelial transition (MET) by restoring E-cadherin, reducing vimentin expression, and inhibiting cell invasion in vitro. Based on these findings, it can be concluded that targeting the oncoprotein Bmi-1 might provide a potential new strategy to prevent EC progression.

Proto-oncogene activation represents a critical component in the intrinsic pathway of cancer-related inflammation. In this context, mutations in *RAS* genes play an important role in tumorigenesis of sarcoma. Overall, up to 30 % of all human tumors harbor mutations in canonical *RAS* genes (*KRAS, HRAS, NRAS*). Remarkably, these oncogenic mutations predominantly affect the *KRAS* locus, with oncogenic *KRAS* mutations being detected in 25–30 % of all screened tumor samples (Forbes et al. 2011). Activating *RAS* mutations are also present in up to 44 % of human STS (Yoo et al. 1999) and in up to 35 % of human embryonal RMS (Martinelli et al. 2009). The high frequency of *KRAS* mutations and their appearance in early tumor stages argue for a causative role of the K-Ras protein in human tumorigenesis (Fernandez-Medarde and Santos 2011). Members of the RAS family are crucial for the connection of upstream signals to downstream effector pathways that are functionally related to cell cycle progression, growth, migration, cytoskeletal changes, apoptosis, and senescence. In tumor cells, activation of mutated Ras is followed by the induction of several intracellular signaling pathways including the Raf/MEK/ERK kinase cascade, the PI3K/AKT/mTOR pathway, and RalGDS proteins (Downward 2009), the latter belonging to the family of nucleotide-exchange factors activating small GTPases such as RalB. RalB stimulates the TANK-binding kinase 1 (TBK-1) resulting in NF-κB activation. NF-κB not only functions as crucial regulator of inflammatory and immune responses as well as of cell survival, but it has also been implicated in cellular transformation and tumorigenesis. In cancer cells, a constitutive activation of this pathway, via chronic RalB activation, restricts the initiation of apoptosis after oncogenic stress (Chien et al. 2006). Beside NF-κB activation, TBK-1 activates the transcription factors IRF-3 and IRF-7 (Hacker and Karin 2006), leading to the production of growth and inflammatory mediators. Previously, it has been shown that oncogenic K-Ras is a direct inducer of pro-inflammatory IL-6 and pro-angiogenic IL-8 in vitro required for the initiation of tumor-associated inflammation and neovascularization promoting tumor growth (Sparmann and Bar-Sagi 2004; Ancrile et al. 2007). Since TBK-1 and NF-κB signaling have been identified as being essential in K-Ras mutant tumors (Barbie et al. 2009), it was assumed that targeting the NF-κB signaling pathway might be effective in treating Ras-mutated tumors (Downward 2009). Interestingly, NF-κB inhibition by dehydroxymethylepoxyquinomicin (DHMEQ) inhibited proliferation, decreased the mitotic index, and triggered apoptosis of OS cells HOS and MG-63 (Castro-Gamero et al. 2012) while NF-κB inhibition by the semisynthetic flavonoid 7-mono-O-(β-hydroxyethyl)-rutoside (monoHER) potentiated the anti-tumor activity of doxorubicin in the human LS cell line WLS-160 (Jacobs et al. 2011).

An intriguing aspect in cellular transformation is presented by the group of Bharat Aggarwal, who discussed the potential role of oxidative stress in tumorigenesis (Reuter et al. 2010). As stated by the authors, oxidative stress impacts any stage of tumorigenesis. In the initial phase, oxidative stress induces genetic instability by enhancing the mutation rate of cells and consequently leading to oncogenic transformation (Jackson and Loeb 2001). Apart from mediating genomic destabilization, ROS have been found to activate several intracellular signaling pathways promoting tumor growth and metastasis. In this context, the transcription factor FoxM1, a member of the large evolutionarily conserved family of forkhead box transcription factors involved in activating detoxifying enzymes (e.g., manganese superoxide dismutase), obviously plays a pivotal role in tumorigenesis since it is overexpressed in various human malignancies (Pilarsky et al. 2004). FoxM1 is also expressed in ES (Christensen et al. 2013), neuroblastoma (Wang et al. 2011) and medullablastoma cell lines (Priller et al. 2011). In glioblastoma cells, a high expression of FoxM1 was found to correlate with the tumorigenicity of the tumor cells (van den Boom et al. 2003; Liu et al. 2006).

The glycophosphoprotein osteopontin (OPN) is implicated in several physiological and pathophysiological processes including atherosclerosis, glomerulonephritis, chronic inflammatory diseases, and cancer (Lund et al. 2009). OPN is involved in proliferation, cell adhesion, migration, and invasion via interaction with its receptor, $\alpha v \beta_3$-integrin. It has been shown previously that OPN induction is required for tumor promotor-mediated transformation of preneoplastic mouse epidermal cells (Chang et al. 2003). Chen and coworkers convincingly demonstrated that

OPN enhances the migration of human chondrosarcoma cells JJ012 by increasing MMP-9 expression through $\alpha v\beta_3$ -integrin, FAK (focal adhesion kinase), MEK, ERK, and NF-κB signal transduction pathways (Chen et al. 2009).

11.3.2 Role of Inflammatory Molecules in the Survival of Sarcoma Cells

It has increasingly been recognized during the past years that malignancy not only results from enhanced proliferation but also from decreased apoptosis, a fundamental process in tumor cell kinetics. Cancer cells are extremely dependent on aberrations of the apoptotic pathways to survive. Critical regulators of this pathway include the Bcl-2 family of proteins and p53. In cultured KS tumor cells, flow cytometric and immunoblotting analyses revealed a predominant expression of anti-apoptotic Bcl-x_L over Bcl-2 with no detectable pro-apoptotic Bax or Bcl-x_S (Foreman et al. 1996). Bcl-2 is also expressed in the SS cell line, SN-SY-1 (Noguchi et al. 1997). It has been shown previously that Bcl-2 expression can be induced by VEGF in human dermal microvascular endothelial cells (HDMECs), thereby enhancing endothelial survival and sustaining angiogenesis (Nör et al. 1999). These data suggest that the ability of VEGF to enhance endothelial cell survival might be attributed to its capacity to induce the expression of Bcl-2. Of note, exposure of KS cells to pro-inflammatory IL-1 increased the expression of Bcl-2 and decreased that of Bax without affecting Bcl-x_L expression providing a link between KS cell escape from apoptosis and the immune dysregulation associated with KS (Simonart and Van Vooren 2002). Bcl-2 overexpression has been recently reported in SS in situ (Hirakawa et al. 1996).

Evidence for the role of inflammatory mediators in the survival of sarcoma cells is given by several in vitro studies, revealing that cultured human astrocytes as well as glioblastoma cell lines release GM-CSF that can be enhanced by addition of TNF or IL-1, respectively (Frei et al. 1992; Curran et al. 2011). In human neuroblastoma and glioblastoma cell lines, exposure to GM-CSF showed cytoprotective effects on these cell lines by inhibiting staurosporine-induced apoptosis (Huang et al. 2007; Choi et al. 2007). The same group found out that pretreatment of N2a glioblastoma cells with GM-CSF inhibited staurosporine-induced expression of pro-apoptotic p53 and Bax, while upregulated that of Bcl-2 (Huang et al. 2007). These data imply that the GM-CSF-mediated modulation of pro- and anti-apoptotic gene expression is crucially involved in inflammation-driven sarcomagenesis.

A wide range of pro-survival factors are activated by the essential embryonic sonic hedgehog (Hh) signaling pathway which has been implied in tumor formation and progression of various cancers. Aberrant activation of the Hh signaling pathway has been shown as playing a crucial role in RMS, OS, CS, ES as well as medulloblastoma (Quesada and Amato 2012; Martin Liberal et al. 2012). Upon Hh activation, upregulated expression of several marker genes, e.g., *PTCH1*, *GLI1*, *GLI3*, and *MYF5,* can be observed in embryonal RMS and also in fusion gene-negative alveolar RMS (Zibat et al. 2010). Together with the finding of an elevated Hh signaling in cancer stem cells and nonmalignant stromal cells surrounding malignant tumors, the Hh pathway can be considered as key cofactor in sarcomagenesis (Takebe et al. 2011).

Further critical signaling pathways in sarcomagenesis involve the PI3K/AKT/mTOR as well as the Ras/Raf/MAPK cascade. The study by Sasaki and coworkers detected *RAF1* and *MEK1/2* mRNA in OS and MFH cells (Sasaki et al. 2011). Treatment with the MEK inhibitor U0126 decreased proliferation of OS and MFH cells in a time- and dose-dependent manner. In human SS cells, inhibition of the MAPK pathway by sorafenib led to downregulation of cyclin D1 and pRb, G1 arrest, and induction of apoptosis (Peng et al. 2009). Notably, the work by the group of Hiroki Sakai convincingly demonstrated that the mTORC-2/AKT pathway was constitutively activated in canine hemangiosarcoma (HAS) cell lines and tumors (Murai et al. 2012a, b).

Angiogenin (ANG), a 14-kDa multifunctional pro-angiogenic growth factor, is upregulated in several types of cancers including KSHV-associated cancers such as KS (Sadagopan et al. 2009). ANG mediates its effects in multiple subcellular compartments, including the nucleolus where it directly binds to DNA, thereby inducing 45S rRNA transcription and cell proliferation (Moroianu and Riordan 1994). Studies by the group of Bala Chandran demonstrated that ANG plays a crucial role in the anti-apoptotic state of KSHV-infected cells by suppressing p53 functions (Sadagopan et al. 2012; Paudel et al. 2012). Moreover, ANG expression inhibited pro-apoptotic Bax and $p21^{Waf\text{-}1}$ expression, induced anti-apoptotic Bcl-2 and blocked cell death. ANG was also found to colocalize with the p53 regulator protein Mdm-2 and to increase p53/Mdm-2 interactions suggesting that ANG promotes the inhibition of p53 functions to mediate anti-apoptosis and cell survival (Sadagopan et al. 2012).

The crucial role of FoxM1 in tumorigenesis of sarcomas has already been mentioned. An altered expression and function of FoxM1B as can be found in several human malignancies also has an impact on apoptosis, possibly by regulating the cell cycle repressor protein $p27^{Kip\text{-}1}$ (Liu et al. 2006). $p27^{Kip\text{-}1}$ has been found to modulate apoptosis in various cell types, including glioblastoma multiforme cells (Hiromura et al. 1999; Lee and McCormick 2005). Knockdown of FoxM1 in medulloblastoma cell lines significantly decreased cell viability which was caused by a failure in mitotic spindle formation and caspase-dependent mitotic catastrophe (Priller et al. 2011).

11.3.3 Role of Inflammatory Molecules in the Proliferation of Sarcoma Cells

Tumor cells have to evade various cellular stress factors for proliferation and survival including a markedly increased production of ROS. In this context, the serine/threonine kinase Mirk/Dyrk1B has been reported to be highly expressed in several types of cancer cells, including OS (U2OS, KHOS), uterine sarcoma (MES-SA), CS (CS-1), SS (SS-1), ES (TC-71), and ovarian cancer (SKOV-3) in comparison with normal human osteoblast cell lines (Yang et al. 2010a). The same group clearly demonstrated that Mirk mediates cell proliferation and apoptosis in KHOS cells (Yang et al. 2010a). Mirk knockdown by RNA interference or shRNA induced apoptosis in both, OS cell lines and primary OS cell cultures in vitro. Mirk was also identified as being an active kinase in RMS cells in which its depletion by RNA interference led to apoptosis induction (Mercer et al. 2006). Mirk is known to upregulate the expression of several anti-oxidant genes involved in scavenging ROS by acting as a coactivator for distinct transcription factors and thus mediating cell survival (Deng et al. 2009).

Recent observations suggest a contribution of Mirk to the Hh pathway in sarcomas. As demonstrated previously, Mirk is a downstream effector of oncogenic K-Ras and an active kinase in RMS and OS cells (Jin et al. 2007). Moreover, activating *RAS* mutations can be found in up to 44 % of human STS (Yoo et al. 1999) and in up to 35 % of human embryonal RMS (Martinelli et al. 2009). Since Mirk has been found to enhance Gli1-dependent gene transcription and to act synergistically with sonic Hh in inducing transcription, one can hypothesize that Mirk alters Hh signaling and consequently controls stromal environment of these tumors (Friedman 2011).

As already mentioned, OPN, a secreted phosphorylated chemokine-like protein, plays an important role in proliferation of tumor cells. In particular, the two isoforms of OPN, OPN-A and OPN-B, have been found to stimulate pro-tumorigenic behaviors, such as cell proliferation, migration, invasion, and soft agar colony formation in transiently transfected mesothelioma cell lines (Ivanov et al. 2009).

Evidence for the role of inflammatory mediators in the proliferation of sarcoma cells is further given by several in vitro studies revealing that cultured human astrocytes as well as glioblastoma cell lines release growth-promoting GM-CSF that can be enhanced by addition of TNF or IL-1, respectively (Frei et al. 1992; Curran et al. 2011). Human glioblastoma cell lines and murine OS cell lines secrete TGF-β (Constam et al. 1992; Navid et al. 2000) and IL-1 (Fontana et al. 1984; Lee et al. 1989), the latter has been found to modulate TGF-β secretion from malignant glioma cells (Naganuma et al. 1996). The effect of TGF-β on growth of sarcoma cells remains an open question. While TGF-β obviously did not affect growth of malignant glioma cells exposed to IL-1 (Naganuma et al. 1996), it markedly increased proliferation of murine OS cells (Navid et al. 2000) but decreased that of human RS cells (Ye et al. 2005). TNF, a critical cytokine in tumorigenesis and produced by astrocytes in vitro and in vivo, contrarily affected proliferation of the astrocytoma cells A-172 and U-87, thereby decreasing TGF-β expression in U-87 only (Chen et al. 1993).

Stimulation of human OS cells Saos2 with TNF increased bone sialoprotein (*BSP*), *IL6,* and *PGHS2* mRNA levels (Nakayama et al. 2004). TNF is a pro-inflammatory cytokine crucially involved in cellular proliferation and differentiation. It also contributes to bone remodeling and represents a component of the RANK/RANKL pathway (Silva and Branco 2011). RANKL, a member of the TNF superfamily of cytokines, has been found in a variety of malignant tumor cells where it regulates cell proliferation and migration (Tat et al. 2009). Expression of RANKL could be demonstrated in Paget's sarcoma stromal cells (Sun et al. 2006), OS cells (Mori et al. 2007), bone stromal cells from giant cell tumors (Ng et al. 2010), and ES cells (Taylor et al. 2011). The expression of RANKL increases in response to pro-inflammatory cytokines such as IL-1 in multiple myeloma mesenchymal stromal cells in a MEK/ERK-dependent manner (Fernandez et al. 2010).

PGHS-2 has emerged as another pro-inflammatory mediator in tumorigenesis whose expression is mediated by NF-κB. PGHS-2 is the rate-limiting enzyme involved in the conversion of arachidonic acid to prostanoids acting as key mediators of inflammation. Aberrant or increased expression of PGHS-2 has been shown to be involved in the pathogenesis of several malignancies including OS. PGHS-2 and prostaglandins contribute to carcinogenesis by stimulating cell proliferation, apoptosis, angiogenesis, and metastasis (Aggarwal and Gehlot 2009; Kundu and Surh 2012). Overexpression of PGHS-2 results in the secretion of large amounts of VEGF and therefore is associated with increased tumor cell invasion and poor prognosis (Raut et al. 2004; Ladetto et al. 2005). Our own investigations on the human OS cell line U-2 OS revealed a strong IL-6 and IL-8 production by U2 OS after stimulation with IL-1 (Hönicke et al. 2012). IL-6 is an NF-κB-regulated pleiotropic pro-inflammatory cytokine that enables tumor growth and inhibits apoptosis in numerous human cancers (Rose-John and Schooltink 2007). Similarly, IL-8 increases proliferation and survival of endothelial and cancer cells (Takamori et al. 2000; Li et al. 2003; Yao et al. 2007). In CS cells SW1353, IL-1 exposure strongly induced IL-6 production and upregulated secretion of MMP-1 and MMP-13 (Radons et al. 2006b). Experiments with pharmacological inhibitors clearly demonstrated a contribution of the p38MAPK and/or the PI3K/JNK (c-Jun N-terminal kinase) pathway to IL-1-induced IL-6 secretion in SW1353 cells (Radons et al. 2006a).

Recent investigations of the laboratory of Brooke Mossman demonstrated an increased secretion of inflammatory mediators (IL-13, bFGF, G-CSF, and VEGF) in human malignant mesothelioma (MM) cells LP9/TERT-1 after exposure to asbestos (Hillegass et al. 2010b). Exposure to asbestos fibers is known to induce the development of MM, a rare form of cancer that affects the thin cell wall lining (mesothelium) of the body's internal organs and structures. Using an RNA interference, the asbestos-induced upregulation of IL-1β, IL-13, and G-CSF as well as of growth-promoting PDGF-BB and pro-angiogenic VEGF in LP9/TERT-1 cells could be attributed to an activation of the transcription factor ATF-3 (Shukla et al. 2009). In malignant peripheral nerve sheath tumor (MPNST), a highly aggressive STS without any effective treatment options, PDGF-BB functions as the most effective inducer of MPNST cell proliferation and invasion. As demonstrated by Iwasaki and collaborators, PDGF-BB was found to enhance the invasive activity of MPNST cells via PDGFR phosphorylation which could be blocked by imatinib mesylate in vitro (Iwasaki et al. 2009). In addition, EMMPRIN is a transmembrane glycoprotein expressed on tumor cells and induces the production of MMPs in peritumoral fibroblasts thus promoting tumor growth and invasiveness of human carcinomas. Epithelioid sarcoma cell lines have been shown to express EMMPRIN and to upregulate MMP-2 in fibroblasts in coculture experiments critical for epithelioid sarcoma cell stromal invasion and vascular involvement (Koga et al. 2007). These findings render tumor-associated EMMPRIN a potentially useful target in the therapy of certain STS.

To analyze the functional and potential therapeutic relevance of IGF-1R signaling, Friedrichs and collaborators treated SS cell lines with the IGF-1R inhibitor NVP-AEW541 (Friedrichs et al. 2008). In this study, the IGF-1R antagonist was found to inhibit cell growth through a reduction in phosphorylation of AKT and p44/42 MAPK. Moreover, inhibition of the receptor led to increased apoptosis and diminished mitotic activity. In a recent study, an upregulated expression of IGF-1R, c-Met, HER-2, VEGFR-3, insulin receptor, and PDGFR-β was identified in OS cell lines suggesting a contribution of these receptors to osteosarcomagenesis (Hassan et al. 2012). Further in vitro evidence for the contribution of the MAPK pathway to sarcomagenesis is given by the work of Sasaki and colleagues who detected *RAF1* and *MEK1/2* mRNA expression in several human sarcoma cell lines (Sasaki et al. 2011). Treatment with the MEK inhibitor U0126 resulted in dose- and time-dependent inhibition of cell proliferation and suppression of p-ERK expression (Sasaki et al. 2011). A similar observation was made with the SS cell lines SW982 and HS-SY-II where the Raf inhibitor sorafenib effectively inhibited cell proliferation and phosphorylation of MEK and ERK, downregulated cyclin D1 and pRb levels, caused G1 arrest and S phase decrease, and induced apoptosis (Peng et al. 2009).

Lyn, a member of the SRC family of kinases, is a known regulator of tumor cell proliferation, adhesion, motility, and invasion. Elevated Lyn kinase activity has been found in ES cell lines (Rosen et al. 1986; Guan et al. 2008). Shor et al. (2007) also reported high levels of phosphorylated Src in human OS and ES cell lines. In ES cells, Lyn expression is regulated by EWS/Fli-1 which is known to transform cells by acting as an aberrant transcriptional factor for specific target genes (Guan et al. 2008). In vitro, inhibition of Lyn kinase activity by the small-molecule Src family tyrosine kinase (SFK) inhibitor AP23994 suppressed growth of ES tumor cells TC71, while downregulation of Lyn reduced invasive capacity of the cells (Guan et al. 2008). Activation of Lyn can be induced by the KSHV protein K1 in K1 lymphoma cells leading to production of VEGF and NF-κB activation, both strongly implicated in the development of KSHV-derived disorders (Prakash et al. 2005).

As discussed earlier, FoxM1 is a central player in sarcomagenesis. FoxM1 is exclusively expressed in proliferating cells and critically involved in cell cycle progression (Laoukili et al. 2005; Wang et al. 2005a). FoxM1B overexpression increased the growth of glioma cells both in vitro and in vivo, which was at least partially caused by accelerated glioma cell cycle progression (Liu et al. 2006). Consistent with previous studies (Kalinichenko et al. 2004); FoxM1 overexpression was shown to diminish the expression of nuclear $p27^{Kip-1}$ protein but increased the expression of Skp-2 and cyclin D1 protein. From these observations, the authors conclude that FoxM1 probably regulates $p27^{Kip-1}$ protein expression indirectly by inducing Skp-2 expression, which mediates the degradation of $p27^{Kip-1}$ protein. FoxM1 is also expressed in ES cell lines in which reduction of its expression resulted in diminished potential for anchorage-independent growth (Christensen et al. 2013). FoxM1 is obviously implicated in the pathogenesis of neuroblastoma. In neuroblastoma cell lines, reduction in *FOXM1* expression by siRNA markedly diminished anchorage-independent growth (Wang et al. 2011). Furthermore, neuroblastoma cells with reduced FoxM1 expression underwent spontaneous differentiation with diminished levels of Sox-2. Human OS cells U2 OS expressing hyperactivated AKT are addicted to FoxM1 for proliferation and clonogenic survival as they require continuous presence of FoxM1 for survival (Park et al. 2009). The same study further revealed that expression of FoxM1 is induced by oncogenic Ras requiring ROS and that upregulated FoxM1 counteracts elevated intracellular ROS levels in a negative feedback loop by stimulating the expression of anti-oxidant enzyme genes to protect dividing cells and tumor cells from oxidative stress (Park et al. 2009). Together, these observations indicate a strong reliance of tumor cells on FoxM1.

11.3.4 Role of Inflammatory Molecules in the Invasion, Metastasis, and Angiogenesis of Sarcoma Cells

Angiogenesis, which is essential for tumor growth, is regulated by various pro-angiogenic factors (e.g., VEGF, IL-8, bFGF, EGF, PDGF, MMP-2, Notch-1/-4, and OPN). Among them, VEGF has been identified as a crucial player in sarcomagenesis. As demonstrated by our group, human U2 OS cells spontaneously release high amounts of invasiveness- and angiogenesis-promoting MMP-2, VEGF, and IL-8 that can be further enhanced by pro-inflammatory IL-1 (Hönicke et al. 2012). IL-1 was also found to strongly upregulate secretion of pro-angiogenic IL-8, suggesting a crucial involvement in osteosarcomagenesis. We also detected a massive release of pro-angiogenic MMP-1 and MMP-13 in CS cells SW1353 after exposure to IL-1 highlighting the crucial impact of inflammatory mediators in bone sarcomagenesis (Radons et al. 2006b). Measurement of VEGF levels in cell supernatants of canine HAS cell lines treated with masitinib mesylate demonstrated a statistically significant increased VEGF release in close proximity to the IC_{50} of each cell line followed by a decline back toward baseline levels (Lyles et al. 2012). VEGF blockade induced a significant cell death in human glioblastoma and fibrosarcoma (FS) cell lines, thereby confirming the central role of VEGF in sarcomagenesis (Lee et al. 2011, 2012). Identical to IGF, VEGF binding to its corresponding receptor leads to activation of the PI3K/AKT/mTOR and Ras/Raf/MAPK pathways, promoting not only angiogenesis but also proliferation, differentiation and survival. In this context, stimulation of human CS cells JJ012 with OPN significantly increased expression of invasiveness- and angiogenesis-promoting MMP-9 and activation of FAK, MEK, ERK, and NF-κB (Chen et al. 2009). In addition, treatment of JJ012 cells with the NF-κB inhibitor PDTC, the IκB protease inhibitor TPCK, RGD peptide, anti-$\alpha v \beta_3$ integrin monoclonal antibody or MEK inhibitors (PD98059, U0126) inhibited the OPN-induced MMP-9 upregulation of CS cells providing in vitro evidence for the role of OPN in angiogenesis and invasiveness of sarcoma. Remarkably, transfection of murine neuroblastoma C1300 cells with OPN did not increase VEGF production and did not affect gene expression of other proangiogenic factors confirmed by complementary DNA microarray system suggesting a pro-angiogenic role independent of VEGF, at least in this sarcoma subtype (Takahashi et al. 2002). Other pro-angiogenic factors are differentially upregulated in STS cells such as angiopoietin-2, bFGF, MMP-2, Notch-1/-4, and PDGF (Engin et al. 2009; Lee et al. 2010; Ye et al. 2012; Bai et al. 2012; Hönicke et al. 2012). Some chromosomal translocations and their gene products are able to upregulate the transcription of pro-angiogenic *VEGF, HIF1A*, *MDK*, *CMET*, and *TIMP2* as can be found in the alveolar soft part sarcoma cell line ASPS-1 (Quesada and Amato 2012). In this context, FoxM1 is required for invasion and angiogenesis of glioma cells as VEGF was identified as being a direct transcriptional target of FoxM1B (Zhang et al. 2008). Furthermore, FoxM1 overexpression increased and inhibition of FoxM1 expression suppressed the angiogenic ability of glioma cells. According to Agulnik (2012), the PI3K/AKT/mTOR pathway has an important role in the regulation of angiogenesis mediated by HIF-1α. Preclinical and clinical studies provide further evidence for the anti-angiogenic effects of specific mTOR inhibitors (rapalogs) in sarcoma (see also Table 11.3).

As already mentioned in Sect. 11.3.2, the multifunctional pro-angiogenic growth factor ANG is upregulated in numerous cancers including KS (Sadagopan et al. 2009). Apart from ANG, KSHV infection upregulates the transcription of a broad range of host genes involved in angiogenesis such as *VEGF* and *PGHS2* (Sivakumar et al. 2008; Sharma-Walia et al. 2010). The nuclear location of ANG is a prerequisite not only for its pro-angiogenic and proliferative properties but also for the pro-angiogenic potential of VEGF and bFGF (Kishimoto et al. 2005). In a previous study, the group of Bala Chandran demonstrated robust *PGHS2* expression and high levels of PGE_2 secretion by KSHV during primary infection of human microvascular endothelial cells (HMVEC-d) and human foreskin fibroblast cells (Sharma-Walia et al. 2006). KSHV infection-induced PGHS-2/PGE_2 expression also upregulated Rac1-GTPases in adhering endothelial cells, thereby accelerating cell adhesion (Sharma-Walia et al. 2010). The same study also demonstrated that KSHV infection-induced PGHS-2 potentially modulated survival, proliferation, and angiogenesis of latently infected endothelial cells by inducing secretion of numerous growth (PDGF-BB, IGF-1, G-CSF, and IL-8), angiogenesis (VEGF, ANG, oncostatin, IL-8, and MMP-2), inflammation (IL-1, TNF, RANTES, and IL-8), and invasiveness-promoting factors (MMP-2/-9).

11.4 Role of Inflammatory Molecules in the Development of Sarcoma: Evidence from In Vivo Studies

Increasing evidence suggests a role of the Ras/Raf/MAPK pathway in the pathogenesis of sarcoma. In a xenograft FS model, the MKK inhibitor LeTx (anthrax lethal toxin) was found to suppress tumor growth and vascularization (Ding et al. 2008). Growth inhibition correlated with decreased cellular proliferation and extensive necrosis, and it was accompanied by a decrease in tumor mean vessel density and a reduction in serum expression of angioproliferative cytokines (Ding et al. 2008). Importantly, up to 44 % of human STS and up to 35 % of human embryonal RMS harbor activating *RAS* mutations (Yoo et al. 1999; Martinelli et al. 2009). It has been shown previously that ectopic expression of oncogenic *KRAS* induces RMS in zebrafish (Langenau et al. 2007) and cooperates with the loss of the tumor suppressor p53 to induce RMS in adult mice (Tsumura et al. 2006). Like *RAS*, perturbations of the cyclin-dependent kinase inhibitor 2A (*CDKN2A*) locus, encoding the cell cycle inhibitors $p16^{Ink\text{-}4a}$ and $p19^{Arf}$, also have been linked to sarcoma pathogenesis (Serrano et al. 1996). Alterations in *CDKN2A* and its downstream effectors *RB1* and *TP53* have been noted in human STS (Obana et al. 2003; Kohashi et al. 2008; Rubin et al. 2011). In human RMS, reduced or absent expression of *INK4A* and/or *ARF* mRNA was noted and showed no significant correlation with clinicopathological parameters (Chen et al. 2007). Based on these data, oncogenic *KRAS* and dysregulated *INK4A/ARF* can be considered as clinically relevant sarcoma-associated lesions (Hettmer et al. 2011).

In a transplantable model of murine histiocytic sarcoma (HS), the introduction of oncogenic *KRAS* into tumor suppressor gene-deficient ($INK4A/ARF^{-/-}$) bone marrow cells by ex vivo gene transduction with subsequent injection of these genetically altered cells into the gastrocnemius muscles of NOD/SCID mice led to an upregulated expression of CD47, also known as integrin-associated protein (IAP; Liu et al. 2012b). CD47 protects cells from being eaten, such that cells with high surface expression of CD47 are able to escape integrin-mediated phagocytosis and death (Oldenborg et al. 2001). The group of Yuji Yamanashi recently demonstrated that mice with coincident loss of *DOK1*, *DOK2,* and *DOK3* genes develop highly invasive and transplantable HS endogenously, and $DOK1/2/3^{-/-}$ macrophages demonstrate enhanced proliferation ability (Mashima et al. 2010). The DOK family consists of seven members acting as downstream targets of many TKs. Among them, Dok-1, Dok-2, and Dok-3 have been identified as negative regulators of TK-mediated proliferation and transformation of cells (Lemay et al. 2000; Honma et al. 2006; Ng et al. 2007). HS also has been observed sporadically in *PEUM/RAS* transgenic mice (Haupt et al. 1992), and $INK4A/ARF^{-/-}$ mice develop HS with homozygous loss of the tumor suppressor gene *PTEN,* providing mechanistic insights into the pathogenesis of human HS (Carrasco et al. 2006). Deficiency of *PTEN* culminates in activation of AKT, as well as ERK-1 and ERK-2 in HS cells indicating hyperactivation of the K-Ras/MAPK pathway (Carrasco et al. 2006).

By using a chimeric mouse model in which sarcoma-associated genetic lesions were introduced into discrete, muscle-resident myogenic and mesenchymal cell lineages, the group of Amy Wagers identified a Ras-predominated gene expression signature shared by *KRAS,* $INK4A/ARF^{-/-}$ mouse sarcomas, and human embryonal as well as alveolar RMS, and demonstrated activation of the Ras/Raf/MEK/ERK pathway as well as the mTOR pathway in *KRAS,* $INK4A/ARF^{-/-}$ mouse sarcomas, and in 26–50 % of human RMS and LMS surveyed (Hettmer et al. 2011). Moreover, chemical inhibition of Ras or mTOR signaling arrested the growth of mouse *KRAS, INK4A/ARF*$^{-/-}$ sarcoma, and human RMS cells in vitro and in vivo (Hettmer et al. 2011). Consistent with a central role of Ras signaling in these tumors, inhibition of the Ras/Raf/MEK/ERK signaling cascade diminished the proliferation of mouse and human sarcoma cells (Marampon et al. 2009).

Several other candidate genes have been linked to mTOR signaling including the actin filament-plasma membrane linker ezrin (encoded by *VIL2*) and the homeodomain-containing transcription factor Six-1 (sine oculis-related homeobox-1 homolog) playing essential roles in determining the metastatic fate of RMS cells (Yu et al. 2004). Similarly, phosphorylation of AKT, the upstream effector of mTOR, was reported in approximately 50 % of human embryonal and alveolar RMS (Cen et al. 2007). The findings by Hettmer et al. (2011) are consistent with previous observations made with RMS cell lines and xenografts demonstrating that pharmacological inhibition of mTOR signaling in mouse and human sarcoma cells impaired tumor growth (Petricoin et al. 2007; Houghton et al. 2008). Beneficial effects were also seen in some patients with advanced sarcomas including RMS (Yarber and Agulnik 2011; Agulnik 2012). All these data clearly document the important contribution of aberrant Ras and mTOR signaling to the growth and malignancy of STS.

As already mentioned in Sect. 11.3.1, overexpression of oncogenic K-Ras was found to induce the secretion of pro-inflammatory IL-6 and pro-angiogenic IL-8 in different tumor cell types. The study by Ancrile et al. (2007) revealed that this Ras-driven cytokine production is required for the initiation of tumor-associated inflammation and neovascularization promoting tumor growth in vivo. In theses studies, knock-down of *IL6*, genetic ablation of the *IL6* gene, or treatment with a neutralizing IL-6 antibody retarded K-Ras-driven tumorigenesis in mice (Ancrile et al. 2007). Ras-induced expression of several pro-inflammatory mediators including IL-1, IL-6, and IL-11 as well as pro-angiogenic IL-8 has been demonstrated to promote tumor growth and neovascularization in vivo (Sparmann and Bar-Sagi 2004). In an animal model of human OS, increased IL-1 levels are also reported (Baamonde et al. 2007).

Further evidence for the impact of inflammation in sarcomagenesis comes from a gene profiling approach in canine HAS (Tamburini et al. 2010). HAS, also called malignant hemangioendothelioma or angiosarcoma, is a deadly cancer that originates in the endothelium and invades the blood vessels. HAS is more common in dogs than any other species. The study by Tamburini et al. (2010) clearly identified inflammation and angiogenesis as distinguishing features of canine HAS. Six genes of the IL-8 signaling cascade were found as being enriched in HAS. These genes included *IL8*, *MMP9*, *VEGF*, *VCAM1*, *PGHS2*, and cyclin D1 (*CCND1*) known as being involved in regulating pro-inflammatory and pro-angiogenic responses via the IL-8 receptor-β (Tamburini et al. 2010). In a SCID mouse xenograft model of human MM, Hillegass and colleagues identified an early and sustained neutrophilia accompanied by early detection of cytokines that promote inflammation (IL-6, IL-8, and IL-12), cell proliferation (IL-6, bFGF, IL-8, G-CSF, and PDGF-BB), and angiogenesis (bFGF, IL-8, and VEGF) by human MM in peritoneal lavage fluid (Hillegass et al. 2010a)

Using a xenograft nude mouse model for human glioblastoma, Liu and coworkers convincingly demonstrated that overexpression of FoxM1B directly promotes the growth of human glioma cells in the brain of nude mice, while inhibition of FoxM1 by FoxM1-siRNA significantly suppressed glioma growth in these mice, thus confirming in vitro results of the same study (Liu et al. 2006). Moreover, depletion of FoxM1 inhibited anchorage-independent growth and tumorigenicity of neuroblastoma xenografts (Wang et al. 2011).

The contribution of oxidative stress to sarcomagenesis is proven by investigations on a transgenic Rac-1 model for KS (Ma et al. 2009). The small GTPase Rac-1, a member of the Rho family within the RAS superfamily, triggers ROS production by members of the phagocytic as well as nonphagocytic NOX family (Abo et al. 1991). Expression of a constitutively active Rac-1 (RacCA) in transgenic mice is sufficient to cause KS-like tumors through mechanisms involving ROS-driven proliferation, upregulation of AKT signaling, and HIF-1α-related angiogenesis (Ma et al. 2009). Notably, the use of the ROS-scavenging agent N-acetylcysteine inhibited angiogenesis and completely abrogated transgenic RacCA tumor formation, indicative for the causal role of ROS in sarcomagenesis. These data clearly imply the direct oncogenicity of Rac-1 and ROS and their contribution to a KS-like malignant phenotype, further underscoring the carcinogenic potential of oxidative stress in the context of chronic infection and inflammation (Ma et al. 2009).

In vivo evidence for the crucial role of OPN in sarcomagenesis is given by the work of Liu and colleagues who successfully reduced the tumorigenecity of human osteosarcoma cells OS-732 xenotransplanted into nude mice using an antisense human *OPN* RNA expression vector (Liu et al. 2008). Takahashi and coworkers recently generated a stable OPN transfectant from murine neuroblastoma C1300 cells and demonstrated that culture medium with OPN-transfected C1300 cells significantly stimulates human umbilical vein endothelial cell (HUVEC) migration and induces neovascularization in mice compared to control cells (Takahashi et al. 2002). Further evidence for the pro-angiogenic role of OPN is provided by the same group who found that OPN enhances tumorigenesis and angiogenesis of murine neuroblastoma cells in mice rendering OPN a promising target in sarcoma therapy (Hirama et al. 2003).

Experimental animal models suggest a contribution of the IGF system in tumorigenesis of sarcomas. In addition as being linked to increased cancer risk and certain neoplasias (see Sect. 11.3.1), dysregulated IGF expression has also been demonstrated to have functional consequences. IGF-1 overexpression in basal keratinocytes resulted in increased formation of squamous papillomas in transgenic mice (Wilker et al. 1999). Injection of ES cells carrying dominant negative IGF-IR into nude mice attenuated tumor formation and metastatic abilities of ES cells and increased survival (Scotlandi et al. 2002). Furthermore, transfected clones showed significantly higher sensitivity to doxorubicin, a major drug in the treatment of ES. Ligand overexpression seems to be driven by pathological alterations, particularly in sarcomas. The *EWS/FLI1* translocation is a defining characteristic of ES and has been shown to upregulate IGF-1 expression and downregulate IGFBP-3 expression, enabling an autocrine regulatory loop consisting of IGF-1 and IGF-1R, which can be blocked by IGF-1R targeting agents (Scotlandi et al. 2002; Prieur et al. 2004). In addition, *EWS/FLI1* was shown to upregulate expression of the Src kinase Lyn in athymic nude mice injected with TC71 human ES tumor cells allowing increased bony lysis by creating space for tumor growth, and providing simple access for tumor cells to the bone stroma facilitating metastasis (Guan et al. 2008). Targeting Lyn using siRNA or the pharmacological inhibitor AP23994 resulted in suppression of tumor growth, decreased bony lysis due to tumor cells, and significantly fewer lung metastases in this ES xenograft tumor model.

Current experimental data support the role of the PI3K/AKT/mTOR pathway in sarcomagenesis. In an animal model of STS, intramuscular delivery of an adenovirus carrying Cre recombinase in mice with conditional mutations in *KRAS* and *TRP53* sufficiently initiated high-grade sarcomas with myofibroblastic differentiation similar to RMS (Kirsch et al. 2007). The PI3K/AKT/mTOR pathway also plays a substantial role in smooth muscle transformation and LMS genesis. As demonstrated by the group of Carlos Cordon-Cardo, mice carrying homozygous deletion of *PTEN* alleles developed widespread smooth muscle cell hyperplasia and abdominal LMS (Hernando et al. 2007).

11.5 Evidence from Patients for the Role of Inflammation in Sarcoma

The role of inflammation in human sarcomagenesis has long been overlooked, but emerging evidence suggests its contribution to the malignant process in humans. The subsequent examples highlight the putative role of inflammatory mediators in the pathogenesis of sarcomas. Among the inflammatory mediators present in the tumor microenvironment, IL-1 acts as crucial player in inflammation-associated carcinogenesis (Lin and Karin 2007; Voronov et al. 2007). Elevated levels of IL-1 have been identified in several human tumor entities. Overall, patients harboring IL-1-positive tumors have markedly worse prognoses (Lewis et al. 2006). IL-1 is produced directly by cancer cells or by cells of the mircroenvironment and stimulates other cell types to produce pro-angiogenic and pro-metastatic mediators, thus playing an important role in inflammation-associated carcinogenesis (Lin and Karin 2007; Voronov et al. 2007). In this context, children with MFH showed elevated serum levels of pro-inflammatory IL-1 and TNF (Ishii et al. 1991). Elevated serum levels of TNF and IL-6 were also found in a patient with ovarian FS (Fukuda et al. 2001). Tumor cells from this patient revealed a focally positive immunoreaction for vimentin, IL-6, TNF, and inhibin-α, a subunit of the heterodimeric hormone inhibin produced in the ovary that antagonizes activin signaling and FSH synthesis in the pituitary. Serum TNF levels were also significantly higher in patients with aural cholesteatoma compared to controls correlating with bone destruction (Sastry et al. 1999). Increased levels of IL-1 and TNF were detected in acquired and congenital cholesteatoma tissues as compared to normal skin (Akimoto et al. 2000). Tissue biopsy samples from chronic otitis media patients with cholesteatoma also harbored significantly higher levels of these cytokines compared to cholesteatoma-free patients (Yetiser et al. 2002). Cholesteatoma-derived TNF and IL-1 can lead to bone resorption which can be inhibited by TNF blockage (Akimoto et al. 2000). Both, TNF and IL-1, induce activation of NF-κB, the key orchestrator in tumorigenesis, regulating the expression of several inflammatory mediators promoting tumor growth and invasiveness. Increased serum levels of angioproliferative cytokines, including IL-6, IL-8, M-CSF, bFGF, TNF, and VEGF, have also been reported in sarcoma patients correlating with poor overall survival (Feldman et al. 2001; Rutkowski et al. 2003). In this context, NF-κB-dependent MMP-2/-9 expression in STS biopsies correlated with metastasis and grade in LS, while lack of tissue inhibitor of metalloproteinase 2 (TIMP-2) expression was identified as a poor prognostic factor for disease-free survival in SS (Benassi et al. 2001).

Malignant peripheral nerve sheath tumor (MPNST) is a rare STS with poor prognosis. MPNST occurs frequently in patients with neurofibromatosis type 1 (NF1), in which *NF1* gene deficiency leads to Ras hyperactivation. Ras activation causes the subsequent activation of the PI3K/AKT/mTOR and Ras/Raf/MAPK pathways and regulates cellular functions. Immunohistochemical and Western blotting analyses of 135 tumor specimens revealed that the PI3K/AKT/mTOR and Ras/Raf/MAPK pathways were activated in more than 50 % of NF1-related and sporadic MPNST correlating with poor prognosis (Endo et al. 2013).

In patients with CS, positive expressions of nitric oxide synthase (NOS) 1 and NOS-2 were associated with decreased overall survival rates (Nakagawa et al. 2010). Nitric oxide stimulates the production of PGHS-2, which is linked to inflammation and angiogenesis in tumors. There was a significant association of nitrotyrosine, PGHS-2, and the endothelial cell marker CD34 with histological grades, but not with overall prognosis in CS patients (Nakagawa et al. 2010). Several studies have identified PGHS-2 expression in a variety of sarcomas, including RMS, OS, and CS. Although PGHS-2 overexpression has been associated with poor prognosis and decreased survival in CS and OS, no relationship between PGHS-2 expression and patient outcome has been demonstrated in RMS or adult STS such as SS (Carmody Soni et al. 2011) and uterine carcinosarcoma (Menczer et al. 2010). The analysis of 51 patients with extremity OS who completed standard therapy and obtained complete initial regression of the tumor, however, revealed a correlation between PGHS-2 overexpression in the primary tumor and the occurrence of distant metastasis suggesting an effect on the post-metastatic survival (Urakawa et al. 2009).

Several genetic and chromosomal abnormalities as part of the intrinsic pathway have been found in OS patients including chromosomal amplification and loss of heterozygosity, associated with poor prognosis (Ta et al. 2009; Smida et al. 2010). Additionally, mutations in the tumor suppressor proteins p53 and pRb have been implicated in the oncogenesis of OS enhancing the risk and thus contributing to its poorer prognosis (Longhi et al. 2001; Heinsohn et al. 2007). Also molecular abnormalities in the p53 regulator Mdm-2 have been identified as critical players in sarcoma development (Cordon-Cardo et al. 1994). Aberrant Mdm-2 expression can be found in a variety of sarcomas including LS and OS (Ladanyi et al. 1993;

Leach et al. 1993; Shimada et al. 2006). In the latter, Mdm-2 overexpression occurs with high frequency as a result of an upregulated *MDM2* mRNA expression correlating with disease recurrence and metastasis (Ladanyi et al. 1993; Gisselsson et al. 2002). An upregulated expression of the *FOXM1* mRNA could be detected in neuroblastoma tissue samples compared to noncancerous ganglioneuroma or less aggressive ganglioneuroblastoma (Koch et al. 2008; Hillegass et al. 2010a). FoxM1 is a transcription factor critically involved in cell cycle progression (see Sect. 11.3.1). As demonstrated by Liu et al. (2006), human glioma tissue specimens apparently had a substantially higher level of FoxM1 expression than normal tissue and this expression correlated directly with the grade of the glioma. Together with the in vitro and in vivo findings from the same study, these data suggest the pivotal role of FoxM1 in tumorigenesis of glioma. FoxM1 is also expressed at robust levels in a variety of Ewing tumor specimens (Christensen et al. 2013). Previous studies have shown that nuclear expression of the cell cycle repressor protein $p27^{Kip-1}$ decreases with malignancy in human astrocytic gliomas and that $p27^{Kip-1}$ has independent prognostic value in patients with astrocytomas (Piva et al. 1997; Alleyne et al. 1999; Kirla et al. 2003). In human gliomas, the Skp-2 expression level directly correlated with the tumor grade but inversely correlated with the $p27^{Kip-1}$ level (Schiffer et al. 2002). FoxM1 has also been implicated in the pathogenesis of human medulloblastoma, the most frequent malignant brain tumor in childhood that can derive from cerebellar granule neuron precursors (Priller et al. 2011). As documented in this study, FoxM1 was highly expressed in all subtypes of medulloblastoma tested. Importantly, expression levels of FoxM1 significantly correlated with unfavorable clinical outcome and has been identified as an independent prognostic marker (Priller et al. 2011). Overexpression of FoxM1 has been reported to strongly correlate with metastasis in prostate cancer (Chandran et al. 2007).

Genetic evidence of the cooperative interactions of the *PTEN* and *INK4A* tumor suppressor genes in the development of human histiocytic sarcoma (HS) is provided by Carrasco and coworkers who investigated the Pten and Ink-4A status in human HS, a rare human neoplasm with only a limited number of cases reported in the world literature (Carrasco et al. 2006). Immunohistochemical analyses of a panel of ten cases of human HS revealed a loss of immunoreactivity for either Pten or $p16^{Ink-4A}$ alone in four and five cases, respectively. Three of the ten cases showed concomitant lack of immunostaining for both Pten and $p16^{Ink-4A}$, while four of the ten cases were positive for both proteins. Most human HS cases demonstrated increased levels of pAKT in the histiocytic tumor cells compared to normal cells. These results highlight the general role of AKT phosphorylation in human HS pathogenesis suggesting that additional mechanisms besides Pten inactivation can lead to AKT activation (Carrasco et al. 2006), including changes in Src activity, Pten expression, PI3K activity, or receptor TK signaling (Lu et al. 2003; Nagata et al. 2004; Shekar et al. 2005; Wang et al. 2005b).

The implication of oxidative and nitrative stress in human sarcomagenesis is attributed, for instance, to the work of Fredika Robertson and colleagues on AIDS-related KS, the most prevalent AIDS-related cancer arising under a unique condition that is characterized by a combination of immunosuppression and immunostimulation (Shah et al. 2002; Restrepo and Ocazionez 2011).

According to Mallery et al. (2004), nitrative stress occurred in situ within lesions of AIDS-KS patients. Cultured AIDS-KS cells from these tumors were found to harbor impaired functional activity of the putative tumor suppressor MnSOD as a result of tyrosine nitration, implying a critical contribution of reactive oxygen and nitrogen species to AIDS-KS pathogenesis. Because the fundamental functions of MnSOD comprise, in addition to its function as tumor suppressor, its anti-oxidant capacity, the loss of the cytoprotective activity of MnSOD might facilitate malignant transformation (Mallery et al. 2004).

It is well known that osteopontin (OPN) plays an important role in tumor progression and that a high OPN expression level in several tumor entities correlates with poor prognosis in cancer patients. In STS, elevated OPN protein in serum as well as in tumor tissues correlates with clinical parameters and functions as an important negative prognostic factor (Bache et al. 2010). In female STS patients and those who received curative radiotherapy, high expression levels of *OPN* splice variants were determined as negative prognostic and predictive markers (Hahnel et al. 2012). An upregulation of certain *OPN* splice variants could also be demonstrated in MM peritoneum specimens compared to healthy controls (Ivanov et al. 2009). The putative role of OPN in human sarcomagenesis is further given by the observation that in 90 % of patients with highly aggressive glioblastoma, OPN is upregulated at both, the mRNA and protein level (Atai et al. 2011). Moreover, OPN protein expression was found to colocalize with neutrophils and macrophages, suggesting that OPN promotes migration of cancer cells as well as of leukocytes in tumors (Atai et al. 2011). Increased OPN serum levels were also found in asbestos-induced MM (Pass et al. 2005).

Among other cancers, miR-155 is upregulated in endometrial carcinosarcoma (ECS) which is known to undergo a true EMT. Castilla and collaborators analyzed the miRNA signatures associated to EMT in human ECS and determined their relationships with EMT markers and repressors of E-cadherin transcription (Castilla et al. 2011). This study clearly demonstrated that the loss of epithelial characteristics, including cadherin switching and the acquisition of a mesenchymal phenotype, was accompanied by changes in the profile of miRNA expression and an upregulation of all the E-cadherin repressors analyzed. On the one hand, members of the miR-200 family were downregulated in the mesenchymal part of the ECS as well as miR-23b and miR-29c involved in the inhibition of mesenchymal markers, and miR-203, involved in the inhibition of cell stemness. On the other hand, an upregulated expression of miR-155, miR-369-5p, miR-370, miR-450a, and miR-542-5p has been noted, thus confirming, at least in part, previous in vitro data on LS cell lines (Zhang et al. 2012). These data suggest that in human ECS, the interplay between transcriptional repressors of E-cadherin and miRNAs provides a link between EMT activation and the maintenance of stemness. In contrast, the group of Dirk Dittmer reported that multiple tumor suppressor miRNAs (miR-155, miR-220/221, let-7 family) are downregulated in KSHV-associated cancers, including KS and primary effusion lymphoma (PEL), whereas others (miR-143/145) are upregulated exclusively in KS tumors highlighting the impact of tumor suppressor miRNAs in oncogenic transformation and their clinical utility for tumor classification (O'Hara et al. 2009).

The role of the IGF system as one of the central players in the tumorigenesis of sarcomas has also been validated in humans. SS exhibits characteristic t(X;18) (p11.2;q11.2) translocations that result in enhanced transcription of the *IGF2* gene, hyperactivation of IGF-1R signaling, phosphorylation of AKT, and activation of p44/42 MAPK (Friedrichs et al. 2008). SS cell migration was found to depend on signals transmitted by the IGF-1R, rendering the IGF-1R a promising therapeutic target in SS. Together with the in vitro data of the same group, it can be postulated that IGF-1R obviously plays a central role in neoplastic transformation and metastasis in a number of cancers, and pathological alterations in the pathway may be particularly important in certain cancers including sarcoma. There is a wealth of evidence illustrating the central role of the PI3K/AKT/mTOR pathway in human sarcomagenesis. Abnormal activation of this pathway via several growth factor receptors triggers the development of various sarcomas (Vemulapalli et al. 2011). Hyperactivation of mTOR in humans can also result from *PTEN* inactivation, lack of the tumor suppressor kinase Lkb-1, and loss of inhibitory function of the tuberous sclerosis complex proteins (Hogendoorn et al. 2004; Wan and Helman 2007; Yang and Guan 2007).

It is well known that numerous TKs are crucially involved in sarcomagenesis. Understanding the mode of their activation may help to develop new targeted therapies. *EWS/FLI1* is the most common translocation found in ES tumors. The oncogene has been shown to transform cells by acting as a transcriptional factor to modulate a cohort of target genes including the Src TK *LYN* (Guan et al. 2008). Meanwhile, elevated Lyn kinase activity was demonstrated in numerous KS and glioblastoma patient samples (Prakash et al. 2005; Stettner et al. 2005), suggesting that Lyn activity plays a seminal role in promoting the malignant phenotype in these cancers and further supporting the consideration of Lyn as being a potential therapeutic target for the treatment of patients with these sarcoma subtypes. A characteristic translocation in alveolar soft part sarcoma (ASPS) results in a novel fusion of the *ASPSCR1* (previously designated *ASPL*) and *TFE3* genes (*ASPSCR1/TFE3*), leading to the formation of a functional transcription factor inducing unregulated transcription of TFE3-regulated genes (Lazar et al. 2007). In this study, ASPS biopsy specimen overexpressed a unique array of pro-angiogenic TFE3-regulated genes and proteins including midkine, Jag-1, and ANG. Elevated serum levels of ANG and VEGF can also be found in OS and ES patients (Kushlinskii et al. 2000). As KSHV infection upregulates ANG secretion in primary HMVEC-d cells (Sadagopan et al. 2009), ANG upregulation can be considered as a crucial player in inflammation-associated tumorigenesis of certain sarcomas.

11.6 Inhibitors of Inflammation for the Prevention and Treatment of Sarcoma

Several lines of evidence indicate that inflammation has been implicated in sarcomagenesis leading to the activation of the key transcription factors NF-κB, STAT-3, and HIF-1 involved in a complex inflammatory network. These factors regulate the expression of a broad panel of tumorigenic factors affecting proliferation, migration, survival, angiogenesis, invasiveness, metastasis as well as radio- and chemoresistance of tumors. Thus, inhibitors of pro-inflammatory pathways have enormous potential. Some of them have been evaluated in clinical trials (Table 11.3). Most of the chemopreventive agents have been found to suppress NF-κB and STAT-3 (Yu et al. 2009; Chaturvedi et al. 2011). Moreover, lifestyle-related agents derived from different sources, including fruits, legumes, vegetables, grains, spices, and exercise, are also able to inhibit NF-κB, including berberine, curcumin, resveratrol, and piperazine (Aggarwal and Gehlot 2009). With respect to sarcoma, the selective PGHS-2/NF-κB inhibitor celecoxib induced apoptosis and reduced β-catenin protein required for cell survival in the human osteosarcoma cell line MG-63 via downregulation of PI3K/AKT (Xia et al. 2010; Hönicke et al. 2012; Liu et al. 2012a). Genes downstream of STAT-3 (*BCL2*, *BIRC5*, and *CCND1*) were downregulated by celecoxib in RMS cells (Reed et al. 2011). Celecoxib prevented lung metastasis in a murine model of ES with no effect on tumor size or neovascularization (Gendy et al. 2011). Clinical trials with celecoxib for treatment of sarcomas are rare. In a phase II study, the combination of low-dose anti-angiogenic vinblastine/celecoxib with standard multiagent chemotherapy for patients with metastatic ES was found as being feasible with a better 24-month event-free survival for those with isolated pulmonary metastases (Felgenhauer et al. 2013). Interestingly, the anti-microbial fish peptide pardaxin exhibited anti-tumor activity toward murine FS by downregulating STAT-3 and p65/RelA (Wu et al. 2012). A clinical phase II study with metastatic cancer patients, evaluating the protective effects of the semisynthetic flavonoid 7-mono-O-(β-hydroxyethyl)-rutoside (monoHER) on doxorubicin-induced cardiotoxicity, revealed a 75 % response rate in STS patients (Bruynzeel et al. 2007), most probably via inhibition of NF-κB (Jacobs et al. 2011). Curcumin from *Curcuma longa* inhibited growth of LMS and OS cells via inhibition of the PI3K/AKT/mTOR and Notch-1 pathway, respectively (Wong et al. 2011; Li et al. 2012). It also induced apoptosis and cell cycle arrest in the ES cell line SK-NEP-1 highlighting its therapeutic potential (Singh et al. 2010). In human OS cells, green tea polyphenols induced apoptosis by decreasing amount and activity of NF-κB, downregulating Bcl-2 and upregulating Bax (Hafeez et al. 2006). Combinatorial treatment of human OS cells with the IL-1 inhibitor IL-1Ra (IL-1 receptor antagonist, anakinra™) and the green tea catechin epigallocatechin-3 gallate (EGCG) resulted in a more pronounced inhibition of IL-1-induced tumorigenic factors rendering this combined administration a promising approach as an adjuvant therapy in OS patients (Hönicke et al. 2012). However, clinical trials with anti-oxidants such as EGCG and curcumin are lacking due to their low bioavailability in humans.

Despite its history as a human teratogen, thalidomide is emerging as a putative treatment for cancer including sarcoma. Thalidomide has been shown to suppress urokinase receptor (uPAR) expression via NF-κB inhibition in CS cells in vitro and to decrease progressive tumor growth and ascites formation in an animal model of human ovarian cancer (Kobayashi et al. 2005). Thalidomide treatment of patients with refractory uterine carcinosarcoma prolonged progression-free survival at six months (McMeekin et al. 2012). However, based on results with thalidomide analogs, the activity was insufficient to strengthen additional investigations.

Novel approaches in limiting sarcoma growth include monoclonal antibodies directed against c-Kit (Edris et al. 2013) and IGFR (Tolcher et al. 2009; Olmos et al. 2010); Cdk inhibitors such as roscovitine (seliciclib; Lambert et al. 2008), flavopiridol (Luke et al. 2012), and dinacliclib (Fu et al. 2011); the EGFR inhibitor erlotinib (Abraham et al. 2011; Xie et al. 2011); and the c-Met inhibitor tivantinib (ARQ197; Wagner et al. 2012). In this context, several phase II trials with anti-IGFR-1 antibodies are currently being conducted. Preliminary data of treatment with cixutumumab in patients with advanced or metastatic STS and ES revealed clinical benefit being achieved in adipocytic sarcoma patients (Schoffski et al. 2011a).

A further option in the treatment of sarcomas represents targeting specific chromosomal translocations as can be found in about 30 % of sarcomas. For instance, clear cell sarcoma (CCS) is associated with a specific chromosomal translocation in most cases, t(12;22)(q13;q12), leading to the activation of c-Met critically involved in angiogenesis and invasiveness. A partial response in a CCS patient with the c-MET inhibitor tivantinib has recently been demonstrated in a phase II trial (Wagner et al. 2012).

Inhibition of molecular chaperones such as Hsp90 is supposed to lead to proteasomal degradation of activated c-Kit, thereby decreasing gene transcription and increasing apoptosis sensitivity. In refractory GIST, Hsp90 inhibition has been assumed to downregulate expression of activated c-Kit and shows in vitro activity against GIST. Based on these observations, several clinical phase I-III trials have been conducted to assess the efficacy of the Hsp90 inhibitor retaspimycin hydrochloride (IPI-504) with contradictory outcomes. Despite these less encouraging results, Hsp90 inhibitors continue to be evaluated in sarcoma patients. For instance, a phase II trial of BIIB021 led to objective responses in refractory GIST patients with mild-to-moderate adverse effects (Dickson et al. 2013). These data warrant further investigations with respect to the development of novel approaches as an adjuvant therapy in certain sarcomas.

11.7 Conclusions and Future Directions

Sarcomas represent a heterogeneous group of tumors with diverse pathologically and clinically overlapping features. It is a rarely curable disease, and their management requires a multidisciplinary team approach. Despite their low incidence in comparison with other tumor entities, the development of novel effective therapeutic approaches is essential. In the past years, an increasing number of new targets have been identified in the treatment of sarcomas forming the basis for the development of targeted therapies. In this context, targeting inflammatory pathways has emerged as a promising option. Although inflammation has been identified as one of the hallmarks of cancer, its contribution to sarcomagenesis has been overlooked for so long. The evidence described here clearly demonstrates that inflammatory pathways are critical targets in both, prevention and therapy of sarcomas. Despite the progress in characterizing the complex oncogenic pathways involved in sarcomagenesis, little progress had been made to translate these findings into effective clinical strategies. The identification of novel key effector molecules in sarcomagenesis has resulted in the development of an increasing number of drugs that need to be tested. As already discussed, aberrant activation of the Hh pathway has been shown in certain sarcomas such as RMS, OS, CS, and ES. Moreover, the aggressiveness of RMS and OS appears to be related to the Notch pathway (Tanaka et al. 2009; Roma et al. 2011). Clinical trials of the Hh inhibitor GDC-0449 and the Notch inhibitor RO4929097 as well as the histone deacetylase inhibitor vorinostat are ongoing with no results up to date.

Another protein related to sarcomas is anaplastic lymphoma kinase (ALK) upregulated in approximately half of inflammatory myofibroblastic tumor (IMT). A phase I trial reported a sustained partial response to the ALK inhibitor crizotinib (PF-02341066) in a patient with ALK-translocated IMT, suggesting a therapeutic strategy for genomically identified patients with this aggressive STS (Butrynski et al. 2010).

It should be kept in mind that cancers including sarcomas are caused by dysregulation of multiple pathways due to cross talk between the pathways. It therefore seems reasonable that agents interfering with multiple pathways are likely as being more effective. The best outcome might be achieved by combining agents with distinct modes of action. Natural products such as nutraceuticals are a reasonable choice due to their safety and ability to suppress multiple targets including NF-κB, STAT-3, and Notch. The strategy of inhibiting multiple pathways simultaneously in sarcoma is currently under investigation. Ongoing studies explore, for instance, the efficacy of a combination of targeted agents alone or together with chemotherapy. An intriguing novel approach in sarcoma treatment relates to oncolytic virotherapy. Preclinical data revealed that oncolytic viruses exhibit potent direct oncolytic effects against human sarcoma in vitro and in vivo (Li et al. 2011; He et al. 2012). As the knowledge of the molecular pathways involved in sarcomagenesis is increasing, individualized targeted therapies aiming to cure sarcomas are not illusive.

References

Abo A, Pick E, Hall A et al (1991) Activation of the NADPH oxidase involves the small GTP-binding protein p21rac1. Nature 353:668–670

Abraham J, Nelon LD, Kubicek CB et al (2011) Preclinical testing of erlotinib in a transgenic alveolar rhabdomyosarcoma mouse model. Sarcoma 2011:130484. doi:10.1155/2011/130484

Aggarwal BB, Gehlot P (2009) Inflammation and cancer: how friendly is the relationship for cancer patients? Curr Opin Pharmacol 9:351–369

Agulnik M (2012) New developments in mammalian target of rapamycin inhibitors for the treatment of sarcoma. Cancer 118:1486–1497

Agulnik M, Yarber JL, Okuno SH et al (2013) An open-label, multicenter, phase II study of bevacizumab for the treatment of angiosarcoma and epithelioid hemangioendotheliomas. Ann Oncol 24:257–263

Akimoto R, Pawankar R, Yagi T et al (2000) Acquired and congenital cholesteatoma: determination of tumor necrosis factor-alpha, intercellular adhesion molecule-1, interleukin-1-alpha and lymphocyte functional antigen-1 in the inflammatory process. ORL J Otorhinolaryngol Relat Spec 62:257–265

Alleyne CH Jr, He J, Yang J et al (1999) Analysis of cyclin dependent kinase inhibitors in malignant astrocytomas. Int J Oncol 14:1111–1116
Ancrile B, Lim KH, Counter CM (2007) Oncogenic Ras-induced secretion of IL6 is required for tumorigenesis. Genes Dev 21:1714–1719
Atai NA, Bansal M, Lo C et al (2011) Osteopontin is up-regulated and associated with neutrophil and macrophage infiltration in glioblastoma. Immunology 132:39–48
Baamonde A, Curto-Reyes V, Juarez L et al (2007) Antihyperalgesic effects induced by the IL-1 receptor antagonist anakinra and increased IL-1beta levels in inflamed and osteosarcoma-bearing mice. Life Sci 81:673–682
Bache M, Kappler M, Wichmann H et al (2010) Elevated tumor and serum levels of the hypoxia-associated protein osteopontin are associated with prognosis for soft tissue sarcoma patients. BMC Cancer 10:132. doi:10.1186/1471-2407-10-132
Bai Y, Li J, Fang B et al (2012) Phosphoproteomics identifies driver tyrosine kinases in sarcoma cell lines and tumors. Cancer Res 72:2501–2511
Barbie DA, Tamayo P, Boehm JS et al (2009) Systematic RNA interference reveals that oncogenic KRAS-driven cancers require TBK1. Nature 462:108–112
Bassuk AG, Leiden JM (1997) The role of Ets transcription factors in the development and function of the mammalian immune system. Adv Immunol 64:65–104
Bay JO, Ray-Coquard I, Fayette J et al (2006) Docetaxel and gemcitabine combination in 133 advanced soft-tissue sarcomas: a retrospective analysis. Int J Cancer 119:706–711
Benassi MS, Gamberi G, Magagnoli G et al (2001) Metalloproteinase expression and prognosis in soft tissue sarcomas. Ann Oncol 12:75–80
Bernstein-Molho R, Kollender Y, Issakov J et al (2012) Clinical activity of mTOR inhibition in combination with cyclophosphamide in the treatment of recurrent unresectable chondrosarcomas. Cancer Chemother Pharmacol 70:855–860
Birchmeier C, Birchmeier W, Gherardi E et al (2003) Met, metastasis, motility and more. Nat Rev Mol Cell Biol 4:915–925
Bond GL, Hu W, Bond EE et al (2004) A single nucleotide polymorphism in the MDM2 promoter attenuates the p53 tumor suppressor pathway and accelerates tumor formation in humans. Cell 119:591–602
Bruynzeel AM, Niessen HW, Bronzwaer JG et al (2007) The effect of monohydroxyethylrutoside on doxorubicin-induced cardiotoxicity in patients treated for metastatic cancer in a phase II study. Br J Cancer 97:1084–1089
Burningham Z, Hashibe M, Spector L et al (2012) The epidemiology of sarcoma. Clin Sarcoma Res 2:14. doi:10.1186/2045-3329-2-14
Butrynski JE, D'Adamo DR, Hornick JL et al (2010) Crizotinib in ALK-rearranged inflammatory myofibroblastic tumor. N Engl J Med 363:1727–1733
Butz H, Liko I, Czirjak S et al (2010) Down-regulation of Wee1 kinase by a specific subset of microRNA in human sporadic pituitary adenomas. J Clin Endocrinol Metab 95:E181–E191
Calvert GT, Randall RL, Jones KB et al (2012) At-risk populations for osteosarcoma: the syndromes and beyond. Sarcoma 2012:152382. doi:10.1155/2012/152382
Carmody Soni EE, Miller BJ, Scarborough MT et al (2011) Cyclooxygenase-2 expression is not associated with clinical outcome in synovial sarcoma. Oncol Rep 26:1513–1517
Carrasco DR, Fenton T, Sukhdeo K et al (2006) The PTEN and INK4A/ARF tumor suppressors maintain myelolymphoid homeostasis and cooperate to constrain histiocytic sarcoma development in humans. Cancer Cell 9:379–390
Castilla MA, Moreno-Bueno G, Romero-Perez L et al (2011) Micro-RNA signature of the epithelial-mesenchymal transition in endometrial carcinosarcoma. J Pathol 223:72–80
Castro-Gamero AM, Borges KS, da Silva Silveira V et al (2012) Inhibition of nuclear factor-kappaB by dehydroxymethylepoxyquinomicin induces schedule-dependent chemosensitivity to anticancer drugs and enhances chemoinduced apoptosis in osteosarcoma cells. Anticancer Drugs 23:638–650
Cen L, Hsieh FC, Lin HJ et al (2007) PDK-1/AKT pathway as a novel therapeutic target in rhabdomyosarcoma cells using OSU-03012 compound. Br J Cancer 97:785–791

Chandran UR, Ma C, Dhir R et al (2007) Gene expression profiles of prostate cancer reveal involvement of multiple molecular pathways in the metastatic process. BMC Cancer 7:64. doi:10.1186/1471-2407-7-64

Chang PL, Cao M, Hicks P (2003) Osteopontin induction is required for tumor promoter-induced transformation of preneoplastic mouse cells. Carcinogenesis 24:1749–1758

Chaturvedi MM, Sung B, Yadav VR et al (2011) NF-κB addiction and its role in cancer: 'one size does not fit all'. Oncogene 30:1615–1630

Chawla SP, Staddon AP, Baker LH et al (2012) Phase II study of the mammalian target of rapamycin inhibitor ridaforolimus in patients with advanced bone and soft tissue sarcomas. J Clin Oncol 30:78–84

Chen TC, Hinton DR, Apuzzo ML et al (1993) Differential effects of tumor necrosis factor-alpha on proliferation, cell surface antigen expression, and cytokine interactions in malignant gliomas. Neurosurgery 32:85–94

Chen Y, Takita J, Mizuguchi M et al (2007) Mutation and expression analyses of the MET and CDKN2A genes in rhabdomyosarcoma with emphasis on MET overexpression. Genes Chromosom Cancer 46:348–358

Chen YJ, Wei YY, Chen HT et al (2009) Osteopontin increases migration and MMP-9 up-regulation via alphavbeta3 integrin, FAK, ERK, and NF-kappaB-dependent pathway in human chondrosarcoma cells. J Cell Physiol 221:98–108

Chien Y, Kim S, Bumeister R et al (2006) RalB GTPase-mediated activation of the IkappaB family kinase TBK1 couples innate immune signaling to tumor cell survival. Cell 127:157–170

Choi JK, Choi BH, Ha Y et al (2007) Signal transduction pathways of GM-CSF in neural cell lines. Neurosci Lett 420:217–222

Christensen L, Joo J, Lee S et al (2013) FOXM1 Is an oncogenic mediator in Ewing sarcoma. PLoS ONE 8:e54556

Chugh R, Griffith KA, Brockstein B et al (2012) Phase I study of doxorubicin (D) plus anti-insulin-like growth factor 1 receptor (IGF-1R) antibody cixutumumab (IMC-A12) in advanced soft tissue sarcoma (STS). J Clin Oncol 30:10028

Colotta F, Allavena P, Sica A et al (2009) Cancer-related inflammation, the seventh hallmark of cancer: links to genetic instability. Carcinogenesis 30:1073–1081

Constam DB, Philipp J, Malipiero UV et al (1992) Differential expression of transforming growth factor-beta 1, -beta 2, and -beta 3 by glioblastoma cells, astrocytes, and microglia. J Immunol 148:1404–1410

Cordon-Cardo C, Latres E, Drobnjak M et al (1994) Molecular abnormalities of mdm2 and p53 genes in adult soft tissue sarcomas. Cancer Res 54:794–799

Cortes J, Montero AJ, Gluck S (2012) Eribulin mesylate, a novel microtubule inhibitor in the treatment of breast cancer. Cancer Treat Rev 38:143–151

Cortes J, O'Shaughnessy J, Loesch D et al (2011) Eribulin monotherapy versus treatment of physician's choice in patients with metastatic breast cancer (EMBRACE): a phase 3 open-label randomised study. Lancet 377:914–923

Crago AM, Singer S (2011) Clinical and molecular approaches to well differentiated and dedifferentiated liposarcoma. Curr Opin Oncol 23:373–378

Curran CS, Evans MD, Bertics PJ (2011) GM-CSF production by glioblastoma cells has a functional role in eosinophil survival, activation, and growth factor production for enhanced tumor cell proliferation. J Immunol 187:1254–1263

D'Adamo DR, Anderson SE, Albritton K et al (2005) Phase II study of doxorubicin and bevacizumab for patients with metastatic soft-tissue sarcomas. J Clin Oncol 23:7135–7142

Das P, Kotilingam D, Korchin B et al (2007) High prevalence of p53 exon 4 mutations in soft tissue sarcoma. Cancer 109:2323–2333

Datta SR, Brunet A, Greenberg ME (1999) Cellular survival: a play in three Akts. Genes Dev 13:2905–2927

Davis AM, O'Sullivan B, Turcotte R et al (2005) Late radiation morbidity following randomization to preoperative versus postoperative radiotherapy in extremity soft tissue sarcoma. Radiother Oncol 75:48–53

Debiec-Rychter M, Dumez H, Judson I et al (2004) Use of c-KIT/PDGFRA mutational analysis to predict the clinical response to imatinib in patients with advanced gastrointestinal stromal tumours entered on phase I and II studies of the EORTC Soft Tissue and Bone Sarcoma Group. Eur J Cancer 40:689–695

Demetri GD, Chawla SP, von Mehren M et al (2009a) Efficacy and safety of trabectedin in patients with advanced or metastatic liposarcoma or leiomyosarcoma after failure of prior anthracyclines and ifosfamide: results of a randomized phase II study of two different schedules. J Clin Oncol 27:4188–4196

Demetri GD, Heinrich MC, Fletcher JA et al (2009b) Molecular target modulation, imaging, and clinical evaluation of gastrointestinal stromal tumor patients treated with sunitinib malate after imatinib failure. Clin Cancer Res 15:5902–5909

Demetri GD, von Mehren M, Blanke CD et al (2002) Efficacy and safety of imatinib mesylate in advanced gastrointestinal stromal tumors. N Engl J Med 347:472–480

Deng X, Ewton DZ, Friedman E (2009) Mirk/Dyrk1B maintains the viability of quiescent pancreatic cancer cells by reducing levels of reactive oxygen species. Cancer Res 69:3317–3324

Dickson MA, Okuno SH, Keohan ML et al (2013) Phase II study of the HSP90-inhibitor BIIB021 in gastrointestinal stromal tumors. Ann Oncol 24:252–257

Ding Y, Boguslawski EA, Berghuis BD et al (2008) Mitogen-activated protein kinase kinase signaling promotes growth and vascularization of fibrosarcoma. Mol Cancer Ther 7:648–658

Dong P, Kaneuchi M, Watari H et al (2011) MicroRNA-194 inhibits epithelial to mesenchymal transition of endometrial cancer cells by targeting oncogene BMI-1. Mol Cancer 10:99. doi:10.1186/1476-4598-10-99

Douglas JL, Gustin JK, Moses AV et al (2010) Kaposi sarcoma pathogenesis: a triad of viral infection, oncogenesis and chronic inflammation. Transl Biomed 1:pii 172

Downward J (2009) Cancer: a tumour gene's fatal flaws. Nature 462:44–45

Edris B, Willingham SB, Weiskopf K et al (2013) Anti-KIT monoclonal antibody inhibits imatinib-resistant gastrointestinal stromal tumor growth. Proc Natl Acad Sci USA 110:3501–3506

Efeyan A, Sabatini DM (2010) mTOR and cancer: many loops in one pathway. Curr Opin Cell Biol 22:169–176

Ellis SR, Gleizes PE (2011) Diamond Blackfan anemia: ribosomal proteins going rogue. Semin Hematol 48:89–96

Enders GH (2010) Gauchos and ochos: a Wee1-Cdk tango regulating mitotic entry. Cell Div 5:12. doi:10.1186/1747-1028-5-12

Endo M, Yamamoto H, Setsu N et al (2013) Prognostic Significance of AKT/mTOR and MAPK Pathways and Antitumor Effect of mTOR Inhibitor in NF1-Related and Sporadic Malignant Peripheral Nerve Sheath Tumors. Clin Cancer Res 19:450–461

Engin F, Bertin T, Ma O et al (2009) Notch signaling contributes to the pathogenesis of human osteosarcomas. Hum Mol Genet 18:1464–1470

Fasanaro P, Capogrossi MC, Martelli F (2010) Regulation of the endothelial cell cycle by the ubiquitin-proteasome system. Cardiovasc Res 85:272–280

Fata F, O'Reilly E, Ilson D et al (1999) Paclitaxel in the treatment of patients with angiosarcoma of the scalp or face. Cancer 86:2034–2037

Feldman AL, Pak H, Yang JC et al (2001) Serum endostatin levels are elevated in patients with soft tissue sarcoma. Cancer 91:1525–1529

Felgenhauer JL, Nieder ML, Krailo MD et al (2013) A pilot study of low-dose anti-angiogenic chemotherapy in combination with standard multiagent chemotherapy for patients with newly diagnosed metastatic Ewing sarcoma family of tumors: A Children's Oncology Group (COG) Phase II study NCT00061893. Pediatr Blood Cancer 60:409–414

Fernandez M, Pino AM, Figueroa P et al (2010) The increased expression of receptor activator of nuclear-kappaB ligand (RANKL) of multiple myeloma bone marrow stromal cells is inhibited by the bisphosphonate ibandronate. J Cell Biochem 111:130–137

Fernandez-Medarde A, Santos E (2011) Ras in cancer and developmental diseases. Genes Cancer 2:344–358
Ferrari A, Sultan I, Huang TT et al (2011) Soft tissue sarcoma across the age spectrum: a population-based study from the surveillance epidemiology and end results database. Pediatr Blood Cancer 57:943–949
Fletcher O, Easton D, Anderson K et al (2004) Lifetime risks of common cancers among retinoblastoma survivors. J Natl Cancer Inst 96:357–363
Fontana A, Hengartner H, de Tribolet N et al (1984) Glioblastoma cells release interleukin 1 and factors inhibiting interleukin 2-mediated effects. J Immunol 132:1837–1844
Forbes SA, Bindal N, Bamford S et al (2011) COSMIC: mining complete cancer genomes in the Catalogue of Somatic Mutations in Cancer. Nucleic Acids Res 39:D945–D950
Foreman KE, Wrone-Smith T, Boise LH et al (1996) Kaposi's sarcoma tumor cells preferentially express Bcl-xL. Am J Pathol 149:795–803
Frei K, Piani D, Malipiero UV et al (1992) Granulocyte-macrophage colony-stimulating factor (GM-CSF) production by glioblastoma cells. Despite the presence of inducing signals GM-CSF is not expressed in vivo. J Immunol 148:3140–3146
Friedman E (2011) The role of mirk kinase in sarcomas. Sarcoma 2011:260757. doi:10.1155/2011/260757
Friedrichs N, Kuchler J, Endl E et al (2008) Insulin-like growth factor-1 receptor acts as a growth regulator in synovial sarcoma. J Pathol 216:428–439
Fu W, Ma L, Chu B et al (2011) The cyclin-dependent kinase inhibitor SCH 727965 (dinacliclib) induces the apoptosis of osteosarcoma cells. Mol Cancer Ther 10:1018–1027
Fukuda T, Yamaguchi T, Yamaki T et al (2001) Ovarian fibrosarcoma producing multiple cytokines. Pathol Int 51:739–743
Fuller CK, Charlson JA, Dankle SK et al (2010) Dramatic improvement of inoperable angiosarcoma with combination paclitaxel and bevacizumab chemotherapy. J Am Acad Dermatol 63:e83–e84
Garcia K, Stumpff J, Duncan T et al (2009) Tyrosines in the kinesin-5 head domain are necessary for phosphorylation by Wee1 and for mitotic spindle integrity. Curr Biol 19:1670–1676
Garcia-Carbonero R, Supko JG, Manola J et al (2004) Phase II and pharmacokinetic study of ecteinascidin 743 in patients with progressive sarcomas of soft tissues refractory to chemotherapy. J Clin Oncol 22:1480–1490
Gardner K, Judson I, Leahy M et al (2009) Activity of cediranib, a highly potent and selective VEGF signaling inhibitor, in alveolar soft part sarcoma. J Clin Oncol 27:10523. http://meeting.ascopubs.org/cgi/content/abstract/27/15S/10523?sid=cbb771a3-21c0-4634-955b-60ff724c1f3a
Gendy AS, Lipskar A, Glick RD et al (2011) Selective inhibition of cyclooxygenase-2 suppresses metastatic disease without affecting primary tumor growth in a murine model of Ewing sarcoma. J Pediatr Surg 46:108–114
Gennatas C, Michalaki V, Kairi PV et al (2012) Successful treatment with the mTOR inhibitor everolimus in a patient with perivascular epithelioid cell tumor. World J Surg Oncol 10:181
George S, Blay JY, Casali PG et al (2009) Clinical evaluation of continuous daily dosing of sunitinib malate in patients with advanced gastrointestinal stromal tumour after imatinib failure. Eur J Cancer 45:1959–1968
Gisselsson D, Palsson E, Hoglund M et al (2002) Differentially amplified chromosome 12 sequences in low- and high-grade osteosarcoma. Genes Chromosom Cancer 33:133–140
Giuffrida AY, Burgueno JE, Koniaris LG et al (2009) Chondrosarcoma in the United States (1973–2003): an analysis of 2,890 cases from the SEER database. J Bone Joint Surg Am 91:1063–1072
Grignani G, Palmerini E, Dileo P et al (2012) A phase II trial of sorafenib in relapsed and unresectable high-grade osteosarcoma after failure of standard multimodal therapy: an Italian Sarcoma Group study. Ann Oncol 23:508–516
Grimer R, Athanasou N, Gerrand C et al (2010a) UK guidelines for the management of bone sarcomas. Sarcoma 2010:317462. doi:10.1155/2010/317462

Grimer R, Judson I, Peake D et al (2010b) Guidelines for the management of soft tissue sarcomas. Sarcoma 2010:506182. doi:10.1155/2010/506182
Gronchi A, Blay JY, Trent JC (2010) The role of high-dose imatinib in the management of patients with gastrointestinal stromal tumor. Cancer 116:1847–1858
Gronchi A, Bui BN, Bonvalot S et al (2012) Phase II clinical trial of neoadjuvant trabectedin in patients with advanced localized myxoid liposarcoma. Ann Oncol 23:771–776
Guan H, Zhou Z, Gallick GE et al (2008) Targeting Lyn inhibits tumor growth and metastasis in Ewing's sarcoma. Mol Cancer Ther 7:1807–1816
Guertin DA, Sabatini DM (2005) An expanding role for mTOR in cancer. Trends Mol Med 11:353–361
Gupta AA, Yao X, Verma S et al (2013) Systematic chemotherapy for inoperable, locally advanced, recurrent, or metastatic uterine leiomyosarcoma: a systematic review. Clin Oncol (R Coll Radiol) 25:346–355
Hacker H, Karin M (2006) Regulation and function of IKK and IKK-related kinases. Sci STKE 2006:re13
Hafeez BB, Ahmed S, Wang N et al (2006) Green tea polyphenols-induced apoptosis in human osteosarcoma SAOS-2 cells involves a caspase-dependent mechanism with downregulation of nuclear factor-kappaB. Toxicol Appl Pharmacol 216:11–19
Hahnel A, Wichmann H, Greither T et al (2012) Prognostic impact of mRNA levels of osteopontin splice variants in soft tissue sarcoma patients. BMC Cancer 12:131. doi:10.1186/1471-2407-12-131
Hansen MF, Koufos A, Gallie BL et al (1985) Osteosarcoma and retinoblastoma: a shared chromosomal mechanism revealing recessive predisposition. Proc Natl Acad Sci USA 82:6216–6220
Harbitz F (1924) Chronische und akute Entzündungen als Ursache für Sarkom. Acta Pathol Microbiol Scand 1:438–447
Harbour JW (2001) Molecular basis of low-penetrance retinoblastoma. Arch Ophthalmol 119:1699–1704
Hashimoto O, Shinkawa M, Torimura T et al (2006) Cell cycle regulation by the Wee1 inhibitor PD0166285, pyrido [2,3-d] pyimidine, in the B16 mouse melanoma cell line. BMC Cancer 6:292. doi:10.1186/1471-2407-6-292
Hassan SE, Bekarev M, Kim MY et al (2012) Cell surface receptor expression patterns in osteosarcoma. Cancer 118:740–749
Haupt Y, Harris AW, Adams JM (1992) Retroviral infection accelerates T lymphomagenesis in E mu-N-ras transgenic mice by activating c-myc or N-myc. Oncogene 7:981–986
He S, Li P, Chen CH et al (2012) Effective oncolytic vaccinia therapy for human sarcomas. J Surg Res 175:e53–e60
Heinrich MC, Corless CL, Demetri GD et al (2003a) Kinase mutations and imatinib response in patients with metastatic gastrointestinal stromal tumor. J Clin Oncol 21:4342–4349
Heinrich MC, Corless CL, Duensing A et al (2003b) PDGFRA activating mutations in gastrointestinal stromal tumors. Science 299:708–710
Heinrich MC, Maki RG, Corless CL et al (2008) Primary and secondary kinase genotypes correlate with the biological and clinical activity of sunitinib in imatinib-resistant gastrointestinal stromal tumor. J Clin Oncol 26:5352–5359
Heinsohn S, Evermann U, Zur SU et al (2007) Determination of the prognostic value of loss of heterozygosity at the retinoblastoma gene in osteosarcoma. Int J Oncol 30:1205–1214
Hensley ML, Blessing JA, Degeest K et al (2008a) Fixed-dose rate gemcitabine plus docetaxel as second-line therapy for metastatic uterine leiomyosarcoma: a Gynecologic Oncology Group phase II study. Gynecol Oncol 109:323–328
Hensley ML, Blessing JA, Mannel R et al (2008b) Fixed-dose rate gemcitabine plus docetaxel as first-line therapy for metastatic uterine leiomyosarcoma: a Gynecologic Oncology Group phase II trial. Gynecol Oncol 109:329–334
Hernando E, Charytonowicz E, Dudas ME et al (2007) The AKT-mTOR pathway plays a critical role in the development of leiomyosarcomas. Nat Med 13:748–753

Hettmer S, Liu J, Miller CM et al (2011) Sarcomas induced in discrete subsets of prospectively isolated skeletal muscle cells. Proc Natl Acad Sci USA 108:20002–20007
Hillegass JM, Shukla A, Lathrop SA et al (2010a) Inflammation precedes the development of human malignant mesotheliomas in a SCID mouse xenograft model. Ann NY Acad Sci 1203:7–14
Hillegass JM, Shukla A, MacPherson MB et al (2010b) Utilization of gene profiling and proteomics to determine mineral pathogenicity in a human mesothelial cell line (LP9/TERT-1). J Toxicol Environ Health A 73:423–436
Hirakawa N, Naka T, Yamamoto I et al (1996) Overexpression of bcl-2 protein in synovial sarcoma: a comparative study of other soft tissue spindle cell sarcomas and an additional analysis by fluorescence in situ hybridization. Hum Pathol 27:1060–1065
Hirama M, Takahashi F, Takahashi K et al (2003) Osteopontin overproduced by tumor cells acts as a potent angiogenic factor contributing to tumor growth. Cancer Lett 198:107–117
Hiromura K, Pippin JW, Fero ML et al (1999) Modulation of apoptosis by the cyclin-dependent kinase inhibitor p27(Kip1). J Clin Invest 103:597–604
Hisaoka M, Matsuyama A, Nagao Y et al (2011) Identification of altered MicroRNA expression patterns in synovial sarcoma. Genes Chromosom Cancer 50:137–145
Ho AL, Vasudeva SD, Lae M et al (2012) PDGF receptor alpha is an alternative mediator of rapamycin-induced Akt activation: implications for combination targeted therapy of synovial sarcoma. Cancer Res 72:4515–4525
Hogendoorn PC, Collin F, Daugaard S et al (2004) Changing concepts in the pathological basis of soft tissue and bone sarcoma treatment. Eur J Cancer 40:1644–1654
Hoki Y, Hiraku Y, Ma N et al (2007a) iNOS-dependent DNA damage in patients with malignant fibrous histiocytoma in relation to prognosis. Cancer Sci 98:163–168
Hoki Y, Murata M, Hiraku Y et al (2007b) 8-Nitroguanine as a potential biomarker for progression of malignant fibrous histiocytoma, a model of inflammation-related cancer. Oncol Rep 18:1165–1169
Hönicke AS, Ender SA, Radons J (2012) Combined administration of EGCG and IL-1 receptor antagonist efficiently downregulates IL-1-induced tumorigenic factors in U-2 OS human osteosarcoma cells. Int J Oncol 41:753–758
Honma M, Higuchi O, Shirakata M et al (2006) Dok-3 sequesters Grb2 and inhibits the Ras-Erk pathway downstream of protein-tyrosine kinases. Genes Cells 11:143–151
Houghton PJ, Morton CL, Kolb EA et al (2008) Initial testing (stage 1) of the mTOR inhibitor rapamycin by the pediatric preclinical testing program. Pediatr Blood Cancer 50:799–805
Huang HY, Kang HY, Li CF et al (2006) Skp2 overexpression is highly representative of intrinsic biological aggressiveness and independently associated with poor prognosis in primary localized myxofibrosarcomas. Clin Cancer Res 12:487–498
Huang X, Choi JK, Park SR et al (2007) GM-CSF inhibits apoptosis of neural cells via regulating the expression of apoptosis-related proteins. Neurosci Res 58:50–57
Hussain SP, Harris CC (2007) Inflammation and cancer: an ancient link with novel potentials. Int J Cancer 121:2373–2380
Ishii E, Ohga S, Aoki T et al (1991) Prognosis of children with virus-associated hemophagocytic syndrome and malignant histiocytosis: correlation with levels of serum interleukin-1 and tumor necrosis factor. Acta Haematol 85:93–99
Italiano A, Delcambre C, Hostein I et al (2010) Treatment with the mTOR inhibitor temsirolimus in patients with malignant PEComa. Ann Oncol 21:1135–1137
Ivanov SV, Ivanova AV, Goparaju CM et al (2009) Tumorigenic properties of alternative osteopontin isoforms in mesothelioma. Biochem Biophys Res Commun 382:514–518
Iwasaki H, Nabeshima K, Nishio J et al (2009) Pathology of soft-tissue tumors: daily diagnosis, molecular cytogenetics and experimental approach. Pathol Int 59:501–521
Jackson AL, Loeb LA (2001) The contribution of endogenous sources of DNA damage to the multiple mutations in cancer. Mutat Res 477:7–21
Jacobs H, Bast A, Peters GJ et al (2011) The semisynthetic flavonoid monoHER sensitises human soft tissue sarcoma cells to doxorubicin-induced apoptosis via inhibition of nuclear factor-kappaB. Br J Cancer 104:437–440

Jin K, Park S, Ewton DZ et al (2007) The survival kinase Mirk/Dyrk1B is a downstream effector of oncogenic K-ras in pancreatic cancer. Cancer Res 67:7247–7255

Juergens H, Daw NC, Geoerger B et al (2011) Preliminary efficacy of the anti-insulin-like growth factor type 1 receptor antibody figitumumab in patients with refractory Ewing sarcoma. J Clin Oncol 29:4534–4540

Kalinichenko VV, Major ML, Wang X et al (2004) Foxm1b transcription factor is essential for development of hepatocellular carcinomas and is negatively regulated by the p19ARF tumor suppressor. Genes Dev 18:830–850

Kansara M, Thomas DM (2007) Molecular pathogenesis of osteosarcoma. DNA Cell Biol 26:1–18

Kasper B, Ouali M, van Glabbeke M et al (2013) Prognostic factors in adolescents and young adults (AYA) with high risk soft tissue sarcoma (STS) treated by adjuvant chemotherapy: a study based on pooled European Organisation for Research and Treatment of Cancer (EORTC) clinical trials 62771 and 62931. Eur J Cancer 49:449–456

Keller SA, Hernandez-Hopkins D, Vider J et al (2006) NF-kappaB is essential for the progression of KSHV- and EBV-infected lymphomas in vivo. Blood 107:3295–3302

Kirla RM, Haapasalo HK, Kalimo H et al (2003) Low expression of p27 indicates a poor prognosis in patients with high-grade astrocytomas. Cancer 97:644–648

Kirsch DG, Dinulescu DM, Miller JB et al (2007) A spatially and temporally restricted mouse model of soft tissue sarcoma. Nat Med 13:992–997

Kishimoto K, Liu S, Tsuji T et al (2005) Endogenous angiogenin in endothelial cells is a general requirement for cell proliferation and angiogenesis. Oncogene 24:445–456

Knudson AG Jr (1971) Mutation and cancer: statistical study of retinoblastoma. Proc Natl Acad Sci USA 68:820–823

Kobayashi H, Yagyu T, Kondo T et al (2005) Suppression of urokinase receptor expression by thalidomide is associated with inhibition of nuclear factor kappaB activation and subsequently suppressed ovarian cancer dissemination. Cancer Res 65:10464–10471

Koch M, Nielsen GP, Yoon SS (2008) Malignant tumors of blood vessels: angiosarcomas, hemangioendotheliomas, and hemangioperictyomas. J Surg Oncol 97:321–329

Koga K, Nabeshima K, Aoki M et al (2007) Emmprin in epithelioid sarcoma: expression in tumor cell membrane and stimulation of MMP-2 production in tumor-associated fibroblasts. Int J Cancer 120:761–768

Koga K, Nabeshima K, Nishimura N et al (2005) Microvessel density and HIF-1alpha expression correlate with malignant potential in fibrohistiocytic tumors. Eur J Dermatol 15:465–469

Kohashi K, Oda Y, Yamamoto H et al (2008) Alterations of RB1 gene in embryonal and alveolar rhabdomyosarcoma: special reference to utility of pRB immunoreactivity in differential diagnosis of rhabdomyosarcoma subtype. J Cancer Res Clin Oncol 134:1097–1103

Koshiji M, To KK, Hammer S et al (2005) HIF-1α induces genetic instability by transcriptionally downregulating MutSalpha expression. Mol Cell 17:793–803

Kraljevic Pavelic S, Sedic M, Bosnjak H et al (2011) Metastasis: new perspectives on an old problem. Mol Cancer 10:22. doi:10.1186/1476-4598-10-22

Kuhnen C, Herter P, Muller O et al (2000) Beta-catenin in soft tissue sarcomas: expression is related to proliferative activity in high-grade sarcomas. Mod Pathol 13:1005–1013

Kummar S, Strassberger A, Monks A et al (2011) An evaluation of cediranib as new agent for alveolar soft part sarcoma (ASPS). J Clin Oncol 29:10001. http://meeting.ascopubs.org/cgi/content/abstract/29/15_suppl/10001?sid=629fd0d8-f8f1-4905-816e-134f8d1ad715

Kundu JK, Surh YJ (2008) Inflammation: gearing the journey to cancer. Mutat Res 659:15–30

Kundu JK, Surh YJ (2012) Emerging avenues linking inflammation and cancer. Free Radic Biol Med 52:2013–2037

Kushlinskii NE, Babkina IV, Solov'ev YN et al (2000) Vascular endothelium growth factor and angiogenin in the serum of patients with osteosarcoma and Ewing's tumor. Bull Exp Biol Med 130:691–693

Ladanyi M, Cha C, Lewis R et al (1993) MDM2 gene amplification in metastatic osteosarcoma. Cancer Res 53:16–18

Ladetto M, Vallet S, Trojan A et al (2005) Cyclooxygenase-2 (COX-2) is frequently expressed in multiple myeloma and is an independent predictor of poor outcome. Blood 105:4784–4791

Lahat G, Lazar A, Lev D (2008) Sarcoma epidemiology and etiology: potential environmental and genetic factors. Surg Clin North Am 88:451–481
Lahat G, Zhang P, Zhu QS et al (2011) The expression of c-Met pathway components in unclassified pleomorphic sarcoma/malignant fibrous histiocytoma (UPS/MFH): a tissue microarray study. Histopathology 59:556–561
Lambert LA, Qiao N, Hunt KK et al (2008) Autophagy: a novel mechanism of synergistic cytotoxicity between doxorubicin and roscovitine in a sarcoma model. Cancer Res 68:7966–7974
Langenau DM, Keefe MD, Storer NY et al (2007) Effects of RAS on the genesis of embryonal rhabdomyosarcoma. Genes Dev 21:1382–1395
Laoukili J, Kooistra MR, Bras A et al (2005) FoxM1 is required for execution of the mitotic programme and chromosome stability. Nat Cell Biol 7:126–136
Launonen V, Vierimaa O, Kiuru M et al (2001) Inherited susceptibility to uterine leiomyomas and renal cell cancer. Proc Natl Acad Sci USA 98:3387–3392
Lazar AJ, Das P, Tuvin D et al (2007) Angiogenesis-promoting gene patterns in alveolar soft part sarcoma. Clin Cancer Res 13:7314–7321
Le Cesne A, Ray-Coquard I, Bui BN et al (2010) Discontinuation of imatinib in patients with advanced gastrointestinal stromal tumours after 3 years of treatment: an open-label multicentre randomised phase 3 trial. Lancet Oncol 11:942–949
Leach FS, Tokino T, Meltzer P et al (1993) p53 Mutation and MDM2 amplification in human soft tissue sarcomas. Cancer Res 53:2231–2234
Lee HJ, Kim SA, Lee HJ et al (2010) Paeonol oxime inhibits bFGF-induced angiogenesis and reduces VEGF levels in fibrosarcoma cells. PLoS ONE 5:e12358
Lee J, Ku T, Yu H et al (2012) Blockade of VEGF-A suppresses tumor growth via inhibition of autocrine signaling through FAK and AKT. Cancer Lett 318:221–225
Lee J, Lee J, Yu H et al (2011) Differential dependency of human cancer cells on vascular endothelial growth factor-mediated autocrine growth and survival. Cancer Lett 309:145–150
Lee JC, Simon PL, Young PR (1989) Constitutive and PMA-induced interleukin-1 production by the human astrocytoma cell line T24. Cell Immunol 118:298–311
Lee SH, McCormick F (2005) Downregulation of Skp2 and p27/Kip1 synergistically induces apoptosis in T98G glioblastoma cells. J Mol Med (Berl) 83:296–307
Lehtonen HJ, Kiuru M, Ylisaukko-oja SK et al (2006) Increased risk of cancer in patients with fumarate hydratase germline mutation. J Med Genet 43:523–526
Leidner RS, Aboulafia DM (2005) Recrudescent Kaposi's sarcoma after initiation of HAART: a manifestation of immune reconstitution syndrome. AIDS Patient Care STDS 19:635–644
Lemay S, Davidson D, Latour S et al (2000) Dok-3, a novel adapter molecule involved in the negative regulation of immunoreceptor signaling. Mol Cell Biol 20:2743–2754
Lewis AM, Varghese S, Xu H et al (2006) Interleukin-1 and cancer progression: the emerging role of interleukin-1 receptor antagonist as a novel therapeutic agent in cancer treatment. J Transl Med 4:48. doi:10.1186/1479-5876-4-48
Li A, Dubey S, Varney ML et al (2003) IL-8 directly enhanced endothelial cell survival, proliferation, and matrix metalloproteinases production and regulated angiogenesis. J Immunol 170:3369–3376
Li FP, Fraumeni JF Jr (1969) Soft-tissue sarcomas, breast cancer, and other neoplasms. A familial syndrome? Ann Intern Med 71:747–752
Li G, Kawashima H, Ogose A et al (2011) Efficient virotherapy for osteosarcoma by telomerase-specific oncolytic adenovirus. J Cancer Res Clin Oncol 137:1037–1051
Li Y, Zhang J, Ma D et al (2012) Curcumin inhibits proliferation and invasion of osteosarcoma cells through inactivation of Notch-1 signaling. FEBS J 279:2247–2259
Lin WW, Karin M (2007) A cytokine-mediated link between innate immunity, inflammation, and cancer. J Clin Invest 117:1175–1183
Lipton JM, Federman N, Khabbaze Y et al (2001) Osteogenic sarcoma associated with Diamond-Blackfan anemia: a report from the Diamond-Blackfan Anemia Registry. J Pediatr Hematol Oncol 23:39–44
Liu B, Qu L, Yang Z et al (2012a) Cyclooxygenase-2 inhibitors induce anoikis in osteosarcoma via PI3K/Akt pathway. Med Hypotheses 79:98–100

Liu J, Hettmer S, Milsom MD et al (2012b) Induction of histiocytic sarcoma in mouse skeletal muscle. PLoS ONE 7:e44044
Liu M, Dai B, Kang SH et al (2006) FoxM1B is overexpressed in human glioblastomas and critically regulates the tumorigenicity of glioma cells. Cancer Res 66:3593–3602
Liu SJ, Zhang DQ, Sui XM et al (2008) The inhibition of in vivo tumorigenesis of osteosarcoma (OS)-732 cells by antisense human osteopontin RNA. Cell Mol Biol Lett 13:11–19
Liu X, Newton RC, Scherle PA (2010) Developing c-MET pathway inhibitors for cancer therapy: progress and challenges. Trends Mol Med 16:37–45
Longhi A, Benassi MS, Molendini L et al (2001) Osteosarcoma in blood relatives. Oncol Rep 8:131–136
Lu Y, Yu Q, Liu JH et al (2003) Src family protein-tyrosine kinases alter the function of PTEN to regulate phosphatidylinositol 3-kinase/AKT cascades. J Biol Chem 278:40057–40066
Luke JJ, D'Adamo DR, Dickson MA et al (2012) The cyclin-dependent kinase inhibitor flavopiridol potentiates doxorubicin efficacy in advanced sarcomas: preclinical investigations and results of a phase I dose-escalation clinical trial. Clin Cancer Res 18:2638–2647
Lund SA, Giachelli CM, Scatena M (2009) The role of osteopontin in inflammatory processes. J Cell Commun Signal 3:311–322
Lyles SE, Milner RJ, Kow K et al (2012) In vitro effects of the tyrosine kinase inhibitor, masitinib mesylate, on canine hemangiosarcoma cell lines. Vet Comp Oncol 10:223–235
Ma Q, Cavallin LE, Yan B et al (2009) Antitumorigenesis of antioxidants in a transgenic Rac1 model of Kaposi's sarcoma. Proc Natl Acad Sci USA 106:8683–8688
Maeyama H, Hidaka E, Ota H et al (2001) Familial gastrointestinal stromal tumor with hyperpigmentation: association with a germline mutation of the c-kit gene. Gastroenterology 120:210–215
Maki RG, D'Adamo DR, Keohan ML et al (2009) Phase II study of sorafenib in patients with metastatic or recurrent sarcomas. J Clin Oncol 27:3133–3140
Maki RG, Wathen JK, Patel SR et al (2007) Randomized phase II study of gemcitabine and docetaxel compared with gemcitabine alone in patients with metastatic soft tissue sarcomas: results of sarcoma alliance for research through collaboration study 002 (corrected). J Clin Oncol 25:2755–2763
Malempati S, Weigel B, Ingle AM et al (2012) Phase I/II trial and pharmacokinetic study of cixutumumab in pediatric patients with refractory solid tumors and Ewing sarcoma: a report from the Children's Oncology Group. J Clin Oncol 30:256–262
Malkin D, Li FP, Strong LC et al (1990) Germ line p53 mutations in a familial syndrome of breast cancer, sarcomas, and other neoplasms. Science 250:1233–1238
Mallery SR, Pei P, Landwehr DJ et al (2004) Implications for oxidative and nitrative stress in the pathogenesis of AIDS-related Kaposi's sarcoma. Carcinogenesis 25:597–603
Mantovani A, Allavena P, Sica A et al (2008) Cancer-related inflammation. Nature 454:436–444
Marampon F, Bossi G, Ciccarelli C et al (2009) MEK/ERK inhibitor U0126 affects in vitro and in vivo growth of embryonal rhabdomyosarcoma. Mol Cancer Ther 8:543–551
Marees T, Moll AC, Imhof SM et al (2008) Risk of second malignancies in survivors of retinoblastoma: more than 40 years of follow-up. J Natl Cancer Inst 100:1771–1779
Martin Liberal J, Lagares-Tena L, Sainz-Jaspeado M et al (2012) Targeted therapies in sarcomas: challenging the challenge. Sarcoma 2012:626094. doi:10.1155/2012/626094
Martinelli S, McDowell HP, Vigne SD et al (2009) RAS signaling dysregulation in human embryonal Rhabdomyosarcoma. Genes Chromosom Cancer 48:975–982
Mashima R, Honda K, Yang Y et al (2010) Mice lacking Dok-1, Dok-2, and Dok-3 succumb to aggressive histiocytic sarcoma. Lab Invest 90:1357–1364
May WA, Gishizky ML, Lessnick SL et al (1993) Ewing sarcoma 11; 22 translocation produces a chimeric transcription factor that requires the DNA-binding domain encoded by FLI1 for transformation. Proc Natl Acad Sci USA 90:5752–5756
McMeekin DS, Sill MW, Darcy KM et al (2012) A phase II trial of thalidomide in patients with refractory uterine carcinosarcoma and correlation with biomarkers of angiogenesis: a Gynecologic Oncology Group study. Gynecol Oncol 127:356–361

Melhem MF, Meisler AI, Saito R et al (1993) Cytokines in inflammatory malignant fibrous histiocytoma presenting with leukemoid reaction. Blood 82:2038–2044
Menczer J, Schreiber L, Sukmanov O et al (2010) COX-2 expression in uterine carcinosarcoma. Acta Obstet Gynecol Scand 89:120–125
Mercer SE, Ewton DZ, Shah S et al (2006) Mirk/Dyrk1b mediates cell survival in rhabdomyosarcomas. Cancer Res 66:5143–5150
Mesri EA, Cesarman E, Boshoff C (2010) Kaposi's sarcoma and its associated herpesvirus. Nat Rev Cancer 10:707–719
Meta-analysis (2010) Comparison of two doses of imatinib for the treatment of unresectable or metastatic gastrointestinal stromal tumors: a meta-analysis of 1,640 patients. J Clin Oncol 28:1247–1253
Minobe S, Todo Y, Suzuki Y et al (2011) Mesna, doxorubicin, ifosfamide and dacarbazine chemotherapy for uterine leiomyosarcoma: a report of two cases. J Obstet Gynaecol Res 37:645–649
Mirabello L, Troisi RJ, Savage SA (2009) Osteosarcoma incidence and survival rates from 1973 to 2004: data from the Surveillance, Epidemiology, and End Results Program. Cancer 115:1531–1543
Mita MM, Poplin E, Britten CD et al (2013) Phase I/IIa trial of the mammalian target of rapamycin inhibitor ridaforolimus (AP23573; MK-8669) administered orally in patients with refractory or advanced malignancies and sarcoma. Ann Oncol 24:1104–1111
Mollapour M, Tsutsumi S, Neckers L (2010) Hsp90 phosphorylation, Wee1 and the cell cycle. Cell Cycle 9:2310–2316
Momand J, Zambetti GP, Olson DC et al (1992) The mdm-2 oncogene product forms a complex with the p53 protein and inhibits p53-mediated transactivation. Cell 69:1237–1245
Mori K, Berreur M, Blanchard F et al (2007) Receptor activator of nuclear factor-kappaB ligand (RANKL) directly modulates the gene expression profile of RANK-positive Saos-2 human osteosarcoma cells. Oncol Rep 18:1365–1371
Moroianu J, Riordan JF (1994) Nuclear translocation of angiogenic proteins in endothelial cells: an essential step in angiogenesis. Biochemistry 33:12535–12539
Muftuoglu M, Oshima J, von Kobbe C et al (2008) The clinical characteristics of Werner syndrome: molecular and biochemical diagnosis. Hum Genet 124:369–377
Multhoff G, Molls M, Radons J (2012) Chronic inflammation in cancer development. Front Immunol 2:98. doi:10.3389/fimmu.2011.00098
Multhoff G, Radons J (2012) Radiation, inflammation, and immune responses in cancer. Front Oncol 2:58. doi:10.3389/fonc.2012.00058
Murai A, Abou AS, Kodama A et al (2012a) Immunohistochemical analysis of the Akt/mTOR/4E-BP1 signalling pathway in canine haemangiomas and haemangiosarcomas. J Comp Pathol 147:430–440
Murai A, Asa SA, Kodama A et al (2012b) Constitutive phosphorylation of the mTORC2/Akt/4E-BP1 pathway in newly derived canine hemangiosarcoma cell lines. BMC Vet Res 8:128. doi:10.1186/1746-6148-8-128
Naganuma H, Sasaki A, Satoh E et al (1996) Modulation of transforming growth factor-beta secretion from malignant glioma cells by interleukin-1 beta. Neurol Med Chir (Tokyo) 36:145–150
Nagata Y, Lan KH, Zhou X et al (2004) PTEN activation contributes to tumor inhibition by trastuzumab, and loss of PTEN predicts trastuzumab resistance in patients. Cancer Cell 6:117–127
Naing A, LoRusso P, Fu S et al (2012) Insulin growth factor-receptor (IGF-1R) antibody cixutumumab combined with the mTOR inhibitor temsirolimus in patients with refractory Ewing's sarcoma family tumors. Clin Cancer Res 18:2625–2631
Nakagawa SA, Lopes A, de Lopes CA et al (2010) Nitric oxide synthases, cyclooxygenase-2, nitrotyrosine, and angiogenesis in chondrosarcoma and their relation to prognosis. J Bone Joint Surg Am 92:1738–1746
Nakayama Y, Kato N, Nakajima Y et al (2004) Effect of TNF-alpha on human osteosarcoma cell line Saos2–TNF-alpha regulation of bone sialoprotein gene expression in Saos2 osteoblast-like cells. Cell Biol Int 28:653–660

Navid F, Letterio JJ, Yeung CL et al (2000) Autocrine transforming growth factor-beta growth pathway in murine osteosarcoma cell lines associated with inability to affect phosphorylation of retinoblastoma protein. Sarcoma 4:93–102

Ng CH, Xu S, Lam KP (2007) Dok-3 plays a nonredundant role in negative regulation of B-cell activation. Blood 110:259–266

Ng PK, Tsui SK, Lau CP et al (2010) CCAAT/enhancer binding protein beta is up-regulated in giant cell tumor of bone and regulates RANKL expression. J Cell Biochem 110:438–446

Noguchi SI, Ueki T, Kawauchi S et al (1997) Establishment and characterization of a new synovial sarcoma cell line, SN-SY-1: special reference to bcl-2 protein and SYT-SSX1 hybrid transcripts. Int J Cancer 72:995–1002

Nör JE, Christensen J, Mooney DJ et al (1999) Vascular endothelial growth factor (VEGF)-mediated angiogenesis is associated with enhanced endothelial cell survival and induction of Bcl-2 expression. Am J Pathol 154:375–384

O'Hara AJ, Wang L, Dezube BJ et al (2009) Tumor suppressor microRNAs are underrepresented in primary effusion lymphoma and Kaposi sarcoma. Blood 113:5938–5941

O'Sullivan B, Davis AM, Turcotte R et al (2002) Preoperative versus postoperative radiotherapy in soft-tissue sarcoma of the limbs: a randomised trial. Lancet 359:2235–2241

Obana K, Yang HW, Piao HY et al (2003) Aberrations of p16INK4A, p14ARF and p15INK4B genes in pediatric solid tumors. Int J Oncol 23:1151–1157

Ohshima H, Sawa T, Akaike T (2006) 8-nitroguanine, a product of nitrative DNA damage caused by reactive nitrogen species: formation, occurrence, and implications in inflammation and carcinogenesis. Antioxid Redox Signal 8:1033–1045

Oldenborg PA, Gresham HD, Lindberg FP (2001) CD47-signal regulatory protein alpha (SIRPalpha) regulates Fcgamma and complement receptor-mediated phagocytosis. J Exp Med 193:855–862

Olmos D, Postel-Vinay S, Molife LR et al (2010) Safety, pharmacokinetics, and preliminary activity of the anti-IGF-1R antibody figitumumab (CP-751,871) in patients with sarcoma and Ewing's sarcoma: a phase 1 expansion cohort study. Lancet Oncol 11:129–135

Park HJ, Carr JR, Wang Z et al (2009) FoxM1, a critical regulator of oxidative stress during oncogenesis. EMBO J 28:2908–2918

Park MS, Patel SR, Ludwig JA et al (2011) Activity of temozolomide and bevacizumab in the treatment of locally advanced, recurrent, and metastatic hemangiopericytoma and malignant solitary fibrous tumor. Cancer 117:4939–4947

Pass HI, Lott D, Lonardo F et al (2005) Asbestos exposure, pleural mesothelioma, and serum osteopontin levels. N Engl J Med 353:1564–1573

Paudel N, Sadagopan S, Chakraborty S et al (2012) Kaposi's sarcoma-associated herpesvirus latency-associated nuclear antigen interacts with multifunctional angiogenin to utilize its antiapoptotic functions. J Virol 86:5974–5991

Peng CL, Guo W, Ji T et al (2009) Sorafenib induces growth inhibition and apoptosis in human synovial sarcoma cells via inhibiting the RAF/MEK/ERK signaling pathway. Cancer Biol Ther 8:1729–1736

Pervaiz N, Colterjohn N, Farrokhyar F et al (2008) A systematic meta-analysis of randomized controlled trials of adjuvant chemotherapy for localized resectable soft-tissue sarcoma. Cancer 113:573–581

Petricoin EFI, Espina V, Araujo RP et al (2007) Phosphoprotein pathway mapping: Akt/mammalian target of rapamycin activation is negatively associated with childhood rhabdomyosarcoma survival. Cancer Res 67:3431–3440

Petrioli R, Coratti A, Correale P et al (2002) Adjuvant epirubicin with or without ifosfamide for adult soft-tissue sarcoma. Am J Clin Oncol 25:468–473

Pilarsky C, Wenzig M, Specht T et al (2004) Identification and validation of commonly overexpressed genes in solid tumors by comparison of microarray data. Neoplasia 6:744–750

Piva R, Cavalla P, Bortolotto S et al (1997) p27/kip1 expression in human astrocytic gliomas. Neurosci Lett 234:127–130

Pollak M (2008) Insulin and insulin-like growth factor signalling in neoplasia. Nat Rev Cancer 8:915–928

Pollard P, Wortham N, Barclay E et al (2005a) Evidence of increased microvessel density and activation of the hypoxia pathway in tumours from the hereditary leiomyomatosis and renal cell cancer syndrome. J Pathol 205:41–49
Pollard PJ, Briere JJ, Alam NA et al (2005b) Accumulation of Krebs cycle intermediates and over-expression of HIF1alpha in tumours which result from germline FH and SDH mutations. Hum Mol Genet 14:2231–2239
Postel-Vinay S, Veron AS, Tirode F et al (2012) Common variants near TARDBP and EGR2 are associated with susceptibility to Ewing sarcoma. Nat Genet 44:323–327
Prakash O, Swamy OR, Peng X et al (2005) Activation of Src kinase Lyn by the Kaposi sarcoma-associated herpesvirus K1 protein: implications for lymphomagenesis. Blood 105:3987–3994
Prieur A, Tirode F, Cohen P et al (2004) EWS/FLI-1 silencing and gene profiling of Ewing cells reveal downstream oncogenic pathways and a crucial role for repression of insulin-like growth factor binding protein 3. Mol Cell Biol 24:7275–7283
Priller M, Poschl J, Abrao L et al (2011) Expression of FoxM1 is required for the proliferation of medulloblastoma cells and indicates worse survival of patients. Clin Cancer Res 17:6791–6801
Purohit S, Bhise R, Appachu S et al (2011) Systemic therapy in soft tissue sarcomas: past, present and future. Indian J Surg Oncol 2:327–331
Quek R, Wang Q, Morgan JA et al (2011) Combination mTOR and IGF-1R inhibition: phase I trial of everolimus and figitumumab in patients with advanced sarcomas and other solid tumors. Clin Cancer Res 17:871–879
Quesada J, Amato R (2012) The molecular biology of soft-tissue sarcomas and current trends in therapy. Sarcoma 2012:849456. doi:10.1155/2012/849456
Radons J, Bosserhoff AK, Grassel S et al (2006a) p38MAPK mediates IL-1-induced down-regulation of aggrecan gene expression in human chondrocytes. Int J Mol Med 17:661–668
Radons J, Falk W, Schubert TE (2006b) Interleukin-10 does not affect IL-1-induced interleukin-6 and metalloproteinase production in human chondrosarcoma cells, SW1353. Int J Mol Med 17:377–383
Rao PK, Missiaglia E, Shields L et al (2010) Distinct roles for miR-1 and miR-133a in the proliferation and differentiation of rhabdomyosarcoma cells. FASEB J 24:3427–3437
Raut CP, Nawrocki S, Lashinger LM et al (2004) Celecoxib inhibits angiogenesis by inducing endothelial cell apoptosis in human pancreatic tumor xenografts. Cancer Biol Ther 3:1217–1224
Ray-Coquard I, Italiano A, Bompas E et al (2012) Sorafenib for patients with advanced angiosarcoma: a phase II Trial from the French Sarcoma Group (GSF/GETO). Oncologist 17:260–266
Reed S, Li H, Li C et al (2011) Celecoxib inhibits STAT3 phosphorylation and suppresses cell migration and colony forming ability in rhabdomyosarcoma cells. Biochem Biophys Res Commun 407:450–455
Restrepo CS, Ocazionez D (2011) Kaposi's sarcoma: imaging overview. Semin Ultrasound CT MR 32:456–469
Reuter S, Gupta SC, Chaturvedi MM et al (2010) Oxidative stress, inflammation, and cancer: how are they linked? Free Radic Biol Med 49:1603–1616
Riggi N, Suva ML, De Vito C et al (2010) EWS-FLI-1 modulates miRNA145 and SOX2 expression to initiate mesenchymal stem cell reprogramming toward Ewing sarcoma cancer stem cells. Genes Dev 24:916–932
Roma J, Masia A, Reventos J et al (2011) Notch pathway inhibition significantly reduces rhabdomyosarcoma invasiveness and mobility in vitro. Clin Cancer Res 17:505–513
Rose-John S, Schooltink H (2007) Cytokines are a therapeutic target for the prevention of inflammation-induced cancers. Recent Results Cancer Res 174:57–66
Rosen A, Thimon S, Ternant D et al (2010) Partial response to bevacizumab of an extensive cutaneous angiosarcoma of the face. Br J Dermatol 163:225–227
Rosen N, Bolen JB, Schwartz AM et al (1986) Analysis of pp60c-src protein kinase activity in human tumor cell lines and tissues. J Biol Chem 261:13754–13759

Ross KA, Smyth NA, Murawski CD et al (2013) The biology of Ewing sarcoma. ISRN Oncol 2013:759725. doi:10.1155/2013/759725

Rubin AI, Stiller MJ (2002) A listing of skin conditions exhibiting the Koebner and pseudo-Koebner phenomena with eliciting stimuli. J Cutan Med Surg 6:29–34

Rubin BP, Heinrich MC, Corless CL (2007) Gastrointestinal stromal tumour. Lancet 369:1731–1741

Rubin BP, Nishijo K, Chen HI et al (2011) Evidence for an unanticipated relationship between undifferentiated pleomorphic sarcoma and embryonal rhabdomyosarcoma. Cancer Cell 19:177–191

Rutkowski P, Kaminska J, Kowalska M et al (2003) Cytokine and cytokine receptor serum levels in adult bone sarcoma patients: correlations with local tumor extent and prognosis. J Surg Oncol 84:151–159

Sadagopan S, Sharma-Walia N, Veettil MV et al (2009) Kaposi's sarcoma-associated herpesvirus upregulates angiogenin during infection of human dermal microvascular endothelial cells, which induces 45S rRNA synthesis, antiapoptosis, cell proliferation, migration, and angiogenesis. J Virol 83:3342–3364

Sadagopan S, Veettil MV, Chakraborty S et al (2012) Angiogenin functionally interacts with p53 and regulates p53-mediated apoptosis and cell survival. Oncogene 31:4835–4847

Sandau KB, Faus HG, Brune B (2000) Induction of hypoxia-inducible-factor 1 by nitric oxide is mediated via the PI 3K pathway. Biochem Biophys Res Commun 278:263–267

Sarcoma Meta-analysis Collaboration (1997) Adjuvant chemotherapy for localised resectable soft-tissue sarcoma of adults: meta-analysis of individual data. Sarcoma Meta-analysis Collaboration. Lancet 350:1647–1654

Sasaki K, Hitora T, Nakamura O et al (2011) The role of MAPK pathway in bone and soft tissue tumors. Anticancer Res 31:549–553

Sasaki M, Ikeda H, Itatsu K et al (2008) The overexpression of polycomb group proteins Bmi1 and EZH2 is associated with the progression and aggressive biological behavior of hepatocellular carcinoma. Lab Invest 88:873–882

Sastry KV, Sharma SC, Mann SB et al (1999) Aural cholesteatoma: role of tumor necrosis factor-alpha in bone destruction. Am J Otol 20:158–161

Savage SA, Mirabello L (2011) Using epidemiology and genomics to understand osteosarcoma etiology. Sarcoma 2011:548151. doi:10.1155/2011/548151

Scheidler S, Fredericks WJ, Rauscher FJ III et al (1996) The hybrid PAX3-FKHR fusion protein of alveolar rhabdomyosarcoma transforms fibroblasts in culture. Proc Natl Acad Sci USA 93:9805–9809

Schiffer D, Cavalla P, Fiano V et al (2002) Inverse relationship between p27/Kip.1 and the F-box protein Skp2 in human astrocytic gliomas by immunohistochemistry and Western blot. Neurosci Lett 328:125–128

Schoffski P, Adkins D, Blay J et al (2011a) Phase II trial of anti-IGF-IR antibody cixutumumab in patients with advanced or metastatic soft-tissue sarcoma and Ewing family of tumors. J Clin Oncol 29:10004. http://meeting.ascopubs.org/cgi/content/abstract/29/15_suppl/10004?sid=a6464a16-77fd-4537-baa7-c98ad3b1e0bc

Schoffski P, Ray-Coquard IL, Cioffi A et al (2011b) Activity of eribulin mesylate in patients with soft-tissue sarcoma: a phase 2 study in four independent histological subtypes. Lancet Oncol 12:1045–1052

Schuetze SM, Zhao L, Chugh R et al (2012) Results of a phase II study of sirolimus and cyclophosphamide in patients with advanced sarcoma. Eur J Cancer 48:1347–1353

Schwartz GK, Maki RG, Undevia SD et al (2011) Brivanib (BMS-582664) in advanced soft-tissue sarcoma (STS): biomarker and subset results of a phase II randomized discontinuation trial. J Clin Oncol 29:1000

Schwartz GK, Tap WD, Qin LX et al (2012) A phase II multicenter study of the IGF-1 receptor antibody cixutumumab (A12) and the mTOR inhibitor temsirolimus (TEM) in patients (pts) with refractory IGF-1R positive (+) and negative (−) bone and soft tissue sarcomas (STS).

J Clin Oncol 30:10003. http://meeting.ascopubs.org/cgi/content/abstract/30/15_suppl/10003?sid=80ce8716-8c84-4aa3-a0db-6843813c51d1

Scotlandi K, Avnet S, Benini S et al (2002) Expression of an IGF-I receptor dominant negative mutant induces apoptosis, inhibits tumorigenesis and enhances chemosensitivity in Ewing's sarcoma cells. Int J Cancer 101:11–16

Serrano M, Lee H, Chin L et al (1996) Role of the INK4a locus in tumor suppression and cell mortality. Cell 85:27–37

Shah MH, Porcu P, Mallery SR et al (2002) AIDS-associated malignancies. Cancer Chemother Biol Response Modif 20:633–664

Sharma-Walia N, Paul AG, Bottero V et al (2010) Kaposi's sarcoma associated herpes virus (KSHV) induced COX-2: a key factor in latency, inflammation, angiogenesis, cell survival and invasion. PLoS Pathog 6:e1000777

Sharma-Walia N, Raghu H, Sadagopan S et al (2006) Cyclooxygenase 2 induced by Kaposi's sarcoma-associated herpesvirus early during in vitro infection of target cells plays a role in the maintenance of latent viral gene expression. J Virol 80:6534–6552

Shekar SC, Wu H, Fu Z et al (2005) Mechanism of constitutive phosphoinositide 3-kinase activation by oncogenic mutants of the p85 regulatory subunit. J Biol Chem 280:27850–27855

Shen Z, Hoffman JD, Hao F et al (2012) More than just skin deep: faciocutaneous clues to genetic syndromes with malignancies. Oncologist 17:930–936

Shimada S, Ishizawa T, Ishizawa K et al (2006) The value of MDM2 and CDK4 amplification levels using real-time polymerase chain reaction for the differential diagnosis of liposarcomas and their histologic mimickers. Hum Pathol 37:1123–1129

Shor AC, Keschman EA, Lee FY et al (2007) Dasatinib inhibits migration and invasion in diverse human sarcoma cell lines and induces apoptosis in bone sarcoma cells dependent on SRC kinase for survival. Cancer Res 67:2800–2808

Shukla A, MacPherson MB, Hillegass J et al (2009) Alterations in gene expression in human mesothelial cells correlate with mineral pathogenicity. Am J Respir Cell Mol Biol 41:114–123

Silva I, Branco JC (2011) Rank/Rankl/opg: literature review. Acta Reumatol Port 36:209–218

Simonart T, Van Vooren JP (2002) Interleukin-1 beta increases the BCL-2/BAX ratio in Kaposi's sarcoma cells. Cytokine 19:259–266

Singh M, Pandey A, Karikari CA et al (2010) Cell cycle inhibition and apoptosis induced by curcumin in Ewing sarcoma cell line SK-NEP-1. Med Oncol 27:1096–1101

Sinkovics JG (2007a) Adult human sarcomas. I. Basic science. Expert Rev Anticancer Ther 7:31–56

Sinkovics JG (2007b) Adult human sarcomas. II. Medical oncology. Expert Rev Anticancer Ther 7:183–210

Sinkovics JG (2012) Molecular biology of oncogenic inflammatory processes. I. Non-oncogenic and oncogenic pathogens, intrinsic inflammatory reactions without pathogens, and microRNA/DNA interactions (Review). Int J Oncol 40:305–349

Sivakumar R, Sharma-Walia N, Raghu H et al (2008) Kaposi's sarcoma-associated herpesvirus induces sustained levels of vascular endothelial growth factors A and C early during in vitro infection of human microvascular dermal endothelial cells: biological implications. J Virol 82:1759–1776

Skubitz KM, Haddad PA (2005) Paclitaxel and pegylated-liposomal doxorubicin are both active in angiosarcoma. Cancer 104:361–366

Sleijfer S, Ouali M, van Glabbeke M et al (2010) Prognostic and predictive factors for outcome to first-line ifosfamide-containing chemotherapy for adult patients with advanced soft tissue sarcomas: an exploratory, retrospective analysis on large series from the European Organization for Research and Treatment of Cancer-Soft Tissue and Bone Sarcoma Group (EORTC-STBSG). Eur J Cancer 46:72–83

Sleijfer S, Ray-Coquard I, Papai Z et al (2009) Pazopanib, a multikinase angiogenesis inhibitor, in patients with relapsed or refractory advanced soft tissue sarcoma: a phase II study from

the European organisation for research and treatment of cancer-soft tissue and bone sarcoma group (EORTC study 62043). J Clin Oncol 27:3126–3132
Smida J, Baumhoer D, Rosemann M et al (2010) Genomic alterations and allelic imbalances are strong prognostic predictors in osteosarcoma. Clin Cancer Res 16:4256–4267
Sparmann A, Bar-Sagi D (2004) Ras-induced interleukin-8 expression plays a critical role in tumor growth and angiogenesis. Cancer Cell 6:447–458
Spurrell EL, Fisher C, Thomas JM et al (2005) Prognostic factors in advanced synovial sarcoma: an analysis of 104 patients treated at the Royal Marsden Hospital. Ann Oncol 16:437–444
Stacchiotti S, Dagrada GP, Morosi C et al (2012a) Extraskeletal myxoid chondrosarcoma: tumor response to sunitinib. Clin Sarcoma Res 2:22. doi:10.1186/2045-3329-2-22
Stacchiotti S, Negri T, Libertini M et al (2012b) Sunitinib malate in solitary fibrous tumor (SFT). Ann Oncol 23:3171–3179
Stettner MR, Wang W, Nabors LB et al (2005) Lyn kinase activity is the predominant cellular SRC kinase activity in glioblastoma tumor cells. Cancer Res 65:5535–5543
Stiller CA, Trama A, Serraino D et al (2013) Descriptive epidemiology of sarcomas in Europe: report from the RARECARE project. Eur J Cancer 49:684–695
Stojadinovic A, Leung DH, Hoos A et al (2002) Analysis of the prognostic significance of microscopic margins in 2,084 localized primary adult soft tissue sarcomas. Ann Surg 235:424–434
Sturgis EM, Potter BO (2003) Sarcomas of the head and neck region. Curr Opin Oncol 15:239–252
Subramanian S, Lui WO, Lee CH et al (2008) MicroRNA expression signature of human sarcomas. Oncogene 27:2015–2026
Suhasini AN, Brosh RM Jr (2013) DNA helicases associated with genetic instability, cancer, and aging. Adv Exp Med Biol 767:123–144
Sun SG, Lau YS, Itonaga I et al (2006) Bone stromal cells in pagetic bone and Paget's sarcoma express RANKL and support human osteoclast formation. J Pathol 209:114–120
Ta HT, Dass CR, Choong PF et al (2009) Osteosarcoma treatment: state of the art. Cancer Metastasis Rev 28:247–263
Takahashi F, Akutagawa S, Fukumoto H et al (2002) Osteopontin induces angiogenesis of murine neuroblastoma cells in mice. Int J Cancer 98:707–712
Takamori H, Oades ZG, Hoch OC et al (2000) Autocrine growth effect of IL-8 and GROα on a human pancreatic cancer cell line, Capan-1. Pancreas 21:52–56
Takebe N, Harris PJ, Warren RQ et al (2011) Targeting cancer stem cells by inhibiting Wnt, Notch, and Hedgehog pathways. Nat Rev Clin Oncol 8:97–106
Tamburini BA, Phang TL, Fosmire SP et al (2010) Gene expression profiling identifies inflammation and angiogenesis as distinguishing features of canine hemangiosarcoma. BMC Cancer 10:619. doi:10.1186/1471-2407-10-619
Tanaka M, Setoguchi T, Hirotsu M et al (2009) Inhibition of Notch pathway prevents osteosarcoma growth by cell cycle regulation. Br J Cancer 100:1957–1965
Tap WD, Demetri G, Barnette P et al (2012) Phase II study of ganitumab, a fully human anti-type-1 insulin-like growth factor receptor antibody, in patients with metastatic Ewing family tumors or desmoplastic small round cell tumors. J Clin Oncol 30:1849–1856
Tat SK, Pelletier JP, Velasco CR et al (2009) New perspective in osteoarthritis: the OPG and RANKL system as a potential therapeutic target? Keio J Med 58:29–40
Taulli R, Bersani F, Foglizzo V et al (2009) The muscle-specific microRNA miR-206 blocks human rhabdomyosarcoma growth in xenotransplanted mice by promoting myogenic differentiation. J Clin Invest 119:2366–2378
Taylor R, Knowles HJ, Athanasou NA (2011) Ewing sarcoma cells express RANKL and support osteoclastogenesis. J Pathol 225:195–202
Thomas ES, Gomez HL, Li RK et al (2007) Ixabepilone plus capecitabine for metastatic breast cancer progressing after anthracycline and taxane treatment. J Clin Oncol 25:5210–5217
Tili E, Michaille JJ, Wernicke D et al (2011) Mutator activity induced by microRNA-155 (miR-155) links inflammation and cancer. Proc Natl Acad Sci USA 108:4908–4913

Tolcher AW, Sarantopoulos J, Patnaik A et al (2009) Phase I, pharmacokinetic, and pharmacodynamic study of AMG 479, a fully human monoclonal antibody to insulin-like growth factor receptor 1. J Clin Oncol 27:5800–5807

Tomlinson IP, Alam NA, Rowan AJ et al (2002) Germline mutations in FH predispose to dominantly inherited uterine fibroids, skin leiomyomata and papillary renal cell cancer. Nat Genet 30:406–410

Toretsky JA, Gorlick R (2010) IGF-1R targeted treatment of sarcoma. Lancet Oncol 11:105–106

Toro JR, Travis LB, Wu HJ et al (2006) Incidence patterns of soft tissue sarcomas, regardless of primary site, in the surveillance, epidemiology and end results program, 1978–2001: an analysis of 26,758 cases. Int J Cancer 119:2922–2930

Tsumura H, Yoshida T, Saito H et al (2006) Cooperation of oncogenic K-ras and p53 deficiency in pleomorphic rhabdomyosarcoma development in adult mice. Oncogene 25:7673–7679

Urakawa H, Nishida Y, Naruse T et al (2009) Cyclooxygenase-2 overexpression predicts poor survival in patients with high-grade extremity osteosarcoma: a pilot study. Clin Orthop Relat Res 467:2932–2938

Valero V, Vrdoljak E, Xu B et al (2012) Maintenance of clinical efficacy after dose reduction of ixabepilone plus capecitabine in patients with anthracycline- and taxane-resistant metastatic breast cancer: a retrospective analysis of pooled data from 2 phase III randomized clinical trials. Clin Breast Cancer 12:240–246

van den Boom J, Wolter M, Kuick R et al (2003) Characterization of gene expression profiles associated with glioma progression using oligonucleotide-based microarray analysis and real-time reverse transcription-polymerase chain reaction. Am J Pathol 163:1033–1043

van der Graaf WT, Blay JY, Chawla SP et al (2012) Pazopanib for metastatic soft-tissue sarcoma (PALETTE): a randomised, double-blind, placebo-controlled phase 3 trial. Lancet 379:1879–1886

van Oosterom AT, Mouridsen HT, Nielsen OS et al (2002) Results of randomised studies of the EORTC Soft Tissue and Bone Sarcoma Group (STBSG) with two different ifosfamide regimens in first- and second-line chemotherapy in advanced soft tissue sarcoma patients. Eur J Cancer 38:2397–2406

Vemulapalli S, Mita A, Alvarado Y et al (2011) The emerging role of mammalian target of rapamycin inhibitors in the treatment of sarcomas. Target Oncol 6:29–39

Verma S, Younus J, Stys-Norman D et al (2008) Meta-analysis of ifosfamide-based combination chemotherapy in advanced soft tissue sarcoma. Cancer Treat Rev 34:339–347

Verweij J, Baker LH (2010) Future treatment of soft tissue sarcomas will be driven by histological subtype and molecular aberrations. Eur J Cancer 46:863–868

Verweij J, Casali PG, Zalcberg J et al (2004) Progression-free survival in gastrointestinal stromal tumours with high-dose imatinib: randomised trial. Lancet 364:1127–1134

Virchow R (1859) Die Cellularpathologie in ihrer Begründung auf physiologische und pathologische Gewebelehre. August Hirschwald, Berlin

Virchow R (1863) Die krankhaften Geschwülste. August Hirschwald, Berlin

von Mehren M, Rankin C, Goldblum JR et al (2012) Phase 2 Southwest Oncology Group-directed intergroup trial (S0505) of sorafenib in advanced soft tissue sarcomas. Cancer 118:770–776

Voronov E, Carmi Y, Apte RN (2007) Role of IL-1-mediated inflammation in tumor angiogenesis. Adv Exp Med Biol 601:265–270

Wagner AJ, Goldberg JM, Dubois SG et al (2012) Tivantinib (ARQ 197), a selective inhibitor of MET, in patients with microphthalmia transcription factor-associated tumors: results of a multicenter phase 2 trial. Cancer 118:5894–5902

Wan X, Helman LJ (2007) The biology behind mTOR inhibition in sarcoma. Oncologist 12:1007–1018

Wang IC, Chen YJ, Hughes D et al (2005a) Forkhead box M1 regulates the transcriptional network of genes essential for mitotic progression and genes encoding the SCF (Skp2-Cks1) ubiquitin ligase. Mol Cell Biol 25:10875–10894

Wang J, Ouyang W, Li J et al (2005b) Loss of tumor suppressor p53 decreases PTEN expression and enhances signaling pathways leading to activation of activator protein 1 and nuclear factor kappaB induced by UV radiation. Cancer Res 65:6601–6611

Wang LL, Gannavarapu A, Kozinetz CA et al (2003) Association between osteosarcoma and deleterious mutations in the RECQL4 gene in Rothmund-Thomson syndrome. J Natl Cancer Inst 95:669–674

Wang Z, Park HJ, Carr JR et al (2011) FoxM1 in tumorigenicity of the neuroblastoma cells and renewal of the neural progenitors. Cancer Res 71:4292–4302

Wardelmann E, Losen I, Hans V et al (2003) Deletion of Trp-557 and Lys-558 in the juxtamembrane domain of the c-kit protooncogene is associated with metastatic behavior of gastrointestinal stromal tumors. Int J Cancer 106:887–895

Wilker E, Bol D, Kiguchi K et al (1999) Enhancement of susceptibility to diverse skin tumor promoters by activation of the insulin-like growth factor-1 receptor in the epidermis of transgenic mice. Mol Carcinog 25:122–131

Wong FL, Boice JD Jr, Abramson DH et al (1997) Cancer incidence after retinoblastoma. Radiation dose and sarcoma risk. JAMA 278:1262–1267

Wong TF, Takeda T, Li B et al (2011) Curcumin disrupts uterine leiomyosarcoma cells through AKT-mTOR pathway inhibition. Gynecol Oncol 122:141–148

Wu SP, Huang TC, Lin CC et al (2012) Pardaxin, a fish antimicrobial peptide, exhibits antitumor activity toward murine fibrosarcoma in vitro and in vivo. Mar Drugs 10:1852–1872

Xia JJ, Pei LB, Zhuang JP et al (2010) Celecoxib inhibits beta-catenin-dependent survival of the human osteosarcoma MG-63 cell line. J Int Med Res 38:1294–1304

Xia SJ, Barr FG (2005) Chromosome translocations in sarcomas and the emergence of oncogenic transcription factors. Eur J Cancer 41:2513–2527

Xie X, Ghadimi MP, Young ED et al (2011) Combining EGFR and mTOR blockade for the treatment of epithelioid sarcoma. Clin Cancer Res 17:5901–5912

Yaich S, Charfeddine K, Zaghdane S et al (2012) Sirolimus for the treatment of Kaposi sarcoma after renal transplantation: a series of 10 cases. Transpl Proc 44:2824–2826

Yan D, Dong XE, Chen X et al (2009) MicroRNA-1/206 targets c-Met and inhibits rhabdomyosarcoma development. J Biol Chem 284:29596–29604

Yang C, Ji D, Weinstein EJ et al (2010a) The kinase Mirk is a potential therapeutic target in osteosarcoma. Carcinogenesis 31:552–558

Yang MH, Hsu DS, Wang HW et al (2010b) Bmi1 is essential in Twist1-induced epithelial-mesenchymal transition. Nat Cell Biol 12:982–992

Yang Q, Guan KL (2007) Expanding mTOR signaling. Cell Res 17:666–681

Yao C, Lin Y, Chua MS et al (2007) Interleukin-8 modulates growth and invasiveness of estrogen receptor-negative breast cancer cells. Int J Cancer 121:1949–1957

Yarber JL, Agulnik M (2011) Targeted therapies in bone sarcomas: current approach and future directions. Expert Opin Investig Drugs 20:973–979

Ye F, Lattif AA, Xie J et al (2012) Nutlin-3 induces apoptosis, disrupts viral latency and inhibits expression of angiopoietin-2 in Kaposi sarcoma tumor cells. Cell Cycle 11:1393–1399

Ye L, Zhang HY, Wang H et al (2005) Effects of transforming growth factor beta 1 on the growth of rhabdomyosarcoma cell line RD. Chin Med J 118:678–686 (Engl)

Yetiser S, Satar B, Aydin N (2002) Expression of epidermal growth factor, tumor necrosis factor-alpha, and interleukin-1alpha in chronic otitis media with or without cholesteatoma. Otol Neurotol 23:647–652

Yoo J, Robinson RA, Lee JY (1999) H-ras and K-ras gene mutations in primary human soft tissue sarcoma: concomitant mutations of the ras genes. Mod Pathol 12:775–780

Yovine A, Riofrio M, Blay JY et al (2004) Phase II study of ecteinascidin-743 in advanced pretreated soft tissue sarcoma patients. J Clin Oncol 22:890–899

Yu H, Pardoll D, Jove R (2009) STATs in cancer inflammation and immunity: a leading role for STAT3. Nat Rev Cancer 9:798–809

Yu Y, Khan J, Khanna C et al (2004) Expression profiling identifies the cytoskeletal organizer ezrin and the developmental homeoprotein Six-1 as key metastatic regulators. Nat Med 10:175–181

Zha J, Lackner MR (2010) Targeting the insulin-like growth factor receptor-1R pathway for cancer therapy. Clin Cancer Res 16:2512–2517

Zhang P, Bill K, Liu J et al (2012) MiR-155 is a liposarcoma oncogene that targets casein kinase-1alpha and enhances beta-catenin signaling. Cancer Res 72:1751–1762

Zhang Y, Zhang N, Dai B et al (2008) FoxM1B transcriptionally regulates vascular endothelial growth factor expression and promotes the angiogenesis and growth of glioma cells. Cancer Res 68:8733–8742

Zibat A, Missiaglia E, Rosenberger A et al (2010) Activation of the hedgehog pathway confers a poor prognosis in embryonal and fusion gene-negative alveolar rhabdomyosarcoma. Oncogene 29:6323–6330

Chapter 12
The Role of Inflammation in Lymphoma

Antonino Carbone, Claudio Tripodo, Carmelo Carlo-Stella, Armando Santoro and Annunziata Gloghini

Abstract Human lymphomas usually develop in specialized tissue microenvironments characterized by different populations of accessory stromal and lymphoid cells that interact with malignant cells. A clinical role of the tumor microenvironment has recently emerged, bringing new knowledge and suggesting new ideas and targets for treatment. This chapter analyzes the microenvironment in human lymphomas highlighting the role of inflammation in their pathogenesis. Microenvironmental specificity is detailed according to different models including classic Hodgkin lymphoma (HL), follicular lymphoma (FL), diffuse large B-cell lymphoma (DLBCL), peripheral T-cell lymphoma, unspecified and angioimmunoblastic T-cell lymphoma (AITL).

12.1 Introduction

Genetic alterations and abnormal microenvironmental factors are involved in tumor development, cell growth, and disease progression. The tumor microenvironment contains accessory cells that within individual organs work through cell–cell contacts

A. Carbone (✉)
Department of Pathology, Centro di Riferimento Oncologico Aviano, Istituto Nazionale Tumori, IRCCS, Via Franco Gallini, 2, 33081 Aviano, Italy
e-mail: acarbone@cro.it

C. Tripodo
Tumor Immunology Unit, Human Pathology Section, Department of Health Sciences, University of Palermo, Palermo, Italy

C. Carlo-Stella · A. Santoro
Department of Oncology and Hematology, Humanitas Cancer Center, Humanitas Clinical and Research Center, Rozzano, Milano, Italy

A. Gloghini
Department of Diagnostic Pathology and Laboratory Medicine, Fondazione IRCCS Istituto Nazionale dei Tumori, Milano, Italy

B. B. Aggarwal et al. (eds.), *Inflammation and Cancer*, Advances in Experimental Medicine and Biology 816, DOI: 10.1007/978-3-0348-0837-8_12, © Springer Basel 2014

and active molecular cross talk. Inflammatory cells and soluble mediators, i.e., cytokines and chemokines, are essential microenvironmental factors that sustain cell growth and invasion, induce angiogenesis, and suppress antitumor immune functions (Mantovani et al. 2008).

Lymphomas usually develop in specialized tissue microenvironments characterized by different populations of accessory stromal and lymphoid cells that interact with malignant cells. In multidimensional studies on hematolymphoid malignancies, a relevant clinical role of the tumor microenvironment has recently emerged, bringing new knowledge and suggesting new ideas and targets for treatment (Burger et al. 2009; Dave et al. 2004; Lenz et al. 2007; Steidl et al. 2010).

12.2 The Microenvironment of Human Lymph Node

The human lymph node is a complex tissue resulting from the microenvironmental organization of different cell populations (lymphoid cells, accessory or non-lymphoid cells, and stromal cells) linked by topographical and/or functional relationships. The follicle is a structure made of B and T lymphoid cells within a network of follicular dendritic cells (FDCs). Germinal centers (GCs) contain different microenvironmental zones (i.e., the "dark" zone [DZ] and the "light" zone [LZ]). There is a sharp demarcation around the whole follicle center, which is highlighted by fibroblastic reticulum cells (FRCs) (Gloghini et al. 1990). Tingible body macrophages (TBMs) are located throughout the GCs (Gloghini and Carbone 1993; MacLennan 1994).

The GC in lymphoid organs is a dynamic and a complex cellular microenvironment where B cells undergo repeated rounds of mutation and selection. Three major cellular components appear necessary for the GC reaction: The FDCs that define the locus of GC formation and serve as antigen-retaining cells for GC B cells (GCBs), antigen-specific T cells, and antigen-specific B cells. GCBs take up antigen from FDC, process it, and present it to antigen-specific T cells. GC T cells that recognize the antigens presented by centrocytes deliver two types of stimuli that result in the proliferation and differentiation of B cells: contact-mediated stimuli and activating cytokines.

12.3 Interactions Between Microenvironment of Secondary Lymphoid Organs and Lymphoma Cells in Human Lymph Nodes and Other Secondary Lymphoid Organs

The principal molecules involved in contact-mediated B-cell stimulation are CD40 on B cells and CD40 ligand on activated T cells. CD40-mediated signals to B cells are well known to strongly upregulate B-cell proliferation and differentiation into either memory B cells or plasma cells. CD40 receptor engagement, usually caused in vivo by the interaction of GC lymphocytes with surrounding T cells at the terminal stages of GC reaction, leads to NFKB-mediated transcriptional activation of the *IRF4* gene (Klein and Dalla-Favera 2008; Lossos 2007). Regarding lymphoid malignancies, in classic Hodgkin lymphoma (HL), CD40 receptor engagement is caused by the interaction of the Reed-Sternberg (RS) cells with surrounding CD40L-positive T cells and leads to NFKB activation of IRF4 (Aldinucci et al. 2011).

Moving to B-cell trafficking between the DL and the LZ in GC physiology, it is regulated by a complex mechanism that is based on the interplay of specialized chemokines and their relative receptors. Centroblasts express CXC receptor 4 (CXCR4) and migrate toward a gradient of CXC chemokine ligand 12 (CXCL12 or SDF1) originating in the LZ and mostly produced by stromal cells (Allen et al. 2004). Centrocytes instead express CXCR5, which attracts cells toward a gradient of CXCL13 produced in the DZ. FDCs have been identified as the main cellular source of this chemokine in lymphoid organs (Ansel et al. 2000). In GC-derived lymphomas, CXCL13 has also been shown to be secreted by follicular lymphoma (FL) cells, which also express CXCR4 and 5 (Husson et al. 2002). CXCL13 expression has been described in angioimmunoblastic T-cell lymphoma (AITL) cases (Dupuis et al. 2006).

12.4 Relationships Between Lymphoma Cells and Microenvironment

The relationships between lymphomas and microenvironment appear to follow 3 major patterns: (1) an independent, largely autonomous pattern, (2) a dependent on deregulated interactions pattern, (3) a dependent on regulated coexistence pattern (Burger et al. 2009). A typical example of the first pattern is Burkitt lymphoma where all tumor cells proliferate because of permanent c-*myc* gene activation. This pattern may be referred to as loss of interconnection with the microenvironmental network, which occurs when transformed cells have proliferation advantage that is largely autonomous and independent of microenvironmental signals (Burger et al. 2009). A typical example of the second pattern is classic HL, where RS cells escape the regulated cell growth and proliferation control. This pattern may be referred to a dysfunctional environment, where the neoplastic cells engage in deregulated interactions with the supportive environment that provide the malignant cells with growth signals (Aldinucci et al. 2010). A typical example of the third pattern is FL and mucosa-associated lymphoid tissue (MALT) lymphomas. In this pattern, a regulated coexistence of the malignant cells and the microenvironment resembles the pattern that the normal counterpart B cells engage in with their respective microenvironments. At least initially, tumor development and cell growth largely dependent on external signals from the microenvironment, such as antigens, cytokines, and cell–cell interactions (Carbone et al. 2009).

12.5 Microenvironmental Specificity According to Different Models

12.5.1 Classic HL

A well-studied model of tumor–microenvironment interactions is classical HL, in which the RS tumor cells (Kuppers 2009) are regulated by interactions with reactive cells in HL-involved tissues. These reactive cells, recruited and/or induced to proliferate by RS tumor cells, produce soluble or membrane-bound molecules involved in tumor cell growth and survival. Moreover, the abnormal cytokine/chemokine network seems to contribute not only to RS cells proliferation but also to the maintenance of an environment in which an effective host immune response to RS cells cannot be achieved (reviewed in Aldinucci et al. 2010).

12.5.1.1 Microenvironmental Cell Types

Classic HL is a monoclonal B-cell neoplasm, composed of mononuclear Hodgkin cells and multinucleated RS cells residing in a reactive cellular microenvironment. Based on the characteristics of the reactive cellular infiltrate, several histological subtypes have been traditionally distinguished (Lukes and Butler 1966). At present, four subtypes have been recognized: lymphocyte-rich HL, nodular sclerosis HL, mixed cellularity HL, and lymphocyte-depleted HL (Stein et al. 2008).

In most HL cases, RS cells represent the minority of the tumor burden and are dispersed among reactive elements comprising mixture of inflammatory cells, stromal cells, and a predominance of Th2 cells between the various subpopulations of lymphoid cells. Microenvironmental cell types include non-neoplastic B and T small lymphocytes, plasma cells, eosinophils, mast cells, histiocytes/macrophages, fibroblast-like cells, and interdigitating reticulum cells.

12.5.1.2 Recruitment of HL Microenvironment

Numerous molecules (see below) (Aldinucci et al. 2010) are involved directly or indirectly in the recruitment and/or proliferation of cells constituting the classic HL microenvironment.

An abnormal network of cytokines and chemokines and/or their receptors in RS cells are involved in the attraction of many of the microenvironmental cells into the lymphoma background (see below). RS cells are surrounded by CD40L-expressing rosetting T cells (Carbone et al. 1995) and are dependent on survival signals received from other cells, such as CD40L-expressing T cells (Carbone et al. 1995), CD30L+ mast cells and eosinophils, or by a proliferation-inducing ligand (APRIL)-producing neutrophils (Kuppers 2009).

A considerable fraction of infiltrating $CD4^+$ T cells is regulatory T (Treg) cells, which have been shown to have immunosuppressive activity on HL-infiltrating cytotoxic T cells (Schreck et al. 2009). Recently, it was suggested that Treg cells and programmed death 1 (PD-1)+ T cells also interact with RS cells (Marshall et al. 2004; Schreck et al. 2009; Yamamoto et al. 2008), which produce the Treg attractant galectin-1 and the PD-1 ligand (PDL-1).

$CD4^+$ T helper (TH) cells are attracted by RS cells through secretion of chemokines, including regulated on activation, normal T cell expressed, and secreted (RANTES)/CC chemokine ligand 5 (CCL5). CCL5 has an additional role in the recruitment of eosinophils and mast cells (Aldinucci et al. 2008).

Polarized Th1 and Th2 cells represent two subgroups of helper T cells. On the contrary to Th1 cells, the Th2 cells produce IL-4, IL-5, IL-10, and IL-13, which are responsible for strong antibody production and inhibition of several macrophage functions, thus providing phagocyte-independent protective responses.

A whole plethora of soluble mediators synthesized by RS cells with chemotactic activity such as the cytokines and chemokines IL-5, IL-8, IL-9, CCL-5, and CCL-28 are involved in the recruitment of granulocytes, mast cells, and macrophages, whereas IL-7, CCL-5, CCL-17, CCL-20, and CCL-22 were effectors of lymphocyte recruitment and expansion (Aldinucci et al. 2010).

Recruitment of infiltrating immune cells is also boosted by reactive cells themselves and particularly by macrophages and mast cells synthesizing CCL-3, CCL-4, and CCL-8 chemokines (Aldinucci et al. 2010; Poppema 1989, 2005). Chemokine receptors, CXCR3, CXCR4, and CCR7, and adhesion molecules including CD62 ligand were found to be expressed on most T cells within HL tissues, while the corresponding ligands were expressed on malignant cells and vascular endothelium.

12.5.2 Nodular Lymphocyte-Predominant Hodgkin Lymphoma

NLPHL is a monoclonal B-cell neoplasm characterized by a nodular, or a nodular and diffuse, proliferation of RS cell variants, known as popcorn or lymphocyte-predominant cells (LP cells). LP cells reside within nodules consisting of spherical meshworks of FDCs that are filled with non-neoplastic inflammatory cells (Schmitz et al. 2009). Inflammatory cells include small B cells, T cells, and histiocytes. Furthermore, the nodules of NLPHL are characterized by an increase in GC-derived $CD57^+$, $IRF4^+$, and PD-1^+ T cells that are closely associated with, and surround, the neoplastic LP cells (Carbone et al. 2002; Kraus and Haley 2000; Nam-Cha et al. 2008; Poppema et al. 2008; Timens et al. 1986).

LP cells of NLPHL clearly resemble GCBs in many phenotypic and genetic aspects and proliferate in association with a cellular microenvironment that retains key features of a normal primary follicle.

12.5.3 Follicular Lymphoma

Morphologically, FL is defined as a proliferation of malignant GCBs that are admixed with non-malignant cells such as T cells, FDCs, and macrophages and whose normal counterparts, i.e., centrocytes and centroblasts, represent the predominant cell types of the GC reaction (WHO). FLs are derived from GCBs and maintain the gene expression programme of this stage of differentiation (Dave et al. 2004). Unlike normal GCBs, roughly 85 % of FLs express BCL2 as a result of the characteristic t(14;18) translocation.

It has become increasingly clear that development and progression in FL are driven not only by genetic changes but also by the close interaction with the immune microenvironment and stromal cells. Classes of $CD4^{+}$ T cells, including follicular helper T cells and regulatory T cells, are the major players in regulating the delicate balance of effector populations (de Jong and Fest 2011). In FL, the tumor cells reside and proliferate in follicular structures in close association with FDCs (Manconi et al. 1988), even when the infiltrate localize in the bone marrow and in non-lympoid organs (Burger et al. 2009; Carbone et al. 1985). Therefore, the lymphoma cells seem to require the cellular interactions in the GC-like environment for their proliferation and to retain key features of normal GCBs including the interaction with T cells and FDCs in the follicular microenvironment (Carbone et al. 1995). A relevant role of the microenvironment on the final outcome of the disease has been demonstrated by gene expression profiling analysis showing that survival of patients with FL might be associated with "immune response" signatures expressed by non-malignant cells, such as T cells and macrophages (Dave et al. 2004).

The fact that FL is a malignancy primarily related to defects in the induction of apoptosis and is widely accepted, judging from the clinical course and the in vivo data. Evidence from in vitro studies points to a possible role of CD40 and its interactions with CD40L in the pathogenesis of FL. This interaction plays a very important role in GC physiology. The initiation of GC response depends critically on the interactions between co-stimulatory B-cell surface receptors and ligands expressed by T cells or antigen-presenting cells. The most important of them involves the tumor necrosis factor (TNF) receptor family member CD40, which is expressed by all B cells, and its ligand CD40L (or CD154), expressed by Th cells

A proposed model of the interplay between microenvironment and FL hypothesizes that beneficial signals for growth and survival include cytokines such as IL-4 and IL-21, which bind to interleukin receptors on lymphoma cells (IL-4R/IL-21R) or CXCL12 and CXCL13 secreted by stromal cell subsets. BCR signaling occurs through stimulation of the BCR by the innate immune system through N-glycans or by specific antigen presentation through FDCs. Tumor cells subvert the anti-tumor immune response from T helper cells, CTLs, and macrophages. Immune cell subsets that suppress an efficient immunological response against the tumor include Tregs and M2-polarized macrophages (TAMs) (Kridel et al. 2012).

Regarding disease progression, FL may have a pure follicular pattern (in situ or in early FL), or at least partially follicular pattern (in FL associated with diffuse lymphoma). The factors determining which individuals carrying t(14;18) develop

FL and the genetic events underlying the progression from in situ FL to overt FL and to diffuse lymphoma are totally unknown. There is a wide spectrum of genetic abnormalities identified in FL, such as genomic copy number changes and somatic mutation of the histone modifying genes including *EZH2* (7 %) (Morin et al. 2010), *MLL2* (89 %) (Morin et al. 2011), *MEF2B* (15 %) (Morin et al. 2010), *CREBBP* (33 %) (Pasqualucci et al. 2011), and *EP300* (8.7 %) (Pasqualucci et al. 2011), and inactivation of TNFRSF14 (18 %) (Cheung et al. 2010). It remains to be investigated whether these genetic changes are driver mutations and cooperate with t(14;18) in malignant transformation. In other words, in some cases, FL "transforms" into an aggressive lymphoma resembling diffuse large B-cell lymphoma (DLBCL), and this transformation can be associated with a variety of oncogenic changes (Lossos and Levy 2003). Accumulation of genomic alterations and clonal selection account for subsequent FL progression and transformation. However, a role for the immunological microenvironment of FL in determining clinical behavior and prognosis of the disease has also recently been substantiated.

In addition to genetic events, microenvironment factors could underlie the FL progression. The interaction between lymphoid tumor cells and their tissue microenvironment may promote dissemination and progression from in situ lymphoma to early or overt FL.

The molecular pathways of cross talk between the lymphoma cells and their nursing stroma of the follicular mantle (Hopken and Rehm 2012; Skibinski et al. 2001) might be mediated by factors expressed by mantle fibroblasts, also known as FRCs (Gloghini et al. 1990). It is known that invasion requires active movement on the part of the tumor cells. Movement of tumor cells through stromal tissues is mediated in part by a "scatter factor" that is synthesized and secreted by fibroblasts (Woolf 1998). Scatter factor, also known as hepatocyte growth factor (HGF), is a multifunctional cytokine whose activities mainly include stimulation of epithelial cell motility and invasiveness (reviewed in Skibinski et al. 2001). Its receptor is a transmembrane tyrosine kinase encoded by the proto-oncogene, c-met (reviewed in Skibinski et al. 2001), which can also be expressed, or induced, on normal B cells (reviewed in Skibinski et al. 2001). Furthermore, B cells, when appropriately stimulated, express the HGF receptor c-met, creating the potential for functional interaction between mesenchymal and lymphoid cells (Skibinski et al. 2001; Weimar et al. 1997). We suggest that these functional interactions may influence lymphoid cell motility and invasiveness. Microenvironmental factors should be further investigated to clarify their role in the progression from in situ FL to early FL or overt FL.

12.5.4 Diffuse Large B-Cell Lymphoma Related to Inflammation

DLBCL is the most common B-cell lymphoid neoplasm. DLBCL associated with chronic inflammation, defined as DLBCL arising in the context of long-standing chronic inflammation, is associated with Epstein–Barr virus (EBV) infection or HCV infection.

12.5.4.1 DLBCL Associated with Chronic Inflammation Related to EBV Infection

DLBCL associated with chronic inflammation most commonly involves body cavities. The prototype for this category is pyothorax-associated lymphoma (PAL). PAL was first reported in 1987 in patients who were treated for tuberculosis with the induction of an artificial pneumothorax and is EBV positive about 70 % of the time (Aozasa 2006; Fukayama et al. 1993). Patients present with fever, chest/back pain, and cough with a latency period of 10–64 years after the onset of the original inflammatory effusion and are often found to have a very large tumor (often > 10 cm) confined to the thoracic cavity. Other cases of DLBCL occurring in the setting of chronic inflammation (such as chronic skin ulcers or osteomyelitis) are also frequently positive for EBV. Interferon-inducible (IFI) protein 27 is differentially expressed in PAL cell lines compared to bystander cells (Aozasa 2006). The function of IFI27 is not known, but it can be induced in B cells by the stimulation of interferon. The presence of inflammation itself plays a dual role in PAL with EBV inducing B-cell transformation and escape from cytotoxic T cells.

12.5.4.2 Lymphomatoid Granulomatosis Related to EBV Infection

Lymphomatoid granulomatosis (LYG) is a rare angiodestructive EBV-driven lymphoproliferative disease comprised of atypical clonal EBV^{+} B cells in an inflammatory background. Patients usually do not have an overt immunodeficiency prior to diagnosis, but many patients show evidence of immune dysregulation. It is recognized, however, that patients with known immunodeficiency are at increased risk (Wilson et al. 1996). EBV transformation of B cells and chemokine induction is currently believed to be at the center of all the pathological and clinical features of LYG (Jaffe and Wilson 1997). Histologically, LYG is comprised of a small number of EBV^{+} B cells admixed with a prominent inflammatory background comprised of T cells, plasma cells, and histiocytes. The malignant B cells usually are large in size and express CD20, LMP1, and EBER by in situ hybridization. They are variably positive for CD30 and usually negative for CD15. Vascular changes and angiodestruction are distinctive features with intimal thickening of blood vessels and accompanying necrosis in many cases. LYG mostly involves extranodal sites with the lung virtually always being involved. Patients present with multiple bilateral pulmonary nodules of varying size. These nodules are usually localized in the mid- and lower lung fields. Often the nodules show evidence of central necrosis and/or cavitation.

Other common sites of extranodal involvement include the central nervous system and skin in up to 20 % of patients (Jaffe and Wilson 1997). One striking feature of LYG is that lymph nodes and spleen are almost always spared at initial diagnosis and only involved at late stages of disease.

12.5.4.3 B-Cell Lymphomas Associated with Chronic Inflammation Related to HCV Infection

Many studies have provided evidence that HCV infection is associated with development of lymphoplasmacytoid lymphoma (immunocytoma) and with other indolent and aggressive B-cell NHL (Mele et al. 2003; Germanidis et al. 1999; Sansonno et al. 2007). However, a case–control study of patients with various B-cell NHL subtypes indicated that HCV infection was detected most frequently among those with DLBCL (Talamini et al. 2004). In contrast, the finding from several case–control studies did not support a notable effect of HCV on T-cell lymphomas (reviewed in IARC). The similarities shared by rearranged Ig genes present in B cells from patients with type II MC and malignant B cells from HCV-positive patients with B-cell NHL support the possibility that the antigens that promote type II MC and B-cell NHL in HCV-positive patients are the same (De Vita et al. 1995; Sansonno et al. 1996). These similarities also suggest that type II MC may be a precursor of B-cell NHL (Dammacco et al.1998). Type II MC probably plays a central role in the development of B-cell lymphoma in HCV-positive patients with Sjögren's syndrome (SS) (Mariette 2001).

The liver is the main target of HCV infection and the major site of inflammatory events, including recruitment of inflammatory cells. An emerging area of research is directed to the definition of effective signals that enhance the survival of immunocompetent cells (Taneda et al. 2001). Uncontrolled and inappropriate survival signals are known to underlie many autoimmune disorders. The B-cell-activating factor of the TNF family (BAFF), in particular, is a fundamental survival factor (Mackay and Browing 2002; Schneider and Tschopp 2003).

Occurrence of HCV enrichment in intrahepatic inflammatory infiltrates supports the notion that HCV is directly involved in the emergence and maintenance of these B-cell expansions (Sansonno et al. 2004). Intrahepatic B-cell clonalities are invariably associated with extrahepatic manifestations of HCV infection, frank B-cell NHL.

Molecular mechanisms of HCV-associated lymphoma development are still poorly understood. Three general theories have emerged to understand the HCV-induced lymphomagenesis: (1) continuous external stimulation of lymphocyte receptors by viral antigens and consecutive proliferation; (2) direct role of HCV replication and expression in infected B cells; (3) permanent B-cell damage, e.g., mutation of tumor suppressor genes, caused by a transiently intracellular virus ("hit and run" theory) (IARC 2012; Peveling-Oberhag et al. 2013).

Other non-exclusive hypotheses have been proposed over the past two decades. These hypotheses have variously emphasized the important role played by chromosomal aberrations, cytokines, or microRNA molecules (Zignego et al. 2012). However, the mechanisms by which B-cell lymphomas are induced by HCV remain the subject of debate.

12.5.5 Peripheral T-Cell Lymphomas, Unspecified and AITLs

Our understanding of the biology of T-cell lymphomas is growing along with the development of new tools for molecular profiling of T-cell clones. Lymphomas of peripheral T cells (PTCLs) are commonly burdened by phenotypic aberrancies implying antigenic losses, which impair specification of neoplastic T-cell differentiation. Yet, gaining insight into the functional skewing of the neoplastic clone is a fundamental step toward the correct interpretation of microenvironment biological influence. It is conceivable that T cell clones with diverse Th or Tc polarization would differently prime the surrounding immunological and stromal milieu and differently respond to the environment feedback. To date, we have limited but significant evidence that PTCLs can originate from, or at least reproduce, functionally differentiated T cells (Piccaluga et al. 2007; Iqbal et al. 2010). A notable example is AITL, which has been demonstrated to derive from follicular helper T cells (Tfh), a specific subset of T cells providing key help to B-cell responses under the fringes of GC programs. Tfh cell differentiation and function are strictly reliant on IL-21/IL-21R axis, and they express the stigmata of GC-associated lymphocytes such as BCL-6, CD10, CXCL13, CXCR5, PD1, and ICOS expression. According to their Tfh differentiation, AITL neoplastic cells display the Tfh phenotype and also synthesize IL-21 and CXCL13. Signs of AITCl clone deregulated Tfh function can be identified in the associated microenvironment such as the exuberant proliferation of FDC network and abundant B- and plasma cell infiltration. FDC expansion can be directly induced by AITL cells through IL-21 and CXCL13 release and is also sustained by the release of pro-inflammatory mediators by bystander myeloid cells. Reactive B cells infiltrating the AITL microenvironment classically display an activated phenotype and signs of EBV infection. These cells have been implicated in the arousal of AITL-associated B-cell malignancies and in the orchestration of autoimmune humoral responses. Abundant CXCL13 and IL-21 release by AITL cells are effective stimuli favoring B-cell attraction and activation, which warn about interpretation of the actual role of EBV in AITL-associated B-cell expansion. Actually, EBV-infected B cells can be more susceptible to CXCL13 attraction owing to the upregulation of CXCR5, and this event could underlie the enrichment of EBV-infected B cells in the AITL milieu even in the absence of a trigger role for EBV in B-cell expansion. The influence of AITL clone also extends to bystander T cells via the activity of myeloid effectors. By CXCL13 release, AITL cells recruit overly inflammatory mast cells eventually inducing Treg skewing toward Th17 differentiation by IL-6 and OX40/OX40L interaction. The induction of a Th17-prone background further contributes to magnifying myeloid cell accrual and fostering the autoimmune diathesis of AITL cases (Tripodo et al. 2010).

The pressure exerted by the neoplastic clone over the mesenchymal components of AITL-infiltrated lymphoid tissues also results in the induction of the characteristic vascular proliferation. AITL angiogenic response is not mere expression of the vascular remodeling associated with an expanding lymphoid clone, rather it reflects the outcome of the uncontrolled release of pro-angiogenic factors such as the prototypical VEGF-A, which is constitutively synthesized and released by neoplastic cells. Moreover, the angiogenic loop is further boosted through the engendering of pro-inflammatory conditions to which mast cells, macrophages, neutrophils, and eosinophils largely contribute. Notably, endothelial cells of AITL newly formed vessels, which are characterized by BCL2 expression, give rise to a bidirectional cross talk with neoplastic lymphocytes via the VEGF-A axis toward lymphoma progression. Overall, the AITL model well explains the integrated effort of clonal T cells and reactive lymphoid, myeloid, and mesenchymal elements to the orchestration of a vicious homeostasis and provides a precious insight into the influence of T-cell clone polarization in the specification of the associated environment. Recently, PTCLs other than AITL have been reported to be characterized by T cell clones with Tfh phenotype. In these cases of PTCL, typical features of the AITL microenvironment could be variably identified thus suggesting that the nature of the neoplastic T-cell population and the quality of the microenvironment are both determinant in the outcome of the lymphomagenesis. Accordingly, different polarizing environments can be associated with the establishment of diverse T-cell lymphoma histotypes. The induction of a Th-22 polarizing milieu has been reported to favor CTCL development (Miyagaki T et al. 2011) while establishment of a Th-17-skewed environment characterizes some anaplastic T-cell lymphoma (ALCL) cases. The dynamics of induction of Th-17 skewing in ALCL is particularly interesting being mediated by the NPM–ALK translocation via upregulation of miR-135 and Th-2 program repression and thus indicating posttranscriptional regulation of neoplastic T-cell fate as further element of complexity in PTCL biology.

12.6 Inflammation in Human Lymphomas: Prognostic and Therapeutic Implications

Lymphomas represent a heterogeneous group of tumors with pathologically and clinically overlapping features. Although a substantial proportion of cases is cured by currently available multidisciplinary treatment strategies, management of relapsed or refractory patients still represents an unmet medical need requiring the development of effective therapeutical approaches based on the use of molecularly targeted agents (Reeder and Ansell 2011). Over the last decades, genetic alterations that induce cell cycle perturbations, antiapoptotic signaling, block of terminal differentiation, and constitutive activation of intracellular signaling pathways have been increasingly identified as the leading causes in lymphomagenesis as well as attractive therapeutic targets (Nogai et al. 2011). More recently, however, tumor microenvironment has emerged as a critical player in the pathogenesis and progressions of human lymphomas due to its role in providing nutrients to tumor cells, stimulating angiogenesis and triggering immune deregulation (Steidl et al. 2011; Coupland 2011). The microenvironment may also create niches that promote drug resistance and cancer stem cell maintenance (Nakasone et al. 2012). A large body of evidences suggests that tumor microenvironment may play a significant prognostic and also therapeutic role in human lymphomas. Indeed, clinical data regarding biological agents that target the microenvironment, such as lenalidomide, anti-CD137 antibodies, antiangiogenic molecules, and immunocytokines, have shown promising therapeutic activity in the setting of refractory lymphomas, supporting the concept that disrupting the growth-promoting interactions or cross talk between neoplastic and non-neoplastic cells may eventually become a treatment option even in the upfront setting (Lenz and Staudt 2010; Witzig et al. 2011). Despite their complexity and heterogeneity, DLBCL, FL, and cHL are attractive disease models allowing to dissect the prognostic and therapeutic role of tumor microenvironment.

Although a variety of well-defined genetic alterations have been pathogenetically implicated in DLBCL, cross talk between the neoplastic B cells and the microenvironment is currently appreciated as an important aspect of the biology of DLBCL (Gascoyne and Steidl 2011). Tumor microenvironment of DLBCL comprises a wide spectrum of non-neoplastic cells, including benign B cells, regulatory T cells, Th1 cells, Th2 cells, Th17 cells, natural killer cells, antigen-presenting cells, stromal elements, and vascular endothelial cells (Steidl et al. 2011). Cells of tumor microenvironment are mixed in a three-dimensional network with neoplastic B cells (Nelson 2010), and their content, distribution, and function are likely to change in response to therapy (Burger et al. 2009). Important information on the microenvironment in DLBCL was provided a decade ago by a gene expression profiling (GEP) study (Rosenwald et al. 2002). This study demonstrated that a lymph node signature and a MHC class II signature could be used as molecular predictors in DLBCL patients treated with CHOP-like chemotherapy. Interestingly, immunohistochemistry (IHC) correlates of MHC class II loss were shown to be prognostic in DLBCL and related lymphoma subtypes (Rimsza et al. 2004; Roberts et al. 2006). Subsequently, the Lymphoma/Leukemia Molecular Profiling Project (LLMPP) analyzed 181 de novo cases of DLBCL treated with CHOP and 233 de novo cases of DLBCL treated with R-CHOP using GEP and confirmed that three gene expression signatures—termed "GC B cell," "stromal-1," and "stromal-2" – predicted survival both in patients who received CHOP and patients who received R-CHOP, further supporting the role of the microenvironment in DLBCL pathogenesis (Lenz et al. 2008). The whole-section GEP data were complemented by data derived from magnetic bead separations of CD19-positive B cells versus CD19-negative cells from DLBCL biopsies that convincingly showed that two new signatures *stromal-1* and *stromal-2* were clearly derived from non-neoplastic CD19-negative cells in the tumor microenvironment. The *stromal-1* signature conferred a favorable outcome and revealed genes suggesting extracellular matrix deposition and histiocytic infiltration. The *stromal-2* gene signature was associated with inferior survival and revealed genes involved in endothelial cell biology and adipocyte function. Overall, these data strongly establish an important role for non-neoplastic cells in the pathogenesis of DLBCL and suggest that treatment approaches that target both the malignant B cells and the non-neoplastic cells in the microenvironment should be explored to improve the efficacy of first-line therapy in selected subsets of patients with DLBCL.

FL is characterized by a substantial molecular, histological, and clinical heterogeneity with no agreement on optimal initial therapy. Studies aimed at evaluating the prognostic impact of microenvironment parameters, such as analysis of lymphoma-associated macrophages and microvessel density (MVD), have provided conflicting results. Increased numbers of macrophages in diagnostic biopsies of FL have been associated with inferior survival (Farinha et al. 2005; Canioni et al. 2008). However, addition of rituximab to chemotherapy was shown to overcome the negative prognostic impact of macrophages (Canioni et al. 2008) and indeed was associated with a survival advantage (Taskinen et al. 2007). Analysis of MVD found a correlation of increased MVD with favorable outcome in FL patients treated with CVP and interferon (IFN)-alpha followed by maintenance IFN-α (Koster et al. 2005), while conflicting result emerged from FL patients treated with BP-VACOP (Farinha et al. 2010). Whether or not these differences in the prognostic impact of MVD can be interpreted as related to IFN-α, a drug known to have some antiangiogenic effects, remains an open issue. The role of the microenvironment in histologic transformation of FL to DLBCL has been addressed by several studies with conflicting results. A frequency of programmed cell death 1 (PD-1)-positive cells $\leq$5 % has been associated with a higher risk of transformation, whereas a high content of PD-1-positive cells predicted favorable outcome of FL patients (Carreras et al. 2009). In contrast, a recent study from Mayo Clinic (Smeltzer et al. 2013) has identified the pattern of PD-1^{+} cells and the localization of CD14+ cells to the follicle as associated with inferior time to transformation (TTT) and overall survival (OS). Interestingly, after accounting for FLIPI score, both these factors remained significant, thus identifying two independent predictors of the rate of transformation in FL and suggesting that location rather than quantity of CD14^{+} or PD-1^{+} cells may influence clinical outcome. Overall, these conflicting results do not allow to reach any definitive conclusion on the prognostic role of microenvironment in FL rather they clearly show that several issues still require to be accurately addressed by the prospective analysis of homogeneously treated large cohorts of patients. These studies should combine conventional approaches, such as immunohistochemistry and cell separation techniques, with genomic technologies including DNA sequencing and analysis of the transcriptional profiles.

cHL represents a paradigm of tumor cell–microenvironment interactions, as the neoplastic HRS cells typically represent <5 % of the total infiltrate in lymph node biopsies, whereas >95 %of the total infiltrate consists of a mixture of inflammatory and immune cells. Both HRS cells and non-neoplastic cells within the microenvironment pathogenetically contribute to the pathological process by secreting cytokines and chemokines that allow the neoplastic HRS cells to survive and evade antitumor immune mechanisms. cHL microenvironment allows HRS cells to grow in a Th2 milieu where HRS cells produce a variety of factors, including among others galectin-1, PD-L1, CSF-1, and TARC that create a peculiar microenvironment leading to the recruitment of macrophages and regulatory T cells that further contribute to immune privilege. Several GEP studies performed using whole biopsy sections have explored the contribution of the microenvironment to disease outcome (Steidl et al. 2010; Sanchez-Aguilera et al. 2006; Scott et al. 2013). These studies consistently implicate macrophages, benign B cells and specific T-cell subsets in predicting the success of first-line therapy in patients with cHL. The study by Steidl and colleagues (Steidl et al. 2010) analyzed 130 cases of cHL including 38 primary treatment failures and 92 treatment successes. In this study, macrophage signatures were associated with treatment failure. Validation of this results using an unrelated clinical cohort and a IHC-based approach using CD68 expression showed that increased CD68-positive macrophages at the time of diagnosis were associated with treatment failure and interestingly were also associated with failure following salvage therapy. Based on these results, targeting the microenvironment might be a useful strategy in the treatment of selected subsets of cHL patients (Germano et al. 2013). The availability of biological agents such as brentuximab vedotin targeting CD30-positive HRS cells combined with agents that can disrupt the cross talk with the non-neoplastic cells in the microenvironment (e.g., lenalidomide) might represent important new strategies for the treatment of refractory cHL patients.

A variety of therapeutic targets are emerging from studies investigating lymphoma microenvironment. However, the translation of our current knowledge of tumor microenvironment into hypothesis-driven clinical trials remains a challenging issue. The concept that the tumor microenvironment might be a promising therapeutic target involves not only the use of biological agents but also that of conventional molecules, such as the pyrimidine analog gemcitabine, a cytotoxic agent reported to be effective in relapsed cHL and known to specifically target regulatory T cells(Correale et al. 2008). Inflammation has been implicated in lymphomagenesis because it may lead to the activation of the key transcriptional factors NF-κB and STAT-3 which are involved in a complex inflammatory network. These transcriptional factors regulate oncogenic factors affecting proliferation, migration, angiogenesis, invasiveness, as well as drug resistance of tumors. Since cancers including lymphomas are caused by dysregulation of multiple pathways, it seems reasonable that agents interfering with multiple pathways are likely as being more effective. In conclusion, therapies targeting cells of the microenvironment or disrupting microenvironment-dependent signaling in the malignant cells might have a positive impact on patients with relapsed lymphomas. Current clinical trials focusing on the combination of targeted agents with classical chemotherapy agents as well as randomized trials comparing these novel agents with the current standard of care for first- and second-line therapies will ultimately determine their significance in the overall landscape of lymphoma treatment.

References

Aldinucci D, Lorenzon D, Cattaruzza L, Pinto A, Gloghini A, Carbone A, Colombatti (2008) Expression of CCR5 receptors on Reed-Sternberg cells and Hodgkin lymphoma cell lines: involvement of CCL5/RANTES in tumour cell growth and microenvironmental interactions. Int J Cancer 122(4):769–776

Aldinucci D, Gloghini A, Pinto A, De Filippi R, Carbone A (2010) The classical Hodgkin's lymphoma microenvironment and its role in promoting tumour growth and immune escape. J Pathol 221(3):248–263

Aldinucci D, Celegato M, Borghese C, Colombatti A, Carbone A (2011) IRF4 silencing inhibits Hodgkin lymphoma cell proliferation, survival and CCL5 secretion. Br J Haematol 152(2):182–190

Allen CD, Ansel KM, Low C, Lesley R, Tamamura H, Fujii N et al (2004) Germinal center dark and light zone organization is mediated by CXCR4 and CXCR5. Nat Immunol 5(9):943–952

Ansel KM, Ngo VN, Hyman PL, Luther SA, Forster R, Sedgwick JD et al (2000) A chemokine-driven positive feedback loop organizes lymphoid follicles. Nature 406(6793):309–314

Aozasa K (2006) Pyothorax-associated lymphoma. J Clin Exp Hematop 46(1):5–10

Burger JA, Ghia P, Rosenwald A, Caligaris-Cappio F (2009) The microenvironment in mature B cell malignancies: a target for new treatment strategies. Blood 114(16):3367–3375

Canioni D, Salles G, Mounier N, Brousse N, Keuppens M, Morchhauser F, Lamy T, Sonet A, Rousselet MC, Foussard C, Xerri L (2008) High numbers of tumor-associated macrophages have an adverse prognostic value that can be circumvented by rituximab in patients with follicular lymphoma enrolled onto the GELA-GOELAMS FL-2000 trial. J Clin Oncol 26(3):440–446. doi:10.1200/JCO.2007.12.8298

Carbone A, Manconi R, Poletti A, Volpe R (1985) Practical importance of immunostaining paraffin-embedded biopsy samples of small lymphocytic and follicle centre cell lymphomas for S100 protein. Lancet 2(8455):617

Carbone A, Gloghini A, Gruss HJ, Pinto A (1995) CD40 ligand is constitutively expressed in a subset of T cell lymphomas and on the microenvironmental reactive T cells of follicular lymphomas and Hodgkin's disease. Am J Pathol 147(4):912–922

Carbone A, Gloghini A, Aldinucci D, Gattei V, Dalla-Favera R, Gaidano G (2002) Expression pattern of MUM1/IRF4 in the spectrum of pathology of Hodgkin's disease. Br J Haematol 117(2):366–372

Carbone A, Gloghini A, Cabras A, Elia G (2009) The Germinal centre-derived lymphomas seen through their cellular microenvironment. Br J Haematol 145(4):468–480

Carreras J, Lopez-Guillermo A, Roncador G, Villamor N, Colomo L, Martinez A, Hamoudi R, Howat WJ, Montserrat E, Campo E (2009) High numbers of tumor-infiltrating programmed cell death 1-positive regulatory lymphocytes are associated with improved overall survival in follicular lymphoma. J Clin Oncol 27(9):1470–1476. doi:10.1200/JCO.2008.18.0513

Cheung KJ, Johnson NA, Affleck JG, Severson T, Steidl C, Ben-Neriah S et al (2010) Acquired TNFRSF14 mutations in follicular lymphoma are associated with worse prognosis. Cancer Res 70(22):9166–9174

Correale P, Del Vecchio MT, La Placa M, Montagnani F, Di Genova G, Savellini GG, Terrosi C, Mannucci S, Giorgi G, Francini G, Cusi MG (2008) Chemotherapeutic drugs may be used to enhance the killing efficacy of human tumor antigen peptide-specific CTLs. J Immunother 31(2):132–147. doi:10.1097/CJI.0b013e31815b69c8

Coupland SE (2011) The challenge of the microenvironment in B-cell lymphomas. Histopathology 58(1):69–80. doi:10.1111/j.1365-2559.2010.03706.x

Dammacco F, Gatti P, Sansonno D (1998) Hepatitis C virus infection, mixed cryoglobulinemia, and non-Hodgkin's lymphoma: an emerging picture. Leuk Lymphoma 31(5–6):463–476

Dave SS, Wright G, Tan B, Rosenwald A, Gascoyne RD, Chan WC et al (2004) Prediction of survival in follicular lymphoma based on molecular features of tumor-infiltrating immune cells. N Engl J Med 351(21):2159–2169

de Jong D, Fest T (2011) The microenvironment in follicular lymphoma. Best Pract Res Clin Haematol 24(2):135–146. doi:10.1016/j.beha.2011.02.007. (Epub 2011 May 17)

De Vita S, Sansonno D, Dolcetti R, Ferraccioli G, Carbone A, Cornacchiulo V et al (1995) Hepatitis C virus within a malignant lymphoma lesion in the course of type II mixed cryoglobulinemia. Blood 86(5):1887–1892

Dupuis J, Boye K, Martin N, Copie-Bergman C, Plonquet A, Fabiani B et al (2006) Expression of CXCL13 by neoplastic cells in angioimmunoblastic T-cell lymphoma (AITL): a new diagnostic marker providing evidence that AITL derives from follicular helper T cells. Am J Surg Pathol 30(4):490–494

Farinha P, Masoudi H, Skinnider BF, Shumansky K, Spinelli JJ, Gill K, Klasa R, Voss N, Connors JM, Gascoyne RD (2005) Analysis of multiple biomarkers shows that lymphoma-associated macrophage (LAM) content is an independent predictor of survival in follicular lymphoma (FL). Blood 106(6):2169–2174. doi:10.1182/blood-2005-04-1565

Farinha P, Kyle AH, Minchinton AI, Connors JM, Karsan A, Gascoyne RD (2010) Vascularization predicts overall survival and risk of transformation in follicular lymphoma. Haematologica 95(12):2157–2160. doi:10.3324/haematol.2009.021766

Fukayama M, Ibuka T, Hayashi Y, Ooba T, Koike M, Mizutani S (1993) Epstein-Barr virus in pyothorax-associated pleural lymphoma. Am J Pathol 143(4):1044–1049

Gascoyne RD, Steidl C (2011) VII. The role of the microenvironment in lymphoid cancers. Ann Oncol 22 (Suppl 4):iv47–iv50. doi:10.1093/annonc/mdr173

Germanidis G, Haioun C, Dhumeaux D, Reyes F, Pawlotsky JM (1999) Hepatitis C virus infection, mixed cryoglobulinemia, and B-cell non-Hodgkin's lymphoma. Hepatology 30(3):822–823

Germano G, Frapolli R, Belgiovine C, Anselmo A, Pesce S, Liguori M, Erba E, Uboldi S, Zucchetti M, Pasqualini F, Nebuloni M, van Rooijen N, Mortarini R, Beltrame L, Marchini S, Fuso Nerini I, Sanfilippo R, Casali PG, Pilotti S, Galmarini CM, Anichini A, Mantovani A, D'Incalci M, Allavena P (2013) Role of macrophage targeting in the antitumor activity of trabectedin. Cancer Cell 23(2):249–262. doi:10.1016/j.ccr.2013.01.008

Gloghini A, Carbone A (1993) The nonlymphoid microenvironment of reactive follicles and lymphomas of follicular origin as defined by immunohistology on paraffin-embedded tissues. Hum Pathol 24(1):67–76

Gloghini A, Volpe R, Carbone A (1990) Vimentin immunostaining in fibroblastic reticulum cells within human reactive and neoplastic lymphoid follicles. Hum Pathol 21(8):792–798

Hopken UE, Rehm A (2012) Homeostatic chemokines guide lymphoma cells to tumor growth-promoting niches within secondary lymphoid organs. J Mol Med 90(11):1237–1245

Husson H, Freedman AS, Cardoso AA, Schultze J, Munoz O, Strola G et al (2002) CXCL13 (BCA-1) is produced by follicular lymphoma cells: role in the accumulation of malignant B cells. Br J Haematol 119(2):492–495

IARC (2012) Monographs on the evaluation of carcinogenic risks to humans. In: ARC monographs on the evaluation of carcinogenic risks to humans, vol 100B. Biological Agents, Lyon, France

Iqbal J, Weisenburger DD, Greiner TC, Vose JM, McKeithan T, Kucuk C et al (2010) Molecular signatures to improve diagnosis in peripheral T-cell lymphoma and prognostication in angioimmunoblastic T-cell lymphoma. Blood 115(5):1026–1036

Jaffe ES, Wilson WH (1997) Lymphomatoid granulomatosis: pathogenesis, pathology and clinical implications. Cancer Surv 30:233–248

Klein U, Dalla-Favera R (2008) Germinal centres: role in B-cell physiology and malignancy. Nat Rev Immunol 8(1):22–33

Koster A, van Krieken JH, Mackenzie MA, Schraders M, Borm GF, van der Laak JA, Leenders W, Hebeda K, Raemaekers JM (2005) Increased vascularization predicts favorable outcome in follicular lymphoma. Clin Cancer Res 11(1):154–161

Kraus MD, Haley J (2000) Lymphocyte predominance Hodgkin's disease: the use of bcl-6 and CD57 in diagnosis and differential diagnosis. Am J Surg Pathol 24(8):1068–1078

Kridel R, Sehn LH, Gascoyne RD (2012) Pathogenesis of follicular lymphoma. J Clin Invest 122(10):3424–3431

Kuppers R (2009) The biology of Hodgkin's lymphoma. Nat Rev Cancer 9(1):15–27

Lenz G, Staudt LM (2010) Aggressive lymphomas. N Eng J Med 362(15):1417–1429. doi:10.1056/NEJMra0807082; [pii] 362/15/1417

Lenz G, Wright G, Dave S, Kohlmann A, Xiao W, Powell J et al (2007) Gene expression signatures predict overall survival in diffuse large B cell lymphoma treated with Rituximab and Chop-like chemotherapy. Blood 110(11):348 (ASH Annual Meeting Abstracts)

Lenz G, Wright G, Dave SS, Xiao W, Powell J, Zhao H, Xu W, Tan B, Goldschmidt N, Iqbal J, Vose J, Bast M, Fu K, Weisenburger DD, Greiner TC, Armitage JO, Kyle A, May L, Gascoyne RD, Connors JM, Troen G, Holte H, Kvaloy S, Dierickx D, Verhoef G, Delabie J, Smeland EB, Jares P, Martinez A, Lopez-Guillermo A, Montserrat E, Campo E, Braziel RM, Miller TP, Rimsza LM, Cook JR, Pohlman B, Sweetenham J, Tubbs RR, Fisher RI, Hartmann E, Rosenwald A, Ott G, Muller-Hermelink HK, Wrench D, Lister TA, Jaffe ES, Wilson WH, Chan WC, Staudt LM (2008) Stromal gene signatures in large-B-cell lymphomas. N Engl J Med 359(22):2313–2323. doi:10.1056/NEJMoa0802885 (Lymphoma/Leukemia Molecular Profiling P)

Lossos IS (2007) The endless complexity of lymphocyte differentiation and lymphomagenesis: IRF-4 downregulates BCL6 expression. Cancer Cell 12(3):189–191

Lossòs IS, Levy R (2003) Higher grade transformation of follicular lymphoma: phenotypic tumor progression associated with diverse genetic lesions. Sem Cancer Biol 13(3):191–202

Lukes RJ, Butler JJ (1966) The pathology and nomenclature of Hodgkin's disease. Cancer Res 26(6):1063–1083

Mackay F, Browning JL (2002) BAFF: a fundamental survival factor for B cells. Nat Rev Immunol 2(7):465–475

MacLennan IC (1994) Germinal centers. Annu Rev Immunol 12:117–139

Manconi R, Poletti A, Volpe R, Sulfaro S, Carbone A (1988) Dendritic reticulum cell pattern as a microenvironmental indicator for a distinct origin of lymphoma of follicular mantle cells. Br J Haematol 68(2):213–218

Mantovani A, Allavena P, Sica A, Balkwill F (2008) Cancer-related inflammation. Nature 454(7203):436–444

Mariette X (2001) Lymphomas complicating Sjogren's syndrome and hepatitis C virus infection may share a common pathogenesis: chronic stimulation of rheumatoid factor B cells. Ann Rheum Dis 60(11):1007–1010

Marshall NA, Christie LE, Munro LR, Culligan DJ, Johnston PW, Barker RN et al (2004) Immunosuppressive regulatory T cells are abundant in the reactive lymphocytes of Hodgkin lymphoma. Blood 103(5):1755–1762

Mele A, Pulsoni A, Bianco E, Musto P, Szklo A, Sanpaolo MG et al (2003) Hepatitis C virus and B-cell non-Hodgkin lymphomas: an Italian multicenter case-control study. Blood 102(3):996–999

Miyagaki T, Sugaya M, Suga H, Kamata M, Ohmatsu H, Fujita H et al (2011) IL-22, but not IL-17, dominant environment in cutaneous T-cell lymphoma. Clin Cancer Res 17(24):7529–7538

Morin RD, Johnson NA, Severson TM, Mungall AJ, An J, Goya R et al (2010) Somatic mutations altering EZH2 (Tyr641) in follicular and diffuse large B-cell lymphomas of germinal-center origin. Nat Genet 42(2):181–185

Morin RD, Mendez-Lago M, Mungall AJ, Goya R, Mungall KL, Corbett RD et al (2011) Frequent mutation of histone-modifying genes in non-Hodgkin lymphoma. Nature 476(7360):298–303

Nakasone ES, Askautrud HA, Kees T, Park JH, Plaks V, Ewald AJ, Fein M, Rasch MG, Tan YX, Qiu J, Park J, Sinha P, Bissell MJ, Frengen E, Werb Z, Egeblad M (2012) Imaging tumor-stroma interactions during chemotherapy reveals contributions of the microenvironment to resistance. Cancer Cell 21(4):488–503. doi:10.1016/j.ccr.2012.02.017

Nam-Cha SH, Roncador G, Sanchez-Verde L, Montes-Moreno S, Acevedo A, Dominguez-Franjo P et al (2008) PD-1, a follicular T-cell marker useful for recognizing nodular lymphocyte-predominant Hodgkin lymphoma. Am J Surg Pathol 32(8):1252–1257

Nelson BH (2010) CD20+ B cells: the other tumor-infiltrating lymphocytes. J Immunol 185(9):4977–4982. doi:10.4049/jimmunol.1001323

Nogai H, Dorken B, Lenz G (2011) Pathogenesis of non-Hodgkin's lymphoma. J Clin Oncol 29(14):1803–1811. doi:10.1200/JCO.2010.33.3252

Pasqualucci L, Dominguez-Sola D, Chiarenza A, Fabbri G, Grunn A, Trifonov V et al (2011) Inactivating mutations of acetyltransferase genes in B-cell lymphoma. Nature 471(7337):189–195

Peveling-Oberhag J, Arcaini L, Hansmann ML, Zeuzem S (2013) Hepatitis C-associated B-cell non-Hodgkin lymphomas. Epidemiology, molecular signature and clinical management. J Hepatol 59(1):169–177

Piccaluga PP, Agostinelli C, Califano A, Carbone A, Fantoni L, Ferrari S et al (2007) Gene expression analysis of angioimmunoblastic lymphoma indicates derivation from T follicular helper cells and vascular endothelial growth factor deregulation. Cancer Res 67(22):10703–10710

Poppema S (1989) The nature of the lymphocytes surrounding Reed-Sternberg cells in nodular lymphocyte predominance and in other types of Hodgkin's disease. Am J Pathol 135(2):351–357

Poppema S (2005) Immunobiology and pathophysiology of Hodgkin lymphomas. Hematol Am Soc Hematol Educ Program (1):231–238

Poppema S, Delsol G, Pileri SA, Stein H (2008) Nodular lymphocyte predominant Hodgkin lymphoma. In: Swerdlow SH, Campo E, Harris NL, Jaffe ES, Pileri SA, Stein H et al (eds) WHO classification of tumours of haematopoietic and lymphoid tissues. IARC, Lyon, pp 323–325

Reeder CB, Ansell SM (2011) Novel therapeutic agents for B-cell lymphoma: developing rational combinations. Blood 117(5):1453–1462. doi:10.1182/blood-2010-06-255067

Rimsza LM, Roberts RA, Miller TP, Unger JM, LeBlanc M, Braziel RM, Weisenberger DD, Chan WC, Muller-Hermelink HK, Jaffe ES, Gascoyne RD, Campo E, Fuchs DA, Spier CM, Fisher RI, Delabie J, Rosenwald A, Staudt LM, Grogan TM (2004) Loss of MHC class II gene and protein expression in diffuse large B-cell lymphoma is related to decreased tumor immunosurveillance and poor patient survival regardless of other prognostic factors: a follow-up study from the Leukemia and Lymphoma Molecular Profiling Project. Blood 103(11):4251–4258. doi:10.1182/blood-2003-07-2365

Roberts RA, Wright G, Rosenwald AR, Jaramillo MA, Grogan TM, Miller TP, Frutiger Y, Chan WC, Gascoyne RD, Ott G, Muller-Hermelink HK, Staudt LM, Rimsza LM (2006) Loss of major histocompatibility class II gene and protein expression in primary mediastinal large B-cell lymphoma is highly coordinated and related to poor patient survival. Blood 108(1):311–318. doi:10.1182/blood-2005-11-4742

Rosenwald A, Wright G, Chan WC, Connors JM, Campo E, Fisher RI, Gascoyne RD, Muller-Hermelink HK, Smeland EB, Giltnane JM, Hurt EM, Zhao H, Averett L, Yang L, Wilson WH, Jaffe ES, Simon R, Klausner RD, Powell J, Duffey PL, Longo DL, Greiner TC, Weisenburger DD, Sanger WG, Dave BJ, Lynch JC, Vose J, Armitage JO, Montserrat E, Lopez-Guillermo A, Grogan TM, Miller TP, LeBlanc M, Ott G, Kvaloy S, Delabie J, Holte H, Krajci P, Stokke T, Staudt LM (2002) The use of molecular profiling to predict survival after chemotherapy for diffuse large-B-cell lymphoma. N Engl J Med 346(25):1937–1947. doi:10.1056/NEJMoa012914 (Lymphoma/Leukemia Molecular Profiling P)

Sanchez-Aguilera A, Montalban C, de la Cueva P, Sanchez-Verde L, Morente MM, Garcia-Cosio M, Garcia-Larana J, Bellas C, Provencio M, Romagosa V, de Sevilla AF, Menarguez J, Sabin P, Mestre MJ, Mendez M, Fresno MF, Nicolas C, Piris MA, Garcia JF (2006) Tumor microenvironment and mitotic checkpoint are key factors in the outcome of classic Hodgkin lymphoma. Blood 108(2):662–668. doi:10.1182/blood-2005-12-5125 (Spanish Hodgkin Lymphoma Study G)

Sansonno D, De Vita S, Cornacchiulo V, Carbone A, Boiocchi M, Dammacco F (1996) Detection and distribution of hepatitis C virus-related proteins in lymph nodes of patients with type II mixed cryoglobulinemia and neoplastic or non-neoplastic lymphoproliferation. Blood 88(12):4638–4645

Sansonno D, Lauletta G, De Re V, Tucci FA, Gatti P, Racanelli V et al (2004) Intrahepatic B cell clonal expansions and extrahepatic manifestations of chronic HCV infection. Eur J Immunol 34(1):126–136

Sansonno D, Carbone A, De Re V, Dammacco F (2007) Hepatitis C virus infection, cryoglobulinaemia, and beyond. Rheumatology 46(4):572–578

Schmitz R, Stanelle J, Hansmann ML et al (2009) Pathogenesis of classical and lymphocyte-predominant Hodgkin lymphoma. Annu Rev Pathol 4:151–174

Schneider P, Tschopp J (2003) BAFF and the regulation of B cell survival. Immunol Lett 88(1):57–62

Schreck S, Friebel D, Buettner M, Distel L, Grabenbauer G, Young LS et al (2009) Prognostic impact of tumour-infiltrating Th2 and regulatory T cells in classical Hodgkin lymphoma. Hematol Oncol 27(1):31–39

Scott DW, Chan FC, Hong F, Rogic S, Tan KL, Meissner B, Ben-Neriah S, Boyle M, Kridel R, Telenius A, Woolcock BW, Farinha P, Fisher RI, Rimsza LM, Bartlett NL, Cheson

BD, Shepherd LE, Advani RH, Connors JM, Kahl BS, Gordon LI, Horning SJ, Steidl C, Gascoyne RD (2013) Gene expression-based model using formalin-fixed paraffin-embedded biopsies predicts overall survival in advanced-stage classical Hodgkin lymphoma. J Clin Oncol 31(6):692–700. doi:10.1200/JCO.2012.43.4589

Skibinski G, Skibinska A, James K (2001) The role of hepatocyte growth factor and its receptor c-met in interactions between lymphocytes and stromal cells in secondary human lymphoid organs. Immunol 102(4):506–514

Smeltzer LP, Jones JM, Ziesmer S, Grote D, Yang ZZ, Novak A, Xiu B, Ristow K, Ansell SM (2013) Changes in the tumor microenvironment associated with transformation in follicular lymphoma. J Clin Oncol 31:(suppl; abstr 8538)

Steidl C, Lee T, Shah SP, Farinha P, Han G, Nayar T et al (2010) Tumor-associated macrophages and survival in classic Hodgkin's lymphoma. N Engl J Med 362(10):875–885

Steidl C, Connors JM, Gascoyne RD (2011) Molecular pathogenesis of Hodgkin's lymphoma: increasing evidence of the importance of the microenvironment. J Clin Oncol 29(14):1812–1826. doi:10.1200/JCO.2010.32.8401

Stein H, Delsol G, Pileri SA, Weiss LM, Poppema S, Jaffe ES (2008) Classical Hodgkin lymphoma, introduction. In: Swerdlow SH, Campo E, Harris NL, Jaffe ES, Pileri SA, Stein H et al (eds) WHO classification of tumours of haematopoietic and lymphoid tissues, 4th edn. IARC, Lyon, pp 326–329

Talamini R, Montella M, Crovatto M, Dal Maso L, Crispo A, Negri E et al (2004) Non-Hodgkin's lymphoma and hepatitis C virus: a case-control study from northern and southern Italy. Int J Cancer 110(3):380–385

Taneda S, Segerer S, Hudkins KL, Cui Y, Wen M, Segerer M et al (2001) Cryoglobulinemic glomerulonephritis in thymic stromal lymphopoietin transgenic mice. Am J Pathol 159(6):2355–2369

Taskinen M, Karjalainen-Lindsberg ML, Nyman H, Eerola LM, Leppa S (2007) A high tumor-associated macrophage content predicts favorable outcome in follicular lymphoma patients treated with rituximab and cyclophosphamide-doxorubicin-vincristine-prednisone. Clin Cancer Res 13(19):5784–5789. doi:10.1158/1078-0432.CCR-07-0778

Timens W, Visser L, Poppema S (1986) Nodular lymphocyte predominance type of Hodgkin's disease is a germinal center lymphoma. Lab Invest 54(4):457–461

Tripodo C, Gri G, Piccaluga PP, Frossi B, Guarnotta C, Piconese S et al (2010) Mast cells and Th17 cells contribute to the lymphoma-associated pro-inflammatory microenvironment of angioimmunoblastic T-cell lymphoma. Am J Pathol 177(2):792–802

Weimar IS, de Jong D, Muller EJ, Nakamura T, van Gorp JM, de Gast GC et al (1997) Hepatocyte growth factor/scatter factor promotes adhesion of lymphoma cells to extracellular matrix molecules via alpha 4 beta 1 and alpha 5 beta 1 integrins. Blood 89(3):990–1000

Wilson WH, Kingma DW, Raffeld M, Wittes RE, Jaffe ES (1996) Association of lymphomatoid granulomatosis with Epstein-Barr viral infection of B lymphocytes and response to interferon-alpha 2b. Blood 87(11):4531–4537

Witzig TE, Vose JM, Zinzani PL, Reeder CB, Buckstein R, Polikoff JA, Bouabdallah R, Haioun C, Tilly H, Guo P, Pietronigro D, Ervin-Haynes AL, Czuczman MS (2011) An international phase II trial of single-agent lenalidomide for relapsed or refractory aggressive B-cell non-Hodgkin's lymphoma. Ann Oncol 22 (7):1622–1627. doi:10.1093/annonc/mdq626; [pii] mdq626

Woolf N (1998) Relationship of neoplastic cells with their environment: tumor spread. In: Pathology basic and systemic. WB Sanders Company LTD, London, pp 249–260

Yamamoto R, Nishikori M, Kitawaki T, Sakai T, Hishizawa M, Tashima M et al (2008) PD-1-PD-1 ligand interaction contributes to immunosuppressive microenvironment of Hodgkin lymphoma. Blood 111(6):3220–3224

Zignego AL, Gragnani L, Giannini C, Laffi G (2012) The hepatitis C virus infection as a systemic disease. Int Emerg Med 7(Suppl 3):S201–S208

Chapter 13
The Role of Inflammation in Leukaemia

Janusz Krawczyk, Michael O'Dwyer, Ronan Swords, Ciara Freeman and Francis J Giles

Abstract Acute leukaemias are a group of malignancies characterised by the invasion of the bone marrow by immature haematopoietic precursors and differentiation arrest at various maturation steps. Multiplicity of intrinsic and extrinsic factors influences the transformation and progression of leukaemia. The intrinsic factors encompass genetic alterations of cellular pathways leading to the activation of, among others, inflammatory pathways (such as nuclear factor kappa B). The extrinsic components include, among others, the inflammatory pathways activated by the bone marrow microenvironment and include chemokines, cytokines and adhesion molecules. In this chapter, we review the role of inflammatory processes in the transformation, survival and proliferation of leukaemias, particularly the role of nuclear factor kappa B and its downstream signalling in leukaemias and the novel therapeutic strategies that exploit potentially unique properties of inflammatory signalling that offer interesting options for future therapeutic interventions.

An erratum to this chapter is available at 10.1007/978-3-0348-0837-8_18

J. Krawczyk
Department of Haematology, Galway University Hospital, Galway, Ireland

M. O'Dwyer
Biosciences, National University of Ireland Galway, Upper Newcastle, Galway, Ireland

R. Swords
Sylvester Comprehensive Cancer Center, University of Miami, Miami, USA

C. Freeman
Department of Haematology, Barts and the Royal London NHS Trust, London, UK

F. J. Giles (✉)
Northwestern Medicine Developmental Therapeutics Institute, Robert H. Lurie Comprehensive Cancer Center of Northwestern University, Chicago, USA
e-mail: frankgiles@aol.com

13.1 Introduction

Leukaemia is a broad category of haematological neoplasms. Based on clinical criteria, leukaemias are grouped into acute and chronic. Based on pathological criteria, leukaemias are grouped into myeloid and lymphoid. In adults, the most common types of leukaemia are chronic lymphocytic leukaemia (CLL) and acute myeloid leukaemia (AML). Chronic myeloid leukaemia (CML) and acute lymphoid leukaemia (ALL) are less frequent. AML is a heterogeneous group of disorders characterised by the uncontrolled proliferation of myeloid progenitors with a reduced potential to differentiate into mature cells. Laboratory data suggest that AML originates from a population of rare cells, termed leukaemic stem cells (LSCs), which are capable of self-renewal, proliferation and differentiation. These cells may persist after treatment and are probably responsible for disease relapse. Molecular alterations underlying the development of leukaemia, typically involve the disruption of tumour suppressor genes (point mutations, chromosomal deletions), activation of proto-oncogenes or the formation of oncogenic fusion proteins. In AML, several chromosomal abnormalities and mutations have been identified. The t(8;21), t(16;16) and inv(16) mutations are associated with a better prognosis. Mutation in the FLT3 tyrosine kinase receptor gene is the most common mutation in AML and is associated with poor clinical outcomes. Mutations in the DNA methyltransferase gene, DNMT3A, are also associated with poor prognosis and are recurrent in patients with intermediate-risk AML. The presence of any DNMT3A mutation, either alone or in combination with the FLT3 internal tandem duplication (ITD) mutation, is associated with a significantly shorter overall survival rate. Tables 13.1 and 13.2 present the key chromosomal and molecular prognostic factors in AML. The incidence of AML is 3.7 per 100,000 per year (Dohner et al. 2010). Over the past several decades, better chemotherapeutic regimens have improved the outcomes in both acute leukaemias. The primary goal of therapy in AML is to achieve and maintain a complete remission (CR), as it significantly improves survival (Freireich et al. 1961). The patients who remain in CR for 3 years have a low (<10 %) probability of relapse (de Lima et al. 1997). Standard remission induction chemotherapy for AML consists of a combination of anthracycline and cytarabine (known as 3 + 7 regimen). Despite an initial sensitivity to chemotherapy, long-term disease-free survival in AML remains low mostly due to the frequency of relapses. In the USA, the overall 5-year relative survival rate for 2002–2008 from Surveillance Epidemiology and End Results (SEER) database was 23.4 % (NCI 2013). Although more than one-half of adult patients achieve CR, relapses occur frequently as result of the expansion of leukaemic cells that have escaped chemotherapy. Minimal residual disease (MRD), which is detected by immunophenotyping or molecular analyses, identifies malignant cells that have survived chemotherapy. The level of MRD after chemotherapy has a strong prognostic impact and may provide a surrogate endpoint or provide assistance in assessing the clinical efficacy of new targeted therapies. For younger patients, despite the improved protocols of treatment developed in the last years, the survival rate remains unsatisfactory, and the curative options for relapse after allogeneic HSCT are poor.

Table 13.1 AML cytogenetic risk groups

Karyotype	Frequency (%)	Complete remission (%)	Event-free survival (%)
Favourable			
t(8;21)	5–10	90	60–70
inv(16)	5–10	90	60–70
t(15;17)	5–10	80–90	70
Intermediate			
Diploid, -Y	40–50	70–80	30–40
Unfavourable			
−5/−7	20–30	50	5–10
+8	10	60	10–20
11q23, 20q−, other	10–20	60	10

Table 13.2 Prognostic factors in AML

Factor	Relapse rate	Survival
↑ *BAACL*		↓
*FLT*3 ITD/mutation	↑	↓
MLL PTD	↑	
↑ *BCL*2 and *WT*1 mRNA	↑	↓
↑ *EVI*1 mRNA	↑	↓
*p*53 mutation		↓
CEBPA mutation	↓	↑
c-kit mutation	↑	↓

Limiting factors in the treatment of AML include the development of drug resistance, the relatively high treatment-related mortality and the long-term side effects. Immunotherapy holds great promise to sustain AML remission once the disease has been bulk-reduced with chemotherapy. Despite recent improvements in the treatment of AML, the frequency of relapses and the difficulty to completely eradicate the disease warrant the search for innovative therapies.

The age-adjusted incidence of ALL is 1.7 per 100,000 persons, with a median age at diagnosis of 13 years. ALL is the most common childhood acute leukaemia, representing approximately 80 % of childhood leukaemia cases, although it represents only 20 % of adult leukaemias. The aetiology of ALL remains unknown in most cases. Chromosomal translocations have been suggested as the primary cause for paediatric ALL; some genetic disorders are associated with a higher risk of ALL (trisomy 21, XXY). Some studies have suggested possible infectious aetiologies. Therapy of ALL is one of the most complex types of anti-cancer programs. Multiple drugs are combined into regimen-specific sequences in order to reconstitute normal haematopoiesis, prevent resistance, provide adequate prophylaxis of sanctuary sites and eliminate MRD through postremission consolidation and maintenance therapy.

CLL is a common monoclonal B-cell lymphoproliferative disease, derived from antigen-experienced B lymphocytes. The CLL cells depend on external factors for survival and proliferation. B-cell receptor stimulation and activation of a variety of signalling pathways, including PI3K/AKT, NF-κB, MAPK/ERK, WNT and

NOTCH, have also been associated with CLL cell survival, with the incidence of three cases per 100,000 individuals, and it accounts for 35 % of all leukaemias diagnosed in the United States. Currently, several cytogenetic and molecular markers have an established prognostic value, including among others, chromosomal abnormalities (especially deletions of 11q and 17p, beta-2-microglobulin, IgVH mutation status, CD38 expression and ZAP70). The introduction of purine analogues, monoclonal antibodies and other targeted therapies has shifted the treatment paradigm for CLL in recent years. These modern therapies commonly achieve CRs and even eradication of MRD—endpoints that were essentially impossible in the past (NCI 2013). Despite these advances, it remains an incurable disease.

CML is a clonal disorder of a pluripotent stem cell that affects myeloid, erythroid, megakaryocytic lineages and lymphocytes. The age-adjusted annual incidence of CML in the United States is 1.6/100,000 (NCI 2013). CML is characterised by the presence of Philadelphia chromosome and the BCR-ABL oncogene. The expression of the chimeric BCR-ABL gene in CML led to development of agents specifically targeted at inhibiting the resulting tyrosine kinase that have significantly changed the natural history of the disease.

13.2 Key Links Between Inflammation and Leukaemia

The development of leukaemia is a multistep process, where genetic alterations confer specific growth advantages driving a progressive transformation from normal to malignant cells. In haematological malignancies, mutations occur in somatic cells expressing oncogenic proteins that disrupt the equilibrium between cell proliferation and cell death. Chronic inflammation is considered of to be one of the hallmarks of malignancy (Colotta et al. 2009). The connection between inflammation and cancer is based on two mechanisms. The extrinsic mechanism involves immune and microenvironment factors, where a constant inflammatory state contributes to the initiation and progression of the cancer. The intrinsic mechanism includes acquired genetic alterations affecting oncogenes, tumour suppressors and genome stability genes that contribute to the activation of the inflammatory pathways. Several molecular and cellular signalling pathways have been identified as links between inflammatory processes and cancer development (Aggarwal and Gehlot 2009). Key molecular regulators include innate immune cells, cytokines, chemokines and members of molecular pathways including NF-κB and STAT3 and others.

13.3 Tumour-Associated Macrophages

The presence of tumour-associated macrophages (TAMs) correlates with improved prognosis in patients with solid tumours. Recent studies have shown that AML cells express CD47, a protective marker against TAMs. In a mouse model, the administration of a blocking antibody to CD47 induced macrophage-mediated phagocytosis of AML stem cells and inhibited their engraftment. The treatment of human AML LSC-engrafted mice with anti-CD47 antibody depleted AML and targeted AML LSCs (Majeti et al. 2009; Jaiswal et al. 2009; Chao et al. 2010). These observations suggest that macrophage mediated tumour immune-surveillance is an important factor in survival of leukemia stem cells (LSCs). Further identification and characterisation of distinct sets of receptor/ligands on phagocytic macrophages may be an ideal strategy with which to investigate the interaction of cancer stem cells and TAM and may lead to the exploration of new therapeutic targets against cancer stem cells.

The development of CLL is delayed in the absence of macrophage migration inhibitory factor (MIF)—a proinflammatory and immunoregulatory cytokine. Macrophages are the primary source of MIF, but also other cells of the immune system can secrete it. The absence of MIF delays the development and progression of CLL by reducing the survival of CLL cells and the number and migratory capacity of macrophages in leukaemic homing organs. This may serve as a potential new therapeutic strategy (Reinart et al. 2013).

13.3.1 Cytokines and Chemokines in Leukaemia

In normal hematopoietic cells, the activation of cell surface receptors by cytokines, chemokines and growth factors regulate signal transduction activity and the interaction between cells and the bone marrow microenvironment (Ferretti et al. 2012). The relative frequency of the activation of signal transduction in AML exceeds the frequency of mutations or genetic alterations found in the pathways or receptors, suggesting an alternative mechanism of stimulation that can include extracellular signalling. This provides leukaemic cells with proliferative and survival advantages by inhibiting apoptosis, stimulating proliferation and blocking differentiation. The abnormal cytokine signalling can be a result of an autocrine secretion, modulation of receptor expression, receptor mutations, activation of specific oncogenes or the deregulation of transcription factors. The drop in cytokine levels in patients with leukaemia in remission is well documented, suggesting that cytokine levels depend on AML activity, possibly due to autonomous blast cytokine secretion (Van Etten 2007).

The evidence for abnormal cyto- and chemokine regulation in AML is mainly based on single cytokine serum level analysis. For example, a high level of transcription factor MEF2C induces over-expression of CCL2, CCL3 and CCL4 (Schwieger et al. 2009). A series of individual regulatory axes were studied. However, the most comprehensive study so far is the analysis of serum cytokine levels in patients with AML, MDS, including a panel of 27 cyto- and chemokines. In this study, the levels of CCL5, IL-8, IL-2, CCL4 and IL-5 were predictive for survival in AML, while IL-4 and CCL3 were predictive for survival in MDS. Patients who achieved remission were more likely to have increased levels of CCL5, IL-2/4/5/10, and decreased levels of CCL2 and tumour necrosis factor (TNF). The long-time survival rate was only associated with increased levels of CCL5 and IL-2/5 and decreased levels of CCL4 and CXCL8. A panel of 11 cyto- and chemokines (including CCL3 and CCL5) allowed for the separation of patients into favourable, intermediate and unfavourable remission groups with significantly different median survival rates (52 vs. 32 vs. 16 weeks, $p = 0.003$). The effect of chemo- and cytokines in leukaemia is complex, as the level of receptor expression, the presence of receptor mutations, para- and autocrine secretion and abnormalities in signalling pathways activation modulate the effected cytokines (Kornblau et al. 2010).

One of the best-characterised chemokine is stromal-derived factor 1α, SDF-1α (CXCL12). It is constitutively secreted by marrow stromal cells and binds to C-X-C chemokine receptor type 4 (CXCR4), also known as CD184 (Koblas et al. 2007). The main role of this axis is the homing of hematopoietic progenitors and leukaemia cells within the bone marrow. CXCL12/CXCR4 mediates the adhesion of leukaemic cells to marrow stromal cells, influences survival and proliferation, protects AML cells from the effects of chemotherapy in vitro and in vivo and activates ERK and PI3K pathways (Tilton et al. 2000; Nebreda and Gavin 1999; Datta et al. 1999). In primary AML samples, the increased CXCR4 expression was found in 64 % of samples and was an independent poor prognostic factor for relapse and survival (Spoo et al. 2007). In ALL, a high expression of CXCR4 was strongly predictive for extramedullary organ involvement (Crazzolara et al. 2001).

The chemokine receptor CCR7 is an essential adhesion signal required for the targeting of leukaemic T cells into the CNS. Ccr7 gene expression is controlled by the activity of the Notch1 oncogene and is expressed in human tumours carrying Notch1-activating mutations. The silencing of either CCR7 or its chemokine ligand CCL19 in an animal model of T-ALL specifically inhibits CNS infiltration. In a murine model, CNS-targeting by human T-ALL cells depended on the expression of CCR7 (Buonamici et al. 2009).

13.3.2 NF-κB in Leukaemia

Family of nuclear factor kappa B (NF-κB) transcription factors is the key signalling pathway linking cancer and inflammation. NF-κB activates more than 200 genes including the expression of inflammatory cytokines, adhesion molecules, key enzymes in the prostaglandin synthase pathway (COX-2), nitric oxide (NO) synthase and angiogenic factors. In addition, by inducing anti-apoptotic genes (e.g. Bcl2), it promotes survival in malignant cells. In resting cells, the majority of NF-κB complexes are bound to the Inhibitor-κB (IκB) and remain sequestered in cytoplasm. The classical activation pathway of NF-κB in response to pro-inflammatory cytokines and chemokines, DNA damaging agents, Toll-like receptors (TLRs) ligands or viruses starts with the activation of inhibitor kappa B kinase (IKK) that phosphorylates IκB and frees NF-κB complexes to enter the nucleus. The non-classical signalling responds to the subset of TNF receptors and depends on the processing of a precursor protein p100 into a mature NF-κB subunit (p52) (Sun 2011).

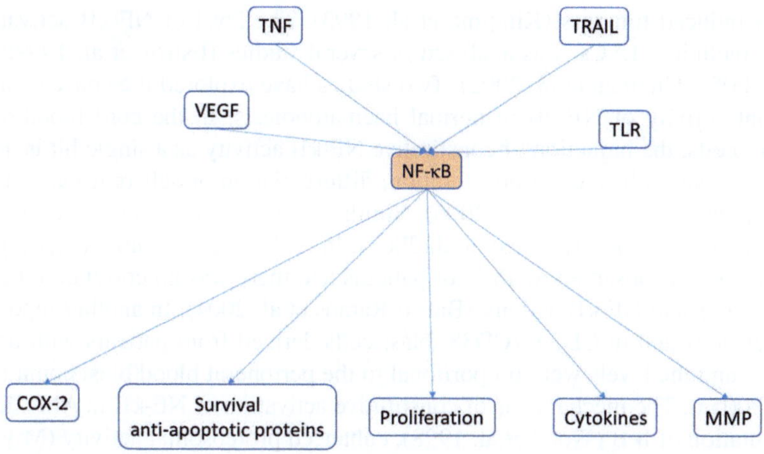

Fig. 13.1 The central role of NF-κB in signal crosstalk between inflammation and leukaemia; only pathways with proven significance are shown (*MMP* matrix metalloproteases, *TLR* Toll-like receptors, *TRAIL* tumour necrosis factor-related apoptosis-inducing ligand, *TNF* tumour necrosis factor, *VEGF* vascular endothelial growth factor, *NF-κB* nuclear factor kappa B)

Activated NF-κB can be downregulated through multiple pathways including being exported to cytoplasm by newly synthesised proteins. Constitutive activation NF-κB is frequent in malignant cell lines and primary tumours samples. It is rare in normal cells, with the exception of immune cells (proliferating T cells, B cells, thymocytes, monocytes and astrocytes). In addition, NF-κB activation can be the result of cell-autonomous genetic alterations (amplification, mutations or deletions) in cancer cells. In both malignant and inflammatory cells, NF-κB is activated downstream to the TLR-MyD88 pathway (sensing microbes and tissue damage) or the inflammatory cytokines, including TNF and IL-1β. Alternatively, NF-κB activation can be the result of genetic alterations (amplification, mutations or deletions) in cancer cells. Figure 13.1 shows the essential NF-κB-related signalling pathways with proven significance in leukaemias.

The evidence supporting the potential role for NF-κB in leukaemogenesis is based mainly on in vitro data. NF-κB is required for leukaemogenesis initiated by the Bcr-Abl chimeric protein (a deregulated tyrosine kinase) in CML (Reuther et al. 1998). The activation or expression of NF-κB was also observed in T- and B-cell lymphocyte leukaemia (Bargou et al. 1996). Consequently, a role for NF-κB in the leukaemogenesis is highly possible. It is still unclear whether over-activation or excessive expression of NF-κB in these transformed cells is a primary event or whether NF-κB provides only an accessory signal for the transformation. In HTLV-1-induced T cell acute lymphoblastic leukaemias, NF-κB is activated by Tax—a protein (encoded by HTLV-1 virus)—and it can be a mediator for viral-induced tumourigenesis (Hiscott et al. 1997). Indirect evidence to support this hypothesis is provided by the observation that mice treated with anti-sense oligonucleotides to relA (NF-κB p65) have a reduced incidence of Tax-induced tumours (Kitajima et al. 1993). The level of NF-κB activation in AML, including LSCs, was analysed in several studies (Estrov et al. 1999; Frelin et al. 2005a; Guzman et al. 2002). Two studies have explored the consequences of aberrant activity of NF-κB in normal haematopoiesis. In the cord blood-derived $CD34^+$ cells, the induction of constitutive NF-κB activity as a single hit is not sufficient to cause changes in proliferation, differentiation or self-renewal in normal haemopoiesis (Schepers et al. 2006). Similar results were also reported in adult-derived $CD34^+$ cells (Romano et al. 2003). In AML, the constitutive activation of the NF-κB was observed in 46 % of patients and there was no correlation between blast counts and NF-κB activity (Bueso-Ramos et al. 2004). In another report, NF-κB was activated in $CD34^+/CD38^-$ blast cells derived from patients with de novo AML—and the levels were proportional to the peripheral blood blast count (Frelin et al. 2005a). The mechanisms of constitutive activation of NF-κB in AML include the mutation of IκB (Wood et al. 1998), enhanced proteosomal activity (Miyamoto et al. 1994) or the enhanced inflammatory cytokine expression (O'Connell et al. 1995). It is also likely that autocrine production of cytokines may play a role in stimulating NF-κB in leukaemia. This is supported by observations of spontaneous expression of IL-1β and IL-6 in AML blast cells, as well as elevated levels of IL-6 in the serum of most patients with AML (Dokter et al. 1995). In AML, the constitutive NF-κB activity is observed in LSC and not in the normal hematopoietic stem cells (Guzman et al. 2001b). Because LSCs are responsible for disease relapse, these cells are promising targets for future therapies with IKK inhibitors (Frelin et al. 2005a). The treatment of blast cells with NF-κB or proteasome inhibitors in vitro has led to apoptosis (Guzman et al. 2001a). Interestingly, these effects are more selective on leukaemic cells, producing minor effects on normal stem cell populations. The proteasome inhibitor that blocks NF-κB but also other signalling pathways has shown selective toxicity for LSCs rather than for haematopoiesis in vitro.

In MDS, the degree of NF-κB activation correlated with the risk of progression to AML, with bone marrow blast counts and the high level of activation (Braun et al. 2006); two mechanisms can explain significant NF-κB activation. A combined immunohistochemical detection of p65 and FISH detection of common MDS-associated cytogenetic abnormalities revealed that NF-κB activation was restricted to malignant stem cells (as opposed to non-mutated stroma cells), suggesting that the intrinsic mechanism of activation is dependent on acquired mutations. An alternative mechanism of paracrine NF-κB activation via TNF is suggested in another study that described the correlation between the relative expression level of two TNF-R subunits (R1 or p55 versus R2 or p75) and the degree of NF-κB activation in MDS. The patients with predominately R1 expression of the NF-κB activation were the highest [65]. It is also possible that both intrinsic and TNF-dependent mechanisms coexist. Possibly, genetic abnormalities could lead to both NF-κB activation and differential TNF-α-R subunit expression as independent consequences, or alternatively the mutational profile of MDS blast would change the TNF-R subunit expression balance, which in turn would increase the intrinsic capacity of MDS blasts to activate NF-κB.

Constitutive activation of Bcr-Abl kinase in CML signals down to many survival pathways, including NF-κB and STAT, among others (Steelman et al. 2004). The NF-κB activation may be as a result of the increase in nuclear translocation as well as an increase in the potential of transactivation. Bcr-Abl activates NF-κB-dependent gene expression, at least partially, via Ras pathway, which transactivates the p65. IKK activation is not enhanced in primary CML cells (Lounnas et al. 2009). NF-κB is also important in malignant transformation by Bcr-Abl as shown both in vivo (nude mice) and in vitro experiments. The activation of NF-κB mediates proliferation, transformation and resistance to apoptosis in Bcr-Abl-positive cells. The key genes regulated by NF-κB include c-myc, necessary for Bcr-Abl transformation as well as many surface molecules mediating cell adhesion and cellular interactions. Studies demonstrated an intrinsic activity of NF-κB in Bcr-Abl-positive cells is increasing during the progression of the disease from the chronic phase to more advanced stages.

In CLL, the NF-κB activity is increased, in comparison to non-malignant B cells. The activity was further increased by the ligation of CD40 by the physiological ligand CD154, a critical pathway for CLL cell survival. In $CD154^+$ CLL samples, the addition of a neutralising anti-154 mAb resulted in the inhibition of NF-κB activity associated with subsequent cell death. As expected, the anti-apoptotic proteins TRAF1 and TRAF2 were upregulated in CLL cells, but it is unclear whether this occurs through a NF-κB-dependent mechanism. In CLL, many other factors, including AKT activation, B-cell receptor signalling and interleukin-4 (IL-4), have been demonstrated to increase NF-κB activity and enhance CLL cell survival. The constitutive high NF-κB in CLL was found in primary CLL samples taken from untreated patients. The activity of NF-κB was modulated with cytokines (IL-4 and IL-13 increased and TGF-β reduced) (Zaninoni et al. 2003). NF-κB in CLL was linked with fludarabine resistance (Hewamana et al. 2008). In primary ALL samples, a constitutive NF-κB activity was found in Ph+ samples, while in Ph- primary samples and B-precursor cell lines both had normal NF-κB activity. The constitutive NF-κB activity in Ph+ blasts was not related to elevated endogenous IKK activity (Munzert et al. 2004).

13.3.3 STAT3 in Leukaemia

The signal transducer and activator of transcription 3 (STAT3) is a transcription factor responding to various inflammatory and non-inflammatory cytokines and growth factors [interferons, epidermal growth factor, IL-5, IL-6, leukaemias inhibitory factor (LIF), IL-10] and regulating cell growth and apoptosis. STAT3 and NF-κB can co-regulate the expression of target genes (including those encoding PAI-1, Bcl-3 and Bcl-2). In some cases, resistance to tyrosine kinase inhibitors (TKI) can be attributed to the increased activity of the STAT3 pathway, and the STAT3 inhibition restores TKI sensitivity (Zhou et al. 2009).

In AML, STAT3 was constitutively activated in most of the cell lines and nearly half of the primary paediatric samples (Redell et al. 2011). STAT proteins are involved in the hematopoietic cytokine receptor signalling pathways that regulate cell proliferation, differentiation and survival. STATs are dysregulated in AML; mechanisms of dysregulation include constitutive activation and truncation of the C-terminal transactivation domain; the latter results in a beta isoform that has a trans-dominant negative effect on gene induction, mediated by the full-length STAT alpha form. A constitutive STAT3 activity in AML was associated with poor prognosis (Benekli et al. 2002), possibly due to the resistance to chemotherapy. Disease-free survival (DFS) was significantly shorter in patients with constitutive STAT3 activity (median 8.7 vs. 20.6 months; $P = 0.01$). The overall survival rate did not differ significantly. The subgroup of patients with constitutive STAT3 activity and the STAT3 beta isoform had the shortest DFS ($P = 0.006$) and the shorter overall survival rate ($P = 0.049$) than all other patients. It is not clear whether adverse treatment outcomes are attributable to constitutive STAT activity or to a process that leads to constitutive STAT activity (Benekli et al. 2002). The constitutive serine phosphorylation of STAT1 and STAT3 is present, although the physiologic significance of these modifications remains to be determined (Frank et al. 1997). CLL cells have high levels of unphosphorylated STAT-3 (USTAT-3). It was confirmed that USTAT-3 USTAT-3/NF-κB complexes bind to DNA and activate NF-κB-regulated genes in CLL cells (Liu et al. 2011).

13.3.4 NF-κB Modulators in Leukaemia

13.3.4.1 Vascular Endothelial Growth Factor

One of the newly discovered NF-κB activators is vascular endothelial growth factor (VEGF). In AML, the number of vessels in the bone marrow biopsies was significantly increased at diagnosis, compared with normal bone marrow ($P = 0.019$) and was restored to normal levels after achieving CR. The expression of VEGF correlated with a degree of neoangiogenesis. These results suggest that malignant cell proliferation, angiogenesis and VEGF expression are linked in AML and might contribute to the growth advantage of the malignant clone (de Bont et al. 2001). In CLL, VEGF mediates neovascularization in bone marrow. B-CLL lymphocytes produced VEGF in vitro, and increased VEGF levels were found in primary samples. Elevated VEGF receptor (VEGFR)-2 had a negative prognostic impact on survival. Also VEGF stimulates NF-κB in malignant B-CLL cells. The downstream transcriptional targets of NF-κB activation in CLL are also likely to be diverse, but certainly include the inhibitor of apoptosis proteins (IAPs) and anti-apoptotic members of the Bcl-2 family of proteins, for example, Bcl-2, Bcl-XL and Bfl1/A1.

13.3.4.2 Tumour Necrosis Factor

TNF is a monocyte-derived cytotoxin promoting the inflammatory response and signalling via three pathways, an anti-apoptotic NF-κB (one of the most potent activators), generally pro-apoptotic MAPK and a relatively weak induction of death signalling (via caspase-8). The overall effects of TNF activation are multiple and frequently conflicting. In AML, a high serum TNF level was found in approximately 50 % of the cases and was an adverse prognostic factor for survival in patients with untreated AML or high-risk MDS (Tsimberidou et al. 2008). In the in vitro studies, TNF has had a potent anti-tumour and proapoptotic activity in AML cell lines as a single agent and after pre-treatment with interferon or IL-2 (Katschinski et al. 1999). Interestingly, the TNF gene polymorphisms are associated with poor prognosis in various haematological malignancies, including CLL (Lech-Maranda et al. 2013). In primary CLL samples, TNF levels were significantly higher than in a controlled population and when correlated with adverse prognostic factors such as ZAP-70 and CD38 (Bojarska-Junak et al. 2008).

13.3.4.3 Tumour Necrosis Factor-Related Apoptosis-Inducing Ligand

TNF-related apoptosis-inducing ligand (TRAIL) is a promising anti-cancer cytokine as it mediates apoptosis via the caspase-8-dependent pathway, primarily in tumour cells, by binding to death receptors and not in normal cells (Kaufmann and Steensma 2005). TRAIL binds to membrane receptors including proapoptotic TRAIL-R1 (DR4), TRAIL-R2 (DR5) containing the death domain and mediating apoptosis, anti-apoptotic TRAIL-R3 and TRAIL-R4 without a complete cytoplasmic death domain that cannot mediate apoptosis upon ligand binding (Schulze-Osthoff et al. 1998). In cells expressing TRAIL-R4, TRAIL also activates NF-κB and promotes inflammation. The normal bone marrow progenitors show no significant increase in apoptosis when exposed to TRAIL (Zang et al. 2001).

The initial experiments on AML-derived cell lines showed significant sensitivity to TRAIL-induced apoptosis (Wen et al. 2000). In the primary samples, however, a very low sensitivity of AML cells to TRAIL-induced apoptosis was observed (Jones et al. 2003) and this was likely related to the expression of TRAIL decoy receptors (Riccioni et al. 2005). A recent report has related the poor response of AML to the simultaneous expression of death and decoy receptors (Inukai et al. 2006), whereas co-expression of death receptors with the decoy receptor TRAIL-R3 resulted in significant shortened overall survival of AML patients (Chamuleau et al. 2011). Several strategies were tested in order to overcome TRAIL resistance in AML. The combination of TRAIL with classic chemotherapeutic agents (fludarabine, cytosine arabinoside or daunorubicin) shows additive or synergistic caspase-related pro-apoptotic effects. The initial results of in vitro testing of a combination of TRAIL and histone deacetylase inhibitors (HDACis) showed significant apoptosis and upregulation of the TRAIL-R2 expression. The AKT inhibitors showed upregulation of TRAIL-R2 and increased sensitivity of AML to TRAIL. Bortezomib was also found to increase sensitivity of primary AML blasts to TRAIL. A combination of TRAIL and Nutlin-3 (a potent activator of the p53 pathway) has shown synergistic effects in the induction of apoptosis both in AML cell lines and primary AML samples with wild-type p53 status (Impicciatore et al. 2010).

The activity of TRAIL in primary ALL samples is much lower than in the cell lines (29 % killing efficiency vs. 75 % in Jurkat cell line) (Clodi et al. 2000). In T-ALL cell lines and primary samples of childhood T-ALL, soluble rTRAIL has failed to demonstrate efficacy, likely due to the low cell surface expression levels of TRAIL-R1 and TRAIL-R2. Mature normal neutrophils show low sensitivity to TRAIL (Meurette et al. 2006). Single-agent TRAIL significantly reduces the number of myeloid colonies and clusters in primary CML samples, while normal human stem cells treated with high doses of TRAIL maintain a proliferation potential when transplanted into NOD/SCID mice (Zang et al. 2001). It was also recently demonstrated that the loss of Bcr-Abl, in imatinib-resistant CML cells, lead to an increase in TRAIL sensitivity, suggesting that TRAIL could be an effective strategy for the treatment of imatinib-resistant CML with the loss of Bcr-Abl (Park et al. 2009). Preliminary studies carried out on cell lines and on a number of primary samples have shown a low cytotoxic activity of TRAIL on B-CLL (MacFarlane et al. 2002). In consistence with this hypothesis, the combination of TRAIL with anti-CD95 ligand has proved effective in inducing apoptosis of CD40-activated B-CLL cells. A more recent study identified a different TRAIL sensitivity of Zap-70 low and Zap-70 high B-CLL subsets, proposing this negative prognostic marker as being responsible to redirect TRAIL signalling from pro-apoptotic to pro-inflammatory pathway (Richardson et al. 2005).

13.3.4.4 Toll-Like Receptors

TLRs are pattern recognition receptors and take part, among others, in the initiation of inflammation. They are involved in innate and adaptive immune responses when activated by pathogen-associated molecular patterns (PAMPS), and they mediate the secretion of cytokines. TLRs display both pro- and anti-tumour properties. TLRs after the recognition of a specific ligand signal down through adapter protein MyD88. MyD88 mediates the classical pathway of the NF-κB activation. Pro-tumourigenic effects of endotoxin occur through TLR4-mediated NF-κB activation. The focus of recent research has been aimed at activation of the immune system in order to inhibit cancer cell growth and induce cancer cell apoptosis. TLRs, therefore, offer a unique target for cancer therapy. TLR3 is an intracellular, type 1 trans-membrane receptor and is an important "danger" signalling receptor that takes part in the control of the balance between tolerance and inflammation on the one hand and inflammation and disease on the other hand. In cytogenetically normal, but high-risk AML (based on FLT3–ITD, a wild-type NPM1, or expression of both genes), the microRNA expression profiling revealed increased TLR2, TLR4 and TLR8 expression (Marcucci et al. 2008). On the contrary, the reduced expression of TLR4 was reported in both CLL and AML in comparison with normal controls (Webb et al. 2009). Further studies are needed to explain whether the decreased TLR4 expression contributes to the pathogenesis of leukaemia through impaired immune surveillance and whether TLR4 agonists might serve to effectively strengthen the response of the immune system in battling the leukaemic burden.

13.3.4.5 Matrix Metalloproteases

NF-κB regulates matrix metalloproteases (MMP). In AML, variable expression levels of MMP-2 and MMP-9 were detected in myeloid cell lines. The matrigel invasion assay has shown a dependence on MMP-2 but not on MMP-9 (Sawicki et al. 1998). A decrease in the MMP-9 expression was observed in primary AML samples at diagnosis, with normalisation at remission and a decrease at relapse (Lin et al. 2002). The lower levels in active leukaemia can be explained by the fact that most of MMP-9 is secreted by stromal, endothelial cell fibroblasts. Patients with lower MMP-9 levels tend to have longer survival times [185]. MMP-2-positive patients have survived for over 3 years, whereas all MMP-2-negative patients relapsed within 13.5 months of their diagnosis (Kuittinen et al. 1999). In ALL, MMP-2 expression of lymphoblastic cell lines correlated with the ability to invade matrigel in vitro and with the capacity to invade and metastasise in a SCID mouse model (Hendrix et al. 1992). MMP-9 expression in lymphoblastic cell lines was found to be important for the invasion and metastasis (Ivanoff et al. 1999). In adults, 65 % of ALL cases were positive for MMP-2 and 25 % for MMP-9. MMP-2 expression correlated with an extramedullary disease pattern. In addition, a trend towards a worse survival rate has been observed in MMP-9-positive cases (Qu et al. 2011). Those results suggest a possible role of MMPs as surrogate markers of remission status and in risk assessment.

13.3.5 Other Signalling Pathways

COX2 has emerged as another major mediator of inflammation, and over-expression has been observed in many malignancies. In leukaemias, increased COX-2 expression was noted in chronic phase CML (76.32 %) and CLL (75.86 %). In addition, the expression of COX-2 may correlate with the prognosis in those chronic leukaemias (Bao et al. 2007).

Inducible nitric oxide synthase (iNOS) expression is regulated by NF-κB and mediates the production of NO. In AML and ALL cell lines, IFN-gamma induced iNOS expression and generated high levels of NO production that induced apoptosis (Siripin et al. 2011). CML cells are also sensitive to the anti-proliferative effect of NO (Ferry-Dumazet et al. 2002).

13.4 Role of Inflammatory Molecules in the Development of Leukaemia

In the last few years, studies have also clearly demonstrated that leukaemia populations are highly heterogeneous and that the disease is propagated by a subpopulation of LSC. LSCs, like normal hematopoietic stem cells, possess a range of biological characteristics that enable for their long-term survival. Therefore, LSCs reside in a mostly quiescent state, and as a consequence, the overall activity of many chemotherapeutic agents that function by targeting cycling cells is possibly reduced (Konopleva and Jordan 2011). Although some studies have indicated a role for NF-κB in quiescent cells, the activation of NF-κB is an acquired phenomenon. Unstimulated human $CD34^{+}$ progenitor cells do not express NF-κB, while primary AML cells display readily detectable NF-κB activity. NF-κB is highly activated in leukaemic cells, which suggests that an intrinsic aspect of AML biology resides in the constitutive activation of various pathways. Furthermore, detailed analyses of enriched AML stem cells (CD341/CD382/CD1231) indicate that NF-κB is also active in the LSC population. Interestingly, leukaemic cells showed a rapid apoptotic response while stimulated by a NF-κB inhibitor (MG-132), whereas normal CD341/CD382 cells showed a limited effect. Taken together, these data indicate that primitive AML cells aberrantly express NF-κB and that the presence of this factor may provide unique opportunities to preferentially ablate LSCs (Guzman et al. 2001a).

T-cell acute lymphoblastic leukaemia (T-ALL) is associated with an increased risk of central nervous system (CNS) relapse. Little is known about the mechanism of leukaemic cell infiltration of the CNS. In an animal T-ALL model, chemokine receptor, CCR7, was shown to be an essential adhesion signal required for the targeting of leukaemic T cells into the CNS. The CCR7 gene expression is controlled by the activity of the T-ALL oncogene Notch1 and is expressed in human tumours carrying Notch1-activating mutations. The silencing of either CCR7 or its chemokine ligand CCL19 (Bellosillo et al. 1998) in an animal model of T-ALL specifically inhibits CNS infiltration. These studies identify a single chemokine-receptor interaction as a CNS "entry" signal and open the way for future pharmacological targeting. The targeted inhibition of CNS involvement in T-ALL could potentially decrease the intensity of CNS-targeted therapy, thus reducing its associated short- and long-term complications (Buonamici et al. 2009).

13.5 Evidence from Patients for the Role of Inflammation in Leukaemia

Direct, patient-derived evidence supporting the role of inflammation in the development of leukaemia is limited. Epidemiological studies give insight into the role of the inflammatory processes in the development of different leukaemias.

The aetiology of leukaemias remains largely undetermined. Smoking was identified as a major risk factor in AML, ionising radiation in AML and CML and exposure to benzene in AML and CLL (Khalade et al. 2010). The possible association between the development of leukaemia and chronic inflammation is illustrated in a series of epidemiological studies. In a Swedish nationwide cohort of patients with ulcerative colitis, there was a moderately increased relative risk of AML, while in the Crohn's disease, there was no increase observed (Askling et al. 2005). In another Swedish study, the standardised incidence ratio (SIR) of leukaemias was analysed in a cohort of patients hospitalised for autoimmune diseases. SIR for AML was significantly increased in rheumatoid arthritis (SIR = 1.92), systemic lupus (SIR = 4.63), polymyalgia (SIR = 2.53), pernicious anaemia (SIR = 4.08) and Wegener granulomatosis (SIR = 2.83). SIRs in Crohn's disease and ulcerative colitis were not significantly increased (Hemminki et al. 2013). Similar associations were reported in a study based on US SEER data (Anderson et al. 2009). Interestingly, for CML, association with Crohn's disease and ulcerative colitis were reported in Swedish studies but were not replicated in US-based study. In another large, population-based study, the risk of AML and MDS associated with a prior history of a broad range of infections or autoimmune diseases were analysed. In total, 9,219 patients with AML, 1,662 patients with MDS and 42,878 matched controls were included. Overall, a history of any infectious disease was associated with a significantly increased risk of both AML (overall risk (OR) = 1.3) and MDS (OR = 1.3). A previous history of any autoimmune disease was associated with a 1.7-fold increased risk for AML and 2.1-fold increased risk for MDS. Similar to previous reports, conditions were associated with AML and MDS (Kristinsson et al. 2011). Studies on the use of NSAID and the development of leukaemia have showed interesting results. A prospective cohort study of over 28,000 postmenopausal women in Iowa (Kasum et al. 2003) reported a 55 % decreased risk of leukaemia (mostly AML and CLL) in women who reported usage of aspirin two or more times weekly in comparison with women who never used aspirin. A case-control study of acute leukaemia involving 169 cases and 676 controls showed only modest decreases in the risk of leukaemia in aspirin users as opposed to a moderate increase in paracetamol (acetaminophen) users (Weiss et al. 2006). In another prospective, cohort study (VITAL), no statistically significant effect of aspirin use on haematological malignancies was reported (Walter et al. 2011). The above studies show no convincing epidemiological evidence of the protective effect of aspirin against leukaemia; however, there is the possibility of a weak protective effect. The mechanistic explanation of the role of aspirin is still lacking, but the observations can be explained by anti-inflammatory properties or caspase activation by aspirin observed in vitro in AML cell lines (Klampfer et al. 1999). The epidemiological data show a chronological association between leukaemias and autoimmune disorders or infections; however, it does not provide an insight into underlying mechanism. The possible explanations for the epidemiological observations include the possibility that autoimmune conditions or infections are caused by the immune dysfunction that precedes the development of leukaemia. The findings may also be related to immune- or inflammation-driven tumourigenesis from autoimmune conditions that lead to leukaemia. In addition, the therapies for autoimmune disorders can contribute to the development of leukaemia. Overall, the evidence currently available suggests an association between chronic inflammation and development of leukaemias. The confirmation of this association through a large, prospective study is required.

13.6 Inhibitors of Inflammation for the Prevention and Treatment of Leukaemia

As has been mentioned above, various inflammatory pathways are activated in leukaemias; therefore, modulation of those pathways may have the potential for treatment and possibly the prevention of leukaemias. Complete inhibition of a single pathway is more likely to be toxic and less likely to be effective. Partial downregulation of several pathways is more likely to inhibit the deregulated inflammatory signalling and be less toxic and more efficient in therapy. The key agents modulating inflammatory pathways include steroids, proteasome inhibitors, TNF inhibitors, NF-κB inhibitors and COX2 inhibitors, TRAIL, chemokine modulators and others. Another group of interesting agents is the naturally occurring modifiers of NF-κB activation.

13.6.1 Cytokine-Based Interventions

Modifying CXCL12/CXCR4 axis is very attractive clinically. Currently, a CXCL12 analogue (plerixafor) is used for the mobilisation of haematopoietic progenitor. Data from murine models of AML demonstrated that plerixafor could mobilise AML blasts into the peripheral circulation. Furthermore, the addition of plerixafor-sensitised leukaemic blasts to the effects of cytotoxic chemotherapy increased the overall survival of leukaemic mice treated with the combination of plerixafor and chemotherapy compared to chemotherapy alone. Feasibility of plerixafor use in relapsed/refractory AML was demonstrated in a phase I/II study in combination with mitoxantrone, etoposide and cytarabine. The encouraging remission rate was also noted. Interestingly, in this study, neither symptomatic leukostasis nor delayed hematopoietic recovery was observed (Uy et al. 2012). The polypeptide RCP168 seems to have a strong antagonistic effect on the stromal cell-induced chemotaxis of leukaemic cells. Furthermore, RCP168 blocked the binding of anti-CXCR4 monoclonal antibody 12G5 to the surface CXCR4 in a concentration-dependent manner and inhibited SDF-1alpha-induced AKT and extracellular signal-regulated kinase phosphorylation. Equivalent results were obtained with the small-molecule CXCR4 inhibitor AMD3465. A second-generation CXCR4 inhibitor, AMD3465, antagonized SDF-1α and stroma-induced chemotaxis and suppressed stroma-activated PI3K/AKT and MEK/ERK pathways, which effectively mobilised leukaemia cells and stem cells into circulation and enhanced the sensitivity to chemotherapy or FLT3-inhibitor-induced cell death. Other antagonists have also been investigated. One of them, RCP168, had a strong antagonistic effect on chemotaxis of leukaemic cells. Another candidate molecule, E-4031, a specific hERG1K(+) channel inhibitor and CXCL12 blocker, inhibited the migration of leukaemic cell-induced G0/G1 arrest, impaired proliferation and apoptosis of AML cells.

It was also found that ubiquitin is a natural ligand of CXCR4. Ubiquitin is a small, highly conserved protein; it primarily targets intracellular proteins for degradation via the ubiquitin proteasome system. Evidence in numerous animal models suggests that extracellular ubiquitin is an anti-inflammatory immune modulator and an endogenous opponent of pro-inflammatory damage-associated molecular pattern molecules. It is speculated this interaction may be through CXCR4 mediated signalling pathways and regulatory effects on the growth of various leukaemia cell lines (Majetschak 2011).

13.6.2 Inhibition of NF-κB Pathway in Leukaemia

NF-κB inhibition can be accomplished by upstream blocking of the NF-κB activators or direct competitive inhibitors. Upstream inhibition includes proteasome inhibitors (bortezomib), IKK inhibitors (non-steroidal anti-inflammatory drugs [NSAIDs], sulphasalazine, curcumin and parthenolide analogues) and antioxidants (disulfiram and glutathione). Direct targeting strategies include the use of peptide inhibitors, decoy oligodeoxynucleotides and anti-sense oligonucleotide. In in vitro experiments, bortezomib induced apoptosis in primary AML samples (Guzman et al. 2001a; Frelin et al. 2005b), with a relatively selective effect on leukaemic cells and was sparing of normal haematopoiesis. These results provide the rational for Phase I/II clinical trials for the treatment of refractory or relapsed AML patients with proteasome inhibitors (Cortes et al. 2004). The clinical efficacy of a single-agent bortezomib is limited. In phase II trial, there was no CR or PR and only a limited decrease in the blast count was observed after the administration to 14 high-risk AML patient (Sarlo et al. 2013). Similarly, in CLL, bortezomib had cytotoxic effects in vitro and it enhanced the effects of fludarabine. The treatment of CLL patients with single-agent bortezomib is, however, not effective. The inhibition of IKK2 (AS602868) has led to the apoptosis in primary AML samples. The effect was dose dependent and affected both patients at diagnosis or under treatment, demonstrating a strong pro-survival potential for NF-κB in AML cells (Frelin et al. 2005b). Aspirin and other NSAIDs (ibuprofen, indomethacin and SDX-308) suppress NF-κB by inhibition of IKK activation and IκBα degradation. Aspirin has induced apoptosis in a dose and time-dependent manner in primary CLL cells, an effect not observed with other NSAIDs probably mediated by cyclooxygenase-independent mechanisms (Bellosillo et al. 1998). Sulphasalazine, a synthetic anti-inflammatory and immunosuppressive agent, has also inhibited NF-κB activation via the direct inhibition of IKK and IKK leading to apoptosis in primary CLL.

Curcumin (diferuloylmethane) is a polyphenol derived from the plant Curcuma longa with antioxidant, anti-inflammatory, anti-angiogenic and anti-tumour activity. It has induced apoptosis in CLL cells via the inhibition of NF-κB and other pathways (STAT3 and AKT). Interestingly, there was synergism between curcumin and epigallocatechin-3 gallate (green tea extract). Resveratrol (another naturally occurring polyphenol) was shown to be a potent inhibitor of NF-κB activation and NF-κB-dependent gene expression through its ability to inhibit IKK activity.

Bortezomib induced proliferation arrest and apoptosis in imatinib-sensitive and imatinib-resistant CML cell lines (Gatto et al. 2003), which provides a rationale for the use of this drug in the subset of patients resistant to imatinib. In addition, a combination of bortezomib and flavopiridol (a cyclin-dependent kinase inhibitor) has shown synergism in apoptosis induction in CML cells resistant to imatinib through both Bcr-Abl-dependent and Bcr-Abl-independent mechanisms (Dai et al. 2004). These findings suggest that a combination of bortezomib and other drugs including flavopiridol is promising in CML. The IKK inhibitor PS1145 (Millennium, Cambridge, USA) in CML cells was shown to induce growth arrest and apoptosis synergistically with imatinib in cell lines and in bone marrow cells from CML patients (Cilloni et al. 2006). The combinations of imatinib plus the IKK inhibitors or bortezomib represent a valid approach to be tested in vivo for the treatment of CML patients resistant to imatinib therapy.

13.6.3 Other Therapeutic Options

The approved inhibitors of TNF—etanercept (a recombinant extracellular TNF-binding portion of the TNF receptor linked to the Fc portion of IgG1) and infliximab (a chimeric monoclonal anti-TNF antibody). Both agents showed haematological responses in small clinical trials in MDS. No results of trials of the inhibition of TNF in AML or CLL were reported. The analysis of cytokine levels will allow identification of patients with high TNF level. This group of patients could be candidates for combination therapies including anti-TNF agent.

A novel small-molecule Stat3 inhibitor (C188-9) inhibited G-CSF-induced Stat3 phosphorylation and apoptosis in AML cell lines and primary samples. It also inhibited AML blast colony formation at low micro molar range concentrations (Redell et al. 2011). The agents used in combination with TRAIL either enhance TRAIL-R1/-R2 expression or decrease the expression of anti-apoptotic proteins (c-FLIP, X-IAP, Bcl-2). A number of receptor-specific TRAIL variants and agonistic antibodies have been recently developed. Some of these agents targeting TRAIL-R1 and/or TRAIL-R2 (TRAIL receptor agonists) are progressing to phase I/II clinical trials. A number of natural compounds stimulate TRAIL and NF-κB-mediated apoptosis in leukaemia cells. Wogonin (derived from a popular Chinese herb) sensitises TNF-resistant T-cell leukaemia cell line to TNF and TRAIL-induced apoptosis. Wogonin does not affect the viability of normal peripheral blood T cells (Fas et al. 2006). Curcumin (derived from turmeric) upregulates

TRAIL-R2 expression and inactivates NF-κB in a ROS-dependent manner. Taken together, these findings demonstrate that non-genotoxic natural molecules or small compounds enhance TRAIL-mediated killing of leukaemia cells with reduced side effects compared to conventional chemotherapy.

13.7 Conclusions and Future Directions

Inflammation represents a link between intrinsic (oncogenes, tumour suppressors and genome stability genes) and extrinsic (immune and microenvironment) factors contributing to tumour development. Despite the fact that currently available therapies have significantly improved clinical outcomes in a variety of leukaemias, they are not always efficient and are usually associated with significant toxicities. To improve outcomes, the novel therapeutic strategies should include agents capable of eliminating quiescent cells or must include cell cycle activation of LSCs.

The new strategies should utilise the unique properties of the microenvironment to permit more selective and efficient eradication of LSC. In most cancers, a variety of chemokine ligands are observed. Their exact role is not characterised. The comprehensive study of chemokines and receptors in leukaemia will be crucial to the further understanding of the chemokine network. Chemokines are important for survival, proliferation and the homing of leukaemic cells. The importance of CXCR4 has been well demonstrated, and the targeting of the mechanisms that mediate LSC adhesion within BM niches and stimulation of niche-induced pro-survival and self-renewal pathways both appear to be useful strategies. Profiling the current and new experimental agents from the point of view of interference with the CXCR4 receptor should help to design rational drug combinations that will possibly eradicate LSCs.

From the perspective of interphase of the inflammation and leukaemia, the increased constitutive activation of NF-κB appears to be the most promising target. NF-κB is a major regulator of cell survival, and it is closely involved in carcinogenesis. As presented, NF-κB acts together with other important oncogenic signalling pathways. As a non-selective inhibition of NF-κB is likely to cause significant adverse effects, identification of selective modifiers of NF-κB responses may be a rational approach leading to the utilisation of NF-κB in the therapy of malignancy as well as in chronic inflammatory diseases. Characterisation of the interaction between those mechanisms will have an important role in the identification of future biomarkers and planning of therapeutic combinations. For example, as IKK inhibitors are under study in therapy of leukaemia and inflammatory diseases, full understanding of the structure and function will be important for the rational design of combination protocols. The data presented provide sufficient evidence that inflammatory pathways are a critical mediator of proliferation and survival of leukaemic clones. It suggests that purpose-designed biomarkers based on inflammatory pathways can have role in diagnostic and prognostic evaluation of different leukaemias. Although numerous cell culture and animal studies have identified several natural anti-inflammatory agents, their true potential will only be recognised through well-controlled clinical trials. They are likely not to be utilised as single agents, but rather as a part of multidrug protocols that can lead to a successful therapy for different haematological malignancies

Further understanding of interactions between inflammation and leukaemia will reveal novel targets for monitoring and novel therapies in combination with conventional treatments. Therapeutic modifications of inflammatory pathways in leukaemias will possibly improve the clinical efficacy. A better identification of bone marrow and leukaemia-specific inflammatory mechanisms will allow personalisation of therapeutic strategies. Therapeutic manipulation of inflammatory pathways is likely to change the inflammatory microenvironment into an anti-cancer microenvironment. Taking into account the relevance of inflammatory networking in leukaemia, it would be very important to incorporate inflammatory parameters into traditional classification schemes to provide new prognostic tools. The challenges for the future are to investigate the activation, function and prognostic value of inflammatory pathways in leukaemia, as well as to evaluate the therapeutic potential of novel therapeutic strategies in clinical trials that interfere with inflammatory signalling, including NF-κB. The novel agents interfering with inflammatory pathways look promising and will most likely be a useful addition to the treatments that are currently available for many leukaemias.

In this chapter, we have provided conclusive evidence that inflammatory signalling pathways play an important role in leukaemia. It is, therefore, evident that anti-inflammatory agents should be explored for both the prevention and treatment of leukaemia. Although numerous cell culture and animal studies have identified several natural anti-inflammatory agents, their true potential will be recognised only through well-controlled clinical trials.

References

Aggarwal BB, Gehlot P (2009) Inflammation and cancer: how friendly is the relationship for cancer patients? Curr Opin Pharmacol 9(4):351–369. doi:10.1016/j.coph.2009.06.020

Anderson LA, Pfeiffer RM, Landgren O, Gadalla S, Berndt SI, Engels EA (2009) Risks of myeloid malignancies in patients with autoimmune conditions. Br J Cancer 100(5):822–828. doi: 10.1038/sj.bjc.6604935

Askling J, Brandt L, Lapidus A, Karlen P, Bjorkholm M, Lofberg R, Ekbom A (2005) Risk of haematopoietic cancer in patients with inflammatory bowel disease. Gut 54(5):617–622. doi:10.1136/gut.2004.051771

Bao ZH, Li GL, Yu JH (2007) Expression of cyclooxygenase-2 in bone marrow cells of chronic leukemia and its significance. Zhongguo shi yan xue ye xue za zhi / Zhongguo bing li sheng li xue hui = Journal of experimental hematology / Chinese Association of Pathophysiology 15(5):923–926

Bargou RC, Leng C, Krappmann D, Emmerich F, Mapara MY, Bommert K, Royer HD, Scheidereit C, Dorken B (1996) High-level nuclear NF-kappa B and Oct-2 is a common feature of cultured Hodgkin/Reed-Sternberg cells. Blood 87(10):4340–4347

Bellosillo B, Pique M, Barragan M, Castano E, Villamor N, Colomer D, Montserrat E, Pons G, Gil J (1998) Aspirin and salicylate induce apoptosis and activation of caspases in B-cell chronic lymphocytic leukemia cells. Blood 92(4):1406–1414

Benekli M, Xia Z, Donohue KA, Ford LA, Pixley LA, Baer MR, Baumann H, Wetzler M (2002) Constitutive activity of signal transducer and activator of transcription 3 protein in acute myeloid leukemia blasts is associated with short disease-free survival. Blood 99(1):252–257

Bojarska-Junak A, Hus I, Szczepanek EW, Dmoszynska A, Rolinski J (2008) Peripheral blood and bone marrow TNF and TNF receptors in early and advanced stages of B-CLL in correlation with ZAP-70 protein and CD38 antigen. Leuk Res 32(2):225–233. doi:10.1016/j.leukres.2007.06.007

Braun T, Carvalho G, Fabre C, Grosjean J, Fenaux P, Kroemer G (2006) Targeting NF-kappaB in hematologic malignancies. Cell Death Differ 13(5):748–758. doi:10.1038/sj.cdd.4401874

Bueso-Ramos CE, Rocha FC, Shishodia S, Medeiros LJ, Kantarjian HM, Vadhan-Raj S, Estrov Z, Smith TL, Nguyen MH, Aggarwal BB (2004) Expression of constitutively active nuclear-kappa B RelA transcription factor in blasts of acute myeloid leukemia. Hum Pathol 35(2):246–253

Buonamici S, Trimarchi T, Ruocco MG, Reavie L, Cathelin S, Mar BG, Klinakis A, Lukyanov Y, Tseng JC, Sen F, Gehrie E, Li M, Newcomb E, Zavadil J, Meruelo D, Lipp M, Ibrahim S, Efstratiadis A, Zagzag D, Bromberg JS, Dustin ML, Aifantis I (2009) CCR7 signalling as an essential regulator of CNS infiltration in T-cell leukaemia. Nature 459(7249):1000–1004. doi:10.1038/nature08020

Chamuleau ME, Ossenkoppele GJ, van Rhenen A, van Dreunen L, Jirka SM, Zevenbergen A, Schuurhuis GJ, van de Loosdrecht AA (2011) High TRAIL-R3 expression on leukemic blasts is associated with poor outcome and induces apoptosis-resistance which can be overcome by targeting TRAIL-R2. Leuk Res 35(6):741–749. doi:10.1016/j.leukres.2010.12.032

Chao MP, Alizadeh AA, Tang C, Myklebust JH, Varghese B, Gill S, Jan M, Cha AC, Chan CK, Tan BT, Park CY, Zhao F, Kohrt HE, Malumbres R, Briones J, Gascoyne RD, Lossos IS, Levy R, Weissman IL, Majeti R (2010) Anti-CD47 antibody synergizes with rituximab to promote phagocytosis and eradicate non-Hodgkin lymphoma. Cell 142(5):699–713. doi:10.1016/j.cell.2010.07.044

Cilloni D, Messa F, Arruga F, Defilippi I, Morotti A, Messa E, Carturan S, Giugliano E, Pautasso M, Bracco E, Rosso V, Sen A, Martinelli G, Baccarani M, Saglio G (2006) The NF-kappaB pathway blockade by the IKK inhibitor PS1145 can overcome imatinib resistance. Leukemia (Official Journal of the Leukemia Society of America, Leukemia Research Fund, UK) 20(1):61–67. doi:10.1038/sj.leu.2403998

Clodi K, Wimmer D, Li Y, Goodwin R, Jaeger U, Mann G, Gadner H, Younes A (2000) Expression of tumour necrosis factor (TNF)-related apoptosis-inducing ligand (TRAIL) receptors and sensitivity to TRAIL-induced apoptosis in primary B-cell acute lymphoblastic leukaemia cells. Br J Haematol 111(2):580–586

Colotta F, Allavena P, Sica A, Garlanda C, Mantovani A (2009) Cancer-related inflammation, the seventh hallmark of cancer: links to genetic instability. Carcinogenesis 30(7):1073–1081. doi:10.1093/carcin/bgp127

Cortes J, Thomas D, Koller C, Giles F, Estey E, Faderl S, Garcia-Manero G, McConkey D, Ruiz SL, Guerciolini R, Wright J, Kantarjian H (2004) Phase I study of bortezomib in refractory or relapsed acute leukemias. Clin Cancer Res 10(10):3371–3376. doi:10.1158/1078-0432.CCR-03-0508

Crazzolara R, Kreczy A, Mann G, Heitger A, Eibl G, Fink FM, Mohle R, Meister B (2001) High expression of the chemokine receptor CXCR4 predicts extramedullary organ infiltration in childhood acute lymphoblastic leukaemia. Br J Haematol 115(3):545–553

Dai Y, Rahmani M, Pei XY, Dent P, Grant S (2004) Bortezomib and flavopiridol interact synergistically to induce apoptosis in chronic myeloid leukemia cells resistant to imatinib mesylate through both Bcr/Abl-dependent and -independent mechanisms. Blood 104(2):509–518. doi:10.1182/blood-2003-12-4121

Datta SR, Brunet A, Greenberg ME (1999) Cellular survival: a play in three Akts. Genes Dev 13(22):2905–2927

de Bont ES, Rosati S, Jacobs S, Kamps WA, Vellenga E (2001) Increased bone marrow vascularization in patients with acute myeloid leukaemia: a possible role for vascular endothelial growth factor. Br J Haematol 113(2):296–304 de Lima M, Strom SS, Keating M, Kantarjian H, Pierce S, O'Brien S, Freireich E, Estey E (1997) Implications of potential cure in acute myelogenous leukemia: development of subsequent cancer and return to work. Blood 90(12):4719–4724

Dohner H, Estey EH, Amadori S, Appelbaum FR, Buchner T, Burnett AK, Dombret H, Fenaux P, Grimwade D, Larson RA, Lo-Coco F, Naoe T, Niederwieser D, Ossenkoppele GJ, Sanz MA, Sierra J, Tallman MS, Lowenberg B, Bloomfield CD, European L (2010) Diagnosis and management of acute myeloid leukemia in adults: recommendations from an international expert panel, on behalf of the European LeukemiaNet. Blood 115(3):453–474. doi:10.1182/blood-2009-07-235358

Dokter WH, Tuyt L, Sierdsema SJ, Esselink MT, Vellenga E (1995) The spontaneous expression of interleukin-1 beta and interleukin-6 is associated with spontaneous expression of AP-1 and NF-kappa B transcription factor in acute myeloblastic leukemia cells. Leukemia (Official Journal of the Leukemia Society of America, Leukemia Research Fund, UK) 9(3):425–432

Estrov Z, Manna SK, Harris D, Van Q, Estey EH, Kantarjian HM, Talpaz M, Aggarwal BB (1999) Phenylarsine oxide blocks interleukin-1beta-induced activation of the nuclear transcription factor NF-kappaB, inhibits proliferation, and induces apoptosis of acute myelogenous leukemia cells. Blood 94(8):2844–2853

Fas SC, Baumann S, Zhu JY, Giaisi M, Treiber MK, Mahlknecht U, Krammer PH, Li-Weber M (2006) Wogonin sensitizes resistant malignant cells to TNFalpha- and TRAIL-induced apoptosis. Blood 108(12):3700–3706. doi:10.1182/blood-2006-03-011973

Ferretti E, Cocco C, Airoldi I, Pistoia V (2012) Targeting acute myeloid leukemia cells with cytokines. J Leukoc Biol 92(3):567–575. doi:10.1189/jlb.0112036

Ferry-Dumazet H, Mamani-Matsuda M, Dupouy M, Belloc F, Thiolat D, Marit G, Arock M, Reiffers J, Mossalayi MD (2002) Nitric oxide induces the apoptosis of human BCR-ABL-positive myeloid leukemia cells: evidence for the chelation of intracellular iron. Leukemia (Official Journal of the Leukemia Society of America, Leukemia Research Fund, UK) 16(4):708–715. doi:10.1038/sj.leu.2402404

Frank DA, Mahajan S, Ritz J (1997) B lymphocytes from patients with chronic lymphocytic leukemia contain signal transducer and activator of transcription (STAT) 1 and STAT3 constitutively phosphorylated on serine residues. J Clin Invest 100(12):3140–3148. doi:10.1172/JCI119869

Freireich EJ, Gehan EA, Sulman D, Boggs DR, Frei E 3rd (1961) The effect of chemotherapy on acute leukemia in the human. J Chronic Dis 14:593–608

Frelin C, Imbert V, Griessinger E, Peyron A-C, Rochet N, Philip P, Dageville C, Sirvent A, Hummelsberger M, Berard E, Dreano M, Sirvent N, Peyron J-F (2005a) Targeting NF-kappaB activation via pharmacologic inhibition of IKK2-induced apoptosis of human acute myeloid leukemia cells. Blood 105(2):804–811

Frelin C, Imbert V, Griessinger E, Peyron AC, Rochet N, Philip P, Dageville C, Sirvent A, Hummelsberger M, Berard E, Dreano M, Sirvent N, Peyron JF (2005b) Targeting NF-kappaB activation via pharmacologic inhibition of IKK2-induced apoptosis of human acute myeloid leukemia cells. Blood 105(2):804–811. doi:10.1182/blood-2004-04-1463

Gatto S, Scappini B, Pham L, Onida F, Milella M, Ball G, Ricci C, Divoky V, Verstovsek S, Kantarjian HM, Keating MJ, Cortes-Franco JE, Beran M (2003) The proteasome inhibitor PS-341 inhibits growth and induces apoptosis in Bcr/Abl-positive cell lines sensitive and resistant to imatinib mesylate. Haematologica 88(8):853–863

Guzman ML, Neering SJ, Upchurch D, Grimes B, Howard DS, Rizzieri DA, Luger SM, Jordan CT (2001a) Nuclear factor-kappaB is constitutively activated in primitive human acute myelogenous leukemia cells. Blood 98(8):2301–2307

Guzman ML, Neering SJ, Upchurch D, Grimes B, Howard DS, Rizzieri DA, Luger SM, Jordan CT (2001b) Nuclear factor-kappaB is constitutively activated in primitive human acute myelogenous leukemia cells. Blood 98(8):2301–2307

Guzman ML, Swiderski CF, Howard DS, Grimes BA, Rossi RM, Szilvassy SJ, Jordan CT (2002) Preferential induction of apoptosis for primary human leukemic stem cells. Proc Natl Acad Sci U S A 99(25):16220–16225

Hemminki K, Liu X, Forsti A, Ji J, Sundquist J, Sundquist K (2013) Subsequent leukaemia in autoimmune disease patients. Br J Haematol. doi:10.1111/bjh.12330

Hendrix MJ, Seftor EA, Grogan TM, Seftor RE, Hersh EM, Boyse EA, Liotta LA, Stetler-Stevenson W, Ray CG (1992) Expression of type IV collagenase correlates with the invasion of human lymphoblastoid cell lines and pathogenesis in SCID mice. Mol Cell Probes 6(1):59–65

Hewamana S, Lin TT, Jenkins C, Burnett AK, Jordan CT, Fegan C, Brennan P, Rowntree C, Pepper C (2008) The novel nuclear factor-kappaB inhibitor LC-1 is equipotent in poor prognostic subsets of chronic lymphocytic leukemia and shows strong synergy with fludarabine. Clin Cancer Res 14(24):8102–8111. doi:10.1158/1078-0432.CCR-08-1673

Hiscott J, Beauparlant P, Crepieux P, DeLuca C, Kwon H, Lin R, Petropoulos L (1997) Cellular and viral protein interactions regulating I kappa B alpha activity during human retrovirus infection. J Leukoc Biol 62(1):82–92

Impicciatore G, Sancilio S, Miscia S, Di Pietro R (2010) Nutlins and ionizing radiation in cancer therapy. Curr Pharm Des 16(12):1427–1442

Inukai T, Zhang X, Goto M, Hirose K, Uno K, Akahane K, Nemoto A, Goi K, Sato H, Takahashi K, Honna H, Kagami K, Nakamoto K, Yagita H, Okumura K, Koyama-Okazaki T, Nakazawa S, Sugita K (2006) Resistance of infant leukemia with MLL rearrangement to tumor necrosis factor-related apoptosis-inducing ligand: a possible mechanism for poor sensitivity to antitumor immunity. Leukemia (Official journal of the Leukemia Society of America, Leukemia Research Fund, UK) 20(12):2119–2129. doi:10.1038/sj.leu.2404429

Ivanoff A, Ivanoff J, Hultenby K, Sundqvist KG (1999) Infiltrative capacity of T leukemia cell lines: a distinct functional property coupled to expression of matrix metalloproteinase-9 (MMP-9) and tissue inhibitor of metalloproteinases-1 (TIMP-1). Clin Exp Metastasis 17(8):695–711

Jaiswal S, Jamieson CH, Pang WW, Park CY, Chao MP, Majeti R, Traver D, van Rooijen N, Weissman IL (2009) CD47 is upregulated on circulating hematopoietic stem cells and leukemia cells to avoid phagocytosis. Cell 138(2):271–285. doi:10.1016/j.cell.2009.05.046

Jones DT, Ganeshaguru K, Mitchell WA, Foroni L, Baker RJ, Prentice HG, Mehta AB, Wickremasinghe RG (2003) Cytotoxic drugs enhance the ex vivo sensitivity of malignant cells from a subset of acute myeloid leukaemia patients to apoptosis induction by tumour necrosis factor receptor-related apoptosis-inducing ligand. Br J Haematol 121(5):713–720

Kasum CM, Blair CK, Folsom AR, Ross JA (2003) Non-steroidal anti-inflammatory drug use and risk of adult leukemia. Cancer Epidemiol Biomarkers Prev 12(6):534–537

Katschinski DM, Robins HI, Schad M, Frede S, Fandrey J (1999) Role of tumor necrosis factor alpha in hyperthermia-induced apoptosis of human leukemia cells. Cancer Res 59(14):3404–3410

Kaufmann SH, Steensma DP (2005) On the TRAIL of a new therapy for leukemia. Leukemia (Official Journal of the Leukemia Society of America, Leukemia Research Fund, UK) 19(12):2195–2202. doi:10.1038/sj.leu.2403946

Khalade A, Jaakkola MS, Pukkala E, Jaakkola JJ (2010) Exposure to benzene at work and the risk of leukemia: a systematic review and meta-analysis. Environ Health Glob Access Sci Sour 9:31. doi:10.1186/1476-069X-9-31

Kitajima I, Shinohara T, Bilakovics J, Brown DA, Xu X, Nerenberg M (1993) Ablation of transplanted HTLV-I tax-transformed tumors in mice by antisense inhibition of NF-kappa B. Science 259(5101):1523

Klampfer L, Cammenga J, Wisniewski HG, Nimer SD (1999) Sodium salicylate activates caspases and induces apoptosis of myeloid leukemia cell lines. Blood 93(7):2386–2394

Koblas T, Zacharovova K, Berkova Z, Mindlova M, Girman P, Dovolilova E, Karasova L, Saudek F (2007) Isolation and characterization of human CXCR4-positive pancreatic cells. Folia Biol 53(1):13–22

Konopleva MY, Jordan CT (2011) Leukemia stem cells and microenvironment: biology and therapeutic targeting. J Clin Oncol (Official Journal of the American Society of Clinical Oncology) 29(5):591–599. doi:10.1200/JCO.2010.31.0904

Kornblau SM, McCue D, Singh N, Chen W, Estrov Z, Coombes KR (2010) Recurrent expression signatures of cytokines and chemokines are present and are independently prognostic in acute myelogenous leukemia and myelodysplasia. Blood 116(20):4251–4261. doi:10.1182/blood-2010-01-262071

Kristinsson SY, Bjorkholm M, Hultcrantz M, Derolf ÅR, Landgren O, Goldin LR (2011) Chronic immune stimulation might act as a trigger for the development of acute myeloid leukemia or myelodysplastic syndromes. J Clin Oncol (Official Journal of the American Society of Clinical Oncology) 29(21):2897–2903

Kuittinen O, Savolainen ER, Koistinen P, Turpeenniemi-Hujanen T (1999) Gelatinase A and B (MMP-2, MMP-9) in leukaemia MMP-2 may indicate a good prognosis in AML. Anticancer Res 19(5C):4395–4400

Lech-Maranda E, Mlynarski W, Grzybowska-Izydorczyk O, Borowiec M, Pastorczak A, Cebula-Obrzut B, Klimkiewicz-Wojciechowska G, Wcislo M, Majewski M, Kotkowska A, Robak T, Warzocha K (2013) Polymorphisms of TNF and IL-10 genes and clinical outcome of patients with chronic lymphocytic leukemia. Genes Chromosom Cancer 52(3):287–296. doi:10.1002/gcc.22028

Lin LI, Lin DT, Chang CJ, Lee CY, Tang JL, Tien HF (2002) Marrow matrix metalloproteinases (MMPs) and tissue inhibitors of MMP in acute leukaemia: potential role of MMP-9 as a surrogate marker to monitor leukaemic status in patients with acute myelogenous leukaemia. Br J Haematol 117(4):835–841

Liu Z, Hazan-Halevy I, Harris DM, Li P, Ferrajoli A, Faderl S, Keating MJ, Estrov Z (2011) STAT-3 activates NF-kappaB in chronic lymphocytic leukemia cells. Mol Cancer Res 9(4):507–515. doi:10.1158/1541-7786.MCR-10-0559

Lounnas N, Frelin C, Gonthier N, Colosetti P, Sirvent A, Cassuto JP, Berthier F, Sirvent N, Rousselot P, Dreano M, Peyron JF, Imbert V (2009) NF-kappaB inhibition triggers death of imatinib-sensitive and imatinib-resistant chronic myeloid leukemia cells including T315I Bcr-Abl mutants. Int J Cancer 125(2):308–317. doi:10.1002/ijc.24294

MacFarlane M, Harper N, Snowden RT, Dyer MJ, Barnett GA, Pringle JH, Cohen GM (2002) Mechanisms of resistance to TRAIL-induced apoptosis in primary B cell chronic lymphocytic leukaemia. Oncogene 21(44):6809–6818. doi:10.1038/sj.onc.1205853

Majeti R, Chao MP, Alizadeh AA, Pang WW, Jaiswal S, Gibbs KD Jr, van Rooijen N, Weissman IL (2009) CD47 is an adverse prognostic factor and therapeutic antibody target on human acute myeloid leukemia stem cells. Cell 138(2):286–299. doi:10.1016/j.cell.2009.05.045

Majetschak M (2011) Extracellular ubiquitin: immune modulator and endogenous opponent of damage-associated molecular pattern molecules. J Leukoc Biol 89(2):205–219. doi:10.1189/jlb.0510316

Marcucci G, Radmacher MD, Maharry K, Mrozek K, Ruppert AS, Paschka P, Vukosavljevic T, Whitman SP, Baldus CD, Langer C, Liu CG, Carroll AJ, Powell BL, Garzon R, Croce CM, Kolitz JE, Caligiuri MA, Larson RA, Bloomfield CD (2008) MicroRNA expression in cytogenetically normal acute myeloid leukemia. N Engl J Med 358(18):1919–1928. doi:10.1056/NEJMoa074256

Meurette O, Fontaine A, Rebillard A, Le Moigne G, Lamy T, Lagadic-Gossmann D, Dimanche-Boitrel MT (2006) Cytotoxicity of TRAIL/anticancer drug combinations in human normal cells. Ann N Y Acad Sci 1090:209–216. doi:10.1196/annals.1378.023

Miyamoto S, Maki M, Schmitt MJ, Hatanaka M, Verma IM (1994) Tumor necrosis factor alpha-induced phosphorylation of I kappa B alpha is a signal for its degradation but not dissociation from NF-kappa B. Proc Natl Acad Sci USA 91(26):12740–12744

Munzert G, Kirchner D, Ottmann O, Bergmann L, Schmid RM (2004) Constitutive NF-kappab/Rel activation in philadelphia chromosome positive (Ph+) acute lymphoblastic leukemia (ALL). Leuk Lymphoma 45(6):1181–1184

NCI: National Cancer Institute (2013) SEER Stat fact sheets: acute myeloid leukemia. Available at http://www.seercancergov/statfacts/html/amylhtml. Accessed 14/02/2013

Nebreda AR, Gavin AC (1999) Perspectives: signal transduction. Cell survival demands some Rsk. Science 286(5443):1309–1310

O'Connell MA, Cleere R, Long A, O'Neill LA, Kelleher D (1995) Cellular proliferation and activation of NF kappa B are induced by autocrine production of tumor necrosis factor alpha in the human T lymphoma line HuT 78. J Biol Chem 270(13):7399–7404

Park SJ, Kim MJ, Kim HB, Kang CD, Kim SH (2009) Sensitization of imatinib-resistant CML cells to TRAIL-induced apoptosis is mediated through down-regulation of Bcr-Abl as well as c-FLIP. Biochem J 420(1):73–81. doi:10.1042/BJ20082131

Qu P, Yan C, Du H (2011) Matrix metalloproteinase 12 overexpression in myeloid lineage cells plays a key role in modulating myelopoiesis, immune suppression, and lung tumorigenesis. Blood 117(17):4476–4489. doi:10.1182/blood-2010-07-298380

Redell MS, Ruiz MJ, Alonzo TA, Gerbing RB, Tweardy DJ (2011) Stat3 signaling in acute myeloid leukemia: ligand-dependent and -independent activation and induction of apoptosis by a novel small-molecule Stat3 inhibitor. Blood 117(21):5701–5709. doi:10.1182/blood-2010-04-280123

Reinart N, Nguyen PH, Boucas J, Rosen N, Kvasnicka HM, Heukamp L, Rudolph C, Ristovska V, Velmans T, Mueller C, Reiners KS, von Strandmann EP, Krause G, Montesinos-Rongen M, Schlegelberger B, Herling M, Hallek M, Fingerle-Rowson G (2013) Delayed development of chronic lymphocytic leukemia in the absence of macrophage migration inhibitory factor. Blood 121(5):812–821. doi:10.1182/blood-2012-05-431452

Reuther JY, Reuther GW, Cortez D, Pendergast AM, Baldwin AS Jr (1998) A requirement for NF-kappaB activation in Bcr-Abl-mediated transformation. Genes Dev 12(7):968–981

Riccioni R, Pasquini L, Mariani G, Saulle E, Rossini A, Diverio D, Pelosi E, Vitale A, Chierichini A, Cedrone M, Foa R, Lo Coco F, Peschle C, Testa U (2005) TRAIL decoy receptors mediate resistance of acute myeloid leukemia cells to TRAIL. Haematologica 90(5):612–624

Richardson PG, Mitsiades CS, Hideshima T, Anderson KC (2005) Novel biological therapies for the treatment of multiple myeloma. Best Pract Res Clin Haematol 18(4):619–634. doi:10.1016/j.beha.2005.01.010

Romano MF, Petrella A, Bisogni R, Turco MC, Venuta S (2003) Effect of NF-kappaB/Rel inhibition on spontaneous vs chemotherapy-induced apoptosis in AML and normal cord blood CD34+ cells. Leukemia (Official Journal of the Leukemia Society of America, Leukemia Research Fund, UK) 17(6):1190–1192. doi:10.1038/sj.leu.2402953

Sarlo C, Buccisano F, Maurillo L, Cefalo M, Di Caprio L, Cicconi L, Ditto C, Ottaviani L, Di Veroli A, Del Principe MI, Grasso MA, Nasso D, De Santis G, Amadori S, Venditti A (2013) Phase II study of Bortezomib as a single agent in patients with previously untreated or relapsed/refractory acute myeloid leukemia ineligible for intensive therapy. Leuk Res Treat 2013:705714. doi:10.1155/2013/705714

Sawicki G, Matsuzaki A, Janowska-Wieczorek A (1998) Expression of the active form of MMP-2 on the surface of leukemic cells accounts for their in vitro invasion. J Cancer Res Clin Oncol 124(5):245–252

Schepers H, Eggen BJ, Schuringa JJ, Vellenga E (2006) Constitutive activation of NF-kappa B is not sufficient to disturb normal steady-state hematopoiesis. Haematologica 91(12):1710–1711

Schulze-Osthoff K, Ferrari D, Los M, Wesselborg S, Peter ME (1998) Apoptosis signaling by death receptors. Eur J Biochem/FEBS 254(3):439–459

Schwieger M, Schuler A, Forster M, Engelmann A, Arnold MA, Delwel R, Valk PJ, Lohler J, Slany RK, Olson EN, Stocking C (2009) Homing and invasiveness of MLL/ENL leukemic cells is regulated by MEF2C. Blood 114(12):2476–2488. doi:10.1182/blood-2008-05-158196

Siripin D, Fucharoen S, Tanyong DI (2011) Nitric oxide and caspase 3 mediated cytokine induced apoptosis in acute leukemia. Asian Pac J Allergy Immunol (Launched by the Allergy and Immunology Society of Thailand) 29(1):102–111

Spoo AC, Lubbert M, Wierda WG, Burger JA (2007) CXCR4 is a prognostic marker in acute myelogenous leukemia. Blood 109(2):786–791. doi:10.1182/blood-2006-05-024844

Steelman LS, Pohnert SC, Shelton JG, Franklin RA, Bertrand FE, McCubrey JA (2004) JAK/STAT, Raf/MEK/ERK, PI3 K/Akt and BCR-ABL in cell cycle progression and leukemogenesis. Leukemia (Official Journal of the Leukemia Society of America, Leukemia Research Fund, UK) 18(2):189–218. doi:10.1038/sj.leu.2403241

Sun SC (2011) Non-canonical NF-kappaB signaling pathway. Cell Res 21(1):71–85. doi:10.1038/cr.2010.177

Tilton B, Ho L, Oberlin E, Loetscher P, Baleux F, Clark-Lewis I, Thelen M (2000) Signal transduction by CXC chemokine receptor 4. Stromal cell-derived factor 1 stimulates prolonged protein kinase B and extracellular signal-regulated kinase 2 activation in T lymphocytes. J Exp Med 192(3):313–324

Tsimberidou AM, Estey E, Wen S, Pierce S, Kantarjian H, Albitar M, Kurzrock R (2008) The prognostic significance of cytokine levels in newly diagnosed acute myeloid leukemia and high-risk myelodysplastic syndromes. Cancer 113(7):1605–1613. doi:10.1002/cncr.23785

Uy GL, Rettig MP, Motabi IH, McFarland K, Trinkaus KM, Hladnik LM, Kulkarni S, Abboud CN, Cashen AF, Stockerl-Goldstein KE, Vij R, Westervelt P, DiPersio JF (2012) A phase 1/2 study of chemosensitization with the CXCR4 antagonist plerixafor in relapsed or refractory acute myeloid leukemia. Blood 119(17):3917–3924. doi:10.1182/blood-2011-10-383406

Van Etten RA (2007) Aberrant cytokine signaling in leukemia. Oncogene 26(47):6738–6749. doi:10.1038/sj.onc.1210758

Walter RB, Milano F, Brasky TM, White E (2011) Long-term use of acetaminophen, aspirin, and other nonsteroidal anti-inflammatory drugs and risk of hematologic malignancies: results from the prospective Vitamins and Lifestyle (VITAL) study. J Clin Oncol (Official Journal of the American Society of Clinical Oncology) 29(17):2424–2431. doi:10.1200/JCO.2011.34.6346

Webb RN, Cruse JM, Lewis RE (2009) Decreased TLR4 gene expression in leukemic leukocyte populations. Exp Mol Pathol 87(2):117–126. doi:10.1016/j.yexmp.2009.07.007

Weiss JR, Baker JA, Baer MR, Menezes RJ, Nowell S, Moysich KB (2006) Opposing effects of aspirin and acetaminophen use on risk of adult acute leukemia. Leuk Res 30(2):164–169. doi:10.1016/j.leukres.2005.06.023

Wen J, Ramadevi N, Nguyen D, Perkins C, Worthington E, Bhalla K (2000) Antileukemic drugs increase death receptor 5 levels and enhance Apo-2L-induced apoptosis of human acute leukemia cells. Blood 96(12):3900–3906

Wood KM, Roff M, Hay RT (1998) Defective IkappaBalpha in Hodgkin cell lines with constitutively active NF-kappaB. Oncogene 16(16):2131–2139. doi:10.1038/sj.onc.1201735

Zang DY, Goodwin RG, Loken MR, Bryant E, Deeg HJ (2001) Expression of tumor necrosis factor-related apoptosis-inducing ligand, Apo2L, and its receptors in myelodysplastic syndrome: effects on in vitro hemopoiesis. Blood 98(10):3058–3065

Zaninoni A, Imperiali FG, Pasquini C, Zanella A, Barcellini W (2003) Cytokine modulation of nuclear factor-kappaB activity in B-chronic lymphocytic leukemia. Exp Hematol 31(3):185–190

Zhou J, Bi C, Janakakumara JV, Liu SC, Chng WJ, Tay KG, Poon LF, Xie Z, Palaniyandi S, Yu H, Glaser KB, Albert DH, Davidsen SK, Chen CS (2009) Enhanced activation of STAT pathways and overexpression of survivin confer resistance to FLT3 inhibitors and could be therapeutic targets in AML. Blood 113(17):4052–4062. doi:10.1182/blood-2008-05-156422

Chapter 14
The Role of Inflammatory Cells in Angiogenesis in Multiple Myeloma

Domenico Ribatti and Angelo Vacca

Abstract Both innate and adaptive immune cells are involved in the mechanisms of endothelial cell proliferation, migration and activation, via production and release of a large spectrum of pro-angiogenic mediators, thus creating the specific microenvironment that favors increased rate of tissue vascularization. In this article, we focus on the immune cell component of the angiogenic process occurring during multiple myeloma progression. We also provide information on some anti-angiogenic properties of immune cells that may be applied for a potential pharmacological use as anti-angiogenic agents in the disease treatment.

14.1 Introduction

Inflammatory cells regulate endothelial cell functions related to physiological as well as tumor-associated angiogenesis. The relationship between inflammation and cancer was discovered as early as 1863 by Rudolf Virchow, who first described a leukocyte infiltrate in tumor tissues. In some cancers, inflammation precedes development of malignancy, and it is well known that tumor-infiltrating inflammatory cells produce various cytokines that regulate the inflammatory response

D. Ribatti (✉)
Department of Basic Medical Sciences, Neurosciences and Sensory Organs,
Section of Human Anatomy and Histology, University of Bari Medical School,
Piazza Giulio Cesare, 11, 70124 Bari, Italy
e-mail: domenico.ribatti@uniba.it

A. Vacca
Department of Biomedical Sciences and Human Oncology (DIMO),
Section of Internal Medicine and Clinical Oncology, University of Bari Medical School,
Piazza Giulio Cesare, 11, 70124 Bari, Italy
e-mail: angelo.vacca@uniba.it

D. Ribatti
National Cancer Institute, Giovanni Paolo II, 70124 Bari, Italy

B. B. Aggarwal et al. (eds.), *Inflammation and Cancer*, Advances in Experimental Medicine and Biology 816, DOI: 10.1007/978-3-0348-0837-8_14, © Springer Basel 2014

in tumor-bearing hosts, while inflammatory cells may produce growth factors that suppress the anti-tumor immune response. The most aggressive human cancers are associated with dramatic host inflammatory response, and inflammatory cells act in concert with tumor cells, stromal cells, and endothelial cells to create a microenvironment that is critical for the survival, development, and diffusion of the neoplastic mass. These interactions within the tumor microenvironment may represent important mechanisms for tumor development and metastasis by providing an efficient vascular supply and an easy escape pathway.

Inflammatory cells produce angiogenic cytokines, growth factors, and proteases that contribute to new vessels formation at the site of tumor growth. Conversely, microvascular endothelium activated by a number of cytokines and angiogenic growth factors can express pro-inflammatory molecules involved in leukocyte recruitment and activation (Pober and Sessa 2007). Various chemokines may act both as leukocyte attractants and angiogenic inducers by acting directly on endothelial cells. Several pro-inflammatory cytokines, including interleukin (IL)-1α, IL-1β, IL-6, tumor necrosis factor alpha (TNF-α), and osteopontin, induce vessel formation acting directly on endothelial cells or indirectly by inducing leukocyte and/or endothelial cells to produce pro-angiogenic mediators. Conversely, vascular endothelial growth factor (VEGF) and angiopoietin-1 (Ang-1) may elicit pro-inflammatory responses in endothelial cells by up-regulating the expression of cell-adhesion molecules and inflammatory mediators.

14.2 The Role of Monocyte–Macrophage Cells in Tumor Angiogenesis

Cells belonging to the monocyte–macrophage lineage are a major component of the leukocyte infiltration in tumors (Balkwill and Mantovani 2001). The number of tumor-derived chemoattractants ensures macrophage recruitment, including colony-stimulating factor-1 (CSF-1), the CC chemokines CCL-2, CCL-3, CCL-4, CCL-5, and CCL-8, and VEGF secreted by both tumor and stromal cells (Mantovani et al. 2002). Activated macrophages are generally categorized into two types, called M1 ("classically activated") and M2 ("alternatively activated") (Balkwill and Mantovani 2001). M1 macrophages are able to kill microorganisms as well as tumor cells and secrete high levels of pro-inflammatory cytokines and tumoricidal agents (TNF-α and IL-12), as well as reactive nitrogen and oxygen intermediates (RNI, ROI) (Balkwill et al. 2005).

In the tumor microenvironment, macrophages are mainly represented by M2 cells, derived from tumor-associated macrophages (TAMs) upon local exposure to IL-4 and IL-10 (Mantovani et al. 2002), which have poor attitude to destroy tumor cells but are better adapted to promoting angiogenesis, repairing and remodeling wounded or damaged tissues, and suppressing adaptive immunity (Sica et al. 2006). In regressing and non-progressing tumors, TAMs mainly resemble the M1 type and exhibit anti-tumor activity. Worth of note is that in malignant and advanced tumors, TAMs are biased toward the M2 phenotype that favors tumor malignancy (Qian and Pollard 2010).

The molecular mechanisms that promote M1 or M2 subsets within the tumor microenvironment are not completely understood. Unique cell surface markers that distinguish the M1 and M2 TAM phenotypes remain elusive, and expression of M1/M2 associated molecules is highly dependent on tumor type and stage, intratumoral localization, hypoxia, and other microenvironmental signals (Mantovani et al. 2002). The phenotype of polarized M1/M2 macrophages has the potential to be reversed (Guiducci et al. 2005).

Numerous studies have examined the association of TAMs with patient prognosis, survival, and angiogenesis in human tumors. Extensive TAM infiltration correlates with poor prognosis for breast, prostate, cervix, and bladder cancer patients (Talmadge et al. 2007). Besides killing tumor cells once activated by interferon-γ (IFN-γ) and IL-12, these TAMs produce several pro-angiogenic cytokines, including VEGF, TNF-α, IL-8, and FGF-2, as well as extracellular matrix-degrading enzymes, including matrix metalloproteinase-2 (MMP-2), MMP-7, MMP-9, MMP-12, and cycloxygenase-2 (COX-2) (Naldini and Carraro 2005; Klimp et al. 2001).

A close relationship between macrophage infiltrate or depletion and angiogenesis has been established in different experimental models. In a model of subcutaneous melanoma, both angiogenesis and growth rate correlate with tumor infiltration by macrophages expressing angiotensin I receptor and VEGF (Egami et al. 2003). Lewis lung carcinoma cells expressing IL-1β develop neovasculature with macrophage infiltration and enhance tumor growth in wild type but not in monocyte chemotactic protein-1 (MCP-1)-deficient mice, suggesting that macrophage involvement might be a prerequisite for neovascularization and tumor progression (Nakao et al. 2005). In a murine model of mammary carcinoma, deficiency of macrophage colony-stimulating factor (M-CSF), an inductor of macrophage recruitment in tumor tissues, reduces progression to invasive carcinoma and metastasis and angiogenesis (Lin et al. 2001). In polyoma middle-T (PyMT)-induced mouse mammary tumors, accumulation of macrophages in pre-malignant lesions precedes the angiogenic switch and progression into invasive tumors (Lin et al. 2007). Up-regulation of angiogenic activity in TAMs is stimulated by hypoxia and acidosis (Bingle et al. 2002). Moreover, activated macrophages synthesize and release inducible nitric oxide synthase, which increases blood flow and promotes angiogenesis (Jenkins et al. 1995). The angiogenic factors secreted by macrophages stimulate migration of other accessory cells that potentiate angiogenesis, in particular mast cells (Gruber et al. 1995). Osteopontin deeply affects the pro-angiogenic potential of human monocytes (Denhardt et al. 2001) and may affect angiogenesis by acting directly on endothelial cells and/or indirectly via mononuclear phagocyte engagement, enhancing the expression of TNF-α and IL-1β in mononuclear cells (Leali et al. 2003; Naldini et al. 2006).

Macrophages are producers of IL-12, which causes tumor regression and reduces metastasis in animal models, through the promotion of anti-tumor immunity, and also to the significant inhibition of angiogenesis (Colombo and Trinchieri 2002). The anti-angiogenic activity is mediated by IFN-γ production, which in turn induces the chemokine IFN-γ-inducible protein-10 (Angiolillo et al. 1995; Romagnani et al. 2001). Moreover, IL-12 inhibits VEGF production by breast cancer cells and regulates stromal cell interactions, leading to decreased MMP-9 and increased tissue inhibitor of metalloproteinase-1 (TIMP-1) production (Dias et al. 1998). Using a transgenic mouse which develops mammary cancer (PyMT mice), Lin et al. (2006) demonstrated that both the angiogenic switch and the progression to malignancy are regulated by infiltrated macrophages. Moreover, inhibition of macrophage homing into the tumor microenvironment delayed the angiogenic switch, whereas genetic restoration of macrophages rescued the vascular phenotype. In addition, mice deficient in hypoxia inducible factor-2 alpha (HIF-2α) in myeloid cells displayed reduced TAM infiltration in both murine hepatocellular and colitis-associated colon carcinoma models (Imtiyaz et al. 2010). Moreover, mouse mammary tumors exhibited enriched M2-like TAMs in hypoxic tumor areas, with increased pro-angiogenic phenotype in vivo, and TAMs counts increasing as the tumor progressed (Movahedi et al. 2010). The developing vasculature in tumors lacking myeloid-cell-derived VEGF-A was less tortuous, with increased pericyte coverage (indicating enhanced maturation), and decreased vessel length, with evidence of vascular normalization and increased susceptibility to chemotherapeutic agents (Stockman et al. 2008).

De Palma et al. (2005) identified a subpopulation of monocytes expressing the Tie-2 receptor [Tie-2-expressing monocytes (TEMs)], which were selectively recruited to spontaneous and orthotopic tumors, promoted angiogenesis in a paracrine manner, and accounted for the majority of pro-angiogenic activity induced by myeloid cells in these tumors. Moreover, TEMs knockout completely prevented human glioma neovascularization in the mouse brain and induced tumor regression, and their gene expression profile was highly related to TAMs (Pucci et al. 2009). Finally, Ang-2 (a Tie-2 ligand) blockade did not inhibit recruitment of TEMs to the tumor microenvironment, but abrogated their up-regulation of Tie-2 expression, association with blood vessels, and their ability to restore angiogenesis in tumors (Mazzieri et al. 2008).

A significant relationship between the number of TAMs and the density of blood vessels has been established in human tumors, including breast carcinoma, melanoma, glioma, squamous cell carcinoma of the esophagus, bladder carcinoma, and prostate carcinoma (Lewis et al. 1995; Leek et al. 1996; Makitie et al. 2001; Nishie et al. 1999; Koide et al. 2004; Hanada et al. 2000; Lissbrant et al. 2000). Depletion of TAMs reduces to about 50 % tumor vascular density, leading to areas of necrosis by loss of blood supply within the tumor mass, and macrophages accumulate particularly in such necrotic and hypoxic areas in different neoplasia, such as human endometrial, breast, prostate, and ovarian carcinomas (Ohno et al. 2004; Leek et al. 1999).

14.3 Mast Cells and Angiogenesis in Tumors

Mast cells are bone marrow-derived tissue-homing leukocytes which were first described by Paul Ehrlich in 1878. They appear as highly versatile cells playing an important role in a large spectrum of biological settings, including inflammation, angiogenesis, tissue repair and remodeling, and cancer. As concerns the role of mast cells in tumor growth, although some evidence suggests that these cells can promote tumorigenesis and tumor progression, there are some clinical data as well as experimental tumor models in which mast cells seem to have functions that favor the host (Ribatti and Crivellato 2009). Mast cells are attracted into the microenvironment by stem cell factor (SCF) secreted by tumor cells and produce several angiogenic factors as well as MMPs, which promote, respectively, tumor vascularization and invasiveness (Ribatti and Crivellato 2009). Mast cells are capable of suppressing immune reactions by releasing histamine (which can induce tumor cell proliferation through H1 receptors and suppress the immune system through H2 receptors), TNF-α (Ullrich et al. 2007), and inhibitory cytokines, such as IL-10, and are essential in promoting the immune tolerance mediated by regulatory T cells (Treg) which, in their turn, stimulate immune tolerance and tumor promotion (Grimbaldenston et al. 2007). By contrast, mast cells may promote inflammation, inhibition of tumor cell growth, and tumor cell apoptosis by releasing cytokines, such as IL-1, IL-4, IL-6, IL-8, MCP-3 and MCP-4, transforming growth factor beta (TGF-β), TNF-α, and chymase. Mast cells also produce chondroitin sulfate and tryptase: chondroitin sulfate may inhibit tumor cells diffusion, while tryptase causes both tumor cell disruption and inflammation through activation of protease-activated receptors (PAR-1 and -2) (Ribatti and Crivellato 2012).

Increased mast cell number has been correlated with a poor prognosis in several human tumors, including melanoma (Ribatti et al. 2003a), oral squamous carcinoma (Wanachantarak 2003), and squamous cell carcinoma of the lip (Rojas et al. 2005). Mast cells produce several pro-angiogenic factors, including FGF-2, VEGF, IL-8, TNF-α, TGF-β, and nerve growth factor (NGF) (Qu et al. 1995, 1998a, b; Grützkau et al. 1998; Aoki et al. 2003; Abdel-Majid et al. 2004; Boesiger et al. 1998; Kanbe et al. 2000; Moller et al. 1993; Walsh et al. 1991; Nilsson et al. 1997). Mast cells migrate in vivo and in vitro in response to VEGF and placental growth factor-1 (PlGF-1) (Detmar et al. 1998; Gruber et al. 1995;Detoraki et al. 2009). Human lung mast cells express VEGF-A, VEGF-B, VEGF-C, and VEGF-D, and supernatants of prostaglandin E2 (PGE2)- and 5′-N-ethylcarboxamido-adenosine (NECA)-activated lung mast cells induced angiogenic response in the chick embryo chorioallantoic membrane (CAM) assay that was inhibited by an anti-VEGF-A antibody (Detoraki et al. 2009). Mast cells store in their secretory granules pre-formed active serine proteases, including tryptase and chymase (Metcalfe et al. 1997). Tryptase stimulates the proliferation of endothelial cells, promotes vascular tube formation in vitro, degrades connective tissue matrix, and activates MMPs and plasminogen activator (PA), which in turn degrade the extracellular matrix with consequent release of VEGF or FGF-2 from their matrix-bound state (Blair et al. 1997). Histamine and heparin stimulate proliferation of endothelial cells in vitro and are angiogenic in the CAM assay (Sörbo et al. 1994; Ribatti et al. 1987). Mast cells contain MMP-2 and MMP-9, and TIMPs, which intervene in regulation of extracellular matrix degradation, allowing release of angiogenic factors. Granulated mast cells and their granules are able to stimulate an intense angiogenic reaction in the CAM assay, partly inhibited by anti-FGF-2 and anti-VEGF antibodies (Ribatti et al. 2001). Moreover, intraperitoneal injection of compound 48/80 causes a vigorous angiogenic response in the rat mesentery window angiogenic assay and in mice (Norrby et al. 1986, 1989).

Mast cells play a direct role in tumor angiogenesis. Mast cell-deficient W/Wv mice exhibit a decreased rate of tumor angiogenesis (Starkey et al. 1988). Heparin facilitates tumor vascularization by a direct pro-angiogenic effect and its anti-clotting effect (Theoharides et al. 2004). An increased number of mast cells have been demonstrated in angiogenesis associated with vascular tumors, such as hemangioma and hemangioblastoma (Glowacki and Mulliken 1982), as well as a number of hematological and solid tumors, including lymphomas (Ribatti et al. 1998, 2000; Fukushima et al. 2001), multiple myeloma (MM) (Ribatti et al. 1999), myelodysplastic syndrome (Ribatti et al. 2002), B-cell chronic lymphocytic leukemia (Ribatti et al. 2003a; Molica et al. 2003), breast cancer (Hartveit et al. 1981; Bowrey et al. 2000), colo-rectal cancer (Lachter et al. 1995), uterine cervix cancer (Graham and Graham, 1996; Bentitez-Bribiesca et al. 2001; Ribatti et al. 2005), and melanoma (Reed et al. 1996; Dvorak et al. 1980), in which mast cell accumulation correlates with increased neovascularization, mast cell VEGF and FGF-2 expression, tumor aggressiveness, and poor prognosis (Tóth-Jakatics et al. 2000; Ribatti et al. 2003b, c). Indeed, a prognostic significance has been attributed to mast cells and microvascular density also in squamous cell cancer of the esophagus (Elpek et al. 2001). An association between VEGF, mast cells, and angiogenesis has been demonstrated in laryngeal carcinoma and in small lung carcinoma (Sawatsubashi et al. 2000; Imada et al. 2000; Takanami et al. 2000; Tomita et al. 2000).

The introduction of novel experimental procedures to induce carcinogenesis in pre-clinical in vivo models contributed to our increased understanding on the role of mast cells in tumor angiogenesis. Development of squamous cell carcinoma in a human papilloma virus (HPV) 16 infected transgenic mouse model of epithelia carcinogenesis provided experimental support for the early participation of mast cells in tumor growth and angiogenesis (Coussens et al. 1999, 2000). Infiltration of mast cells and activation of MMP-9 coincided with the angiogenic switch in pre-malignant lesions through the release of pro-angiogenic molecules from the extracellular matrix. Remarkably, pre-malignant angiogenesis was abrogated in a mast cell-deficient HPV 16 transgenic mouse indicating that neoplastic progression in this model involved infiltration of mast cells in the skin (Coussens et al. 1999, 2000). By using the same in vivo transgenic mouse model, it has been demonstrated that genetic elimination of mature T and B lymphocytes limits neoplastic progression (de Visser et al. 2005; Andreu et al. 2010). Moreover, in prostate tumors derived from both tumor transgenic adenocarcinoma of the mouse prostate (TRAMP) mice and human patients, mast cells promote well-differentiated adenocarcinoma growth (Pittoni et al. 2011).

14.4 Angiogenesis in Multiple Myeloma

In MM, bone marrow angiogenesis measured as microvascular density increases with progression from monoclonal gammopathy of undetermined significance (MGUS) to non-active MM (complete/objective response MM) and active MM (newly diagnosed, relapsed, and resistant MM), and is related with the plasma cell labeling index (Vacca and Ribatti 2006). Myeloma plasma cells induce angiogenesis through the secretion of angiogenic cytokines, including VEGF and FGF-2, by induction of host inflammatory cell infiltration, and secretion of MMP-2 and MMP-9 and urokinase-type plasminogen activator (Vacca and Ribatti 2006). There is also evidence of loss of anti-angiogenic activity on the part of bone marrow plasma cells (Kumar et al. 2004; Mangieri et al. 2008). Moreover, bone marrow MM endothelial cells secrete growth factors, including VEGF and IL-6, which promote MM plasma cell growth (Vacca et al. 2003).

The microenvironment favors angiogenesis in MM. In fact, it is composed by stromal cells (BMSCs), including hematopoietic stem and progenitor cells (HSPCs), fibroblasts, osteoblasts, osteoclasts, adipocytes, endothelial progenitor cells (EPCs), endothelial cells, T cells, macrophages, and mast cells, as well as by extracellular matrix composed by a complex network of proteins such as fibronectin, laminin, and collagen, and a mixture of growth factors, cytokines, and chemokines.

In MM, reciprocal interactions between plasma cells and BMSCs, mediated by several cytokines, receptors, and adhesion molecules, modulate the angiogenic response (Ribatti et al. 2006). BMSCs, osteoclasts, osteoblasts, and endothelial cells secrete several factors, including VEGF, FGF-2, TNF-α, IL-6, B-cell activating factor, stromal cell-derived factor 1α (SDF1α, also known as CXCL12), osteopontin, insulin-like growth factor-1 (IGF-1), and various Notch family members, which are further up-regulated by tumor cell adhesion to extracellular matrix proteins and/or BMSCs (Hideshima et al. 2007).

In this way, BMSCs increase the concentration of angiogenic factors and matrix-degrading enzymes in the bone marrow microenvironment by direct secretion or by stimulation of MM plasma cells or endothelial cells through paracrine interactions. The enhanced invasive and angiogenic capacity of MM cells explain the intramedullary and extramedullary dissemination observed in MM.

14.4.1 The Involvement of Macrophages in MM Neovascularization

In patients with active MM, bone marrow macrophages contribute to neovascularization through a vasculogenic pathway. When these macrophages are exposed to VEGF and FGF-2, which are major angiogenic cytokines secreted by plasma cells (Vacca et al. 1999), and present in the bone marrow microenvironment at 4–5-fold higher levels than in peripheral blood (Di Raimondo et al. 2000), they transform

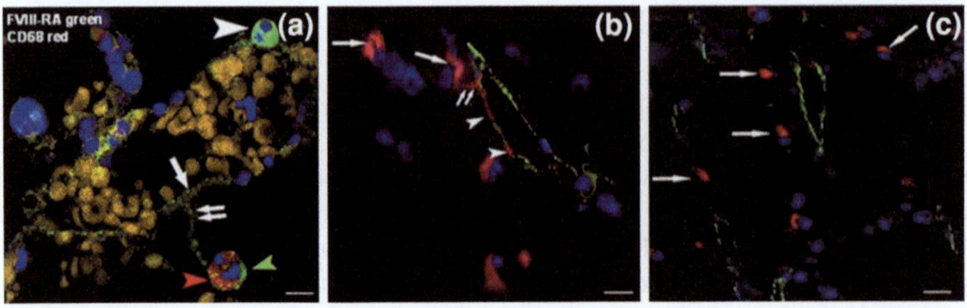

Fig. 14.1 CD68 (*red*) and FVIII-RA (*green*) in (**a**) dual confocal laser microscopy, and (**b**, **c**) immunofluorescence of bone marrow biopsies of (**a**, **b**) a patient with multiple myeloma (*MM*) and (**c**) a patient with monoclonal gammopathy of undetermined significance (*MGUS*). In (**a**), a microvessel lined by flattened FVIII-RA-positive endothelial cells (*arrow*) and FVIII-RA positive macrophage (*arrowhead*) showing protrusions connected to endothelial cells; another macrophage containing double-labeled CD68 (*red arrowhead*) and FVIII-RA (*green arrowhead*) granules in the cytoplasm is connected to endothelial cells by a FVIII-RA-positive cytoplasmic protrusion (*double arrowhead*). **b** Another microvessel formed by FVIII-RA-positive (*green*) endothelial cells and CD68-positive (*red*, *arrowheads*) tracts belonging to the cytoplasmic protrusions (*double arrow*) of macrophages, some of which are *arrowed*. **c** The MGUS microvessel is formed only by FVIII-RA-positive endothelial cells: macrophages (*arrows*) are randomly scattered in the tissue. [Reproduced from Scavelli et al. (2008)]

into cells functionally and phenotypically similar to paired MM endothelial cells, and generate capillary-like networks mimicking those of MM endothelial cells (Scavelli et al. 2008). Endothelial cell-like macrophages and apparently typical macrophages contribute sizably to the formation of the neovessel wall in patients with active MM, whereas their vascular supply is minimal in non-active MM and absent in MGUS patients and control patients (Fig. 14.1) (Scavelli et al. 2008). In patients with active MM, FACS analysis on freshly isolated bone marrow mononuclear cells revealed higher percentages of CD14/CD68 double-positive cells than in those with non-active disease and MGUS. Furthermore, in active MM patients, bone marrow biopsies displayed macrophages with both endothelial cell-like (i.e., CD68/FVIII-RA double positive) and apparently typical (i.e., CD68 positive/FVIII-RA negative) features located in the microvessel wall and collaborating with MM endothelial cells to line the vessel lumen. Figures of this type were rare in non-active MM patients and absent in MGUS. Thus, macrophage involvement in the vasculogenic pathway proceeds in step with MM activity and with progression of plasma cell tumors as well (Scavelli et al. 2008).

14.4.2 The Involvement of Mast Cells in MM Neovascularization

Also, mast cells contribute to MM neovascularization. Bone marrow angiogenesis and mast cell counts are highly correlated in patients with non-active and active MM, and in those with MGUS, and both parameters increase simultaneously in

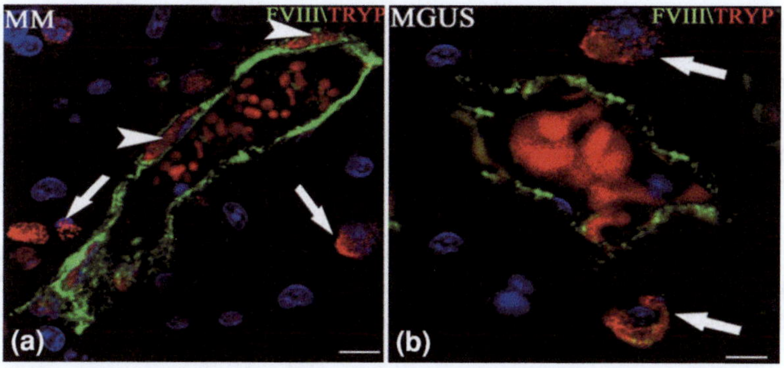

Fig. 14.2 Double FVIII-RA (*green*) and tryptase (*red*) confocal laser microscopy from bone marrow biopsies of patients with (**a**) multiple myeloma (*MM*) and (**b**) monoclonal gammopathy of undetermined significance (MGUS). In (**a**), a vessel is lined by both endothelial cells positive for FVIII-RA and by mast cells positive for tryptase (*arrowheads*). Mast cells containing tryptase-positive granules (*arrows*) are also recognizable on the abluminal side of the vessel. In (**b**), a MGUS vessel is lined only by endothelial cells positive for FVIII-RA and is surrounded by tryptase-positive mast cells (*arrows*). [Reproduced from Nico et al. (2008)]

active MM (Ribatti et al. 1999). Ang-1 is promoter of MM angiogenesis, and experimental evidence indicates that Ang-1 secreted by primary murine mast cells promotes marked neovascularization in an in vivo transplantation assay (Nakayama et al. 2004). Primary mast cells accelerate tumor growth and angiogenesis by established plasmocytoma cell lines, while Ang-1-neutralizing antibodies significantly reduced the growth of plasmocytomas containing mast cells (Nakayama et al. 2004). Vessels from MM biopsies are lined by mast cells whose cytoplasms are filled with numerous and irregularly shaped electron-dense granules (Nico et al. 2008). These findings have been confirmed by confocal laser microscopy using double anti-tryptase (to mark mast cells) and anti-FVIII-RA (to mark endothelial cells) antibodies. Vessels from MM biopsies displayed regions stained by FVIII-RA alternating with regions stained by both tryptase and FVIII-RA. In the MGUS biopsies, the vessels were uniformly stained by the anti-FVIII antibody only, while tryptase-positive mast cells were only recognizable perivascularly (Fig. 14.2) (Nico et al. 2008).

14.5 Immunomodulatory and Anti-inflammatory Molecules in the Treatment of MM

14.5.1 Immunomodulatory Drugs

The Immunomodulatory Drugs (IMiDs) thalidomide, lenalidomide, and pomalidomide, used in the treatment of MM, have direct anti-tumor, immunoregulatory, anti-angiogenic, and anti-inflammatory properties. They specifically trigger caspase-8-mediated apoptosis; decrease binding of tumor cells to bone marrow; inhibit constitutive and MM cell binding-induced secretion of cytokines from bone marrow; and stimulate autologous NK and T-cell immunity to MM cells (Hideshima et al. 2007).

IMiDs inhibit TNF-α, IL-1β, IL-6, IL-12, and TGF-β production. These cytokines enhance growth and survival of myeloma cells, drug resistance, cell migration, and adhesive molecule expression. Moreover, IMiDs increase anti-inflammatory cytokines (IL-10) production. Anti-inflammatory and anti-angiogenic properties of thalidomide are partially controlled by NF-κB transcriptional factor. Moreover, thalidomide significantly inhibits SDF-1α and CXCR4 receptor expression on MM cells leading to decreased IL-6 and VEGF production supporting survival of MM cells.

14.5.2 Cytokines

In MM, both chains of IL-27 receptor are expressed in CD138 positive plasma cells from patients (Cocco et al. 2011). IL-27 inhibits the angiogenic potential of MM cells, down-regulates different angiogenic factors, and up-regulates the anti-angiogenic chemokines CXCL9 and CXCL10 (Cocco et al. 2011). Pre-clinical studies using highly immunodeficient non-obese diabetic/severe combined immunodeficient mice injected with MM plasma cells demonstrated that IL-27 inhibits MM plasma cell growth through inhibition of angiogenesis, thus supporting the concept that IL-27 may represent a novel therapeutic agent for patients with MM.

14.5.3 The Anti-inflammatory Molecule Pentraxin 3

Pentraxin 3 (PTX3) plays an important role in inhibiting the cross talk between BMSCs and plasma cells in MM. Basile et al. (2013) demonstrated that PTX3 inhibits FGF-2-induced angiogenesis of MM endothelial cells through its binding to FGF-2 and exerts a direct impact on FGF-2-induced biological activities on MM fibroblasts, which also support MM cell growth. In particular, PTX3 is cytotoxic on MM cells by inhibiting the activities of endothelial cells and fibroblasts, including cytokine production, and causing loss of adhesive plasma cell capability to these cells.

14.5.4 Other Molecules

Clodronate liposomes depleted macrophages and inhibited tumor angiogenesis in mouse tumor transplantation models (Zeisberger et al. 2006). In the mouse cornea model, killing of COX-2-positive infiltrating macrophages with clodronate liposomes reduces IL-1β-induced angiogenesis and partially inhibits VEGF-induced angiogenesis (Nakao et al. 2005). VEGF inhibitors decrease macrophage recruitment, and this effect may contribute to their anti-angiogenic activity (Giraudo et al. 2004). Specific inhibition of VEGFR-2 decreased tumor macrophage infiltration into orthotopic pancreatic tumors (Dineen et al. 2008). CSF-1 receptor (c-fms) kinase inhibitors exhibit anti-angiogenic and anti-metastatic activity in tumors (Manthey et al. 2009). Anti-CSF-1 antibodies and antisense oligonucleotides suppress macrophage infiltration and xenograft tumor growth in mice (Aharinejad et al. 2002, 2004).

Mast cells might act as a new target for the adjuvant treatment of tumors through the selective inhibition of angiogenesis, tissue remodeling, and tumor promoting molecules, allowing the secretion of cytotoxic cytokines and preventing mast cell-mediated immune-suppression. Pre-clinical studies using anti-cKIT antibodies (Huang et al. 2008), anti-TNF-α antibodies (Gounaris et al. 2007), or the mast cells stabilizer disodium cromoglycate (cromolyn) (Soucek et al. 2007) in mouse models have demonstrated promising results. Thus, identification and targeting of mast cells and macrophages represents an attractive therapeutic approach in cancer. Therapeutic strategies include inhibition of recruitment to the tumor microenvironment and blockade of pro-tumoral effector functions. Chemoprevention with an anti-inflammatory approach has the potential to inhibit neovascularization before the onset of the angiogenic switch, resulting in a significant delay in tumor growth.

14.6 Concluding Remarks

The pathogenesis of most cancers includes complex and mutual interactions that affect the number and phenotype of the tumor cells and host inflammatory cells. In this context, angiogenesis in MM is the result of a complex balance between pro- and anti-angiogenic stimuli generated in the tissue milieu. The evidences summarized highlight the importance of the inflammatory microenvironment during angiogenesis in MM and provide a novel perspective for the complex interplay between several inflammatory and vascular components in the bone marrow microenvironment in MM.

Acknowledgments The research leading to these results has received funding from the European Union Seventh Framework Programme (FP7/2007–2013) under Grant agreement n°278570 to DR and 278706 to AV.

References

Abdel-Majid RM, Marshall JS (2004) Prostaglandin E2 induces degranulation independent production of vascular endothelial growth factor by human mast cells. J Immunol 172:1227–1236

Aharinejad S, Abraham D, Paulus P et al (2002) Colony-stimulating factor-1 antisense treatment suppresses growth of human tumor xenografts in mice. Cancer Res 62:5317–5324

Aharinejad S, Paulus P, Sioud M et al (2004) Colony-stimulating factor-1 blockade by antisense oligonucleotide and small interfering RNAs suppresses growth of human mammary tumor xenograft in mice. Cancer Res 64:5378–5384

Andreu P, Johansson M, Affara NI et al (2010) FcR gamma activation regulates inflammation-associated squamous carcinogenesis. Cancer Cell 17:121–134
Angiolillo AL, Sgadari C, Taub DD et al (1995) Human interferon-inducible protein 10 is a potent inhibitor of angiogenesis in vivo. J Exp Med 182:155–162
Aoki M, Pawankar R, Niimi Y et al (2003) Mast cells in basal cell carcinoma express VEGF, IL-8 and RANTES. Int Arch Allergy Immunol 130:216–223
Balkwill F, Mantovani A (2001) Inflammation and cancer: back to Virchow? Lancet 357:539–545
Balkwill F, Charles KA, Mantovani A (2005) Smoldering and polarized inflammation in the initiation and promotion of malignant disease. Cancer Cell 7:211–217
Basile A, Moschetta M, Ditonno P et al (2013) Pentraxin 3 (PTX3) inhibits plasma cell/stromal cell cross-talk in the bone marrow of multiple myeloma patients. J Pathol 229:87–98
Benitez-Bribiesca L, Wong A, Utrera D et al (2001) The role of mast cell tryptase in neoangiogenesis of premalignant and malignant lesions of the uterine cervix. J Histochem Cytochem 49:1061–1062
Bingle L, Brown NJ, Lewis CE (2002) The role of tumour-associated macrophages in tumour progression: implications for new anticancer therapies. J Pathol 196:254–265
Blair RJ, Meng H, Marchese MJ et al (1997) Human mast cells stimulate vascular tube formation: tryptase is a novel potent angiogenic factor. J Clin Invest 99:2691–2700
Boesiger J, Tsai M, Maurer M et al (1998) Mast cells can secrete vascular permeability factor/vascular endothelial cell growth factor and exhibit enhanced release after immunoglobulin E-dependent upregulation of fc epsilon receptor I expression. J Exp Med 188:1135–1145
Bowrey PF, King J, Magarey C et al (2000) Histamine, mast cells and tumour cell proliferation in breast cancer: does preoperative cimetidine administration have an effect? Br J Cancer 82:167–170
Cocco C, Morandi F, Airoldi J (2011) Interleukin-27 and interleukin-23 modulate human plasma cell functions. J Leukoc Biol 89:729–734
Colombo MP, Trinchieri G (2002) Interleukin-12 in anti-tumor immunity and immunotherapy. Cytokine Growth Factor Rev 13:155–168
Coussens LM, Raymond WW, Bergers G et al (1999) Inflammatory mast cells up-regulate angiogenesis during squamous epithelial carcinogenesis. Genes Dev 13:1382–1397
Coussens LM, Tinkle CL, Hanahan D et al (2000) MMP-9 supplied by bone marrow-derived cells contributes to skin carcinogenesis. Cell 103:481–490
Denhardt DT, Noda M, O'Regan AW et al (2001) Osteopontin as a means to cope with environmental insults: regulation of inflammation, tissue remodeling, and cell survival. J Clin Invest 107:1055–1061
De Palma M, Venneri MA, Galli R et al (2005) Tie2 identifies a hematopoietic lineage of proangiogenic monocytes required for tumor vessel formation and a mesenchymal population of pericyte progenitors. Cancer Cell 8:211–226
Detmar M, Brown LF, Schön MP et al (1998) Increased microvascular density and enhanced leukocyte rolling and adhesionin the skin of VEGF transgenic mice. J Invest Dermatol 111:1–6
Detoraki A, Staiano RI, Granata F et al (2009) Vascular endothelial growth factors synthesized by human lung mast cells exert angiogenic effects. J Allergy Clin Immunol 123:1142–1149
de Visser KE, Korets LV, Coussens LM (2005) De novo carcinogenesis promoted by chronic inflammation is B lymphocyte dependent. Cancer Cell 7:411–423
Dias S, Boyd R, Balkwill F (1998) IL-12 regulates VEGF and MMPs in a murine breast cancer model. Int J Cancer 78:361–365
Dineen SP, Lynn KD, Holloway SE et al (2008) Vascular endothelial growth factor receptor 2 mediates macrophage infiltration into orthotopic pancreatic tumors in mice. Cancer Res 68:4340–4346
Di Raimondo F, Azzaro MP, Palombo G et al (2000) Angiogenic factors in multiple myeloma: higher levels in bone marrow than in peripheral blood. Haematologica 85:800–805
Dvorak AM, Mihm MC Jr, Osage JE et al (1980) Melanoma. An ultrastructural study of the host inflammatory and vascular responses. J Invest Dermatol 75:388–393
Egami K, Murohara T, Shimada T et al (2003) Role of host angiotensin II type 1 receptor in tumor angiogenesis and growth. J Clin Invest 112:67–75

Elpek GO, Gelen T, Aksoy NH et al (2001) The prognostic relevance of angiogenesis and mast cells in squamous cell carcinoma of the esophagus. J Clin Pathol 54:940–944
Fukushima N, Satoh T, Sano M et al (2001) Angiogenesis and mast cells in non-Hodgkin's lymphoma: a strong correlation in angioimmunoblastic T-cell lymphoma. Leuk Lymphoma 42:709–720
Giraudo E, Inoue M, Hanahan D (2004) An aminobisphosphonate targets MMP-9-expressing macrophages and angiogenesis to impair cervical carcinogenesis. J Clin Invest 114:623–633
Glowacki J, Mulliken JB (1982) Mast cells in hemangiomas and vascular malformations. Pediatrics 70:48–51
Gounaris E, Erdman SE, Restaino C et al (2007) Mast cells are an essential hematopoietic component for polyp development. Proc Natl Acad Sci USA 104:19977–19982
Graham R, Graham J (1996) Mast cells and cancer of the cervix. Surg Gynecol Obstet 123:3–9
Grimbaldesnton MA, Nakae S, Kalesnikoff K et al (2007) Mast cell-derived interleukin 10 limits skin pathology in contact dermatitis and chronic irradiation with ultraviolet B. Nat Immunol 38:1095–1104
Gruber BL, Marchese MJ, Kew R (1995) Angiogenic factors stimulate mast cell migration. Blood 86:2488–2493
Grützkau A, Krüger-Krasagakes S, Baumeister H et al (1998) Synthesis, storage, and release of vascular endothelial growth factor/vascular permeability factor (VEGF/VPF) by human mast cells: implications for the biological significance of VEGF206. Mol Biol Cell 9:875–884
Guiducci L, Vicari AP, Sangaletti S et al (2005) Redirecting in vivo elicited tumor infiltrating macrophages and dendritic cells towards tumor rejection. Cancer Res 65:3437–3446
Hanada T, Nakagawa M, Emoto A et al (2000) Prognostic value of tumor-associated macrophage count in human bladder cancer. Int J Urol 7:263–269
Hartveit F (1981) Mast cells and metachromasia in human breast cancer: their occurrence, significance and consequence: a preliminary report. J Pathol 134:7–11
Hideshima T, Mitsiades C, Tonon G et al (2007) Understanding multiple myeloma pathogenesis in the bone marrow to identify new therapeutic targets. Nat Rev Cancer 7:585–598
Huang B, Lei Z, Zhang GM et al (2008) SCF-mediated mast cell infiltration and activation exacerbate the inflammation and immunosuppression in tumor microenvironment. Blood 112:1269–1279
Imada A, Shijubo N, Koijma H et al (2000) Mast cells correlate with angiogenesis and poor outcome in stage I lung adenocarcinoma. Eur Resp J 15:1087–1093
Imtiyaz HZ, Williams EP, Hickey MM et al (2010) Hypoxia-inducible factor 2 alpha regulates macrophage function in mouse models of acute and tumor inflammation. J Clin Invest 120:2699–2714
Jenkins DC, Charles IG, Thomsen LL et al (1995) Roles of nitric oxide in tumor growth. Proc Natl Acad Sci USA 92:4392–4396
Kanbe N, Kurosawa M, Nagata H et al (2000) Production of fibrogenic cytokines by cord blood-derived cultured human mast cells. J Allergy Clin Immunol 106:S85–S90
Klimp AH, Hollema H, Kempinga C et al (2001) Expression of cyclooxygenase-2 and inducible nitric oxide synthase in human ovarian tumors and tumor-associated macrophages. Cancer Res 61:7305–7309
Koide N, Nishio A, Sato T et al (2004) Significance of macrophage chemoattractant protein-1 expression and macrophage infiltration in squamous cell carcinoma of the esophagus. Am J Gastroenterol 99:1667–1674
Kumar S, Witzig TE, Timm M et al (2004) Bone marrow angiogenic ability and expression of angiogenic cytokines in myeloma: evidence favouring loss of marrow angiogenesis inhibitory activity with disease progression. Blood 104:1159–1165
Lachter J, Stein M, Lichting C et al (1995) Mast cells in colorectal neoplasias and premalignant disorders. Dis Colon Rectum 38:290–293
Leali D, Dell'Era P, Stabile H et al (2003) Osteopontin (Eta-1) and fibroblast growth factor-2 cross-talk in angiogenesis. J Immunol 171:1085–1093

Leek RD, Lewis CE, Whitehouse R et al (1996) Association of macrophage infiltration with breast carcinoma. Cancer Res 56:4625–4629

Leek RD, Landers RJ, Harris AL et al (1999) Necrosis correlates with high vascular density and focal macrophage infiltration in invasive carcinoma of the breast. Br J Cancer 79:991–995

Lewis CE, Leek R, Harris A et al (1995) Cytokine regulation of angiogenesis in breast cancer: the role of tumor-associated macrophages. J Leukoc Biol 57:747–751

Lin EY, Nguyen AV, Russel RG et al (2001) Colony-stimulating factor 1 promotes progression of mammary tumors to malignancy. J Exp Med 193:727–740

Lin EY, Li JF, Gnatovskiy L et al (2006) Macrophages regulate the angiogenic switch in a mouse model of breast cancer. Cancer Res 66:11238–11246

Lin EY, Li JF, Bricard G et al (2007) Vascular endothelial growth factor restores delayed tumor progression in tumors depleted of macrophages. Mol Oncol 1:288–302

Lissbrant IF, Stattin P, Wikstrom P et al (2000) Tumor associated macrophages in human prostate cancer: relation to clinicopathological variables and survival. Int J Oncol 17:445–451

Makitie T, Summanen P, Takkanen A et al (2001) Tumor-infiltrating macrophages (CD68+ cells) and prognosis in malignant uveal melanoma. Invest Ophtalmol Vis Sci 42:1414–1421

Mangieri D, Nico B, Benagiano V et al (2008) Angiogenic activity of multiple myeloma endothelial cells in vivo in the chick embryo chorioallantoic membrane assay is associated to a down-regulation in the expression of endogenous endostatin. J Cell Mol Med 12:1023–1028

Manthey CL, Johnson DL, Illig CR et al (2009) JNI-28312141, a novel orally active colony-stimulating factor-1 receptor/FMS-related receptor tyrosine kinase-3 receptor tyrosine kinase inhibitor with potential utility in solid tumors, bone metastases, and acute myeloid leukemia. Mol Cancer Ther 8:3151–3161

Mantovani A, Sozzani S, Locati M (2002) Macrophage polarization: tumor associated macrophages as a paradigm for polarized M2 mononuclear phagocytes. Trends Immunol 23:549–555

Mazzieri R, Pucci F, Moi D et al (2008) Targeting the ANG2/TIE2 axis inhibits tumor growth and metastasis by impairing angiogenesis and disabling rebounds of proangiogenic myeloid cells. Cancer Cell 14:299–311

Metcalfe DD, Baram D, Mekori YA (1997) Mast cells. Physiol Rev 77:1033–1079

Molica S, Vacca A, Crivellato E et al (2003) Tryptase-positive mast cells predict clinical outcome of patients with B-cell chronic lymphocytic leukemia. Eur J Haematol 71:137–139

Moller A, Lippert U, Lessmann D et al (1993) Human mast cells produce IL-8. J Immunol 151:3261–3266

Movahedi K, Laoui D, Gysemans C et al (2010) Different tumor microenvironments contain functionally distinct subsets of macrophages derived from Ly6C(high) monocytes. Cancer Res 70:5728–5739

Nakao S, Kuwano T, Tsutsumi-Miyahara C et al (2005) Infiltration of COX-2-expressing macrophages is a prerequisite for IL-1beta-induced neovascularization and tumor growth. J Clin Inves 115:2979–2991

Nakayama T, Yao L, Tosato G (2004) Mast cell derived angiopoietin-1 plays a role in the growth of plasma cell tumors. J Clin Invest 114:1317–1325

Naldini A, Carraro F (2005) Role of inflammatory mediators in angiogenesis. Curr Drug Targets Inflamm Allergy 4:3–8

Naldini A, Leali D, Pucci A et al (2006) Cutting edge: IL-1beta mediates the proangiogenic activity of osteopontin-activated human monocytes. J Immunol 177:4267–4270

Nico B, Mangieri D, Crivellato E et al (2008) Mast cells contribute to vasculogenic mimicry in multiple myeloma. Stem Cells Dev 17:19–22

Nishie A, Ono M, Shono T et al (1999) Macrophage infiltration and heme oxygenase-1 expression correlate with angiogenesis in human gliomas. Clin Cancer Res 5:1107–1113

Nilsson G, Forsberg-Nilsson K, Xiang Z et al (1997) Human mast cells express functional TrkA and are a source of nerve growth factor. Eur J Immunol 27:2295–2301

Norrby K, Jakobsson A, Sörbo J (1986) Mast cell-mediated angiogenesis: a novel experimental model using the rat mesentery. Virchows Arch B Cell Pathol Mol Pathol 52:195–206

Norrby K, Jakobsson A, Sörbo J (1989) Mast-cell secretion and angiogenesis, a quantitative study in rats and mice. Virchows Arch B Cell Pathol Mol Pathol 57:251–256

Ohno S, Ohno Y, Suzuki N et al (2004) Correlation of histological localization of tumor-associated macrophages with clinicopathological features in endometrial cancer. Anticancer Res 24:3335–3342

Pittoni P, Tripodo C, Piconese S et al (2011) Mast cell targeting hampers prostate adenocarcinoma development but promotes the occurrence of highly malignant neuroendocrine cancers. Cancer Res 71:5987–5997

Pober JS, Sessa WC (2007) Evolving functions of endothelial cells in inflammation. Nat Rev Immunol 7:803–815

Pucci F, Venneri MA, Biziato D et al (2009) A distinguishing gene signature shared by tumor-infiltrating Tie2-expressing monocytes, blood "resident" monocytes, and embryonic macrophages suggests common functions and developmental relationships. Blood 114:901–914

Qian BZ, Pollard JM (2010) Macrophage diversity enhances tumor progression and metastasis. Cell 141:39–51

Qu Z, Liebler JM, Powers MR et al (1995) Mast cells are a major source of basic fibroblast growth factor in chronic inflammation and cutaneous hemangioma. Am J Pathol 147:564–573

Qu Z, Huang X, Ahmadi P et al (1998a) Synthesis of basic fibroblast growth factor by murine mast cells. Regulation by transforming growth factor beta, tumor necrosis factor alpha, and stem cell factor. Int Arch Allergy Immunol 115:47–54

Qu Z, Kayton RJ, Ahmadi P et al (1998b) Ultrastructural immunolocalization of basic fibroblast growth factor in mast cells secretory granules. Morphological evidence for bfgf release through degranulation. J Histochem Cytochem 46:1119–1128

Reed JA, McNutt NS, Bogdany JK et al (1996) Expression of the mast cell growth factor interleukin-3 in the melanocytic lesions correlates with an increased number of mast cells in the perilesional stroma: implications for melanoma progression. J Cutan Pathol 23:495–505

Ribatti D, Roncali L, Nico B et al (1987) Effects of exogenous heparin on the vasculogenesis of the chorioallantoic membrane. Acta Anat 130:257–263

Ribatti D, Nico B, Vacca A et al (1998) Do mast cells help to induce angiogenesis in B-cell non-Hodgkin's lymphomas? Br J Cancer 77:1900–1906

Ribatti D, Vacca A, Nico B et al (1999) Bone marrow angiogenesis and mast cell density increase simultaneously with progression of human multiple myeloma. Br J Cancer 79:451–455

Ribatti D, Vacca A, Marzullo A et al (2000) Angiogenesis and mast cell density with tryptase activity increase simultaneously with pathological progression in B-cell non-Hodgkin's lymphomas. Int J Cancer 85:171–175

Ribatti D, Crivellato E, Candussio L et al (2001) Mast cells and their secretory granules are angiogenic in the chick embryo chorioallantoic membrane. Clin Exp Allergy 31:602–608

Ribatti D, Polimero G, Vacca A et al (2002) Correlation of bone marrow angiogenesis and mast cells with tryptase activity in myelodysplastic syndromes. Leukemia 16:1680–1684

Ribatti D, Vacca A, Ria R et al (2003a) Neovascularization, expression of basic fibroblast growth factor-2, and mast cells with tryptase activity increase simultaneously with pathological progression in human malignant melanoma. Eur J Cancer 39:666–675

Ribatti D, Molica S, Vacca A et al (2003b) Tryptase-positive mast cells correlate positively with bone marrow angiogenesis in B-cell chronic lymphocytic leukemia. Leukemia 17:1428–1430

Ribatti D, Vacca A, Ria R et al (2003c) Neovascularization, expression of fibroblast growth factor-2, and mast cells with tryptase activity increase simultaneously with pathological progression in human malignant melanoma. Eur J Cancer 39:666–674

Ribatti D, Finato N, Crivellato E et al (2005) Neovascularization and mast cells with tryptase activity increase simultaneously with pathological progression in human endometrial cancer. Am J Obstet Gynecol 193:1961–1965

Ribatti D, Nico B, Vacca A (2006) Importance of the bone marrow microenvironment in inducing the angiogenic response in multiple myeloma. Oncogene 25:4257–4266

Ribatti D, Crivellato E (2009) The controversial role of mast cells in tumor growth. Int Rev Cell Mol Biol 275:89–131

Ribatti D, Crivellato E (2012) Mast cells, angiogenesis, and tumor growth. Biochim Biophys Acta Mol Basis Dis 1822:2–8

Rojas IG, Spencer ML, Martinez A et al (2005) Characterization of mast cell subpopulations in lip cancer. J Oral Pathol Med 34:268–273

Romagnani P, Annunziato F, Lasagni L et al (2001) Cell cycle-dependent expression of CXC chemokine receptor 3 by endothelial cells mediates angiostatic activity. J Clin Invest 107:53–63

Sawatsubashi M, Yamada T, Fukushima N et al (2000) Association of vascular endothelial growth factor and mast cells with angiogenesis in laryngeal squamous cell carcinoma. Virchows Arch B Cell Pathol Mol Pathol 436:243–248

Scavelli C, Nico B, Cirulli T et al (2008) Vasculogenic mimicry by bone marrow macrophages in patient with multiple myeloma. Oncogene 27:663–674

Sica A, Schioppa T, Mantovani A et al (2006) Tumour-associated macrophages are a distinct M2 polarised population promoting tumour progression: potential target sof anti-cancer therapy. Eur J Cancer 42:717–727

Sörbo J, Jakobbson A, Norrby K (1994) Mast cell histamine is angiogenic through receptors for histamine 1 and histamine 2. Int J Exp Pathol 75:43–50

Soucek L, Lawlor ER, Soto D et al (2007) Mast cells are required for angiogenesis and macroscopic expansion of Myc-induced pancreatic islet tumors. Nat Med 13:1211–1218

Starkey JR, Crowle PK, Taubenberger S (1988) Mast cell-deficient W/Wv mice exhibit a decreased rate of tumor angiogenesis. Int J Cancer 42:48–52

Stockmann C, Doedens A, Weidemann A et al (2008) Deletion of vascular endothelial growth factor in myeloid cells accelerates tumorigenesis. Nature 456:814–818

Takanami I, Takeuchi K, Naruke M (2000) Mast cell density is associated with angiogenesis and poor prognosis in pulmonary adenocarcinoma. Cancer 88:2686–2692

Talmadge JE, Donkor M, Scholar E (2007) Inflammatory cell infiltration of tumors: Jekyll or Hyde. Cancer Met Rev 26:373–400

Theoharides TC, Conti P (2004) Mast cells: the Jekyll and Hyde of tumor growth. Trends Immunol 25:235–241

Tomita M, Matsuzaki Y, Onitsuka T (2000) Effect of mast cells on tumor angiogenesis in lung cancer. Ann Thorac Surg 69:1686–1689

Tóth-Jakatics R, Jimi S, Takebayashi S et al (2000) Cutaneous malignant melanoma: correlation between neovascularization and peritumoral accumulation of mast cells overexpressing vascular endothelial growth factor. Human Pathol 31:955–960

Ullrich SE, Nghiem DX, Khaskina P (2007) Suppression of an established immune response by UVA-a critical role for mast cells. Photochem Photobiol 83:1095–1100

Vacca A, Ribatti D (2006) Bone marrow angiogenesis in multiple myeloma. Leukemia 20:193–199

Vacca A, Ribatti D, Presta M et al (1999) Bone marrow neovascularization, plasma cell angiogenic potential and matrix metalloproteinase-2 secretion parallel progression of human multiple myeloma. Blood 93:3064–3073

Vacca A, Semeraro F, Merchionne F et al (2003) Endothelial cells in the bone marrow of patients with multiple myeloma. Blood 102:3340–3348

Walsh LJ, Trinchieri G, Waldorf HA et al (1991) Human dermal mast cells contain and release tumor necrosis factor alpha, which induces endothelial leukocyte adhesion molecule 1. Proc Natl Acad Sci USA 88:4220–4224

Wanachantatak S (2003) Increase of mast cells and tumor angiogenesis in oral squamous cell carcinoma. J Oral Pathol Med 23:195–199

Zeisberger SM, Odermatt B, Marty C et al (2006) Clodronate-liposome-mediated depletion of tumour-associated macrophages: a new high and highly effective antiangiogenic therapy approach. Br J Cancer 95:272–281

Chapter 15
The Role of Inflammation in Cervical Cancer

S. Deivendran, K Hezlin Marzook and M. Radhakrishna Pillai

Abstract Knowledge regarding cervical cancer and human papillomavirus is expanding rapidly. Inflammation subsequent to viral infection is a driving force that accelerates cancer development. The infiltrated immune cells and their secretory cytokines along with chemokines and growth factors greatly contribute the malignant traits of cervical cancer. A better understanding of the mechanisms related to inflammation and cancer progression in terms of pathogen survival, cancer development, progression, and metastasis will lead to innovative approach for treating cancer.

15.1 Introduction: Incidence, Survival, Major Gene Products, and Current Therapies for Cervical Cancer

15.1.1 Cervical Cancer Incidence—Worldwide

Cancer is the major health problem and accounts for 14 % of the death worldwide. Cervical cancer is the seventh most common cancer (including both sexes) and accounts for about 4.2 % of the total cancers. It is also third most common among the women and occupies 13 % of female cancer, which is next only to breast cancer. More than 85 % of the cases of cervical cancer are present in the developing countries. Incidence of cervical cancer is highest in Eastern, Western, Southern Africa, and in south-central Asia. Incidence is lowest in Western Asia, Northern America, Australia, and New Zealand, and Western Asia. Cervical cancer remains

S. Deivendran · K. H. Marzook · M. Radhakrishna Pillai (✉)
Cancer Research Program, Rajiv Gandhi Centre for Biotechnology,
Thiruvananthapuram, India
e-mail: mrpillai@rgcb.res.in

B. B. Aggarwal et al. (eds.), *Inflammation and Cancer*, Advances in Experimental Medicine and Biology 816, DOI: 10.1007/978-3-0348-0837-8_15, © Springer Basel 2014

the most common cancer among women only in Eastern Africa, south-central Asia, and Melanesia. Cervical cancer is also the fourth most common cancer causing death next to breast, lung, and colorectal cancer. About 9 % of cancerous people are diagnosed with cervical cancer.

Cervical cancer incidence varied between regions ranging from 5 per 100,000 in Western Asia to 35 per 100,000 in Eastern Africa in 2008. Highest incidence rates were 56 and 53 per 100,000, respectively, in Guinea and Zambia. The UK was 145th highest out of 184 countries worldwide. Cervical cancer is more prevalent in countries where Human Developmental Index is low. Cervical cancer is the second most prevalent cancer in females (present in 37 countries in South and Central America, Southern Africa, and Asia) (Ferlay et al. 2010b).

It was estimated that cervical cancer leads to 275,000 deaths worldwide in 2008, accounting for 8.2 % of all female cancer deaths (3.6 % of the total in men and women). Cervical cancer is the tenth leading cancer in developed countries (76,500 cases), and it shifts to second in case of developing countries (453,300). It also ranks second (242,000) in causing mortality in developing countries which is closely next to breast cancer (268,900 cases). Incidence of cervical cancer is 9.0 % in developed countries, and it rises to 17.8 % in developing countries. Mortality rate is 3.2 % in developed countries, and it increases to threefold in developing countries (9.8 %). Mortality rates were less than 2 per 100,000 in Australia/New Zealand and Northern America and 25 per 100,000 in Eastern Africa in 2008.

15.1.1.1 Cervical Cancer Incidence in Europe

In Europe, the overall incidence rate of cervical cancer is 10.6 per 100,000. Europe continent is diverse, and incidence of cervical cancer varies from region to region. Incidence of cervical cancer in Western Europe is low (6.9/100,000), and it increases to twofold in Central/Eastern Europe. Incidence in Northern Europe and Southern Europe is almost similar with rate of 8.4/100,000 and 8.1/100,000, respectively. Incidence is highest in Romania (23.9/100,000) and lowest in Malta (2.1/100,000). Eastern Europe has increased 4–5 times risk of developing cervical cancer when compared to western countries. The incidence of cervical cancer in some countries in eastern part of Europe is 20 per 100,000. Incidence in Europe has not changed, and it remains almost the same for the past few years (11.05 per 100,000 in 2002; 10.06 per 100,000 in 2008). For the past 10 years, the incidence of cervical cancer in eastern European countries continues to increase. In Europe, mortality due to cervical cancer decreased around 10 % from 5.0 per 100,000 to 4.5 per 100,000 (during the period 2002–2008) (Ferlay et al. 2010a).

15.1.1.2 Cervical Cancer Incidence in Asia–Oceania Region

Asia–Oceania region carries around 50 % burden of cervical cancer worldwide. Every year around 315,000 persons are diagnosed with cervical cancer, and incidence rate is 15.2 per 100,000. Among the region, incidence is higher in Nepal (32 per 100,000), followed by Mongolia (28.4 per 100,000) and India (27 per 100,000). Incidence of cervical cancer is second highest in Asia–Oceania region where the list is headed by breast cancer. Incidence is lowest in Australia, Singapore, and Hong Kong. Mortality rate is around 7.9 per 100,000 in Asia–Oceania region. Every year around 160,000 women dies because of cervical cancer. Mortality rate is highest in Nepal, Papua New Guinea, and India, and lowest in Japan and Australia. Though the incidence of cervical cancer is second highest in Asia–Oceania region, in mortality, it ranks fourth (Garland et al. 2012).

15.1.1.3 Cervical Cancer Incidence in Africa

15.2 % of total cervical cancer burden is from Africa. The incidence of cervical cancer varies from region to region. Incidence is high in Southern and Eastern Africa (40 per 100,000). Incidence is high among Lesotho and Swaziland. Mortality due to cervical cancer in Africa is 19.4 %.

15.1.1.4 Cervical Cancer Incidence in England

Incidence of cervical cancer decreased to one-third from 15.0 to 9.8 (per 100,000 female populations) over the 20 years. United Kingdom has lower mortality rate and ranked 157th among 184 countries worldwide. Mortality rates were higher in the less developed regions of the world. It has been estimated that cervical cancer contributes over 2.7 million years of life lost among women dying between the ages of 25 and 64 years worldwide, some 2.4 million of which occur in the developing countries and only 0.3 million in the developed countries.

15.1.2 Cervical Cancer Survival

In USA, one-year survival rate of cervical patient is 87 %. Five-year survival rate for all stages in cervical cancer is 68 %. Invasive cervical cancer, when detected at early stage, can be successfully treated. In USA, the five-year relative survival rate (measure of survival of cancer patients in comparison with the general population) is 91 % and the rate decreases to 17 % when detected at a later stage. Cancer survival rate varies across the countries. Europe, North America, Australia, and New Zealand have higher survival rate for cervical cancer. Survival data from African, Asian, Caribbean, and Central American countries showed wide variation. Survival rate was lower in Uganda (19 %) and Gambia (23 %), whereas it is higher in Seoul, South Korea (76 %), and Hong Kong (77 %). Survival rate also varied drastically within the countries like India, where the 5-year survival rate for women in Bhopal is 31 % and Chennai is 60 %. Lower cancer survival and higher mortality in the developing countries is attributed to lack of screening facilities. In Singapore, around 81 % of cervical cancer patients are diagnosed at the earlier stages, whereas in Chennai, India, it is only 7 %, similarly with the countries Costa Rica (33 %), Manila, Philippines (35 %), and Cuba (53 %). Survival rate is higher in Singapore when compared to other countries like USA. In China, Singapore, South Korea, and Turkey, the median relative survival for cervical cancer is 63–79 %. One-, three-, and five-year survival in invasive cervix cancer is 83, 61, and 54 %, respectively in Costa Rica (Sankaranarayanan 2011; Coleman et al. 2008).

15.1.3 Major Inflammatory Gene Products in Cervical Cancer

Inflammation is termed as the seventh hall mark of cancer, and chronic inflammation is involved in cellular transformation, survival, proliferation, invasion, and metastasis. Inflammation process involves tissue-remodeling events brought about by alterations to epithelial, vascular, and immune cell function. These events occur by the involvement of cytokines, chemokines, growth factors, and lipid mediators, and also by the activation of transcription factors such as nuclear factor-κB, STAT3, and HIF-1.

15.1.3.1 HPV Infection and Cervical Cancer

Among the identified and categorized HPV's, twelve HPVs namely 16, 18, 31, 33, 35, 39, 45, 51, 52, 56, 58, and 59 are defined as high risk by the World Health Organization (WHO) along with types 68, 73 being as 'possibly' cancer causing. HPV16 and HPV18 are found closely associated with high chances of cervical cancer. Within the consolidated 8 early viral genes (E1–E8), E6 and E7 hold a lead role in driving the HPV infection in the way to cancer. Recently, E5 is also added to the same group considering its expression as a boon for the tumor progression in HPV-infected conditions. Functional differences between high-risk type E6 and E7 with low-risk type accounts for the potential of these viruses to be carcinogenic. After infection, HPV amplifies the HPV E1/L1 genes through its *tat* protein which leads to the viral replication and release of virions. Viral E6 protein binds to p53 and degrades by ubiquitination. E7 protein binds to Rb protein and disrupts the Rb/E2F complex leading to the increase in production of nitric oxide (NO), DNA damage and the activation of the cyclooxygenase 2 (COX-2)/prostaglandin (PG)/PG G receptor inflammatory pathways leading to increased inflammation and tumorigenesis.

15.1.3.2 Inflammatory Molecules in Cervical Cancer

The inflammatory molecules involved in the inflammation-mediated cervical cancers are reactive oxygen species (ROS), tumor necrosis factor-α (TNF-α), interleukin-1 (IL-1), interleukin-6 (IL-6), interleukin-8 (IL-8), interleukin-18 (IL-18), hypoxia-inducing factor (HIF), cyclooxygenase (COX), inducible nitric oxide synthase (iNOS), matrix metalloproteinase-9 (MMP9), and chemokines.

Cyclooxygenase-Prostaglandin Pathway

Cyclooxygenase-prostaglandin (COX-PG) pathway is a major pathway involved in the inflammation of cervical cancer. COX-1 and COX-2 are involved in the process. COX catalyzes the formation of prostaglandins from arachidonic acid through the formation of unstable intermediate PGH2, which in turn is converted by terminal PG synthase enzymes to specific classes of prostaglandins. These prostaglandins can promote metastasis and angiogenesis, and increases the cell proliferation. COX-1 is expressed in normal tissues and catalyzes the formation of prostaglandins from normal physiological functions. COX-2 is absent in normal tissues, and it is induced by inflammatory cytokines, growth factors, and oncogenes. In HPV, 16 E6 and E7 expressing cancer cells, the mRNA, and protein levels of prostaglandin E2 (PGE2) and COX-2 were higher when compared to HPV-negative cell line. So HPV16 stimulates the transcription of COX. After HPV infection and integration into the cervical cancer cells, they increases the expression of COX-2, increases the biosynthesis of PGE2 and E-series prostanoid G protein-coupled receptors (PTGER) expression. These PGE2 regulates the tumor functions through PTGER.

Hypoxia-Inducing Factors

Normally in tissues, oxygen levels are maintained by the homeostatic mechanisms at cellular, organ, and system levels. Percentage of oxygen ranges from 22.5 to 9 % in normal tissues. Under inflamed conditions, the oxygen levels will be decreased to less than 1 % due to large number of infiltrating cells. Inflammatory cytokines and growth factors induce the HIFs. These HIFs are also induced by pro-inflammatory cytokines such as TNF-α and IL-1β. HIF is a heterodimer with oxygen-regulated α subunit and constitutively expressing β subunit, belonging to basic helix-loop-helix/PAS transcription factor family member and HIF-1α with three isoforms. The abundance of HIF1α is regulated by prolyl hydroxylases PHD1, PHD2, and PHD3. In the presence of oxygen, oxygen-dependent degradation (ODD) domain of HIF-1α is hydroxylated. Once HIF is hydroxylated, the von Hippel–Lindau (pVHL) tumor suppressor protein binds to α-subunit and tags them for ubiquitination and proteasomal degradation. In the presence of hypoxia, activity of PHD decreases leading to the stabilization of HIF-1α, which tranlocates to the nucleus and induces the transcription of target genes through hypoxia responsible elements (HREs).

Inflammatory Cytokines

TNF-α, a cytokine plays a major role in the inflammation process. It triggers other inflammatory mediators and proteases involved in the process. It can promote tumorigenesis and plays a major role in cellular transformation, promotion, survival, proliferation, invasion, angiogenesis, and metastasis. In cervical cells, it induces amphiregulin which in turn plays a major role in proliferation. It stimulates the proliferation in immortal cervical cells along with the IL-1α. Interleukins (IL) (namely IL-1, IL-6, IL-8, and IL-18) are involved in the inflammation process. IL-1α promotes the proliferation of cervical cancer cells. IL-1 and IL-6 are involved in the cell growth, metastasis, and tumor development.

15.1.4 Current Therapy for Cervical Cancer

Cervical cancer is treated according to the stages classified by Féderation Internationale de Gynécologieetd'Obstétrique (FIGO). The classification is based on tumor size, vaginal or parametrial involvement, bladder/rectum extension, and distant metastases. Cervical cancer treatment consists of surgery, radiotherapy, or a combination of radiotherapy and chemotherapy.

Stage IA1: Conization (removal of cone-shaped or cylindrical piece of tissue from the cervix and cervical canal) is done to those who wish to preserve their fertility. In the early stage 1A1, extrafascial hysterectomy (removal of cervix and uterus), modified radical trachelectomy (removal of cervix and adjacent tissues), or hysterectomy with pelvic node dissection is recommended. In the presence of lymphovascular space involvement (LVSI), lymphadenectomy (removal of lymph nodes) is done.

Stage 1A2: Stage 1A2 is treated by conization. If LVSI is present, pelvic lymphadenectomy is done with radical trachelectomy or radical hysterectomy. Brachytherapy is also done in patients with surgical contraindications.

Stages IB1 to IIA1: Radial surgery including pelvic lymphadenectomy or radiotherapy is done for stages IB1 to IIA1. Generally, chemotherapy is done for the patients in stages IB1 to IIA1. For lymph node-positive cases, chemotherapy is done. Brachytherapy with or without cisplatin-based chemotherapy is given to patients with stage IB or IIA

Stages IB2 to IVA: Chemoradiation is done for treating the patients in stages from IB2 to IVA. In locally advanced cervical cancer, radiotherapy controls around 88–95 % for stage IB, 70–80 % for stage IIB, and 30–40 % for stage III, and 5-year survival >80 % for stage IB, 65 % for stage IIB, and 40 % for stage III.

Stages IIB to IVA is considered as advanced stages, and the treatment includes chemoradiation and brachytherapy. Chemoradiation therapy includes the administration of cisplatin along with weekly once radiation therapy (minimum 4 cycles; maximum 6 cycles). Sometimes 5-FluroUracil is also administered on days 2–5.

Stage IVB: Cisplatin-based chemotherapy is given to stage IVB patients. Individualized radiation therapy is also performed. Paclitaxel combined with cisplatin or topotecan with cisplatin or paclitaxel is given for stage IV recurrent or metastatic disease. Drugs bevacizumab, docetaxel, gemcitabine, ifosfamide, 5-FU, mitomycin, irinotecan, and topotecan are also given as a second-line therapy for stage IV recurrent or metastatic disease (Colombo et al. 2012).

15.2 Inflammatory Signaling Pathways Associated with Cervical Cancer

Inflammation is regarded as the seventh hallmark of cancer. Unlike the basic function of inflammation as in wound healing to destroy the infectious agents, during cancer, inflammation persists to acquire a chronic condition and fails to undergo healing process leading to a persistent infection. Occurrence of chronic inflammation is accompanied by release if certain agents from the immune response cell that will support the better thriving of the pathogen in the host organism. This enhances the betterment in incorporation of carcinogenic genetic material by the virus to the host machinery. During an HPV infection, the inflammatory signaling pathways mainly include pro-inflammatory cytokine pathway, interferon pathway, TNF-α pathway, NF-κB, and COX-2 in order to link inflammation with carcinogenesis. Thus, the key features of inflammation during a carcinogenesis may include the infiltration of white blood cells, prominently tumor-associated macrophages (TAMs); the presence of polypeptide messengers of inflammation [cytokines such as TNF, IL-1, and IL-6, chemokines such as CCL2 and CXCL8, and the occurrence of tissue remodeling and angiogenesis] (Colotta et al. 2009). A better understanding of inflammation and tumor microenvironment is crucial for the development of new therapeutic strategies based on the nature of tumor development, progression, and metastasis.

15.3 Role of Inflammatory Molecules in the Development of Cervical Cancer: Evidences from In Vitro Studies

Infectious agents have become a common cause for the development of tumor-associated inflammation which triggers the inflammatory molecules in the microenvironment to drive the persistence of tumor and therefore its progress. In majority of the HPV infections, eradication of neoplastic lesions occurs in the initial stages, failure of which may impart the ability for HPV to evade the immune barriers and integrate into the host genome. This whole process ultimately results in a complex role for inflammation to occur during an HPV infection. The main transmission of HPV pathogen to a cervix is via an infected partner's semen during coitus after which the virus resides in the epidermal mucosa with a total cut-off from the connective tissue and paves the way to hide itself from host immune system. Within this period, the virus attains the potential to induce mechanisms to evade the host immune system by deregulating various pathways involving pattern recognition receptor namely the toll-like receptor (TLR)-9 by the host. Mere infection is incapable of inducing tumorigenesis in cervix. Under such instances, oxidative stress induces the pathogen to drive the cell to attain oncogenic property. Oxidative stress modifies the DNA and protein of the cell to provide a platform for neoplastic development and its progress. This condition is further enhanced by iNOS overexpression whose function is further induced by other inflammatory molecules like TNF-α, IL-1β, and NF-κB (De Marco et al. 2012). Infection with HPV may be cofactored by the resident *Chlamydia trachomatis* or *Neisseria gonorrhoeae,* tobacco carcinogens and weak immune system which ultimately leads to inflammation to generate cascade of complex networks involving cytokines, chemokines, IL, growth factors, and prostaglandins. Inflammation initiated by theses cascade networks compels to alter the host immune function along with changes in the epithelial and the vascular nature of the tissue.

Once a pathogen attacks a system, it implies several mechanisms to sustain and multiply. Among such is the inhibition of interferon-stimulated genes (ISG), which will ultimately reduce the pathogen recognition receptors (PRR); the so-called TLR3, RIG-I, and MDA5. This may be directly correlated with the reduced levels of IFNβ, IFNλ, and CCL20, further ensuring the minimized expression of inducible IFN possessing antiviral property such as IFIT1 and MX1 (Reiser et al. 2011). Reports from same laboratory has also shown a reduced CCL20 expression when cell lines were established by immortalization with complete HPV genomes. This may indicate that CCL20 expression is prevented both by reducing PRR levels and by interference at the transcriptional level by HPV. HPV-positive cervical cells also exhibited an inhibition in the constitutive expression of IFNκ (DeCarlo et al. 2010). This inhibition may be one of the causes for the inhibition of ISG in human cervical cancer cells. Recent reports came up with the fact that DNA methylation on the interferon; the IFNκ promoter can regulate the expression of IFNκ gene which may be influenced by the viral proteins. This study was further supported by an observation in HeLa cells where they emphasizes that IFNκ expression is extremely down which can be reverted by DNA methyltransferase inhibitors such as 5-aza-dC (Rincon-Orozco et al. 2009). In this way, the hurdle of IFNκ is managed by the HPV genes such that pathogen acquires more power and support for its growth and survival using the host machineries.

15.3.1 Role of Inflammatory Molecules in the Transformation of Cervical Cancer Cells

Immunosuppressed victims of HPV are more prone to the persistence of infection and develop a high-risk HPV-related cancers. On the onset of infection, release of inflammatory molecules including cytokines occurs at the site of infection from the keratinocytes; the process even more supported by macrophages and NK cells. Role of anti-inflammatory molecules comes into act then, where TNF-α, IL-1, and IFNα/β inhibit transcription of viral oncogenes which was evident from various in vitro studies. Despite all these, certain proportion of infection are capable of establishing infection leading to chronic inflammation.

Activation of interferon pathway is a common response during a viral infection. Interferons are antiviral particles which can induce resistance to viral genome replication in the infected host cell. Initiation of IFN pathways occurs by binding of type I (IFNα/β) and type II (IFNγ) to the specific cell receptors which in turn induces the transcription of IFN-induced genes via JAK-STAT pathway (Chang and Laimins 2000). High-risk E6 and E7 proteins repress the STAT1 expression, which will inhibit its regulatory function on IFN response. It is also found that high-risk E6 and E7 proteins downregulates type 1 IFN expression and absence of influencing signals by these IFN during the process of antigen recognition leads to immune tolerance than expected immune responses (Sasagawa et al. 2012). In vitro studies in support of these observation lead to clinical trials of IFN to accomplish the eradication of viral infection on the onset of the disease. Treatment of type I IFN to cells transfected with HPV31 episomes shows a loss of viral episomes. This property of IFN is attributed to its clinical trials, but later on reports indicated to explain the fact that HPV had gained resistance to overcome the IFN therapy. It is now concluded that IFN response by HPV varies on the type of IFN and also on the type of HPV infected and also cell specificity. Recent reports came up with HPV16 oncoproteins E6 and E7 influencing the interferon pathway. E7 oncoprotein physically interacts with the transcription factor and interferon regulatory factor (IRF) 1, and hinders the binding of IRF1 on the IFNβ promoter, thus inhibiting the transactivating function. This inhibition hinders the heterodimerization of STAT1-STAT2, thus affecting the translocation to nucleus (Park et al. 2000). Likewise, E6 oncoprotein interacts with IRF3 and repress the transactivating function of IFNβ promoter by recruiting HDAC onto the promoter (Ronco et al. 1998). Rincon-Orozco et al. (2009) came up with the regulatory aspects of IFNκ by HPV16 E6 oncoprotein. Clinical sample revealed the information that IFNκ was downregulated in cervical patients compared to that of normal ones. This phenomenon was emphasized with the epigenetic silencing of IFNκ by E6 protein.

Despite the antiviral properties of interferon, there are contradictory reports regarding IFNβ. It is in limelight now that IFNβ facilitates the transcription of HPV16 by promoting the binding of IRF1 to the viral promoters. Interferon also plays a crucial role in proliferation. In vitro studies in HeLa cell lines, an HPV18 cervical cell line is shown to proliferate with the induction of IFNα2b. Evidences from certain studies confirm that IFN-β is able to induce replication of HPV11, HPV16, and HPV31 in human keratinocytes. Moreover, on continual IFN-β treatments, it is reported that cells expressing high-risk type cutaneous HPV38 undergo senescence by the induced expression of the tumor suppressor PML, known to be downstream effector of IFN (Chiantore et al. 2012).

Cytokine production is a remarkable property of viral-induced human cancers. As primary site of HPV infection, the keratinocytes are the immediate source of cytokine. IL and TNF mainly contribute to this aspect. TNF has a definitive role on any inflammation caused due to infection. Basically, TNFs are majorly involved in the regulation of inflammation by binding to its cell-specific TNF receptors (TNFR1 or TNFR2) in order to elicit signaling pathways against a viral infection, induce apoptosis, growth arrest, or aid in cell proliferation. TNF-α plays as a growth stimulator for epidermal growth factor (EGF) or serum-depleted cervical cancer cells (Gaiotti et al. 2000). TNF-α acts as a potent keratinocyte inhibitor during the course of viral entry and onset of inflammation and elicit extrinsic apoptotic pathway (Basile et al. 2001). Extrinsic pathway is initiated by the binding of these cytokines to receptors mainly TNFR1 or TRAIL. It is reported that E6 high-risk type proteins can bind on these TNFR1 or TRAIL and inhibit the downstream pathways (Filippova et al. 2002). More often, it is also found that E6 protein binds on to FADD and caspase8, thus blocking the FAS-mobilized apoptotic response (Filippova et al. 2004; Garnett et al. 2006). In response to intrinsic pathway, E6 plays a crucial role by interacting with Bax and Bak proteins of Bcl2 family of pro-apoptotic proteins, which induces the upregulation of IAP and survivin (Garnett and Duerksen-Hughes 2006). Thus, literature based on TNF gives out the point that they are responsible for growth arrest in an HPV-infected keratinocyte. TNF activates NF-κB pathway to upregulate the expression of $p21^{CIP1/WAF1}$, which is a well-known cyclin-dependent kinase (Cdk) inhibitor. Moreover, TNF is also having a critical function in downregulating certain cell cycle proteins such as cyclinA, cyclinB, cdc2, and so on.

Polymorphism in inflammatory genes has become a common report, and it stands as a potential therapeutic biomarker in cervical carcinomas. Polymorphism detected in an anti-inflammatory gene IL-10 can lead to its underexpression, thus allowing the cancer progression. PCR–RFLP-assay-based cohort studies implicated the potential effect of SNP on TNF-α-238 G/A in reducing the risk of cervical cancer, whereas the multifunctional cytokine IL-10 is not, the polymorphism of which are highly associated with the risk of cervical cancer (Barbisan et al. 2012).

15.3.2 Role of Inflammatory Molecules in the Survival of Cervical Cancer Cells

Persistence of HPV related to age old cervical cancer shows circulating inflammatory cytokines, namely TNF-α and also IL-8 (Kemp et al. 2010). An increasing levels of resistin and Fas was noted in such a condition where an increased levels of resistin, an adipokine, and sFas is observed in HPV-infected older women with decreased immune function (Baker et al. 2011). Complexing of E7 with Rb leaves a compliment by increasing the level of p53, a tumor suppressor gene, which happens to be the intrinsic mechanism of the cell to undergo apoptosis. To protect this adverse situation the viral particle, E6 comes into play which aids in the proteasomal degradation of p53 by recruiting E6AP (E6-associated protein), a HECT domain containing E3 ubiquitin ligase (Huibregtse et al. 1991). In response to IFN stimulus, p53 gains antiproliferative function which is highly tackled by high-risk HPV proteins. Senescence is promoted in HPV16-expressing keratinocytes which is mediated by acetylated p53.

Among the different strategies used by viruses in its survival, a colorful role is engraved by the expression of class I MHC. HPV nonstructural viral proteins like E5 protein have been shown to interact with several cellular processes in order to impair the antigen presenting function of MHC class I expression, thereby suppressing the Th1 pathway to reduce the functional role of IFNγ. It is evident that overexpression of HPV E5 attenuates MHC class I molecules to sequester itself to the Golgi apparatus (Ashrafi et al. 2005). The viral protein, E7, may block the ability of interferon-γ (IFN-γ) to induce IRF-1 expression, in turn inhibiting the expression of downstream genes related to MHC class I antigen processing and presentation. Recent study by Zhou et al. (2011) demonstrated that expression of HPV16 E7 as a transgene product in epithelial cells does not directly impair, but rather slightly increases MHC class I expression.

Direct role of inflammation to survival is evident from the participation of NF-κB by bypassing apoptotic mechanism. NF-κB activation induces several pro-inflammatory cytokines which are prominent in supporting the progression of HPV-induced cancer (Karin 2006). In cervical cancer cell lines, a constitutive activation of NF-κB was studied which is usually seen to be accompanied with p50 and p65, the heterodimeric complex of RelA family of proteins in the nucleus during the course of tumor progression. NF-κB acts in targeting apoptosis, cell cycle, and cell adhesion in the stage of neoplasia. NF-κB competes with p53 for common transcriptional co-activators such as p300 and CBP (Okamoto et al. 2007) and also for the binding to p21 promoter (Ma et al. 2008). Effect of E6 proteins comes in act by degrading p53 via a tripartite complex formation with p53 along with the acetylating agent p300, thus hindering the acetylating property of p53 and suppression in the activation of p53-inducible genes for senescence (Patel et al. 1999). Unlike the high-risk types, low-risk E6 can directly interact with p53 which is an outstanding feature for survival mechanism in low-risk types.

From the development of macrophages from monocytes, there exist severe conditions of hypoxia which is very evident in tumor microenvironment. At this point, there is an upregulation of HIF1α which plays a crucial role in the survival of cells during hypoxia. HIF1α is expressed immensely in the inflammation site leading to support the survival by regulating several angiogenic genes like VEGF. Moreover, studies show that in cervical cancer cell lines, HPV E7 enhances HIF1α regulating the transcription activation of various pro-angiogenic genes by inhibiting HDAC activity (Bodily et al. 2011). Thus, we can see that HPV protein is facilitating the existing microenvironment rendering it favorable for its own survival and proliferation through their epigenetic control.

15.3.3 Role of Inflammatory Molecules in the Proliferation of Cervical Cancer Cells

Chromosomal instability, an abnormal segregation of chromosomes leading to aneuploidy is a common event in HPV-related cancers. Molecular mechanism behind this is incompletely described though many postulates and evidences have come into existence. Inactivation of p53 is the hallmark in creating chromosomal instability, the reason for which is numerous. One of the reasons for chromosomal instability for p53 inactivation is pro-inflammatory cytokine migration inhibitory factor suppressing p53 activity as a transcriptional activator (Hudson et al. 1999). Moreover, IL-6 increases the activity of DNA methyltransferase, resulting in CpG island methylation, which is also associated with p53 mutation (Hodge et al. 2005).

Aneuploidy is one of the reasons for malignancies in high-risk HPV tumors and can be detected in pre-malignant HPV lesions (Schiffman et al. 2007). The centrosomal aberrations led by E7 occur as several rounds of centrosome synthesis during the S phase which is a CDK2-dependent program. In vivo studies revealed that E7 can induce similar effects in the absence of Rb interaction (Duensing and Munger 2003) which is the prime necessity of CDK2 expression (Duensing et al. 2006). In normal condition, Rb interacts with E2F1–E2F5 transcription factors out of the total eight member of the E2F family of proteins (Lammens et al. 2009); which possess a domain for pocket proteins. This binding normally regulates the G1-S phase transition in the process of cell cycle where during the termination of G1, Rb is phosphorylated by CDK and is released from E2F which can now function as an independent transcription factor for the S phase proteins. The beauty of this regulation is disrupted by the interaction of E7 with Rb which result in the constitutive expression of cyclinA and cyclinE necessary to drive S phase and early synthesis of DNA occurs henceforth (DeGregori and Johnson 2006).

15.3.4 Role of Inflammatory Molecules in the Invasion, Metastasis, and Angiogenesis of Cervical Cancer Cells

During a persistent infection with HPV, there occurs tissue injury which paves the way for epigenetic alterations and remodeling of epithelial cellular events promoting angiogenesis, invasion, finally leading to metastasis. Angiogenesis, invasion, and metastasis are a complex network underwent by tumor for the well progression and spreading of the own. In such a condition, an overall remodeling occurs causing the degradation of extracellular matrix (ECM), cell migration, proliferation, and also generation of vasculature. Angiogenesis and inflammation are two mutually dependent processes for which inflammatory molecules come in contact with cells such as the endothelial cells, fibroblast cells, and also the ECM to promote angiogenesis. In cancer cells, angiogenesis occurs as an abnormal process where there is an imbalance between pro- and anti-angiogenic factors requiring the activation of several receptors by growth factors coupled with the triggering of inflammation. Attack of an HPV fires inflammation and lead to the production of monocytes. It is noted that there are two types of macrophages produced during such a condition in which one acts as tumor supportive and the other as tumor suppressive. Tumor-supportive macrophages are greatly involved in angiogenesis. These macrophages are often referred as TAMs. TAM produces a cytokine MCP-1, which is an indication of macrophage accumulation at the tumor site, in turn giving a feedback regulation.

IL-1β can induce angiogenesis from a study involving mouse cornea. It is also noticed that there occurs a downregulation of MMP during the silencing of IL-1β. Studies related to immunological parameters by immunohistochemistry and ELISA revealed that expression of Th2 inflammation-promoting cytokine TSLP and of IDO1 was higher in invasive carcinoma compared to the normal. On the other side, expression of IL-10 was higher in cervical carcinoma in situ and invasive cervical cancer (Feng et al. 2012). TLR expressions in cells are associated with tumorigenesis. In cervical intraepithelial neoplasial (CIN1), a key stage in the development of cervical cancer is a decrease in the expression of TLR4 during the progression of cervicalneoplasia which is highly associated with the expression of p16INK4A, a molecule regarded as a biomarker for HPV integration into host cells.

Another major participation in terms of metastasis is shared by STAT3 which is activated by various growth factors, cytokines as well as viral oncoproteins, thus rendering a constitutive expression to lead invasion. High levels of IL-6 induce the activation of STAT3, via facilitating the phosphorylation of STAT3. STAT3 promotes invasion directly by transcriptional activation of MMPs, mainly MMP1, MMP2, and MMP10 (Xie et al. 2004). On the other hand, STAT3 directly interact with focal adhesion kinases and paxillin to promote invasion. Focal adhesion kinase (FAK) is important in regulating cytoskeletal reorganization by the phosphorylation of FAK and activation of paxillin. HPV E6 protein is capable of binding to paxillin, but the downstream process still remains unelucidated (McCormack et al. 1997). HPV-infected cases show high levels of FAK, and E6 is capable of binding to fibulin 1, an ECM protein indicating the process of transformation and tumor invasion (Du et al. 2002).

15.4 Role of Inflammatory Molecules in the Development of Cervical Cancer: Evidences from In Vivo Studies

Even though the direct relationship between HPV and inflammation remains undecided and contrary, experiments in animal model support to the fact that HPV controls inflammatory pathways in the host. Direct evidences exist describing the role of HPV16 early genes expressed under human keratin 14 promoter which facilitate the induction of the chemokine CCL2 from the neoplastic lesion to recruit macrophage in the tumor microenvironment. In the development of cancer COX-2-derived PGE2 has a direct effect on inflammation. HIV1 infection augmented with HPV infection is associated with increased cervical COX-2 and increased systemic PGE2 levels (Fitzgerald et al. 2012). Findings in human cervical epithelial cells of neoplasia explain that late genes of HPV16 namely E6 and E7 upregulate COX-2 activate COX/PG pathways. The expression of pro-inflammatory cytokine interleukin-32 (IL-32) is very evident in high-risk HPV-positive cervical cancer which is mediated by COX-2 stimulation controlled by E7. There also exist an E7 and COX-2 downregulation in the IL-32γ overexpressing cells suggesting a feedback mechanism by IL-32γ on E7 and COX-2 cervical cancer cells (Lee et al. 2011). In a study related to mouse corneal angiogenesis induced by IL-1β, inhibition of COX-2 almost completely attenuated angiogenesis (Kuwano et al. 2004).

IL-17 is a pro-inflammatory cytokine produced by Th17 cells, found to play a main role in inflammation-triggered oncogenesis. This observation is further supported by studies in vivo that IL-17 overexpressing human cervical cancer shows high oncogenic growth and the functional status of IL-17 is determined to be pro-angiogenic (Tartour et al. 1999). Studies in transgenic mice with defective E6 protein ensures that there is no development of potent tumor in these mice models due to mutated PDZ binding domain which is associated with PDZ protein and in turn a direct target of p53. Mutations linked to the mentioned PDZ binding domain of the E6 protein may lead to ultimate loss of function of the protein in terms of pathogen survival.

15.4.1 Evidence from Patients for the Role of Inflammation in Cervical Cancer

15.4.1.1 Polymorphisms Associated with TNF-α

Macrophages secretes (TNF-α), and their role in risk of cervical cancer remains controversial until meta-analysis was performed by Ding et al. where polymorphism status is studied in 2298 cases and 1903 controls. They found that polymorphism in TNF-α-308 G > A is a risk factor for developing cervical cancer in Asians and whites but not in Africans (Ding et al. 2012). Recently, TNF-α polymorphism rs1800629 was studied in Chinese population, which included three groups with Group 1 consisted of 285 high-risk HPV-positive cervical cancer patients, Group 2 with 225 high-risk HPV-positive patients without cervical cancer, and Group 3 with 318 HPV-negative women with no cervical cancer. They found that TNF-α polymorphism rs1800629 has no association with HPV infection or risk of developing cervical cancer (Wang et al. 2012). Polymorphisms TNFA-308G/A (rs1800629) and -238G/A (rs361525) are associated with the increase in risk in cervical cancer. Association of polymorphisms in pro- and anti-inflammatory cytokines (TNF-α, TNFA, and interleukin, IL-10) with cervical cancer was studied in 2009 (Singh et al. 2009). The study included 150 histopathologically confirmed cervical cancer patients and 162 age, ethnically matched cervical cytology-negative controls. They found that polymorphism in TNFA (-308 G > A) is associated with developing cervical cancer stages early (IB) and advanced stages (III). They have also concluded that polymorphism IL-10 (-819 C > T) is not associated with cervical cancer (Singh et al. 2009). Recently, polymorphisms were analyzed in North Indian population for IL-6 and IL-10, and contradictorily, they found that polymorphism IL-4 Rp1/Rp2 and IL-10 (AC) genotype is associated with risk in cervical cancer (Shekari et al. 2012) which supported the previous results where promoter polymorphism in IL-6 promoter, which regulates inflammation has the association with increase in cervical cancer (Gangwar et al. 2009).

15.4.1.2 Polymorphisms Associated with Interleukin-1β

Interleukin-1β (IL-1β), inflammation-induced cytokine, has several single-nucleotide polymorphisms. Polymorphism in lL-1β gene (IL-1β +3953) in association with increase in cervical cancer risk was reported in a study which analyzed 150 women cervical cancer patients and 200 healthy controls. Increased IL-1β is due to SNP, C-511T which is present in the promoter region. The plasma levels of IL-1β were analyzed in 100 histopathologically confirmed Egyptian women with cervical cancer and 50 age-matched, cervical cytology-negative, healthy controls. The study revealed that there is a significant increase in IL-1β concentration in cervical cancer cases carrying C-511T variant genotypes and associated with increase in cervical cancer risk (Al-Tahhan et al. 2011). Similarly, increase in cervical risk in association with IL-1β polymorphism was also reported earlier in Indian population (Singh et al. 2008), whereas in Korean population, IL-1B-511 C/C genotypes is associated with the decrease in risk of cervical cancer (Kang et al. 2007).

Association between polymorphisms in cytokine genes [TNF-α, TGF-β1, IFN-γ, and IL-10] and cervical cancer in Chinese population was studied in 2011. The study included 186 histopathologically confirmed cases of cervical cancer and 200 healthy controls. They found that no significant association was found in TNF-α-308G/A, TGF-β1 codons 10 and 25 C/C-G/G and IL-10-1082G/A gene polymorphisms and except IFN-γ+874A/T polymorphism, which may be associated with developing cervical cancer (Wang et al. 2011).

15.4.1.3 Polymorphisms Associated with Other Inflammatory Genes

Association of cervical cancer risk with the polymorphism in interleukin-12A (IL-12A) and interleukin-12B (IL-12B) was reported in Chinese population, where they have analyzed in 400 patients along with 404 controls (Chen et al. 2009).

Polymorphisms in toll-like receptors-3 (TLR-3) and (TLR-9) were analyzed in North Indian population in samples collected from 200 histopathologically confirmed cervical cancer patients and 200 unrelated, age, ethnicity matched, healthy female controls. There is no association of cervical cancer risk with polymorphisms in TLR-3 (c.1377C/T) [rs3775290] and TLR-9 (G2848A) [rs352140] in north India (Pandey et al. 2011).

NO and PG play a major role in the cervical cancer inflammation. In Korean population, polymorphism in these genes was analyzed in 176 histologically confirmed invasive cervical cancer patients and in 172 healthy controls. The results demonstrated that there is no significant association between polymorphism of COX-2 and iNOS genes and cervical cancer (Lee et al. 2007).

Inhibitors of inflammation for the prevention and treatment of cervical cancer
Cervical cancer is mainly due to the deregulated inflammation which may be due to HPV, HIV, and also various other infections. Cervical cancer can be prevented by using cervical cancer vaccines. Till date, 148 HPV types are recognized officially from HPV-1 to HPV-152. Few HPV did not fulfill the adequate criteria and they have classified as the subtypes (HPV-46, HPV-55, HPV-64, and HPV-79). High-risk types HPV16 and HPV18 are responsible for 70 % of cervical cancer. HPV6 and HPV11 are regarded as low-risk genotype and are responsible for the development of genital warts and laryngeal squamous cell papillomas of both genders. Two vaccines have been developed a Cervarix®, bivalent vaccine against HPV16 and HPV18 and Gardasil®, quadrivalent vaccine against HPV6, HPV11, HPV16, and HPV18. The efficacy of these vaccines was studied in clinical trials and proved to be safe. Both these vaccines are intramuscularly administrated in three doses over 6 months, though the recommended timing for the second dose varies between the two vaccines. Gardasil is very effective against development of genital warts caused by types HPV6 and HPV11 (Donovan et al. 2011). These two vaccines have been licensed in more than 110 countries, and in more than 40 countries, universal HPV vaccination system have been introduced through national vaccination program. Though the protection duration for the available vaccine is not exactly known, bivalent vaccine protects over 8.4 years and quadrivalent vaccine gives protection for more than over 5 years. Vaccination is done in females belonging to the age group 9–14 years. Though the efficacy is proved by clinical trials, issues regarding the usage of booster dosages and cross-protection remains standstill. So the efforts are being taken for the generation of second-generation HPV vaccines. A nonavalent vaccine, which, in addition to the four HPV types, contains L1 viral-like proteins of HPV-31, HPV-33, HPV-45, HPV-52, and HPV-58, is in the advanced stage of phase III efficacy trials (Poljak 2012).

Nonsteroidal anti-inflammatory drugs (NSAID) are used in the treatment of cancers. They inhibit inflammatory pathways through COX. The class of inhibitors, which inhibits the COX, was designed as coxibs. NSAIDs are more nonspecific in their action, and so it inhibits COX-1 or COX-2 or both. Aspirin also belongs to the NSAID group. Recently, Fitzgerald reported that COX-2/PGE2 inflammatory pathways were activated by HIV infection and they can be reduced by the use of COX-2 inhibitors like aspirin. They insisted that aspirin or aspirin-like agents, which decrease the production of prostaglandins, can minimize the risk of cervical cancer in HIV- and HPV-infected cases. Apart from COX inhibitors, some of the inhibitors which are used for the treatment of other cancers are used in clinical trials for cervical cancer, and the details of the drugs, their action, and the stage in which they are used are given in Table 15.1 adapted from Duenas-Gonzalez et al. 2012.

Table 15.1 Details of drugs in clinical trials, their action

Compound	Company	Structure	Current indication	Stage of development for cervical cancer	Mechanism of action
Bevacizumab	Genentech, Inc	Anti-VEGF mAb	Metastatic colorectal cancer NSCLC, renal cell cancer	Phase III Phase II	Binds VEGF and prevents the interaction of VEGF to its receptors (Flt-1 and KDR) on the surface of endothelial cells
Cetuximab	Merck, Serono	Anti-EGFR mAb	Metastatic colorectal cancer, H&N carcinoma	Phase II	Binds EGFR and competitively inhibits the binding of its ligands
Panitumumab	Amgen, Inc.	Anti-EGFR mAb	Metastatic colorectal cancer	Phase II	Binds EGFR and competitively inhibits the binding of its ligands
Pazopanib	Glaxo Smith Kline	Small molecule	Metastatic renal cell carcinoma	Phase II	Inhibits the tyrosine kinase activity of human VEGFR2 and VEGFR3
Cediranib	Astra Zeneca	Small molecule	Under clinical development for NSCLC	Phase II	Inhibits the tyrosine kinase activity of VEGFR-1, -2, -3, PDGFR, FGFR-1, c-kit
Hydralazine/valproate	Neolpharma S.A. de C.V. Mexico	Repositioned small molecules	CC, myelodysplastic syndrome (MDS) and cutaneous T-cell lymphoma (CTCL)	Phase III	DNA methylation and HDAC inhibitors, respectively
Sorafenib	Bayer	Small molecule	Metastatic renal cell carcinoma, hepatocellular carcinoma	Phase II	Inhibit multiple intracellular (CRAF, BRAF, and mutant BRAF) and cell surface kinases (KIT, FLT-3, RET, VEGFR-1, VEGFR-2, VEGFR-3, and PDGFR-b)
Sunitinib	Pfizer	Small molecule	Renal cell carcinoma, GISTs after disease progression on or intolerance to imatinib	Phase II	Inhibits (PDGFRa and PDGFRb) (VEGFR1, VEGFR2, and VEGFR3), stem cell factor receptor (KIT), Fms-like tyrosine kinase-3 (FLT3)

(continued)

Table 15.1 (continued)

Compound	Company	Structure	Current indication	Stage of development for cervical cancer	Mechanism of action
Temsirulimus	Wyeth pharmaceuticals, Inc.	Small molecule	Renal cell carcinoma	Phase I–II	mTOR inhibitor
Everolimus	Novartis pharmaceuticals Corp.	Small molecule	Metastatic renal cell carcinoma	Phase I–II	mTOR inhibitor
Olaparib	Astra Zeneca	Small molecule	Under clinical development for breast cancer and ovarian cancer	Phase I–II	poly-ADP- ribose polymerase-1 (PARP-1) inhibitor. Inducer of 'synthetic lethality'
Veliparib	Abbott	Small molecule	under clinical development for breast cancer and ovarian cancer	Phase II–I	poly-ADP- ribose polymerase-1 (PARP-1 and PARP-2) inhibitor. Inducer of 'synthetic lethality'
S1	Taiho Pharmaceutical Co.	Cytotoxic	Advanced gastric cancer	Phase II, III	S-1 contains tegafur, a pro-drug of 5-FU, with 5-chloro-2,4-dihydropyrimidine, a competitive inhibitor of DPD plus, potassium oxonate which reduces the gastro-intestinal toxicity of 5-FU
Ixabepilone	Bristol myers squibb co	Cytotoxic	Breast cancer	Phase II	Binding to beta-tubulins, stabilizes microtubules
Exatecan	Daiichi Pharmaceutical Co	Cytotoxic	Under clinical development for several solid tumors	Phase II	Synthetic analog of the topoisomerase I inhibitor binding to topoisomerase 1, inhibits DNA replication
Belotecan	Chong Keun Dang Corp.	Cytotoxic	Under clinical development for several solid tumors	Phase II	Semi-synthetic camptothecin analog
Mapatumumab	Human genome sciences	Fully human mAb	Under clinical development for solid tumors	Phase I, II	TRAIL R1Agonist

(continued)

Table 15.1 (continued)

Compound	Company	Structure	Current indication	Stage of development for cervical cancer	Mechanism of action
Bryostatin-1	Aphios manufactures	Natural compound	Under clinical development for NHL, leukemia	Phase I, II	Toll-like receptor-4 (TLR-4) ligand
Tirapazamine	Chem net	Cytotoxic and radiosensitizer	Under clinical development for advanced head and neck cancer	Phase III	Radiosensitizer. Under hypoxic conditions is reduced to a highly reactive radical that produces strand breaks in the DNA
Triapine	VION Pharmaceuticals, Inc.	Small molecule	Under clinical development for metastatic head and neck cancer	Phase II	Inhibits the enzyme ribonucleotide reductase (RR), resulting in arrest or slowing of DNA synthesis and cellular proliferation

DPD dihydropyrimidine dehydrogenase, *EGF* epidermal growth factor, *EGFR* epidermal growth factor receptor, *(FGFR)-1 and -3* fibroblast growth factor receptor, cytokine receptor (Kit), *mTOR* mammalian target of rapamycin, *NSCLC* non-small-cell lung cancer, *PDGFR* platelet-derived growth factor receptor, *VEGF* vascular endothelial growth factor, *VEGFR* vascular endothelial growth factor receptor

(Adapted from Duenas-Gonzalez et al. 2012)

15.5 Conclusion

HPV infection is the one of the most common causes of sexually transmitted viral disease. Preceded by breast cancer, cervical cancer holds a second position among the most common cancer prevalent in women across the world. The HPV–cervical cancer bond is so strong that among the 30 HPV types identified that can spread through sexual contact to infect primarily the cervix, vagina, vulva and penis; four are most often associated with cervical cancer malignancies. HPV-related cervical cancer is one of the typical examples for the role of viral infection in developing a malignancy. The primary viral particles responsible for this malignancy by altering the cellular intrinsic pathways are E5, E6, and E7 proteins. The complex interplay between the HPV particles and inflammation is well deciphered and their functional and regulatory aspect in the development of malignancy is also highly focused. The molecular studies in HPV-related cervical cancer had solidified its epidemiological side also. This helped in decreasing the incidence of mortality related to cervical cancer and the emergence of Pap smear tests had greatly added to the importance in detecting the cancer at a very early stage which has a significant influence on the morbidity of cervical cancer. Although Pap smear remains the major screening method, HPV-based testing has been more effective than cytology for the detection of cervical cancer precursors and prevention of cervical cancer. Successful designing of effective therapeutics and vaccines has also greatly helped to eradicate the prevalence of HPV infection at least in developed countries and contributed to the control of cervical cancer.

References

Al-Tahhan MA, Etewa RL, el Behery MM (2011) Association between circulating interleukin-1 beta (IL-1beta) levels and IL-1beta C-511T polymorphism with cervical cancer risk in Egyptian women. Mol Cell Biochem 353:159–165

Ashrafi GH, Haghshenas MR, Marchetti B, O'Brien PM, Campo MS (2005) E5 protein of human papillomavirus type 16 selectively downregulates surface HLA class I. Int J Cancer 113:276–283

Baker R, Dauner JG, Rodriguez AC, Williams MC, Kemp TJ, Hildesheim A, Pinto LA (2011) Increased plasma levels of adipokines and inflammatory markers in older women with persistent HPV infection. Cytokine 53:282–285

Barbisan G, Perez LO, Contreras A, Golijow CD (2012) TNF-alpha and IL-10 promoter polymorphisms, HPV infection, and cervical cancer risk. Tumour Biol 33:1549–1556

Basile JR, Zacny V, Munger K (2001) The cytokines tumor necrosis factor-alpha (TNF-alpha) and TNF-related apoptosis-inducing ligand differentially modulate proliferation and apoptotic pathways in human keratinocytes expressing the human papillomavirus-16 E7 oncoprotein. J Biol Chem 276:22522–22528

Bodily JM, Mehta KP, Laimins LA (2011) Human papillomavirus E7 enhances hypoxia-inducible factor 1-mediated transcription by inhibiting binding of histone deacetylases. Cancer Res 71:1187–1195

Chang YE, Laimins LA (2000) Microarray analysis identifies interferon-inducible genes and stat-1 as major transcriptional targets of human papillomavirus type 31. J Virol 74:4174–4182

Chen X, Han S, Wang S, Zhou X, Zhang M, Dong J, Shi X, Qian N, Wang X, Wei Q, Shen H, Hu Z (2009) Interactions of IL-12A and IL-12B polymorphisms on the risk of cervical cancer in Chinese women. Clin Cancer Res 15:400–405

Chiantore MV, Vannucchi S, Accardi R, Tommasino M, Percario ZA, Vaccari G, Affabris E, Fiorucci G, Romeo G (2012) Interferon-beta induces cellular senescence in cutaneous human papilloma virus-transformed human keratinocytes by affecting p53 transactivating activity. PLoS One 7:e36909

Coleman MP, Quaresma M, Berrino F, Lutz JM, de Angelis R, Capocaccia R, Baili P, Rachet B, Gatta G, Hakulinen T, Micheli A, Sant M, Weir HK, Elwood JM, Tsukuma H, Koifman S, Ga ES, Francisci S, Santaquilani M, Verdecchia A, Storm HH, Young JL (2008) Cancer survival in five continents: a worldwide population-based study (CONCORD). Lancet Oncol 9:730–756

Colombo N, Carinelli S, Colombo A, Marini C, Rollo D, Sessa C (2012) On behalf of the Esmo guidelines working group 2012. Cervical cancer: ESMO clinical practice guidelines for diagnosis, treatment and follow-up. Ann Oncol 23, vii27–vii32

Colotta F, Allavena P, Sica A, Garlanda C, Mantovani A (2009) Cancer-related inflammation, the seventh hallmark of cancer: links to genetic instability. Carcinogenesis 30:1073–1081

de Marco F, Bucaj E, Foppoli C, Fiorini A, Blarzino C, Filipi K, Giorgi A, Schinina ME, di Domenico F, Coccia R, Butterfield DA, Perluigi M (2012) Oxidative stress in HPV-driven viral carcinogenesis: redox proteomics analysis of HPV-16 dysplastic and neoplastic tissues. PLoS One 7:e34366

Decarlo CA, Severini A, Edler L, Escott NG, Lambert PF, Ulanova M, Zehbe I (2010) IFN-kappa, a novel type I IFN, is undetectable in HPV-positive human cervical keratinocytes. Lab Invest 90:1482–1491

Degregori J, Johnson DG (2006) Distinct and overlapping roles for E2F family members in transcription, proliferation and apoptosis. Curr Mol Med 6:739–748

Ding B, Fu S, Wang M, Yue C, Wang W, Zhou D, Zhang Z, Han S (2012) Tumor necrosis factor alpha -308 G > A polymorphisms and cervical cancer risk: a meta-analysis. Int J Gynecol Cancer 22:213–219

Donovan B, Franklin N, Guy R, Grulich AE, Regan DG, Ali H, Wand H, Fairley CK (2011) Quadrivalent human papillomavirus vaccination and trends in genital warts in Australia: analysis of national sentinel surveillance data. Lancet Infect Dis 11:39–44

Du M, Fan X, Hong E, Chen JJ (2002) Interaction of oncogenic papillomavirus E6 proteins with fibulin-1. Biochem Biophys Res Commun 296:962–969

Duenas-Gonzalez A, Cetina L, Coronel J, Cervantes-Madrid D (2012) Emerging drugs for cervical cancer. Expert Opin Emerg Drugs 17:203–218

Duensing S, Munger K (2003) Human papillomavirus type 16 E7 oncoprotein can induce abnormal centrosome duplication through a mechanism independent of inactivation of retinoblastoma protein family members. J Virol 77:12331–12335

Duensing A, Liu Y, Tseng M, Malumbres M, Barbacid M, Duensing S (2006) Cyclin-dependent kinase 2 is dispensable for normal centrosome duplication but required for oncogene-induced centrosome overduplication. Oncogene 25:2943–2949

Feng Q, Wei H, Morihara J, Stern J, Yu M, Kiviat N, Hellstrom I, Hellstrom KE (2012) Th2 type inflammation promotes the gradual progression of HPV-infected cervical cells to cervical carcinoma. Gynecol Oncol 127:412–419

Ferlay J, Parkin DM, Steliarova-Foucher E (2010a) Estimates of cancer incidence and mortality in Europe in 2008. Eur J Cancer 46:765–781

Ferlay J, Shin HR, Bray F, Forman D, Mathers C, Parkin DM (2010b) Estimates of worldwide burden of cancer in 2008: GLOBOCAN 2008. Int J Cancer 127:2893–2917

Filippova M, Song H, Connolly JL, Dermody TS, Duerksen-Hughes PJ (2002) The human papillomavirus 16 E6 protein binds to tumor necrosis factor (TNF) R1 and protects cells from TNF-induced apoptosis. J Biol Chem 277:21730–21739

Filippova M, Parkhurst L, Duerksen-Hughes PJ (2004) The human papillomavirus 16 E6 protein binds to Fas-associated death domain and protects cells from Fas-triggered apoptosis. J Biol Chem 279:25729–25744

Fitzgerald DW, Bezak K, Ocheretina O, Riviere C, Wright TC, Milne GL, Zhou XK, Du B, Subbaramaiah K, Byrt E, Goodwin ML, Rafii A, Dannenberg AJ (2012) The effect of HIV and HPV coinfection on cervical COX-2 expression and systemic prostaglandin E2 levels. Cancer Prev Res (Phila) 5:34–40

Gaiotti D, Chung J, Iglesias M, Nees M, Baker PD, Evans CH, Woodworth CD (2000) Tumor necrosis factor-alpha promotes human papillomavirus (HPV) E6/E7 RNA expression and cyclin-dependent kinase activity in HPV-immortalized keratinocytes by a ras-dependent pathway. Mol Carcinog 27:97–109

Gangwar R, Mittal B, Mittal RD (2009) Association of interleukin-6-174G > C promoter polymorphism with risk of cervical cancer. Int J Biol Markers 24:11–16

Garland SM, Bhatla N, Ngan HY (2012) Cervical cancer burden and prevention strategies: Asia Oceania perspective. Cancer Epidemiol Biomarkers Prev 21:1414–1422

Garnett TO, Duerksen-Hughes PJ (2006) Modulation of apoptosis by human papillomavirus (HPV) oncoproteins. Arch Virol 151:2321–2335

Garnett TO, Filippova M, Duerksen-Hughes PJ (2006) Accelerated degradation of FADD and procaspase 8 in cells expressing human papilloma virus 16 E6 impairs TRAIL-mediated apoptosis. Cell Death Differ 13:1915–1926

Hodge DR, Peng B, Cherry JC, Hurt EM, Fox SD, Kelley JA, Munroe DJ, Farrar WL (2005) Interleukin 6 supports the maintenance of p53 tumor suppressor gene promoter methylation. Cancer Res 65:4673–4682

Hudson JD, Shoaibi MA, Maestro R, Carnero A, Hannon GJ, Beach DH (1999) A proinflammatory cytokine inhibits p53 tumor suppressor activity. J Exp Med 190:1375–1382

Huibregtse JM, Scheffner M, Howley PM (1991) A cellular protein mediates association of p53 with the E6 oncoprotein of human papillomavirus types 16 or 18. EMBO J 10:4129–4135

Kang S, Kim JW, Park NH, Song YS, Park SY, Kang SB, Lee HP (2007) Interleukin-1 beta-511 polymorphism and risk of cervical cancer. J Korean Med Sci 22:110–113

Karin M (2006) Nuclear factor-kappaB in cancer development and progression. Nature 441:431–436

Kemp TJ, Hildesheim A, Garcia-Pineres A, Williams MC, Shearer GM, Rodriguez AC, Schiffman M, Burk R, Freer E, Bonilla J, Herrero R, Pinto LA (2010) Elevated systemic levels of inflammatory cytokines in older women with persistent cervical human papillomavirus infection. Cancer Epidemiol Biomarkers Prev 19:1954–1959

Kuwano T, Nakao S, Yamamoto H, Tsuneyoshi M, Yamamoto T, Kuwano M, Ono M (2004) Cyclooxygenase 2 is a key enzyme for inflammatory cytokine-induced angiogenesis. FASEB J 18:300–310

Lammens T, Li J, Leone G, de Veylder L (2009) Atypical E2Fs: new players in the E2F transcription factor family. Trends Cell Biol 19:111–118

Lee TS, Jeon YT, Kim JW, Park NH, Kang SB, Lee HP, Song YS (2007) Lack of association of the cyclooxygenase-2 and inducible nitric oxide synthase gene polymorphism with risk of cervical cancer in Korean population. Ann N Y Acad Sci 1095:134–142

Lee S, Kim JH, Kim H, Kang JW, Kim SH, Yang Y, Kim J, Park J, Park S, Hong J, Yoon DY (2011) Activation of the interleukin-32 pro-inflammatory pathway in response to human papillomavirus infection and over-expression of interleukin-32 controls the expression of the human papillomavirus oncogene. Immunology 132:410–420

Ma S, Tang J, Feng J, Xu Y, Yu X, Deng Q, Lu Y (2008) Induction of p21 by p65 in p53 null cells treated with Doxorubicin. Biochim Biophys Acta 1783:935–940

McCormack SJ, Brazinski SE, Moore JL, Werness BA, Goldstein DJ (1997) Activation of the focal adhesion kinase signal transduction pathway in cervical carcinoma cell lines and human genital epithelial cells immortalized with human papillomavirus type 18. Oncogene 15:265–274

Okamoto T, Sanda T, Asamitsu K (2007) NF-kappa B signaling and carcinogenesis. Curr Pharm Des 13:447–462

Pandey S, Mittal B, Srivastava M, Singh S, Srivastava K, Lal P, Mittal RD (2011) Evaluation of Toll-like receptors 3 (c.1377C/T) and 9 (G2848A) gene polymorphisms in cervical cancer susceptibility. Mol Biol Rep 38:4715–4721

Park JS, Kim EJ, Kwon HJ, Hwang ES, Namkoong SE, Um SJ (2000) Inactivation of interferon regulatory factor-1 tumor suppressor protein by HPV E7 oncoprotein. Implication for the E7-mediated immune evasion mechanism in cervical carcinogenesis. J Biol Chem 275:6764–6769

Patel D, Huang SM, Baglia LA, McCance DJ (1999) The E6 protein of human papillomavirus type 16 binds to and inhibits co-activation by CBP and p300. EMBO J 18:5061–5072

Poljak M (2012) Prophylactic human papillomavirus vaccination and primary prevention of cervical cancer: issues and challenges. Clin Microbiol Infect 18(Suppl 5):64–69

Reiser J, Hurst J, Voges M, Krauss P, Munch P, Iftner T, Stubenrauch F (2011) High-risk human papillomaviruses repress constitutive kappa interferon transcription via E6 to prevent pathogen recognition receptor and antiviral-gene expression. J Virol 85:11372–11380

Rincon-Orozco B, Halec G, Rosenberger S, Muschik D, Nindl I, Bachmann A, Ritter TM, Dondog B, Ly R, Bosch FX, Zawatzky R, Rosl F (2009) Epigenetic silencing of interferon-kappa in human papillomavirus type 16-positive cells. Cancer Res 69:8718–8725

Ronco LV, Karpova AY, Vidal M, Howley PM (1998) Human papillomavirus 16 E6 oncoprotein binds to interferon regulatory factor-3 and inhibits its transcriptional activity. Genes Dev 12:2061–2072

Sankaranarayanan (2011) Cancer survival in Africa, Asia, the Caribbean and Central America. Introduction. IARC Sci Publ, pp 1–5

Sasagawa T, Takagi H, Makinoda S (2012) Immune responses against human papillomavirus (HPV) infection and evasion of host defense in cervical cancer. J Infect Chemother 18:807–815

Schiffman M, Castle PE, Jeronimo J, Rodriguez AC, Wacholder S (2007) Human papillomavirus and cervical cancer. Lancet 370:890–907

Shekari M, Kordi-Tamandani DM, Malekzadeh K, Sobti RC, Karimi S, Suri V (2012) Effect of anti-inflammatory (IL-4, IL-10) cytokine genes in relation to risk of cervical carcinoma. Am J Clin Oncol 35:514–519

Singh H, Sachan R, Goel H, Mittal B (2008) Genetic variants of interleukin-1RN and interleukin-1beta genes and risk of cervical cancer. BJOG 115:633–638

Singh H, Jain M, Sachan R, Mittal B (2009) Association of TNFA (-308G > A) and IL-10 (-819C > T) promoter polymorphisms with risk of cervical cancer. Int J Gynecol Cancer 19:1190–1194

Tartour E, Fossiez F, Joyeux I, Galinha A, Gey A, Claret E, Sastre-Garau X, Couturier J, Mosseri V, Vives V, Banchereau J, Fridman WH, Wijdenes J, Lebecque S, Sautes-Fridman C (1999) Interleukin 17, a T-cell-derived cytokine, promotes tumorigenicity of human cervical tumors in nude mice. Cancer Res 59:3698–3704

Wang Q, Zhang C, Walayat S, Chen HW, Wang Y (2011) Association between cytokine gene polymorphisms and cervical cancer in a Chinese population. Eur J Obstet Gynecol Reprod Biol 158:330–333

Wang N, Yin D, Zhang S, Wei H, Wang S, Zhang Y, Lu Y, Dai S, Li W, Zhang Q (2012) TNF-alpha rs1800629 polymorphism is not associated with HPV infection or cervical cancer in the Chinese population. PLoS One 7:e45246

Xie TX, Wei D, Liu M, Gao AC, Ali-Osman F, Sawaya R, Huang S (2004) Stat3 activation regulates the expression of matrix metalloproteinase-2 and tumor invasion and metastasis. Oncogene 23:3550–3560

Zhou F, Leggatt GR, Frazer IH (2011) Human papillomavirus 16 E7 protein inhibits interferon-gamma-mediated enhancement of keratinocyte antigen processing and T-cell lysis. FEBS J 278:955–963

Chapter 16
The Role of Inflammation in Liver Cancer

Anupam Bishayee

Abstract Persistent inflammation is known to promote and exacerbate malignancy. Primary liver cancer, mostly hepatocellular carcinoma (HCC), is a clear example of inflammation-related cancer as more than 90 % of HCCs arise in the context of hepatic injury and inflammation. HCC represents the fifth most common malignancy and the third leading cause of cancer-related death worldwide with about one million new cases diagnosed every year with almost an equal number of deaths. Chronic unresolved inflammation is associated with persistent hepatic injury and concurrent regeneration, leading to sequential development of fibrosis, cirrhosis, and eventually HCC. Irrespective of the intrinsic differences among various etiological factors, a common denominator at the origin of HCC is the perpetuation of a wound-healing response activated by parenchymal cell death and the resulting inflammatory cascade. Hence, the identification of fundamental inflammatory signaling pathways causing transition from chronic liver injury to dysplasia and HCC could depict new predictive biomarkers and targets to identify and treat patients with chronic liver inflammation. This chapter critically discusses the roles of several major cytokines, chemokines, growth factors, transcription factors, and enzymes as well as a distinct network of inflammatory signaling pathways in the development and progression of HCC. It also highlights and analyzes preclinical animal studies showing innovative approaches of targeting inflammatory mediators and signaling by a variety of natural compounds and synthetic agents to achieve effective therapy as well as prevention of hepatic malignancy. Additionally, current limitations and potential challenges associated with the inhibition of inflammatory signaling as well as future directions of research to accelerate clinical development of anti-inflammatory agents to prevent and treat liver cancer are presented.

A. Bishayee (✉)
Department of Pharmaceutical Sciences, School of Pharmacy,
American University of Health Sciences, 1600 East Hill Street,
Signal Hill, CA 90755, USA
e-mail: abishayee@auhs.edu

B. B. Aggarwal et al. (eds.), *Inflammation and Cancer*, Advances in Experimental Medicine and Biology 816, DOI: 10.1007/978-3-0348-0837-8_16, © Springer Basel 2014

16.1 Introduction

Primary liver cancers can be categorized into angiosarcoma, cholangiocarcinoma, hepatoblastoma, and hepatocellular carcinoma (HCC). The latter is the most dominant form of primary liver cancer, accounting for more than 90 % of this cancer (El-Serag and Rudolph 2007). HCC represents the fifth most common malignancy and the third leading cause of cancer-related death worldwide (Nordenstedt et al. 2010). HCC has a dismal prognosis with a number of HCC-related deaths almost equal to the number of diagnosed cases (more than 600,000) each year (Sherman 2005). The median survival time of HCC patients is 7–8 months from the time of diagnosis (Wilson 2005), and a 5-year survival rate is below 9 % (Sherman 2005). The rate of HCC incidence continues to increase in several low-risk regions of the world, including developed countries in Western Europe, North America, and Oceania, while the rate is declining in several highest-risk countries of Asia (Center and Jemal 2011). The incidence of HCC has dramatically increased in the USA by more than 70 % during the last quarter century (El-Serag 2004), with approximately 31,000 new cases and about 22,000 deaths expected to occur in 2013 alone (Siegel et al. 2013). The annual health care cost associated with HCC in the USA has been estimated to be approximately 455 million dollars (Lang et al. 2009). The overall costs for HCC patients are two- to eightfold higher than those without HCC, and this underscores the huge burden of medical care expense of illness related to hepatic malignancy (White et al. 2012).

HCC is a complex and heterogeneous malignancy caused by a number of risk factors. The major origin of HCC development is viral hepatitis caused by hepatitis B virus (HBV) and HCV (Marrero and Marrero 2007; Schütte et al. 2009; Gao et al. 2012). Other non-viral risk factors include alcohol abuse, non-alcoholic steatohepatitis (NASH), type 2 diabetes mellitus, and hemochromatosis (El-Serag et al. 2006; Blonski et al. 2010). Accumulating evidence showed that obesity is related to both HCC incidence and mortality and represents an independent risk factor for HCC in patients with alcoholic and cryptogenic cirrhosis (Nair et al. 2002; Larsson and Wolk 2007; Gregor and Hotamisligil 2011). Environmental and dietary carcinogens, such as aflatoxin B_1 (AFB_1, a mycotoxin present in corn, soybean and peanuts) and nitrosamines (present in tobacco smoke, cosmetics, gasoline, and various processed foods, including cured meats, salami and fried fish) are known to cause HCC (Bartsch and Montesano 1984; El-Serag and Rudolph 2007). A cohort study conducted in Shanghai (China) showed that the risk of developing HCC in patients with HBV infection and AFB_1 exposure was more than 59-fold that of normal population (Qian et al. 1994). Similar results were reported by another study conducted in Qidong, a high AFB_1 contamination area in China (Ming et al. 2002). Epidemiologic studies have suggested that cigarette smoking is a risk factor for the development of HCC. Results based on a clinical study on Taiwanese patients indicate that 4-aminobiphenyl exposure, which is primarily a result of cigarette smoking, plays a role in the development of HCC in humans (Wang et al. 1998). Several studies have indicated a causal link between the use of oral contraceptives and HCC development (Kenya 1990; Korula et al. 1991). Finally, gender is another risk factor for HCC as men are more susceptible than women with a male-to-female ratio of 2:1–4:1 (El-Serag and Rudolph 2007; Ruggieri et al. 2010).

Current treatment options for patients with HCC are limited. Surgical resection is the treatment of choice for patients with well-preserved hepatic functions. Unfortunately, it involves a high risk of postoperative complications and tumor recurrence. At the present time, liver transplantation is the most effective way to improve the survival of HCC patients (Dutkowski et al. 2010). However, this option has limitation due to inadequate number of qualified donors as well as occurrence of the disease in the transplanted liver. Although various strategies, such as cryoablation, microwave ablation, radio-frequency ablation, trans-catheter arterial chemoembolization, percutaneous ethanol injection, and yttrium-90 microspheres, are available for inoperable patients, difficulty in the management of patients and tumor recurrence remain two significant limitations for these treatments (Senthil et al. 2010). Currently, sorafenib [*N*-(3-trifluoromethyl-4-chlorophenyl)-*N*′-(4-(2-methylcarbamoyl pyridin-4-yl)oxyphenyl)urea, Nexavar®, Bayer] is the only drug approved by the United States Food and Drug Administration for the treatment of advanced HCC based on two large phase III clinical trials (Llovet et al. 2008; Cheng et al. 2009). Nevertheless, only moderate improvement of survival, a number of adverse side effects, and high costs underscore the need for other novel therapeutic as well as preventive approaches for HCC (Je et al. 2009; Lu 2010; Bishayee et al. 2010a; Bishayee 2012).

16.2 Cellular and Molecular Mechanisms of Liver Cancer

The molecular pathogenesis of hepatocellular cancer is very complex. The exact sequence of hepatocarcinogenesis, including the development of preneoplastic lesions and their growth and eventual progression to HCC, is not fully understood (Farazi and DePinho 2006). Several cellular phenomena, including alterations in tumor microenvironment, inflammation, oxidative stress, and hypoxia, act in concert with various molecular events to facilitate liver tumor initiation, progression, and metastasis (Aravalli et al. 2013). Mounting evidence indicates complex genetic and epigenetic alterations, chromosomal aberrations, mutations, abnormal expression of cellular proteins, overexpression of oncogenes, inhibition of tumor-suppressor genes, and altered molecular pathways lead to the development of HCC (Aravalli et al. 2008; Lachenmayer et al. 2010). Studies carried out during the last several decades have identified numerous signaling pathways activated in HCC, such as angiogenic signaling mediated through vascular endothelial growth factor and platelet-derived growth factor; Raf, mitogen-activated protein extracellular kinase (MEK), and extracellular signal-regulated kinase (ERK) (Ras/Raf/MEK/ERK); janus kinase (JAK)/signal transducers, and activators of transcription (STAT) (JAK/STAT); phosphatidylinositol 3-kinase (PI3K)/Akt/mammalian target of rapamycin (mTOR) (PI3K/Akt/mTOR); and Wnt/β-catenin and Hedgehog pathways (Huynh 2010; Hoshida et al. 2010; Whittaker et al. 2010; Nejak-Bowen and Monga 2011; Bishayee 2013).

16.3 Inflammation and Liver Cancer

Numerous epidemiological and clinical studies have provided convincing evidence that chronic inflammation leads to carcinogenesis (Demaria et al. 2010). Various types of cancer arise in the setting of chronic inflammation, indicating a strong link between inflammation and cancer (Mantovani et al. 2008; Grivennikov et al. 2010). It has been estimated that approximately 15 % of all human cancers are associated with inflammation and chronic infections (Coussens and Werb 2002). The development of HCC represents one of the most extensively investigated inflammation-related carcinogenesis events since more than 90 % of HCCs arise in the context of hepatic injury and inflammation (Nakagawa and Maeda 2012). HCC slowly unfolds on a background of chronic inflammation predominantly triggered by exposure to infectious agents, such as hepatotropic viruses, or to toxic compounds, for example, ethanol (Berasain et al. 2009a). Despite the intrinsic differences among various etiological factors for HCC, a common denominator at the origin this malignancy is the perpetuation of a wound-healing response activated by parenchymal cell death and the resulting inflammatory cascade. During chronic viral hepatitis, the host immune responses to HBV or HCV are often not strong enough to completely eradicate the infection, culminating in lingering stimulation of an antigen-specific immune response (Budhu and Wang 2006). The host immune cells are known to kill virus-infected liver cells, resulting in the production of various cytokines and growth factors and consequently inducing compensatory hepatocyte regeneration (Markiewski et al. 2006). The persistent cycle of "necro-inflammation" and hepatocyte regeneration is believed to enhance the risk of genetic mutation in hepatocytes, promoting survival and expansion of initiated cells (Nakagawa and Maeda 2012). All these events ultimately lead to deregulated hepatocytes proliferation which contributes to the development and progression of hepatic cancer. Moreover, oxidative stress through generation of reactive oxygen and nitrogen species in the initiated hepatocytes as well as inflammatory cells accelerate hepatocarcinogenesis through several mechanisms, including transcription and activation of cytokines and growth factors, oxidative DNA damage, DNA methylation, and hepatocyte injury (Tanaka et al. 2008; Chuma et al. 2008; Marra et al. 2011).

16.4 Inflammatory Mediators and Signaling Pathways Associated with Liver Cancer

Chronic inflammation is associated with persistent hepatic injury and concurrent regeneration, leading to sequential development of fibrosis, cirrhosis, and eventually HCC. Hence, the identification and analysis of fundamental inflammatory signaling pathways causing transition from chronic liver injury to dysplasia and HCC could depict new predictive biomarkers and targets to identify and treat patients with chronic liver inflammation (Weber et al. 2011). A growing number of preclinical and clinical studies have identified a plethora of inflammatory mediators and signaling pathways implicated in hepatocellular cancer (Berasain et al. 2009a; Weber et al. 2011; Nakagawa and Maeda 2012; Wai and Kuo 2012; Szabo and Lippai 2012). It is interesting to note that these complex signaling molecules and pathways do not act independently, but are interconnected with extensive crosstalk. The following section highlights several major cytokines, chemokines, transcription factors, and proteins which belong to inflammatory signaling pathways implicated in hepatocarcinogenesis.

16.4.1 Cytokines

Cytokines are synthesized by various cell types in the liver. Hepatocytes also express cell surface receptors for cytokines. Various inflammatory cytokines, such as interleukin-1α (IL-1α), IL-1β, IL-6, IL-8 and tumor necrosis factor-α (TNF-α), participate in chronic hepatic inflammation, and IL-6 is probably the most important and studied one (Budhu and Wang 2006; Naugler and Karin 2008). During chronic hepatitis, activated Kupffer cells produce IL-6 which enhances local inflammatory responses and induce compensatory hepatocyte proliferation resulting in neoplastic transformation of hepatocytes (Naugler and Karin 2008). Elevated serum levels of IL-6 have been found in patients with chronic liver ailments, including alcoholic hepatitis, NASH, and hepatic infections with HBV and HCV (Deviere et al. 1989; Lee et al. 1998; Wieckowska et al. 2008). Moreover, higher serum levels of IL-6 have been found to be associated with increased risk of HCC development in patients with chronic hepatitis B and C infections (Nakagawa et al. 2009; Wong et al. 2009). All these reports underscore the pivotal role of IL-6 in chronic inflammation-mediated hepatocarcinogenesis in humans.

An elegant study conducted by Naugler et al. (2007) investigated the role of IL-6 in liver cancer using IL-6 knockout mouse model. IL-6 knockout mice exhibited a significant reduction of diethylnitrosamine (DENA)-initiated HCC development, suggesting direct involvement of IL-6 signaling in experimental hepatocarcinogenesis. The results from this study also showed the critical role played by the toll-like receptor (TLR) adapter protein MyD88 in the production of IL-6 by Kupffer cells during DENA-induced HCC development. The production of IL-6 by necrotic hepatocytes was reduced considerably in Kupffer cells deficient for MyD88. The ablation of MyD88 also suppressed DENA-induced hepatic tumorigenesis, indicating that IL-6 production by the TLR/MyD88/nuclear factor-kappaB (NF-κB) pathway is critical for HCC development. Another study from the same laboratory found that DENA-induced acute inflammatory response is triggered by IL-1α release from necrotic hepatocytes, and IL-1α stimulates IL-6 production by Kupffer cells (Sakurai et al. 2008). Moreover, the investigators have found that IL-1α released by damaged hepatocytes is essential for the compensatory proliferation which is essential for DENA-initiated hepatocellular carcinogenesis. Rogers et al. (2007) proposed a multistep model linking chronic hepatitis to liver cancer through cytokine-mediated derangement of gender-specific cellular metabolism. This mouse model introduces a novel mechanism of inflammation-related carcinogenesis consistent with male-predominant HCC risk.

Several epidemiological studies reveal a strong link between obesity and development and progression of liver cancer (Nair et al. 2002; Larsson and Wolk, 2007; Gregor and Hotamisligil 2011). The connection between obesity and liver cancer is likely to be mediated, at least in part, by chronic inflammation (Sun and Karin 2012; Shimizu et al. 2013). Hypertropic adipocytes are known to accumulate excess lipids and release free fatty acids, and these cells together with various immune cells secrete a number of proinflammatory cytokines, including IL-6, IL-1β, IL-9, IL-10, IL-17, IL-18, and TNF-α (Sun and Karin 2012). It has been shown that macrophase infiltration into white adipose tissue, which is accompanied by IL-6 and TNF-α production, is an initial contributing event for the development of chronic low-grade systemic inflammation (Weisberg et al. 2003). Elevated concentrations of IL-6 have been found in type 2 diabetes, an inflammatory condition, inducing cellular insulin resistance (Senn et al. 2002; Donath and Shoelson 2011). Among obesity-related pathophysiological conditions that predispose HCC, insulin resistance and subsequent inflammatory cascades are considered to play a crucial role in the occurrence of HCC (Shimizu et al. 2013). Park et al. (2010) reported that dietary-induced or genetically induced obesity promotes DENA-initiated HCC with low-grade inflammation. Interestingly, ablation of IL-6 or TNF-α abolishes the tumor-promoting effects of these cytokines, indicating that IL-6 and TNF-α are required for the promotion of obesity-linked HCC.

IL-1β, another proinflammatory cytokine in hepatocarcinogenesis, is found to promote hepatic stellate cell proliferation, activation, and transdifferentiation into the myofibroblastic phenotype (Han et al. 2004). IL-1β can promote hepatic inflammation by inducing the production of C-reactive protein, a sensitive marker of infection and inflammation, independently of IL-6 (Weinhold and Rüther 1997). c-Jun N-terminal kinase (JNK) activation by IL-1β stimulated the pSmad3L/plasminogen activator inhibitor 1 pathway in facilitating hepatocytic invasion with simultaneous reduction of transforming growth factor-β (TGF-β)-dependent tumor-suppressive activity by the phosphorylated Smad3C/p21(WAF1) pathway (Matsuzaki et al. 2007). It has been reported that the C31T polymorphism in IL-1β could be a genetic marker for the development of hepatitis-associated HCC (Wang et al. 2003). According to a case-control study including 209 incident HCC cases, IL-1β-31T/C polymorphism may modify HCC risk in relation to alcohol intake or smoking (Sakamoto et al. 2008).

16.4.2 NF-κB Pathway

NF-κB, an important transcription factor that regulates innate immunity and inflammation, plays an essential function in the regulation of inflammatory signaling pathways in the liver (Xiao and Ghosh 2005; Muriel 2009). Accumulating knowledge clearly indicate that NF-κB provides a critical link between inflammation and cancer (Karin 2009; DiDonato et al. 2012). Mammalian NF-κB consists of five members, namely RelA (p65), c-Rel, RelB, NF-κB1 (p50/p105), and NF-κB2 (p52/p100) (Ghosh and Karin 2002). Under normal physiologic conditions, p50 and p65 subunits of NF-κB dimerize are kept inactive in the cytoplasm through binding to the inhibitory protein known as inhibitor of NF-κB (IκB) (Hoffmann and Baltimore 2006). In response to various proinflammatory stimuli, including pathogen-derived lipopolysaccharide, viral and bacterial DNA and RNA, TLR-Myd88 signaling, and inflammatory cytokines (such as TNF-α and IL-1β), the IκB kinase (IKK) complex, which consists of two catalytic subunits, IKK-α and IKK-β, and a regulatory subunit, IKK-γ or NF-κB essential modulator (NEMO), phosphorylates IκB and subsequently induces its degradation by the 26S proteasome (Karin and Ben-Neriah 2000; West et al. 2006). Consequently, the activated NF-κB dimer is released and translocates into the nucleus, binds specific DNA sequences, and stimulates transcription of hundreds of target genes involved in inflammation, immune responses, cell proliferation, and cell survival (Pahl 1999; Ghosh and Karin 2002).

NF-κB has been found to be activated in virtually every chronic liver disease, including viral hepatitis, alcoholic liver disease, non-alcoholic fatty liver disease, and biliary liver disease (Luedde and Schwabe 2011). A wealth of information based on recently published studies illustrates a crucial role of NF-κB in connecting inflammation with hepatic oncogenesis (Arsura and Cavin 2005; Luedde and Schwabe 2011; He and Karin 2011). Several animal models have been developed to study the role of IKK/IκB/NF-κB signaling pathways in various cell populations during hepatocarcinogenesis. In Mdr2 knockout mouse model, which is an animal HCC model induced by chronic inflammation, inhibition of NF-κB with inducible IκB super-repressor resulted in decreased liver tumor progression (Mauad et al. 1994). Likewise, inhibition of NF-κB activation in liver parenchymal cells at later stages of hepatocarcinogenesis led to reduced inflammation-linked tumor progression in Mdr2 knockout mouse (Pikarsky et al. 2004). The liver tumor-promoting role of NF-κB has been confirmed by another study using hepatocyte-specific lymphotoxin αβ transgenic mouse model. In this inflammatory HCC model, inhibition of NF-κB via hepatocyte-specific deletion of IKK-β almost completely diminished HCC development (Haybaeck et al. 2009). In contrary, hepatocyte-specific deletion of IKK-β gene and therefore hepatocyte-specific inactivation of NF-κB signaling resulted in higher incidence of HCC in mice following exposure to hepatocarcinogen DENA (Maeda et al. 2005). Similarly, another laboratory found that inhibition of NF-κB through ablation of IKK-γ/NEMO, the regulatory subunit of IKK complex, in liver parenchymal cells led to spontaneous and sequential development of hepatosteatosis, hepatitis, fibrosis, and HCC (Luedde et al. 2007). Based on all these studies presented above, it can be concluded that NF-κB signaling possibly play dual roles in hepatocarcinogenesis depending on cancer model and stage of tumor development. Activation of NF-κB in non-parenchymal cells typically stimulates inflammation, fibrosis, and hepatocarcinogenesis. On the other hand, suppression of NF-κB activation in parenchymal cells accelerates hepatocarcinogenesis in several cancer models and suppresses tumor formation in other models. During early stages of liver tumor development, the cytoprotective role of NF-κB prevails as it prevents hepatocyte death. In late stages, NF-κB promotes tumor cell survival and proliferation.

The influence of NF-κB signaling in myeloid cells has also been investigated utilizing DENA-induced HCC in mice. Ablation of IKK-β in both hepatocytes and myeloid cells (including Kupffer cells) has been found to inhibit DENA-induced HCC development (Maeda et al. 2005). This effect was accompanied by diminished production of proinflammatory cytokines, such as IL-6, TNF-α and hepatocyte growth factor, which are secreted by non-parenchymal cells in response to dying hepatocytes to stimulate compensatory proliferation of remaining hepatocytes (Maeda et al. 2005). Another study showed that IKK-β in myeloid cells, especially in Kupffer cells, has also been involved in the development of metastatic liver malignancy through IL-6 production (Maeda et al. 2009).

Several reports support the notion that NF-κB plays an indispensable role in the promotion of obesity-associated HCC. The effects of obesity-induced activation of NF-κB are believed to be mediated through the synthesis of NF-κB target genes, including IL-1β, IL-6, and TNF-α (Shoelson et al. 2006). Experimental results showed that high-fat diet increased NF-κB activation, resulting in sustained elevation of IKK-related kinase IKK-ε in the liver, adipocytes, and adipose tissue macrophages. Interestingly, IKK-ε ablation was found to reduce the expression of inflammatory cytokines and protected mice from high-fat diet-induced obesity, chronic hepatic inflammation, and hepatic steatosis (Chiang et al. 2009). Wang et al. (2009a) reported that administration of DENA enhanced the development of preneoplastic lesions in the livers of rats fed with a high-fat diet with simultaneous increase in TNF-α/NF-κB signaling and ERK-related hepatocyte proliferation. The role of hepatic NF-κB in obesity-associated liver tumorigenesis has been investigated in mice with liver-specific inactivation of the NF-κB essential modulator gene NEMO exposed to a high-fat diet. Hepatic NEMO deficiency has been found to synergize with high-fat diet in the development of liver steatosis, increased inflammation, and aggravated liver tumorigenesis (Wunderlich et al. 2008).

16.4.3 JAK-STAT Signaling

STAT proteins are known to play vital roles in cytokine signaling pathways involved in cell growth and differentiation in various species, including mammals (Darnell et al. 1994). The STAT family consists of seven members, such as STAT1, STAT2, STAT3, STAT4, STAT5a, STAT5b, and STAT6. Among STAT family proteins, STAT3 has gained substantial attention as a convergent point for a number of oncogenic signaling pathways as well as regulator of signal transduction pathways of several proinflammatory cytokines and growth factors involved in hepatic damage and repair mechanisms (Taub 2003; Costa et al. 2003). Following phosphorylation and activation by JAKs, especially by JAK2, STAT3 undergoes dimerization before entry to nucleus for DNA binding (Yoshimura et al. 2007).

Subramaniam et al. (2013) have recently published an elegant review in which the authors presented an excellent overview of STAT3 signaling cascade and its interacting partners in the initiation of hepatocarcinogenesis and role of various STAT3-regulated genes in inflammation, survival, invasion, and angiogenesis during HCC progression. Based on an impressive number of studies, STAT3 has been recognized as a key player linking inflammation and liver cancer (Pfitzner et al. 2004; He and Karin 2011; Nakagawa and Maeda 2012; Subramaniam et al. 2013). He et al. (2010) have examined a large number of human HCC specimens and detected activated nuclear STAT3 in approximately 60 % of these samples with STAT3-positive tumors being more aggressive. These results are in agreement with a previous report in which STAT3 was found to be activated in the majority of HCC samples with poor prognosis, but not in surrounding non-malignant tissue or normal liver (Calvisi et al., 2006). Although the precise mechanisms of STAT3 activation in human HCC are not fully understood, the elevated expression of IL-6, IL-11, and IL-22 has been proposed to play an important role (He and Karin 2011).

Hepatocyte-specific STAT3-deficient mice have been used to investigate the role of STAT3 in experimental liver tumorigenesis induced by DENA. STAT3-deficient mice were found to exhibit more than sixfold reduction in liver tumor load compared to their normal counterparts (He et al. 2010). The suppressor of cytokine signaling 3 (SOCS3) is known to block STAT3 signaling, and hepatocyte-specific SOCS3 knockout mice have been found to be susceptible to HCC development, possibly due to activation of JAK/STAT and mitogen-activated protein kinase (MAPK) signaling (Ogata et al. 2006). Another study showed that hepatocyte-specific IL-6 and IL-6 receptor transgenic mice spontaneously developed hepatocellular hyperplasia and adenomas, which represent preneoplastic lesions in humans, with concomitant STAT3 activation (Maione et al. 1998). All these studies underscore the importance of IL-6/JAK/STAT3 pathway in the pathophysiology of liver cancer.

Several lines of evidence suggest possible interactions between STAT3 and NF-κB signaling pathways. It is well established that STAT3 and NF-κB coregulate various inflammatory and tumor-promoting genes (Yu et al. 2009). Moreover, STAT3 can directly interact with RelA (p65) subunit of NF-κB, confiding it in the nucleus, and thereby contributing to the constitutive activation of NF-κB in human neoplasm (Lee et al. 2009). In contrast, a separate study revealed that IKK-β/NF-κB signaling in hepatocyte negatively regulated STAT3 activation in DENA HCC animal model (He et al. 2010). Interestingly, similar inverse correlation between STAT3 and NF-κB signaling has also been observed in human HCC samples (He et al. 2010). SHP1 and SHP2, which dephosphorylate JAK2 and STAT3, function as negative regulator of JAK-STAT pathway. Hepatocyte-specific deletion of SHP2 promotes inflammatory signaling through the STAT3 pathway and hepatic inflammation/necrosis, resulting in spontaneous hyperplasia and development of hepatic tumors in aged mice. Additionally, SHP2 ablation dramatically enhanced DENA-induced HCC development, which was abolished by concurrent deletion of SHP2 and STAT3 in hepatocytes (Bard-Chapeau et al. 2011).

16.4.4 Epidermal Growth Factor Receptor Signaling

Epidermal growth factor receptor (EGFR), also known as ErbB1, is a transmembrane glycoprotein (170 kDa) consisting of an extracellular ligand-binding domain, a transmembrane domain, and a cytoplasmic domain that harbors a tyrosine kinase region. EGFR can be activated by a family of ligands, including epidermal growth factor (EGF), TGF-α, heparin-binding EGF (HB-EGF), betacellulin, epiregulin, and amphiregulin. Mounting evidence supports a role for the EGFR system in inflammation-related cell signaling with special emphasis in liver inflammation and HCC (Berasain et al. 2009b). Upregulation of EGFR has been found in human HCC samples, and several investigators have observed correlations between elevated levels of EGFR and poor patient survival (Berasain et al. 2007; Sibilia et al. 2007). Chronic activation of regenerative and wound-healing response mediated by EGFR signaling is thought to contribute tissue degeneration, resulting in chronic inflammation, fibrosis, and neoplastic transformation in the liver (Avila et al. 2006). Murillo et al. (2007) showed that TGF-β induced the expression of EGFR ligands, such as HB-EGF and TGF-α, in isolated fetal rat hepatocytes through the activation of NF-κB. The importance of EGFR in the activation of inflammation-associated NF-κB signaling has also been shown in the liver of transgenic mice overexpressing EGFR ligand TGF-α (Arsura and Cavin 2005).

16.4.5 Cyclooxygenase-Prostaglandin Pathway

One of the best characterized inflammatory pathways implicated in liver cancer is cyclooxygenase-2 (COX-2)-mediated prostaglandin pathway. COX-2, an inducible enzyme responsible for catalyzing the conversion of arachidonic acid to prostaglandins (PGs), plays a significant role in inflammation-associated hepatocarcinogenesis (Shiota et al. 1999). COX-2 has been found to be induced by pro-inflammatory mitogens, cytokines, and tumor promoters (Williams et al. 1999). Since chronic inflammation contributes to hepatocarcinogenesis and the expression of COX-2 has been known to be regulated by several transcription factors and cytokines implicated in inflammation, including NF-κB and IL-6, it is highly likely that inflammation-mediated induction of COX-2 may represent a pivotal step in hepatocellular carcinogenesis. As a matter of fact, it has been found that COX-2 is chronically overexpressed in chronic inflammation and cirrhosis as well experimental and human HCC (Wu 2006). Clinically, the expression of COX-2 in HCC has been found to be upregulated in well-differentiated HCC compared to less-differentiated tumor or histologically normal liver, indicating the involvement of COX-2 in early stages of hepatocarcinogenesis related to the inflammatory phenomena (Cervello and Montalto 2006; Giannitrapani et al. 2009). Additionally, evidence is available in the literature that COX-2 expressions are independent of tumor mass and tumor stage, and COX-2 signaling may play a key role both in early as well as late states of hepatic cancer (Sung et al. 2004; Yildirim et al. 2008). COX-2-derived PG signaling has also been shown to be involved in cholangiocarcinoma, a highly malignant epithelial tumor arising within the biliary tract (Wu 2005).

Experimental evidence supports a close interaction between COX-2 and EGFR signaling pathways. The activation of EGFR in human HCC cells has been found to upregulate COX-2 expression and PGE2 synthesis (Dajani et al. 2008). Likewise, COX-2-derived PGE2 is known to transactivate the EGFR receptor (Wu 2005; Han et al. 2006). Moreover, COX-2-derived prostanoids may be one key signal in the activation of EGFR involved in the early stages of hepatic inflammation and neoplasia (Berasain et al. 2005; Castillo et al. 2006).

16.4.6 Inducible Nitric Oxide Synthase

Another important mediator linking chronic inflammation and liver cancer is nitric oxide (NO), produced by hepatic parenchymal and non-parenchymal cells from L-arginine through the catalytic function of inducible nitric oxide synthase (iNOS), also known as NOS2. NO reacts with superoxide ($O_2^{\cdot -}$) to form peroxynitrite ($ONOO^-$), a highly reactive nitrogen species that causes nitrative and oxidative DNA damage. Oxidative stress is known to elevate iNOS gene transcription and promoter activity in hepatocytes (Kuo et al. 1997). iNOS can bind and *S*-nitrosylate COX-2 protein to increase its activity (Kim et al. 2005). Mounting evidence underscores the vital role that iNOS plays in the development and progression of HCC as this enzyme has been found to be overexpressed in several rodent liver tumor models (Ahn et al. 1999; Denda et al. 2007; Calvisi et al. 2008). Interestingly, iNOS is a target gene for NF-κB and iNOS cross talk with NF-κB and Ha-RAS/ERK cascades influences HCC growth and prognosis (Calvisi et al. 2008). Additionally, iNOS expression has been found in hepatocytes and Kupffer cells in hepatitis, cirrhosis, and HCC (Rahman et al. 2001; McNaughton et al. 2002; Kawanishi et al. 2006).

16.4.7 Inhibitor of Apoptosis

The inhibitor of apoptosis (IAP) represents a family of proteins, including c-IAP1, c-IAP2, ML-IAP and XIAP, with significant roles in cancer-related inflammation and metastasis (Guicciardi et al. 2011; de Almagro and Vucic 2012). Alterations in IAPs have been observed in several types of human malignancies, including HCC, with chemoresistance, accelerated disease progression, and poor prognosis (Gyrd-Hansen and Meier 2010). IAPs are known to function by regulating caspases involved in apoptosis as well as modulate inflammatory signaling through ubiquitin-mediated activation of NF-κB (Silke and Meier 2013). c-IAP1 and c-IAP2 function as key mediators of TNF-α-induced activation of NF-κB (Gyrd-Hansen and Meier 2010). A survivin-XIAP complex has been shown to activate NF-κB and accelerate metastasis in a splenic model of hepatic metastasis (Mehrotra et al. 2010).

16.4.8 Chemokines

Human chemokines are a family of small proteins (45–50 kb) containing a structural homologous conservative family of cysteine residues. Chemokines are classified into four groups, namely CXC, CC, CX3C, and C according to the presence of four cysteine residues in conserved locations. It is known that tumor cells can regulate chemokine expression to recruit inflammatory cells and also use these agents to facilitate tumor growth (Coussens and Werb 2002). Based on current knowledge, chemokines and their receptors, such as CXCL12-CXCR4 axis, CX3CL1-CX3CR1 axis, and CCL20-CCR6 axis, are believed to play intricate roles in HCC progression, growth, and metastasis, and immune response to HCC (Huang and Geng 2010). Activation of innate immune response in hepatocytes following chronic HCV infection leads to infiltration of proinflammatory and antiviral immune effector cells into the liver (Heydtmann and Adams 2009). This response is recruited to the liver, in part, by the chemokine CXCL10, which exerts its effects on resident and infiltrating cells. The deregulation of these cell populations within the liver may lead to chronic hepatic inflammation in HCV-linked HCC (Brownell and Polyak 2013).

16.4.9 MicroRNAs

MicroRNAs (miRNAs) are endogenous, small (20–25 nucleotides) noncoding RNA molecules that posttranscriptionally inhibit the expression of their target genes through mRNA degradation and/or translational inhibition (Bartel 2004). Several miRNAs function as oncogenes by inhibiting tumor suppressors and are overexpressed in cancers, whereas others function as tumor suppressors by inhibiting oncogenes and are downregulated or lost in cancers (Sengupta and Bishayee 2010). Aberrant expression of several miRNAs has been found to be involved in human liver cancer (Gramantieri et al. 2008; Braconi et al. 2011; Wong et al. 2013). Emerging experimental evidence supports the involvement of miRNAs in hepatocarcinogenesis via modulation of inflammatory signaling pathways. Ji et al. (2009) studied miRNAs expression profiles in human HCC samples and observed reduced levels of miR-26 expression as compared with paired non-cancerous tissues. In addition, tumors with reduced miR-26 expression had activation of NF-κB and IL-6 signaling pathways. Another study demonstrated that low miR-26 played an important role in an experimental mouse model of HCC, and administration of this miRNA using adeno-associated virus resulted in inhibition of cancer cell proliferation, induction of tumor-specific apoptosis, and dramatic suppression of HCC development (Kota et al. 2009).

Wang et al. (2009b) showed upregulation of oncogenic miR-155 with concomitant suppression of its tumor-suppressor target CCAAT/enhancer-binding protein β (C/EBPβ) in choline-deficient and amino acid-defined diet (CDAA)-induced NASH that led to hepatocarcinogenesis in mice. The DNA-binding activity of NF-κB (indication of NF-κB activation) that transactivates *miR-155* gene was significantly elevated in the liver of mice fed with CDAA diet. Interestingly, the expression of miR-155 correlated with CDAA-induced hepatic inflammation as evidenced by histopathological changes. Ectopic expression of miR-155 promoted the growth of HCC cells, and its depletion resulted in an inhibition of tumor cell growth. This study also documented upregulation of miR-155 with a concurrent decrease in C/EBPβ level in primary human HCC samples compared with matching liver tissues.

Hepatocyte nuclear factor 4α (HNF4α) is a transcription factor essential for liver development and hepatocyte function. Recently, transient inhibition of HNF4α has been found to initiate hepatocellular transformation through a microRNA-inflammatory feedback loop circuit consisting of miR-124, IL6R, STAT3, miR-24, and miR-629. Moreover, it has been shown that once this circuit is activated, it maintains suppression of HNF4α and sustains hepatic oncogenesis. Finally, systemic administration of miR-124, which modulates inflammatory signaling, was effective in preventing and suppressing hepatocellular carcinogenesis (Hatziapostolou et al. 2011).

16.5 Inhibitors of Inflammation for the Prevention and Treatment of Liver Cancer

Numerous in vitro, in vivo, and clinical studies as described above have validated the critical role of chronic inflammation in the development and progression of liver cancer. Identification of cellular pathways necessary for the initiation and propagation of inflammatory cascade in HCC not only aids in understanding the pathophysiology, progression, and diagnosis but also provides a valuable tool in designing effective prevention and treatment of this disease. Hence, interfering with various inflammatory signaling molecules and pathways may offer potential opportunities for the development of novel drugs for the prevention as well as therapy of HCC. The following section highlights preclinical animal studies showing innovative approaches of targeting inflammatory mediators and signaling by a variety of natural compounds as well as synthetic agents.

16.5.1 Natural Compounds

A wide spectrum of phytochemicals present in fruits, vegetables, nuts, legumes, beverages, spices, and traditional medicinal herbs are endowed with potent anti-inflammatory properties implicated in cancer prevention and treatment (Murakami 2009; Kim et al. 2009; Aravindaram and Yang 2010; Gupta et al. 2010). Studies carried out in our laboratory and elsewhere strongly suggest that a number of bioactive components from dietary and non-dietary sources are capable of exerting liver cancer preventive and therapeutic efficacies through multiple mechanisms (Bishayee et al. 2010a, 2012; Darvesh and Bishayee 2010, 2013); Darvesh et al. 2012. As presented below and highlighted in Table 16.1, several phytoconstituents have been found to modulate various proinflammatory signaling during experimental hepatocarcinogenesis, resulting in liver cancer preventive or therapeutic effect.

N-acetylcysteine (NAC), a water soluble organosulfur compound present in garlic, exhibited chemopreventive potential against 2-amino-3,8-dimethylimidazo[4,5-*f*] quinoxaline (MeIQx)-initiated hepatocarcinogenesis in rats. NAC treatment during the post-initiation stage exhibited decreased number and area of glutathione *S*-transferase-placental form (GST-P)-positive foci by reducing cell proliferation which may involve downregulation of insulin-like growth factor I (IGF-I) and iNOS (Nishikawa-Ogawa et al. 2006).

Berberine, a bioactive alkaloid, is present in the root and bark of *Berberis aristata* or *Coptis chinensis*. Berberine showed antiproliferative effect during the early phase of hepatocarcinogenesis initiated by DENA and promoted with phenobarbital (PB) in rats, and this response was accompanied by inhibition of hepatic iNOS expression (Zhao et al. 2008).

Anthocyanins (glycosides) and anthocyanidins (aglycones) represent the most ample flavonoid pigments of various fruits and vegetables, including berries, grapes, apples, corn, and purple cabbage. Recently, our laboratory has shown that an anthocyanin-rich fraction from black currant (*Ribes nigrum* L.) fruit, containing cyanidin-3-*O*-rutinoside as the principle anthocyanin, significantly reduced the incidence and multiplicity of hepatic nodules during DENA-initiated and PB-promoted hepatocarcinogenesis in rats (Fig. 16.1) (Bishayee et al. 2011a). Subsequent study from our laboratory demonstrated that black currant anthocyanins afforded a striking inhibition of gamma-glutamyl transpeptidase (GGT)-positive preneoplastic foci during DENA/PB-mediated hepatocarcinogenic events by reversal of hepatic over-expression of COX-2 and iNOS and blockade of the nuclear translocation of NF-κB (Fig. 16.1) (Thoppil et al. 2012; Bishayee et al. 2013a).

Murugan et al. (2010) showed that black tea polyphenols (Polyphenon-B) reduced the multiplicity and volume of hepatic tumors in rats induced by *p*-dimethylaminoazobenzene (DAB) in rats with concomitant inhibition of hepatic NF-κB and elevation of IκB.

Chrysin (5,7-dihydoxy-flavone), a flavonoid present in honey, propolis, and several plant extracts, is available as a dietary supplement. This phytochemical has

Table 16.1 Modulation of inflammatory signaling in liver cancer by agents from dietary and non-dietary sources

Agents	Experimental models	Anti-hepatocarcinogenic effects	Anti-inflammatory mechanisms	References
Dietary compounds				
N-acetylcysteine	MeIQx-induced hepatocarcinogenesis in male F344 rats	↓GST-P-positive foci	↓IGF-I; ↓iNOS	Nishikawa-Ogawa et al. (2006)
Berberine	DENA-initiated and PB-promoted hepatocarcinogenesis in male Sprague-Dawley rats	↓hepatic proliferation	↓iNOS	Zhao et al. (2008)
Black currant anthrocyanins	DENA-induced hepatocarcinogenesis in male Sprague-Dawley rats	↓hepatic nodules; ↓GGT-positive foci	↓iNOS; ↓COX-2; ↓NF-κB	Bishayee et al. (2011a, 2013a), Thoppil et al. (2012)
Black tea polyphenols	DAB-induced hepatocarcinogenesis in male Sprague-Dawley rats	↓liver tumors	↓NF-κB; ↑IκB	Murugan et al. (2010)
Chrysin	DENA-induced hepatocarcinogenesis in male Wistar rats	↓hepatic nodules	↓COX-2; ↓NF-κB	Khan et al. (2011)
Curcumin	DENA-induced hepatocarcinogenesis in male Wistar rats	↓liver hyperplasia	↓NF-κB	Chuang et al. (2000)
	HepG2 xenograft in nude BALB/c mice	↓tumor angiogenesis	↓COX-2	Yoysungnoen et al. (2006)
EGCG	DENA-induced hepatocarcinogenesis in male C57BL/KsJ-db/db obese mice	↓foci, adenoma and HCC	↓p-IGF-IR; ↓p-ERK; ↓p-Akt; ↓p-STAT3; ↓p-JNK; ↓TNF-α; ↓IL-6; ↓IL-1β; ↓IL-18	Shimizu et al. (2011a)
Genistein	HepG2 xenograft in male nude BALB/c mice	↓tumor growth	↓COX-2; ↓NF-κB; ↓Akt	Ma et al. (2011)

(continued)

Table 16.1 (continued)

Agents	Experimental models	Anti-hepatocarcinogenic effects	Anti-inflammatory mechanisms	References
Geranylgeraniol	DENA/2-AAF-induced hepatocarcinogenesis in male Wistar rats	↓GST-P-positive foci; ↓hepatic nodules	↓NF-κB	Espindola et al. (2005)
Lycopene	DENA-initiated and NASH-promoted hepatocarcinogenesis in male Sprague-Dawley rats	↓GST-P-positive foci	↓pERK; ↓NF-κB; ↓TNF-α; ↓IL-1β; ↓IL-12	Wang et al. (2010)
Morin	DENA-induced hepatocarcinogenesis in male Wistar rats	↓hepatic ultra-structural changes	↓COX-2; ↓NF-κB; ↓p-Akt; ↓Akt	Sivaramakrishnan and Devaraj (2009, 2010)
Perillyl alcohol	DENA-induced hepatocarcinogenesis in male F344 rats	↓tumor	↑M6P/IGF-IIR; ↑TGF-β; ↑TGF-βB I, II, IIIR	Mills et al. (1995)
Pomegranate phytochemicals	DENA-initiated and PB-promoted hepatocarcinogenesis in male Sprague-Dawley rats	↓GST-P-positive foci; ↓hepatic nodules	↓iNOS; ↓COX-2; ↓NF-κB	Bishayee et al. (2011b, 2013b)
Resveratrol	DENA-initiated and PB-promoted hepatocarcinogenesis in male Sprague-Dawley rats	↓hepatic nodules	↓iNOS; ↓COX-2; ↓NF-κB; ↑TNF-α; ↑IL-1β; ↑IL-6	Bishayee and Dhir (2009), Bishayee et al. (2010b, c), Mbimba et al. (2012)
Saikosaponin-d	DENA-initiated hepatocarcinogenesis in Sprague-Dawley rats	↓hepatic nodules	↓COX-2; ↓C/EBPβ	Lu et al. (2012)
Silibin	HuH7 xenograft in nude mice	↓tumor growth	↓PTEN/p-Akt; ↓ERK; ↓NF-κB	Cui et al. (2009)

(continued)

Table 16.1 (continued)

Agents	Experimental models	Anti-hepatocarcinogenic effects	Anti-inflammatory mechanisms	References
Silymarin	DENA-initiated hepatocarcinogenesis in Wistar male albino rats	↓hepatic nodules	↓COX-2	Ramakrishnan et al. (2006, 2008)
Synthetic agents				
Acyclic retinoid	DENA-induced hepatocarcinogenesis in male *db/db* mice	↓hepatic adenoma	↓TNF-α; ↓IL-1β; ↓IL-6; ↓pERK	Shimizu et al. (2011b)
Aspirin	DENA- and NMOR-induced metastatic HCC in male F344 rats	↓metastasis	↓COX-2	Futakuchi et al. (2002)
Celecoxib	DENA-initiated and 2-AAF-promoted hepatocarcinogenesis in male Sprague-Dawley rats	↓GGT-positive foci	↓Translocation of NF-κB; ↑IκB-α	Márquez-Rosado et al. (2005)
Etodolac	Spontaneously developed HCC in male fatty liver Shionogi mice	↓HCC nodules	↓PGE2	Liu et al. (2006)
Fenretinide	DENA-initiated and 2-AAF-promoted hepatocarcinogenesis in male F344 rats	↓GST-P-positive foci; ↓hepatic nodules and HCCs	↓iNOS; ↑IκB; ↓NF-κB	Simile et al. (2005)
JTE-522	CDAA-induced hepatocarcinogenesis in male Wistar rats	↓GST-P-positive foci; ↓HCC	↓COX-2; ↓PGE2	Yamamoto et al. (2003)
Nimesulide	CDAA-induced hepatocarcinogenesis in male F344 rats	↓GST-P-positive foci; ↓hepatic nodules; ↓HCC	↓COX-2	Denda et al. 2002

(continued)

Table 16.1 (continued)

Agents	Experimental models	Anti-hepatocarcinogenic effects	Anti-inflammatory mechanisms	References
Pitavastatin	DENA-induced hepatocarcinogenesis in male *db/db* mice	↓preneoplastic foci	↓TNF-α; ↓IL-6	Shimizu et al. (2011c)
Roxithromycin	DENA-induced hepatocarcinogenesis in male Wistar rats	↓tumor volume	↓iNOS; ↓NF-κB	Ueno et al. (2005)
SC-236	CDE-induced hepatocarcinogenesis in C57Bl/6 J mice	↓dysplastic lesions; ↓foci; ↓nodular lesions	↓COX-2	Davies et al. (2006)
Sodium selenite	DENA-initiated and 2-AAF-promoted hepatocarcinogenesis in male Sprague-Dawley rats	Reversed histopathological alterations	↓NF-κB	Alwahaibi et al. (2010)
S-trans-trans-farnesylthiosalicylic acid	DENA-induced hepatocarcinogenesis in male Wistar rats	↓hepatic nodules; ↓GST-P-expressing hepatocytes	↓Ras membrane activity; ↓NF-κB; ↓STAT3	Schneider-Merck et al. (2009), Stärkel et al. (2012)
TNP-470	DENA-initiated and 2-AAF-promoted hepatocarcinogenesis in male Wistar rats	↓GST-P; ↓dysplastic nodules	↓iNOS; ↑IκB; ↓NF-κB	Mauriz et al. (2003)

↓, decrease or downregulation; ↑, increase or upregulation

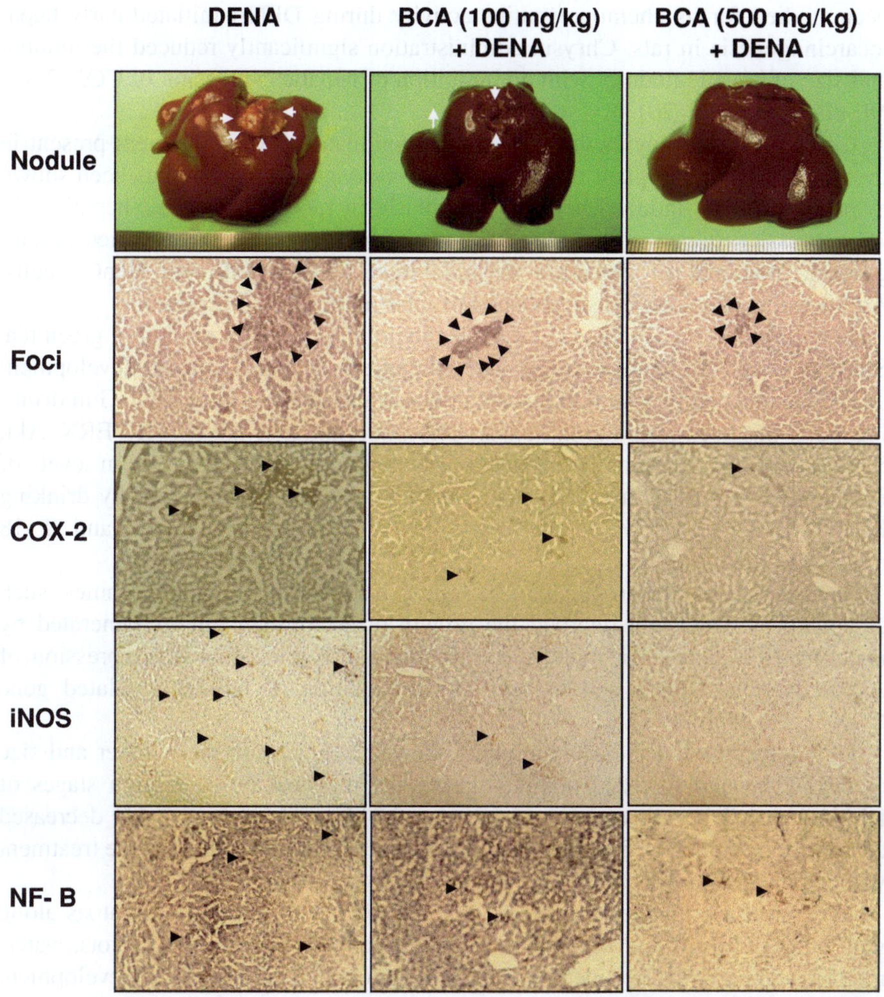

Fig. 16.1 Anti-inflammatory mechanisms implicated in the chemoprevention of rat liver carcinogenesis by black currant anthrocyanins (BCA). Male Sprague-Dawley rats were subjected to diethylnitrosamine (DENA) hepatocarcinogenesis. Rats were treated with BCA in diet (equivalent to 100 or 500 mg/kg body weight), starting the treatment 4 weeks before DENA administration and continued for 18 consecutive weeks following the carcinogenic exposure. Rats were sacrificed 22 weeks following the commencement of the study, and livers were subjected to morphological, histochemical, and immunohistochemical analysis. Chemoprevention of hepatocarcinogenesis by BCA was evidenced by reduced size of macroscopic hepatic nodules (indicated by *white arrows*) and microscopic gamma-glutamyl transpeptidase-positive preneoplastic hepatic foci (indicated by *black arrows*) in various rat groups (magnification: 100x). BCA downregulated hepatic expression of cyclooxygenase-2 (COX-2) and inducible nitric oxide synthase (iNOS) in cytoplasm and reduced the nuclear expression of nuclear factor-kappaB (NF-κB) in a dose-responsive manner, indicating suppression of inflammatory cascade. Reproduced from Bishayee et al. (2011a, 2013a), and Thoppil et al. (2012) with permission

been studied for its chemopreventive activity during DENA-initiated early hepatocarcinogenesis in rats. Chrysin administration significantly reduced the number and size of hepatic nodules with an inhibition of hepatic expression of COX-2 and NF-κB (Khan et al. 2011).

Curcumin (diferuloylmethane) is the predominant active component present in the roots of perennial plant turmeric (*Curcuma longa*). Curcumin has been shown to prevent DENA-induced hepatic hyperplasia in rats with reduced hepatic NF-κB expression (Chuang et al. 2000). Yoysungnoen et al. (2006) reported antiangiogenic potential of curcumin in nude mice xenografted with HepG2 cells. Additional studies showed suppression of intratumor COX-2 expression.

Epigallocatechin-3-gallate (EGCG) is the primary catechin present in green tea. Shimizu et al. (2011a) have investigated the effects of EGCG on the development of DENA-induced liver tumorigenesis in obese and diabetic mice. EGCG in drinking water has been found to inhibit the phosphorylation of the IGF-IR, ERK, Akt, STAT3, and JNK proteins in the livers of experimental mice. The serum levels of insulin, IGF-I, IGF-II, free fatty acid, and TNF-α were all decreased by drinking EGCG, which also lowered the expression of TNF-α, IL-6, IL-1β, and IL-18 mRNAs in the livers.

Genistein, a phytoestrogen, can be found in soybeans and other legumes, such as chickpeas. Genistein retarded the growth of established tumors generated by injecting HepG2 cells in nude mice. Mechanistic results showed suppression of Akt activation, NF-κB activity, and downregulation of NF-κB regulated gene COX-2 (Ma et al. 2011).

Geranylgeraniol, a dietary diterpene, showed reduction in the number and size of GST-P hepatic foci and nodules during the pre- and post-initiation stages of DENA-induced hepatocarcinogenesis in rats. This study also revealed decreased cell proliferation, DNA damage, and NF-κB p65 expression following the treatment with geranylgeraniol (Espindola et al. 2005).

Lycopene, a bright red carotenoid pigment, is mostly found in tomatoes along with other red fruits and vegetables, including red bell peppers, red carrots, watermelons, and papayas. Lycopene as well as tomato extract curtailed the development of GST-P foci in DENA-initiated NASH-promoted hepatocarcinogenesis in rats. Additional results showed reduced activation of ERK and NF-κB and decrease in mRNA expression of proinflammatory cytokines, such as TNF-α, IL-1β, and IL-12 (Wang et al. 2010).

Morin (3,5,7,2′,4′-pentahydroxyflavone), a bioflavonoid, is found in red wine, almonds, figs, and Osage orange. Sivaramakrishnan and Devaraj (2009, 2010) provided evidence for morin-mediated reversal of hepatic ultra-structural changes in DENA-exposed animals via apoptosis induction through modulation of the PI3K/Akt and NF-κB signaling pathways.

Perillyl alcohol, a monoterpene, is found in lavender oil, sage, cherries, orange peel, and peppermint. Mills et al. (1995) showed that dietary perillyl alcohol treatment in rats exposed to DENA inhibited hepatic tumor growth. The mRNA levels of mannose 6-phosphate/insulin-like growth factor-II receptor (M6P/IGF-IIR), and TGF β type I, II, and III receptors (TGF-β I, II, III R) were also significantly increased in the liver tumors of perillyl alcohol-treated rats.

Our laboratory has demonstrated that a pomegranate-based formulation containing various phytochemicals, including caffeic acid, gallic acid, and ellagic acid, exerts a striking chemopreventive activity in rats subjected to DENA-PB hepatocarcinogenesis as evidenced by reduced incidence, number, multiplicity, size, and volume of hepatocyte nodules as well as GGT-positive focal number and area (Bishayee et al. 2011b). We have also reported that pomegranate bioactive phytoconstituents are capable of suppressing DENA-induced inflammatory cascade by reversing the elevated expression of iNOS, COX-2, and NF-κB during experimental hepatocellular carcinogenesis in rats (Bishayee et al. 2013b).

Resveratrol (3,4′,5-trihydroxy-*trans*-stilbene), a naturally occurring antioxidant and anti-inflammatory agent found in grapes, berries, peanuts, plums as well as red wine, has been shown to prevent the development or reduce the growth of tumors in multiple organs (Bishayee 2009). According to our study, dietary resveratrol reduced the incidence, total number, and multiplicity of hepatocyte nodules (Bishayee and Dhir 2009). Ancillary studies showed that resveratrol dose-dependently suppressed DENA-induced elevated expressions of hepatic inflammatory markers, such as iNOS, COX-2, and NF-κB, and attenuated the translocation of NF-κB to the nucleus by stabilizing IκB (Bishayee et al. 2010b, c). Additionally, we have also observed that resveratrol treatment reversed the DENA-induced alteration in the level and expression of hepatic TNF-α, IL-1β, and IL-6 (Mbimba et al. 2012).

Saikosaponin-d, a triterpene saponin, is extracted from *Bupleurum falcatum* L. (Umbelliferae). A recent study has investigated the chemopreventive potential of Saikosaponin-d against hepatocarcinogenesis and its possible molecular mechanism in vivo. The liver nodule formation, tumorous invasion to surrounding organs, and increased cellular atypia induced by DENA were markedly reduced by intraperitoneally injected saikosaponin-d. The immunohistochemical staining demonstrated that the expression of COX-2 and C/EBPβ (a protein involved in inflammation and carcinogenesis) was significantly increased in tumor cells and macrophages of liver tissue from DENA-treated rats, whereas the expression of these two proteins was markedly lowered in the saikosaponin-d plus DENA group (Lu et al. 2012).

Silymarin is a complex mixture of polyphenolic flavonoids present in the seeds of milk thistle (*Silybum marianum* L. Gaertner). Silibinin (also known as silybin) represents the major active component of silymarin. Silibinin reduced the growth transplanted HuH7 tumor through the inhibition of phosphatase and tensin homolog (PTEN)/p-Akt and ERK signaling and reduced the level of NF-κB (Cui et al. 2009). It has been showed time that both pre- and post-treatment of DENA-initiated rats with silymarin significantly inhibited the multiplicity and size of hepatic nodules (Ramakrishnan et al. 2006). A separate study from the same laboratory documented that dietary silymarin supplementation downregulated the hepatic expression of COX-2 during DENA-induced hepatic carcinogenesis (Ramakrishnan et al. 2008).

16.5.2 Synthetic Agents

Shimizu et al. (2011b) examined the effects of acyclic retinoid on the development of DENA-induced liver tumorigenesis in C57BLKS/J- +Lepr^{db}/+Lepr^{db} obese mice. The development of liver cell adenoma was significantly inhibited by acyclic retinoid which also markedly reduced the phosphorylation of ERK. The serum levels of TNF-α and the expression of levels of TNF-α, IL-1β, and IL-6 mRNA in the livers of DENA-treated mice were decreased by acyclic retinoid treatment, indicating attenuation of the chronic inflammation induced by excessive fatty deposits.

Aspirin (acetyl salicylic acid) significantly reduced the degree of highly metastatic HCC developed in rats by sequential treatment with DENA and *N*-nitrosomorpholine (NMOR). This effect was associated with aspirin-mediated downregulation of COX-2 in primary HCC (Futakuchi et al. 2002).

The chemopreventive effect of celecoxib, a specific COX-2 inhibitor, on the development of liver preneoplastic lesions in rats has been evaluated using a medium-term experimental hepatocarcinogenesis protocol. A reduction by 80 and 90 % both in the number and size of altered hepatic foci was observed in the group treated with celecoxib following carcinogen treatment, respectively. Neither COX-2 expression nor PGE2 production has been altered by the hepatocarcinogenic exposure or celecoxib treatment. Interestingly, celecoxib inhibited the translocation of Rel A/p65 to the nucleus from the cytoplasm with significant effect on stability of the repressor IκB-α (Márquez-Rosado et al. 2005).

The effect of etodolac ([±]-1,8-diethyl-1,3,4,9-tetrahydropyrano-[3,4-b] indole-1-acetic acid), a specific COX-2 inhibitor, on spontaneous development of HCC in fatty liver Shionogi mice has been evaluated. The development of HCC has been suppressed slightly in the high-dose group and suppressed markedly in the low-dose group, although the development of fatty liver has not been inhibited in either group. Plasma PGE2 levels were also decreased significantly in the low-dose group, consistent with the suppression of HCC (Liu et al. 2006).

Simile et al. (2005) have investigated the chemopreventive potential and possible mechanisms of action of fenretinide [*N*-(4-hydroxyphenyl)retinamide], a synthetic retinoid, using rats subjected to the "resistant hepatocyte" protocol that included initiation by DENA followed by 2-acetylaminofluorene (2-AAF) treatment and partial hepatectomy. Fenretinide suppressed the development of GST-P-positive foci, nodules, and HCC through inhibition of iNOS and inactivation of NF-κB.

Yamamoto et al. (2003) have investigated the inhibitory effects of JTE-522 [(4-(4-cyclohexyl-2-methyloxazol-5-yl)-2-fluorobenzenesulfonamide], a selective COX-2 inhibitor, on liver fibrosis and carcinogenesis induced by CDAA. JTE-522 significantly inhibited fibrosis and development of preneoplastic lesions in a dose-dependent manner and completely inhibited generation of cirrhosis and HCC at both low and high doses. Mechanistic studies indicated that the CDAA model displayed upregulation of several biomarkers, including COX-2 and PGE2, and increased the proportion of activated hepatic stellate cells, proliferating cell nuclear antigen index, and CD45-positive inflammatory cells in the liver. JTE-522 effectively reversed all these changes.

The chemopreventive efficacy of nimesulide, a specific COX-2 inhibitor, has been tested in CDAA-induced rat hepatocarcinogenesis. Administration of nimesulide through diet decreased the number and size of preneoplastic, enzyme-altered liver foci, multiplicity of neoplastic nodules and hepatocellular carcinomas, and prevented the development of cirrhosis with reduced expression of COX-2 (Denda et al. 2002).

The effects of pitavastatin, a drug used for the treatment of hyperlipidemia, on the development of DENA-induced liver preneoplastic lesions have been examined in C57BL/KsJ-db/db (db/db) obese mice. Feeding of animals with 10 ppm pitavastatin significantly inhibited the development of hepatic premalignant lesions (foci of cellular alteration) as compared to the untreated group through inhibition of cell proliferation and induction of apoptosis. Pitavastatin improved liver steatosis, decreased free fatty acid and aminotransferases levels, while increasing adiponectin levels in the serum. Additionally, the serum levels of TNF-α and the expression of TNF-α and IL-6 mRNAs in the liver were decreased by pitavastatin treatment (Shimizu et al. 2011c).

Roxithromycin, a macrolide antibiotic, inhibited oxidative stress as measured by the level of thiobarbituric acid-reactive substances, NO production, and activation of NF-κB during DENA-induced hepatic carcinogenesis in rats. All these results were associated with a dose-dependent inhibition of hepatic tumor volume in experimental animals (Ueno et al. 2005).

SC-236, a selective COX-2 inhibitor, has been tested for its antihepatocarcinogenic potential using a choline-deficient, ethionine-supplemented (CDE) diet-induced rodent model of HCC. The test compound not only suppressed hepatocyte peri-cellular fibrosis and steatosis, but also inhibited the early stages of HCC (Davies et al. 2006).

Sodium selenite has been found to exert chemoprevention of DENA-initiated and 2-AAF-promoted hepatocarcinogenesis in rats as evidenced from histopathological observations with simultaneous inhibition of hepatic NF-κB expression (Alwahaibi et al. 2010).

Activation of Ras and its downstream signaling pathways are likely to contribute to the development of hepatocarcinoma. It has been shown that intraperitoneal injections of the *S-trans- trans*-farnesylthiosalicylic acid (FTS), a Ras inhibitor, blocks Ras activation and prevents heptocarcinoma development in rats challenged with DENA (Schneider-Merck et al. 2009). A follow-up study from the same laboratory showed that DENA-induced activation of NF-κB and STAT3 has been abrogated by FTS treatment. Although FTS treatment showed no effect on DENA-induced elevation of TNF-α, IL-6, and TLR4, it significantly reduced phosphorylation of the MAPK p38 and of the p70S6 kinase, a surrogate marker for mTOR activation, without affecting ERK and Akt phosphorylation (Stärkel et al. 2012).

TNP-470 (*O*-chloroacetyl-carbamoyl-fumagillol) is a synthetic derivative of fumagillin, a naturally secreted antibiotic from *Aspergillus fumigatus*. The expression of GST-P was significantly reduced in rats with hepatocarcinogenesis receiving TNP-470 when compared to untreated animals. TNP-470 also inhibited oxidative stress, NO production, and NF-κB activation (Mauriz et al. 2003).

16.6 Conclusions and Future Directions

Emerging in vitro, in vivo, and clinical studies carried out during the last decade provide substantial evidence that activation of inflammatory signaling pathways plays a vital role in the pathogenesis and progression of liver cancer. It is also apparent that there are several mechanisms which contribute to the activation of inflammatory cascade in the liver in response to various etiological factors of liver cancer. There also exists the possibility of cross talk between inflammatory pathways and other signaling events in liver cancer. Since various inflammatory pathways are closely regulated at multiple cellular and subcellular levels, these pathways provide opportunities to develop novel preventive and therapeutic strategies for management of liver cancer. Based on current interest in inflammatory signaling pathways in liver cancer, it is conceivable that new signaling molecules and pathways of inflammation-linked HCC would be identified in the near future.

Several animal studies as presented in this chapter clearly demonstrate that various natural and synthetic compounds are capable of disrupting activated inflammatory signaling to halt or reverse the growth of a variety of transplanted HCC cells in vivo and inhibit the development and progression of chemically initiated, dietary-induced, or spontaneously occurring liver tumors in rodents. All these anti-hepatocarcinogenic effects could be possible due to inhibition of upstream activators of key inflammatory regulators, subunits of lead inflammatory mediators, activating kinases or target genes. The unique inflammation-hepatocarcinogenesis sequence in liver cancer clearly indicates that specific inhibitors of inflammatory pathways have the potential to block or disrupt the continuous transition from chronic liver injury to liver neoplasia. It is, indeed, noteworthy that all these structurally dissimilar compounds target nearly all known proinflammatory factors and signaling pathways in hepatic carcinogenesis. Since activation of inflammatory insult occurs during the early as well as late phases of multistage hepatocarcinogenesis, naturally occurring or synthetic anti-inflammatory agents could be effective in both chemoprevention and therapy of liver cancer.

Although a large number of preclinical and clinical studies underscore the importance of inflammation in liver cancer, the direct clinical application of this knowledge has not been fully realized. Similarly, despite the identification of a large number of natural as well as synthetic agents targeting inflammatory pathways during hepatocellular carcinogenesis, there remains a gap in the transition of these impressive results into clinical practice. Hence, future well-controlled clinical studies are needed to validate the promising preclinical results of blocking or diminishing liver cancer by interference with the inflammatory signaling by various natural and synthetic compounds. The safety of these agents also needs to be established by appropriate clinical studies. Moreover, there are certain challenges as well as limitations of targeting inflammatory signaling. Several inflammatory pathways have a wide range of functions with complex cross talk and hence may function differently during hepatocarcinogenesis based on specific cell type and disease stage. Thus, inhibition of a signaling molecule in specific cell type within the liver would be more advantageous than global inhibition of the same target. An example of this premise is NF-κB. The tumor-specific suppression of NF-κB is beneficial. Nevertheless, generalized suppression of this inflammatory regulator may result in serious host toxicity with minimum effect on the tumor (Aggarwal and Sung 2011).

As presented here, various inflammatory signaling pathways are interconnected, and liver cancer may arise due to dysregulation of multiple pathways. Thus, agents that can suppress multiple pathways simultaneously may have better potential as liver cancer preventive and therapeutic drugs. The duration of therapy with anti-inflammatory drugs is another important consideration, and it is related to the extent of liver disease. In patients with severe fibrosis, cirrhosis or HCC, certain anti-inflammatory agents may trigger toxicity due to compromised liver function. Additionally, use of anti-inflammatory drugs in patients undergoing antiviral treatment, such as interferon therapy for HCV infection, may interfere with the clinical outcome of such treatment.

In conclusion, substantial experimental and clinical evidence as presented in this chapter strongly suggests that chronic inflammation fuels the development and progression of liver cancer and various proinflammatory molecules, and signaling pathways represent novel targets for the prevention and therapy of this devastating disease.

Acknowledgements A part of our research on chemoprevention of liver cancer by anti-inflammatory phytoconstituents as presented in this review was carried out at the Northeast Ohio Medical University (Rootstown, OH). I sincerely apologize to those investigators whose contributions were not cited due to space limitation.

References

Aggarwal BB, Sung B (2011) NF-κB in cancer: a matter of life and death. Cancer Discov 1:469–471

Ahn B, Han BS, Kim DJ, Ohshima H (1999) Immunohistochemical localization of inducible nitric oxide synthase and 3-nitrotyrosine in rat liver tumors induced by *N*-nitrosodiethylamine. Carcinogenesis 20:1337–1344

Alwahaibi NY, Budin SB, Mohamed J, Alhamdani A (2010) Nuclear factor-kappa B as a promising target for selenium chemoprevention in rat hepatocarcinogenesis. J Gastroenterol Hepatol 25:786–791

Aravalli RN, Steer CJ, Cressman EN (2008) Molecular mechanisms of hepatocellular carcinoma. Hepatology 48:2047–2063

Aravalli RN, Cressman EN, Steer CJ (2013) Cellular and molecular mechanisms of hepatocellular carcinoma: an update. Arch Toxicol 87:227–247

Aravindaram K, Yang NS (2010) Anti-inflammatory plant natural products for cancer therapy. Planta Med 76:1103–1117

Arsura M, Cavin LG (2005) Nuclear factor-kappaB and liver carcinogenesis. Cancer Lett 229:157–169
Avila MA, Berasain C, Sangro B, Prieto J (2006) New therapies for hepatocellular carcinoma. Oncogene 25:3866–3884
Bard-Chapeau EA, Li S, Ding J, Zhang SS, Zhu HH, Princen F, Fang DD, Han T, Bailly-Maitre B, Poli V, Varki NM, Wang H, Feng GS (2011) Ptpn11/Shp2 acts as a tumor suppressor in hepatocellular carcinogenesis. Cancer Cell 19:629–639
Bartel DP (2004) MicroRNAs: genomics, biogenesis, mechanism, and function. Cell 116:281–297
Bartsch H, Montesano R (1984) Relevance of nitrosamines to human cancer. Carcinogenesis 5:1381–1393
Berasain C, García-Trevijano ER, Castillo J, Erroba E, Lee DC, Prieto J, Avila MA (2005) Amphiregulin: an early trigger of liver regeneration in mice. Gastroenterology 128:424–432
Berasain C, Castillo J, Prieto J, Avila MA (2007) New molecular targets for hepatocellular carcinoma: the ErbB1 signaling system. Liver Int 27:174–185
Berasain C, Castillo J, Perugorria MJ, Latasa MU, Prieto J, Avila MA (2009a) Inflammation and liver cancer: new molecular links. Ann N Y Acad Sci 1155:206–221
Berasain C, Perugorria MJ, Latasa MU, Castillo J, Goñi S, Santamaría M, Prieto J, Avila MA (2009b) The epidermal growth factor receptor: a link between inflammation and liver cancer. Exp Biol Med 234:713–725
Bishayee A (2009) Cancer prevention and treatment with resveratrol: from rodent studies to clinical trials. Cancer Prev Res 2:409–418
Bishayee A (2012) Editorial: recent advances in the prevention and therapy of hepatocellular carcinoma. Curr Cancer Drug Targets 12:1043–1044
Bishayee A (2013) β-Catenin: a novel biomarker and therapeutic target in liver cancer. In: Georgakilas A (ed) Cancer biomarkers. CRC Press, Boca Raton, pp 51–75
Bishayee A, Dhir N (2009) Resveratrol-mediated chemoprevention of diethylnitrosamine-initiated hepatocarcinogenesis: inhibition of cell proliferation and induction of apoptosis. Chem Biol Interact 179:131–144
Bishayee A, Politis T, Darvesh AS (2010a) Resveratrol in the chemoprevention and treatment of hepatocellular carcinoma. Cancer Treat Rev 36:43–53
Bishayee A, Waghray A, Barnes KF, Mbimba T, Bhatia D, Chatterjee M, Darvesh AS (2010b) Suppression of the inflammatory cascade is implicated in resveratrol chemoprevention of experimental hepatocarcinogenesis. Pharm Res 27:1080–1091
Bishayee A, Barnes KF, Bhatia D, Darvesh AS, Carroll RT (2010c) Resveratrol suppresses oxidative stress and inflammatory response in diethylnitrosamine-initiated rat hepatocarcinogenesis. Cancer Prev Res 3:753–763
Bishayee A, Mbimba T, Thoppil RJ, Háznagy-Radnai E, Sipos P, Darvesh AS, Folkesson H, Hohmann J (2011a) Anthocyanin-rich black currant (*Ribes nigrum* L.) extract affords chemoprevention against diethylnitrosamine-induced hepatocellular carcinogenesis in rats. J Nutr Biochem 22:1035–1046
Bishayee A, Bhatia D, Thoppil RJ, Darvesh AS, Nevo E, Lansky EP (2011b) Pomegranate-mediated chemoprevention of experimental hepatocarcinogenesis involves Nrf2-regulated antioxidant mechanisms. Carcinogenesis 32:888–896
Bishayee A, Thoppil RJ, Waghray A, Kruse JA, Novotny NA, Darvesh AS (2012) Dietary phytochemicals in the chemoprevention and treatment of hepatocellular carcinoma: in vivo evidence, molecular targets, and clinical relevance. Curr Cancer Drug Targets 12:1191–1232
Bishayee A, Thoppil RJ, Mandal A, Darvesh AS, Ohanyan V, Meszaros JG, Háznagy-Radnai E, Hohmann J, Bhatia D (2013a) Black currant phytoconstituents exert chemoprevention of diethylnitrosamine-initiated hepatocarcinogenesis by suppression of the inflammatory response. Mol Carcinog 52:304–317
Bishayee A, Thoppil RJ, Darvesh AS, Ohanyan V, Meszaros JG, Bhatia D (2013b) Pomegranate phytoconstituents blunt the inflammatory cascade in a chemically induced rodent model of hepatocellular carcinogenesis. J Nutr Biochem 24:178–187

Blonski W, Kotlyar DS, Forde KA (2010) Non-viral causes of hepatocellular carcinoma. World J Gastroenterol 16:3603–3615
Braconi C, Henry JC, Kogure T, Schmittgen T, Patel T (2011) The role of microRNAs in human liver cancers. Semin Onccol 38:752–763
Brownell J, Polyak SJ (2013) Molecular pathways: hepatitis C virus, CXCL10, and the inflammatory road to liver cancer. Clin Cancer Res 19:1347–1352
Budhu A, Wang XW (2006) The role of cytokines in hepatocellular carcinoma. J Leukoc Biol 80:1197–1213
Calvisi DF, Ladu S, Gorden A, Farina M, Conner EA, Lee JS, Factor VM, Thorgeirsson SS (2006) Ubiquitous activation of Ras and Jak/Stat pathways in human HCC. Gastroenterology 130:1117–1128
Calvisi DF, Pinna F, Ladu S, Pellegrino R, Muroni MR, Simile MM, Frau M, Tomasi ML, De Miglio MR, Seddaiu MA, Daino L, Sanna V, Feo F, Pascale RM (2008) Aberrant iNOS signaling is under genetic control in rodent liver cancer and potentially prognostic for the human disease. Carcinogenesis 29:1639–1647
Castillo J, Erroba E, Perugorría MJ, Santamaría M, Lee DC, Prieto J, Avila MA, Berasain C (2006) Amphiregulin contributes to the transformed phenotype of human hepatocellular carcinoma cells. Cancer Res 66:6129–6138
Center MM, Jemal A (2011) International trends in liver cancer incidence rates. Cancer Epidemiol Biomarkers Prev 20:2362–2368
Cervello M, Montalto G (2006) Cyclooxygenases in hepatocellular carcinoma. World J Gastroenterol 12:5113–5121
Cheng AL, Kang YK, Chen Z, Tsao CJ, Qin S, Kim JS, Luo R, Feng J, Ye S, Yang TS, Xu J, Sun Y, Liang H, Liu J, Wang J, Tak WY, Pan H, Burock K, Zou J, Voliotis D, Guan Z (2009) Efficacy and safety of sorafenib in patients in the Asia-Pacific region with advanced hepatocellular carcinoma: a phase III randomised, double-blind, placebo-controlled trial. Lancet Oncol 10:25–34
Chiang SH, Bazuine M, Lumeng CN, Geletka LM, Mowers J, White NM, Ma JT, Zhou J, Qi N, Westcott D, Delproposto JB, Blackwell TS, Yull FE, Saltiel AR (2009) The protein kinase IKKepsilon regulates energy balance in obese mice. Cell 138:961–975
Chuang SE, Cheng AL, Lin JK, Kuo ML (2000) Inhibition by curcumin of diethylnitrosamine-induced hepatic hyperplasia, inflammation, cellular gene products and cell-cycle-related proteins in rats. Food Chem Toxicol 38:991–995
Chuma M, Hige S, Nakanishi M, Ogawa K, Natsuizaka M, Yamamoto Y, Asaka M (2008) 8-Hydroxy-2'-deoxy-guanosine is a risk factor for development of hepatocellular carcinoma in patients with chronic hepatitis C virus infection. J Gastroenterol Hepatol 23:1431–1436
Costa RH, Kalinichenko VV, Holterman AX, Wang X (2003) Transcription factors in liver development, differentiation, and regeneration. Hepatology 38:1331–1347
Coussens LM, Werb Z (2002) Inflammation and cancer. Nature 420:860–867
Cui W, Gu F, Hu K (2009) Effects and mechanisms of silibinin on human hepatocellular carcinoma xenografts in nude mice. World J Gastroenterol 15:1943–1950
Dajani OF, Meisdalen K, Guren TK, Aasrum M, Tveteraas IH, Lilleby P, Thoresen GH, Sandnes D, Christoffersen T (2008) Prostaglandin E2 upregulates EGF-stimulated signaling in mitogenic pathways involving Akt and ERK in hepatocytes. J Cell Physiol 214:371–380
Darnell JE Jr, Kerr IM, Stark GR (1994) Jak-STAT pathways and transcriptional activation in response to IFNs and other extracellular signaling proteins. Science 264:1415–1421
Darvesh AS, Bishayee A (2010) Selenium in the prevention and treatment of hepatocellular carcinoma. Anticancer Agents Med Chem 10:338–345
Darvesh AS, Bishayee A (2013) Chemopreventive and therapeutic potential of tea polyphenols in hepatocellular cancer. Nutr Cancer 65:329–344
Darvesh AS, Aggarwal BB, Bishayee A (2012) Curcumin and liver cancer: a review. Curr Pharm Biotechnol 13:218–228
Davies RA, Knight B, Tian YW, Yeoh GC, Olynyk JK (2006) Hepatic oval cell response to the choline-deficient, ethionine supplemented model of murine liver injury is attenuated by the administration of a cyclo-oxygenase 2 inhibitor. Carcinogenesis 27:1607–1616

de Almagro MC, Vucic D (2012) The inhibitor of apoptosis (IAP) proteins are critical regulators of signaling pathways and targets for anti-cancer therapy. Exp Oncol 34:200–211

Denda A, Kitayama W, Murata A, Kishida H, Sasaki Y, Kusuoka O, Tsujiuchi T, Tsutsumi M, Nakae D, Takagi H, Konishi Y (2002) Increased expression of cyclooxygenase-2 protein during rat hepatocarcinogenesis caused by a choline-deficient, L-amino acid-defined diet and chemopreventive efficacy of a specific inhibitor, nimesulide. Carcinogenesis 23:245–256

Denda A, Kitayama W, Kishida H, Murata N, Tamura K, Kusuoka O, Tsutsumi M, Nishikawa F, Kita E, Nakae D, Konishi Y, Kuniyasu H (2007) Expression of inducible nitric oxide (NO) synthase but not prevention by its gene ablation of hepatocarcinogenesis with fibrosis caused by a choline-deficient, L-amino acid-defined diet in rats and mice. Nitric Oxide 16:164–176

Demaria S, Pikarsky E, Karin M, Coussens LM, Chen YC, El-Omar EM, Trinchieri G, Dubinett SM, Mao JT, Szabo E, Krieg A, Weiner GJ, Fox BA, Coukos G, Wang E, Abraham RT, Carbone M, Lotze MT (2010) Cancer and inflammation: promise for biologic therapy. J Immunother 33:335–351

Deviere J, Content J, Denys C, Vandenbussche P, Schandene L, Wybran J, Dupont E (1989) High interleukin-6 serum levels and increased production by leucocytes in alcoholic liver cirrhosis. Correlation with IgA serum levels and lymphokines production. Clin Exp Immunol 77:221–225

Donath MY, Shoelson SE (2011) Type 2 diabetes as an inflammatory disease. Nat Rev Immunol 11:98–107

DiDonato JA, Mercurio F, Karin M (2012) NF-κB and the link between inflammation and cancer. Immunol Rev 246:379–400

Dutkowski P, De Rougemont O, Müllhaupt B, Clavien PA (2010) Current and future trends in liver transplantation in Europe. Gastroenterology 138:802–809

El-Serag HB (2004) Hepatocellular carcinoma: recent trends in the United States. Gastroenterology 127:S27–S34

El-Serag HB, Hampel H, Javadi F (2006) The association between diabetes and hepatocellular carcinoma: a systematic review of epidemiologic evidence. Clin Gastroenterol Hepatol 4:369–380

El-Serag HB, Rudolph KL (2007) Hepatocellular carcinoma: epidemiology and molecular carcinogenesis. Gastroenterology 132:2557–2576

Espindola RM, Mazzantini RP, Ong TP, de Conti A, Heidor R, Moreno FS (2005) Geranylgeraniol and β-ionone inhibit hepatic preneoplastic lesions, cell proliferation, total plasma cholesterol and DNA damage during the initial phases of hepatocarcinogenesis, but only the former inhibits NF-κB activation. Carcinogenesis 26:1091–1099

Farazi PA, DePinho RA (2006) Hepatocellular carcinoma pathogenesis: from genes to environment. Nat Rev Cancer 6:674–687

Futakuchi M, Ogawa K, Sano M, Tamano S, Takeshita F, Shirai T (2002) Suppression of lung metastasis by aspirin but not indomethacin in an in vivo model of chemically induced hepatocellular carcinoma. Jpn J Cancer Res 93:1175–1181

Gao J, Xie L, Yang WS, Zhang W, Gao S, Wang J, Xiang YB (2012) Risk factors of hepatocellular carcinoma: current status and perspectives. Asian Pac J Cancer Prev 13:743–752

Ghosh S, Karin M (2002) Missing pieces in the NF-κB puzzle. Cell 109:S81–S96

Giannitrapani L, Ingrao S, Soresi M, Florena AM, La Spada E, Sandonato L, D'Alessandro N, Cervello M, Montalto G (2009) Cyclooxygenase-2 expression in chronic liver diseases and hepatocellular carcinoma: an immunohistochemical study. Ann NY Acad Sci 1155:293–299

Gramantieri L, Fornari F, Callegari E, Sabbioni S, Lanza G, Croce CM, Bolondi L, Negrini M (2008) MicroRNA involvement in hepatocellular carcinoma. J Cell Mol Med 12:2189–2204

Gregor MF, Hotamisligil GS (2011) Inflammatory mechanisms in obesity. Annu Rev Immunol 29:415–445

Grivennikov SI, Greten FR, Karin M (2010) Immunity, inflammation, and cancer. Cell 140:883–899

Gupta SC, Kim JH, Prasad S, Aggarwal BB (2010) Regulation of survival, proliferation, invasion, angiogenesis, and metastasis of tumor cells through modulation of inflammatory pathways by nutraceuticals. Cancer Metastasis Rev 29:405–434

Guicciardi ME, Mott JL, Bronk SF, Kurita S, Fingas CD, Gores GJ (2011) Cellular inhibitor of apoptosis 1 (cIAP-1) degradation by caspase 8 during TNF-related apoptosis-inducing ligand (TRAIL)-induced apoptosis. Exp Cell Res 317:107–116

Gyrd-Hansen M, Meier P (2010) IAPs: from caspase inhibitors to modulators of NF-kappaB, inflammation and cancer. Nat Rev Cancer 10:561–574

Han YP, Zhou L, Wang J, Xiong S, Garner WL, French SW, Tsukamoto H (2004) Essential role of matrix metalloproteinases in interleukin-1-induced myofibroblastic activation of hepatic stellate cell in collagen. J Biol Chem 279:4820–4828

Han C, Michalopoulos GK, Wu T (2006) Prostaglandin E2 receptor EP1 transactivates EGFR/MET receptor tyrosine kinases and enhances invasiveness in human hepatocellular carcinoma cells. J Cell Physiol 207:261–270

Hatziapostolou M, Polytarchou C, Aggelidou E, Drakaki A, Poultsides GA, Jaeger SA, Ogata H, Karin M, Struhl K, Hadzopoulou-Cladaras M, Iliopoulos D (2011) An HNF4α-miRNA inflammatory feedback circuit regulates hepatocellular oncogenesis. Cell 147:1233–1247

Haybaeck J, Zeller N, Wolf MJ, Weber A, Wagner U, Kurrer MO, Bremer J, Iezzi G, Graf R, Clavien PA, Thimme R, Blum H, Nedospasov SA, Zatloukal K, Ramzan M, Ciesek S, Pietschmann T, Marche PN, Karin M, Kopf M, Browning JL, Aguzzi A, Heikenwalder M (2009) A lymphotoxin-driven pathway to hepatocellular carcinoma. Cancer Cell 16:295–308

Heydtmann M, Adams DH (2009) Chemokines in the immunopathogenesis of hepatitis C infection. Hepatology 49:676–688

He G, Karin M (2011) NF-κB and STAT3: key players in liver inflammation and cancer. Cell Res 21:159–168

He G, Yu GY, Temkin V, Ogata H, Kuntzen C, Sakurai T, Sieghart W, Peck-Radosavljevic M, Leffert HL, Karin M (2010) Hepatocyte IKKbeta/NF-kappaB inhibits tumor promotion and progression by preventing oxidative stress-driven STAT3 activation. Cancer Cell 17:286–297

Hoffmann A, Baltimore D (2006) Circuitry of nuclear factor kappaB signaling. Immunol Rev 210:171–186

Hoshida Y, Toffanin S, Lachenmayer A, Villanueva A, Minguez B, Llovet JM (2010) Molecular classification and novel targets in hepatocellular carcinoma: recent advancements. Semin Liver Dis 30:35–51

Huang F, Geng XP (2010) Chemokines and hepatocellular carcinoma. World J Gastroenterol 16:1832–1836

Huynh H (2010) Molecularly targeted therapy in hepatocellular carcinoma. Biochem Pharmacol 80:550–560

Je Y, Schutz FAB, Choueiri TK (2009) Risk of bleeding with vascular endothelial growth factor receptor tyrosine-kinase inhibitors sunitinib and sorafenib: a systematic review and meta-analysis of clinical trials. Lancet Oncol 10:967–974

Ji J, Shi J, Budhu A, Yu Z, Forgues M, Roessler S, Ambs S, Chen Y, Meltzer PS, Croce CM, Qin LX, Man K, Lo CM, Lee J, Ng IO, Fan J, Tang ZY, Sun HC, Wang XW (2009) MicroRNA expression, survival, and response to interferon in liver cancer. N Engl J Med 361:1437–147

Karin M (2009) NF-kappaB as a critical link between inflammation and cancer. Cold Spring Harb Perspect Biol 1:a000141

Karin M, Ben-Neriah Y (2000) Phosphorylation meets ubiquitination: the control of NF-κB activity. Annu Rev Immunol 18:621–663

Kawanishi S, Hiraku Y, Pinlaor S, Ma N (2006) Oxidative and nitrative DNA damage in animals and patients with inflammatory diseases in relation to inflammation-related carcinogenesis. Biol Chem 387:365–372

Kenya PR (1990) Oral contraceptives use and liver tumours: a review. East Afr Med J 67:146–153

Khan MS, Devaraj H, Devaraj N (2011) Chrysin abrogates early hepatocarcinogenesis and induces apoptosis in *N*-nitrosodiethylamine-induced preneoplastic nodules in rats. Toxicol Appl Pharmacol 251:85–94

Kim SF, Huri DA, Snyder SH (2005) Inducible nitric oxide synthase binds, *S*-nitrosylates, and activates cyclooxygenase-2. Science 310:1966–1970
Kim YS, Young MR, Bobe G, Colburn NH, Milner JA (2009) Bioactive food components, inflammatory targets, and cancer prevention. Cancer Prev Res 2:200–208
Kota J, Chivukula RR, O'Donnell KA, Wentzel EA, Montgomery CL, Hwang HW, Chang TC, Vivekanandan P, Torbenson M, Clark KR, Mendell JR, Mendell JT (2009) Therapeutic microRNA delivery suppresses tumorigenesis in a murine liver cancer model. Cell 137:1005–1017
Kuo PC, Abe KY, Schroeder RA (1997) Oxidative stress increases hepatocyte iNOS gene transcription and promoter activity. Biochem Biophys Res Commun 234:289–292
Korula J, Yellin A, Kanel G, Campofiori G, Nichols P (1991) Hepatocellular carcinoma coexisting with hepatic adenoma. Incidental discovery after long-term oral contraceptive use. West J Med 155:416–418
Lachenmayer A, Alsinet C, Chang CY, Llovet JM (2010) Molecular approaches to treatment of hepatocellular carcinoma. Dig Liver Dis 42:S264–S272
Lang K, Danchenko N, Gondek K, Shah S, Thompson D (2009) The burden of illness associated with hepatocellular carcinoma in the United States. J Hepatol 50:89–99
Larsson SC, Wolk A (2007) Overweight, obesity and risk of liver cancer: a meta-analysis of cohort studies. Br J Cancer 97:1005–1008
Lee Y, Park US, Choi I, Yoon SK, Park YM, Lee YI (1998) Human interleukin 6 gene is activated by hepatitis B virus-X protein in human hepatoma cells. Clin Cancer Res 4:1711–1717
Lee H, Herrmann A, Deng JH, Kujawski M, Niu G, Li Z, Forman S, Jove R, Pardoll DM, Yu H (2009) Persistently activated Stat3 maintains constitutive NF-kappaB activity in tumors. Cancer Cell 15:283–293
Liu W, Nakamura H, Tsujimura T, Cheng J, Yamamoto T, Iwamoto Y, Imanishi H, Shimomura S, Yamamoto T, Hirasawa T, Inagaki S, Nishiguchi S, Hada T (2006) Chemoprevention of spontaneous development of hepatocellular carcinomas in fatty liver Shionogi mice by a cyclooxygenase-2 inhibitor. Cancer Sci 97:768–773
Llovet JM, Ricci S, Mazzaferro V, Hilgard P, Gane E, Blanc JF, de Oliveira AC, Santoro A, Raoul JL, Forner A, Schwartz M, Porta C, Zeuzem S, Bolondi L, Greten TF, Galle PR, Seitz JF, Borbath I, Häussinger D, Giannaris T, Shan M, Moscovici M, Voliotis D, Bruix J, SHARP Investigators Study Group (2008) Sorafenib in advanced hepatocellular carcinoma. N Engl J Med 359:378–390
Lu SC (2010) Where are we in the chemoprevention of hepatocellular carcinoma? Hepatology 51:734–736
Lu XL, He SX, Ren MD, Wang YL, Zhang YX, Liu EQ (2012) Chemopreventive effect of saikosaponin-d on diethylinitrosamine-induced hepatocarcinogenesis: involvement of CCAAT/enhancer binding protein β and cyclooxygenase-2. Mol Med Rep 5:637–644
Luedde T, Schwabe RF (2011) NF-κB in the liver: linking injury, fibrosis and hepatocellular carcinoma. Nat Rev Gastroenterol Hepatol 8:108–118
Luedde T, Beraza N, Kotsikoris V, van Loo G, Nenci A, De Vos R, Roskams T, Trautwein C, Pasparakis M (2007) Deletion of NEMO/IKKgamma in liver parenchymal cells causes steatohepatitis and hepatocellular carcinoma. Cancer Cell 11:119–132
Ma Y, Wang J, Liu L, Zhu H, Chen X, Pan S, Sun X, Jiang H (2011) Genistein potentiates the effect of arsenic trioxide against human hepatocellular carcinoma: role of Akt and nuclear factor-κB. Cancer Lett 301:75–84
Maeda S, Kamata H, Luo JL, Leffert H, Karin M (2005) IKKβ couples hepatocyte death to cytokine-driven compensatory proliferation that promotes chemical hepatocarcinogenesis. Cell 121:977–990
Maeda S, Hikiba Y, Sakamoto K, Nakagawa H, Hirata Y, Hayakawa Y, Yanai A, Ogura K, Karin M, Omata M (2009) Ikappa B kinasebeta/nuclear factor-kappaB activation controls the development of liver metastasis by way of interleukin-6 expression. Hepatology 50:1851-1860
Maione D, Di Carlo E, Li W, Musiani P, Modesti A, Peters M, Rose-John S, Della Rocca C, Tripodi M, Lazzaro D, Taub R, Savino R, Ciliberto G (1998) Coexpression of IL-6 and

soluble IL-6R causes nodular regenerative hyperplasia and adenomas of the liver. EMBO J 17:5588–5597
Mantovani A, Allavena P, Sica A, Balkwill F (2008) Cancer-related inflammation. Nature 454:436–444
Markiewski MM, DeAngelis RA, Lambris JD (2006) Liver inflammation and regeneration: two distinct biological phenomena or parallel pathophysiologic processes? Mol Immunol 43:45–56
Márquez-Rosado L, Trejo-Solís MC, García-Cuéllar CM, Villa-Treviño S (2005) Celecoxib, a cyclooxygenase-2 inhibitor, prevents induction of liver preneoplastic lesions in rats. J Hepatol 43:653–660
Marra M, Sordelli IM, Lombardi A, Lamberti M, Tarantino L, Giudice A, Stiuso P, Abbruzzese A, Sperlongano R, Accardo M, Agresti M, Caraglia M, Sperlongano P (2011) Molecular targets and oxidative stress biomarkers in hepatocellular carcinoma: an overview. J Transl Med 9:171
Marrero CR, Marrero JA (2007) Viral hepatitis and hepatocellular carcinoma. Arch Med Res 38:612–620
Matsuzaki K, Murata M, Yoshida K, Sekimoto G, Uemura Y, Sakaida N, Kaibori M, Kamiyama Y, Nishizawa M, Fujisawa J, Okazaki K, Seki T (2007) Chronic inflammation associated with hepatitis C virus infection perturbs hepatic transforming growth factor beta signaling, promoting cirrhosis and hepatocellular carcinoma. Hepatology 46:48–57
Mauad TH, van Nieuwkerk CM, Dingemans KP, Smit JJ, Schinkel AH, Notenboom RG, van den Bergh Weerman MA, Verkruisen RP, Groen AK, Oude Elferink RP et al (1994) Mice with homozygous disruption of the mdr2 P-glycoprotein gene. A novel animal model for studies of nonsuppurative inflammatory cholangitis and hepatocarcinogenesis. Am J Pathol 145:1237–1245
Mauriz JL, Linares P, Macias RI, Jorquera F, Honrado E, Olcoz JL, González P, González-Gallego J (2003) TNP-470 inhibits oxidative stress, nitric oxide production and nuclear factor kappa B activation in a rat model of hepatocellular carcinoma. Free Radic Res 37:841–848
Mbimba T, Awale P, Bhatia D, Geldenhuys WJ, Darvesh AS, Carroll RT, Bishayee A (2012) Alteration of hepatic proinflammatory cytokines is involved in the resveratrol-mediated chemoprevention of chemically-induced hepatocarcinogenesis. Curr Pharm Biotechnol 13:229–234
McNaughton L, Puttagunta L, Martinez-Cuesta MA, Kneteman N, Mayers I, Moqbel R, Hamid Q, Radomski MW (2002) Distribution of nitric oxide synthase in normal and cirrhotic human liver. Proc Natl Acad Sci USA 99:17161–17166
Mehrotra S, Languino LR, Raskett CM, Mercurio AM, Dohi T, Altieri DC (2010) IAP regulation of metastasis. Cancer Cell 17:53–64
Mills JJ, Chari RS, Boyer IJ, Gould MN, Jirtle RL (1995) Induction of apoptosis in liver tumors by the monoterpene perillyl alcohol. Cancer Res 55:979–983
Ming L, Thorgeirsson SS, Gail MH, Lu P, Harris CC, Wang N, Shao Y, Wu Z, Liu G, Wang X, Sun Z (2002) Dominant role of hepatitis B virus and cofactor role of aflatoxin in hepatocarcinogenesis in Qidong, China. Hepatology 36:1214–1220
Murakami A (2009) Chemoprevention with phytochemicals targeting inducible nitric oxide synthase. Forum Nutr 61:193–203
Muriel P (2009) NF-kappaB in liver diseases: a target for drug therapy. J Appl Toxicol 29:91–100
Murillo MM, Carmona-Cuenca I, Del Castillo G, Ortiz C, Roncero C, Sánchez A, Fernández M, Fabregat I (2007) Activation of NADPH oxidase by transforming growth factor-beta in hepatocytes mediates up-regulation of epidermal growth factor receptor ligands through a nuclear factor-kappaB-dependent mechanism. Biochem J 405:251–259
Murugan RS, Priyadarsini RV, Ramalingam K, Hara Y, Karunagaran D, Nagini S (2010) Intrinsic apoptosis and NF-κB signaling are potential molecular targets for chemoprevention by black tea polyphenols in HepG2 cells in vitro and in a rat hepatocarcinogenesis model in vivo. Food Chem Toxicol 48:3281–3287

Nakagawa H, Maeda S (2012) Inflammation- and stress-related signaling pathways in hepatocarcinogenesis. World J Gastroenterol 18:4071–4081

Nakagawa H, Maeda S, Yoshida H, Tateishi R, Masuzaki R, Ohki T, Hayakawa Y, Kinoshita H, Yamakado M, Kato N, Shiina S, Omata M (2009) Serum IL-6 levels and the risk for hepatocarcinogenesis in chronic hepatitis C patients: an analysis based on gender differences. Int J Cancer 125:2264–2269

Nair S, Mason A, Eason J, Loss G, Perrillo RP (2002) Is obesity an independent risk factor for hepatocellular carcinoma in cirrhosis? Hepatology 36:150–155

Naugler WE, Karin M (2008) The wolf in sheep's clothing: the role of interleukin-6 in immunity, inflammation and cancer. Trends Mol Med 14:109–119

Naugler WE, Sakurai T, Kim S, Maeda S, Kim K, Elsharkawy AM, Karin M (2007) Gender disparity in liver cancer due to sex differences in MyD88-dependent IL-6 production. Science 317:121–124

Nejak-Bowen KN, Monga SP (2011) Beta-catenin signaling, liver regeneration and hepatocellular cancer: sorting the good from the bad. Semin Cancer Biol 21:44–58

Nishikawa-Ogawa M, Wanibuchi H, Morimura K, Kinoshita A, Nishikawa T, Hayashi S, Yano Y, Fukushima S (2006) *N*-acetylcysteine and *S*-methylcysteine inhibit MeIQx rat hepatocarcinogenesis in the post-initiation stage. Carcinogenesis 27:982–988

Nordenstedt H, White DL, El-Serag HB (2010) The changing pattern of epidemiology in hepatocellular carcinoma. Dig Liver Dis 42:S206–S214

Ogata H, Kobayashi T, Chinen T, Takaki H, Sanada T, Minoda Y, Koga K, Takaesu G, Maehara Y, Iida M, Yoshimura A (2006) Deletion of the SOCS3 gene in liver parenchymal cells promotes hepatitis-induced hepatocarcinogenesis. Gastroenterology 131:179–193

Pahl HL (1999) Activators and target genes of Rel/NF-kappaB transcription factors. Oncogene 18:6853–6866

Park EJ, Lee JH, Yu GY, He G, Ali SR, Holzer RG, Osterreicher CH, Takahashi H, Karin M (2010) Dietary and genetic obesity promote liver inflammation and tumorigenesis by enhancing IL-6 and TNF expression. Cell 140:197–208

Pfitzner E, Kliem S, Baus D, Litterst CM (2004) The role of STATs in inflammation and inflammatory diseases. Curr Pharm Des 10:2839–2850

Pikarsky E, Porat RM, Stein I, Abramovitch R, Amit S, Kasem S, Gutkovich-Pyest E, Urieli-Shoval S, Galun E, Ben-Neriah Y (2004) NF-kappaB functions as a tumour promoter in inflammation-associated cancer. Nature 431:461–466

Qian GS, Ross RK, Yu MC, Yuan JM, Gao YT, Henderson BE, Wogan GN, Groopman JD (1994) A follow-up study of urinary markers of aflatoxin exposure and liver cancer risk in Shanghai, People's Republic of China. Cancer Epidemiol Biomarkers Prev 3:3–10

Rahman MA, Dhar DK, Yamaguchi E, Maruyama S, Sato T, Hayashi H, Ono T, Yamanoi A, Kohno H, Nagasue N (2001) Coexpression of inducible nitric oxide synthase and COX-2 in hepatocellular carcinoma and surrounding liver: possible involvement of COX-2 in the angiogenesis of hepatitis C virus-positive cases. Clin Cancer Res 7:1325–1332

Ramakrishnan G, Raghavendran HRB, Vinodhkumar R, Devaki T (2006) Suppression of *N*-nitrosodiethylamine induced hepatocarcinogenesis by silymarin in rats. Chem-Biol Interact 161:104–114

Ramakrishnan G, Elinos-Báez CM, Jagan S, Augustine TA, Kamaraj S, Anandakumar P, Devaki T (2008) Silymarin downregulates COX-2 expression and attenuates hyperlipidemia during NDEA-induced rat hepatocellular carcinoma. Mol Cell Biochem 313:53–61

Rogers AB, Theve EJ, Feng Y, Fry RC, Taghizadeh K, Clapp KM, Boussahmain C, Cormier KS, Fox JG (2007) Hepatocellular carcinoma associated with liver-gender disruption in male mice. Cancer Res 67:11536–11546

Ruggieri A, Barbati C, Malorni W (2010) Cellular and molecular mechanisms involved in hepatocellular carcinoma gender disparity. Int J Cancer 127:499–504

Sakamoto T, Higaki Y, Hara M, Ichiba M, Horita M, Mizuta T, Eguchi Y, Yasutake T, Ozaki I, Yamamoto K, Onohara S, Kawazoe S, Shigematsu H, Koizumi S, Tanaka K (2008)

Interaction between interleukin-1β-31T/C gene polymorphism and drinking and smoking habits on the risk of hepatocellular carcinoma among Japanese. Cancer Lett 271:98–104
Sakurai T, He G, Matsuzawa A, Yu GY, Maeda S, Hardiman G, Karin M (2008) Hepatocyte necrosis induced by oxidative stress and IL-1 alpha release mediate carcinogen-induced compensatory proliferation and liver tumorigenesis. Cancer Cell 14:156–165
Schneider-Merck T, Borbath I, Charette N, De Saeger C, Abarca J, Leclercq I, Horsmans Y, Stärkel P (2009) The Ras inhibitor farnesylthiosalicyclic acid (FTS) prevents nodule formation and development of preneoplastic foci of altered hepatocytes in rats. Eur J Cancer 45:2050–2060
Schütte K, Bornschein J, Malfertheiner P (2009) Hepatocellular carcinoma—epidemiological trends and risk factors. Dig Dis 27:80–92
Sengupta S, Bishayee A (2010) MicroRNAs in cancer therapy: from bench to bedside. Curr Cancer Ther Rev 6:157–162
Senn JJ, Klover PJ, Nowak IA, Mooney RA (2002) Interleukin-6 induces cellular insulin resistance in hepatocytes. Diabetes 51:3391–3399
Senthil M, Mailey B, Leong L, Chung V, Yen Y, Chen YJ, Marx H, Kim J (2010) Liver-directed regional therapy in the multi-disciplinary management of hepatocellular cancer. Curr Cancer Ther Rev 6:19–25
Sherman M (2005) Hepatocellular carcinoma: epidemiology, risk factors, and screening. Semin Liver Dis 25:143–154
Shimizu M, Sakai H, Shirakami Y, Yasuda Y, Kubota M, Terakura D, Baba A, Ohno T, Hara Y, Tanaka T, Moriwaki H (2011a) Preventive effects of (-)-epigallocatechin gallate on diethylnitrosamine-induced liver tumorigenesis in obese and diabetic C57BL/KsJ-db/db mice. Cancer Prev Res 4:396–403
Shimizu M, Sakai H, Shirakami Y, Iwasa J, Yasuda Y, Kubota M, Takai K, Tsurumi H, Tanaka T, Moriwaki H (2011b) Acyclic retinoid inhibits diethylnitrosamine-induced liver tumorigenesis in obese and diabetic C57BLKS/J- +(db)/+Lepr(db) mice. Cancer Prev Res 4:128–136
Shimizu M, Yasuda Y, Sakai H, Kubota M, Terakura D, Baba A, Ohno T, Kochi T, Tsurumi H, Tanaka T, Moriwaki H (2011c) Pitavastatin suppresses diethylnitrosamine-induced liver preneoplasms in male C57BL/KsJ-db/db obese mice. BMC Cancer 11:281
Shimizu M, Tanaka T, Moriwaki H (2013) Obesity and hepatocellular carcinoma: targeting obesity-related inflammation for chemoprevention of liver carcinogenesis. Semin Immunopathol 35:191–202
Shiota G, Okubo M, Noumi T, Noguchi N, Oyama K, Takano Y, Yashima K, Kishimoto Y, Kawasaki H (1999) Cyclooxygenase-2 expression in hepatocellular carcinoma. Hepatogastroenterology 46:407–412
Shoelson SE, Lee J, Goldfine AB (2006) Inflammation and insulin resistance. Clin Invest 116:1793–1801
Sibilia M, Kroismayr R, Lichtenberger BM, Natarajan A, Hecking M, Holcmann M (2007) The epidermal growth factor receptor: from development to tumorigenesis. Differentiation 75:770–787
Siegel R, Naishadham D, Jemal A (2013) Cancer statistics, 2013. CA Cancer J Clin 63:11–30
Silke J, Meier P (2013) Inhibitor of apoptosis (IAP) proteins-modulators of cell death and inflammation. Cold Spring Harb Perspect Biol 5: a008730
Simile MM, Pagnan G, Pastorino F, Brignole C, De Miglio MR, Muroni MR, Asara G, Frau M, Seddaiu MA, Calvisi DF, Feo F, Ponzoni M, Pascale RM (2005) Chemopreventive *N*-(4-hydroxyphenyl) retinamide (fenretinide) targets deregulated *NF-κB* and *Mat1A* genes in the early stages of rat liver carcinogenesis. Carcinogenesis 26:417–427
Sivaramakrishnan V, Niranjali Devaraj S (2009) Morin regulates the expression of NF-κB-p65, COX-2 and matrix metalloproteinases in diethylnitrosamine induced rat hepatocellular carcinoma. Chem Biol Interact 180:353–359
Sivaramakrishnan V, Niranjali Devaraj S (2010) Morin fosters apoptosis in experimental hepatocellular carcinogenesis model. Chem Biol Interact 183:284–292

Stärkel P, Charette N, Borbath I, Schneider-Merck T, De Saeger C, Abarca J, Leclercq I, Horsmans Y (2012) Ras inhibition in hepatocarcinoma by *S-trans-trans*-farnesylthiosalicyclic acid: association of its tumor preventive effect with cell proliferation, cell cycle events, and angiogenesis. Mol Carcinog 51:816–825

Subramaniam A, Shanmugam MK, Perumal E, Li F, Nachiyappan A, Dai X, Swamy SN, Ahn KS, Kumar AP, Tan BK, Hui KM, Sethi G (2013) Potential role of signal transducer and activator of transcription (STAT)3 signaling pathway in inflammation, survival, proliferation and invasion of hepatocellular carcinoma. Biochim Biophys Acta 1835:46–60

Sun B, Karin M (2012) Obesity, inflammation, and liver cancer. J Hepatol 56:704–713

Sung YK, Hwang SY, Kim JO, Bae HI, Kim JC, Kim MK (2004) The correlation between cyclooxygenase-2 expression and hepatocellular carcinogenesis. Mol Cells 17:35–38

Szabo G, Lippai D (2012) Molecular hepatic carcinogenesis: impact of inflammation. Dig Dis 30:243–248

Tanaka H, Fujita N, Sugimoto R, Urawa N, Horiike S, Kobayashi Y, Iwasa M, Ma N, Kawanishi S, Watanabe S, Kaito M, Takei Y (2008) Hepatic oxidative DNA damage is associated with increased risk for hepatocellular carcinoma in chronic hepatitis C. Br J Cancer 98:580–586

Taub R (2003) Hepatoprotection via the IL-6/Stat3 pathway. J Clin Invest 112:978–980

Thoppil RJ, Bhatia D, Barnes KF, Háznagy-Radnai E, Hohmann J, Darvesh AS, Bishayee A (2012) Black currant anthocyanins abrogate oxidative stress through Nrf2-mediated antioxidant mechanisms in a rat model of hepatocellular carcinoma. Curr Cancer Drug Targets 12:1244–1257

Ueno S, Aoki D, Kubo F, Hiwatashi K, Matsushita K, Oyama T, Maruyama I, Aikou T (2005) Roxithromycin inhibits constitutive activation of nuclear factor & #x03BA;B by diminishing oxidative stress in a rat model of hepatocellular carcinoma. Clin Cancer Res 11:5645–5650

Wai PY, Kuo PC (2012) Intersecting pathways in inflammation and cancer: hepatocellular carcinoma as a paradigm. World J Clin Oncol 10:15–23

Wang LY, Chen CJ, Zhang YJ, Tsai WY, Lee PH, Feitelson MA, Lee CS, Santella RM (1998) 4-Aminobiphenyl DNA damage in liver tissue of hepatocellular carcinoma patients and controls. Am J Epidemiol 147:315–323

Wang Y, Kato N, Hoshida Y, Yoshida H, Taniguchi H, Goto T, Moriyama M, Otsuka M, Shiina S, Shiratori Y, Ito Y, Omata M (2003) Interleukin-1β gene polymorphisms associated with hepatocellular carcinoma in hepatitis C virus infection. Hepatology 37:65–71

Wang Y, Ausman LM, Greenberg AS, Russell RM, Wang XD (2009a) Nonalcoholic steatohepatitis induced by a high-fat diet promotes diethylnitrosamine-initiated early hepatocarcinogenesis in rats. Int J Cancer 124:540–546

Wang B, Majumder S, Nuovo G, Kutay H, Volinia S, Patel T, Schmittgen TD, Croce C, Ghoshal K, Jacob ST (2009b) Role of microRNA-155 at early stages of hepatocarcinogenesis induced by choline-deficient and amino acid-defined diet in C57BL/6 mice. Hepatology 50:1152–1161

Wang Y, Ausman LM, Greenberg AS, Russell RM, Wang XD (2010) Dietary lycopene and tomato extract supplementations inhibit nonalcoholic steatohepatitis-promoted hepatocarcinogenesis in rats. Int J Cancer 126:1788–1796

Weber A, Boege Y, Reisinger F, Heikenwälder M (2011) Chronic liver inflammation and hepatocellular carcinoma: persistence matters. Swiss Med Wkly 141:w13197

Weinhold B, Rüther U (1997) Interleukin-6-dependent and -independent regulation of the human C-reactive protein gene. Biochem J 327:425–429

Weisberg SP, McCann D, Desai M, Rosenbaum M, Leibel RL, Ferrante AW Jr (2003) Obesity is associated with macrophage accumulation in adipose tissue. J Clin Invest 112:1796–1808

West AP, Koblansky AA, Ghosh S (2006) Recognition and signaling by toll-like receptors. Annu Rev Cell Dev Biol 22:409–437

White LA, Menzin J, Korn JR, Friedman M, Lang K, Ray S (2012) Medical care costs and survival associated with hepatocellular carcinoma among the elderly. Clin Gastroenterol Hepatol 10:547–554

Whittaker S, Marais R, Zhu AX (2010) The role of signaling pathways in the development and treatment of hepatocellular carcinoma. Oncogene 29:4989–5005

Wieckowska A, Papouchado BG, Li Z, Lopez R, Zein NN, Feldstein AE (2008) Increased hepatic and circulating interleukin-6 levels in human nonalcoholic steatohepatitis. Am J Gastroenterol 103:1372–1379

Williams CS, Mann M, DuBois RN (1999) The role of cyclooxygenases in inflammation, cancer, and development. Oncogene 18:7908–7916

Wilson JF (2005) Liver cancer on the rise. Ann Intern Med 142:1029–1032

Wong VW, Yu J, Cheng AS, Wong GL, Chan HY, Chu ES, Ng EK, Chan FK, Sung JJ, Chan HL (2009) High serum interleukin-6 level predicts future hepatocellular carcinoma development in patients with chronic hepatitis B. Int J Cancer 124:2766–2770

Wong CM, Kai AK, Tsang FH, Ng IO (2013) Regulation of hepatocarcinogenesis by microRNAs. Front Biosci 5:49–60

Wu T (2005) Cycloygenase-2 and prostaglandin signaling in cholangiocarcinoma. Biochim Biophys Acta 1755:135–150

Wu T (2006) Cyclooxygenase-2 in hepatocellular carcinoma. Cancer Treat Rev 32:28–44

Wunderlich FT, Luedde T, Singer S, Schmidt-Supprian M, Baumgartl J, Schirmacher P, Pasparakis M, Brüning JC (2008) Hepatic NF-κB essential modulator deficiency prevents obesity-induced insulin resistance but synergizes with high-fat feeding in tumorigenesis. Proc Natl Acad Sci USA 105:1297–1302

Xiao C, Ghosh S (2005) NF-kappaB, an evolutionarily conserved mediator of immune and inflammatory responses. Adv Exp Med Biol 560:41–45

Yamamoto H, Kondo M, Nakamori S, Nagano H, Wakasa K, Sugita Y, Chang-De J, Kobayashi S, Damdinsuren B, Dono K, Umeshita K, Sekimoto M, Sakon M, Matsuura N, Monden M (2003) JTE-522, a cyclooxygenase-2 inhibitor, is an effective chemopreventive agent against rat experimental liver fibrosis. Gastroenterology 125:556–571

Yildirim Y, Ozyilkan O, Bilezikci B, Akcali Z, Haberal M (2008) Lack of influence of cyclooxygenese-2 expression in hepatocellular carcinomas on patient survival. Asian Pac J Cancer Prev 9:295–298

Yoshimura A, Naka T, Kubo M (2007) SOCS proteins, cytokine signalling and immune regulation. Nat Rev Immunol 7:454–465

Yoysungnoen P, Wirachwong P, Bhattarakosol P, Niimi H, Patumraj S (2006) Effects of curcumin on tumor angiogenesis and biomarkers, COX-2 and VEGF, in hepatocellular carcinoma cell-implanted nude mice. Clin Hemorheol Microcirc 34:109–115

Yu H, Pardoll D, Jove R (2009) STATs in cancer inflammation and immunity: a leading role for STAT3. Nat Rev Cancer 9:798–809

Zhao X, Zhang JJ, Wang X, Bu XY, Lou YQ, Zhang GL (2008) Effect of berberine on hepatocyte proliferation, inducible nitric oxide synthase expression, cytochrome P450 2E1 and 1A2 activities in diethylnitrosamine- and phenobarbital-treated rats. Biomed Pharmacother 62:567–572

Chapter 17
The Role of Inflammation in Skin Cancer

Girish B. Maru, Khushboo Gandhi, Asha Ramchandani and Gaurav Kumar

Abstract Cancer is an environmental disease and skin cancer (melanoma and non-melanoma) is the most common of all cancers. Epidemiological and experimental evidence suggest "chronic inflammation" to be one of the hallmarks in solar ultraviolet radiation and several other environmental agent-mediated skin cancers. The identification of transcription factors, mainly nuclear factor-kappa B (NF-κB), signal transducer and activator of transcription 3 (STAT3), hypoxia-inducible factor-1 alpha (HIF-1α) and their gene products i.e. prostaglandins, cyclooxygenase-2 (COX-2), cytokines [tumor necrosis factor- alpha (TNF-α)], chemokines [CXC-chemokine ligand (CXCL)] and chemokine receptors suggest critical role of inflammation in skin carcinogenesis. Considering the potential role of inflammation in tumor initiation and its major role in promotion/progression, as well as tumor angiogenesis and metastasis; inflammatory pathways may become attractive targets for skin cancer prevention. Hence this review focuses on compiling available evidence and understanding the role of chronic inflammation in the development of skin cancer.

17.1 Introduction

Exposure to a wide variety of natural and/or man-made agents/substances in the environment accounts for majority of cases of cancer. These environmental factors include lifestyle choices such as use of tobacco, alcohol, poor diet, and excessive sunlight exposure. Other factors include exposure to certain drugs, hormones, radiation, specific viruses/bacteria, and environmental chemicals that may be present

G. B. Maru (✉) · K. Gandhi · A. Ramchandani · G. Kumar
Maru Lab, Advanced Centre for Treatment, Research and Education in Cancer (ACTREC), Tata Memorial Centre (TMC), Sector-22, Kharghar, Navi Mumbai 410210, India
e-mail: gmaru@actrec.gov.in

B. B. Aggarwal et al. (eds.), *Inflammation and Cancer*, Advances in Experimental Medicine and Biology 816, DOI: 10.1007/978-3-0348-0837-8_17, © Springer Basel 2014

in the air, water, food, and workplace. The chance that an individual will develop cancer in response to exposure to a specific environmental agent depends on complex interactions between environmental and host factors (genetic/acquired susceptibility/protective), how long and how often a person is exposed to a particular substance, exposure to other agents, genetic factors, diet, lifestyle, health, age and gender, etc.

The environmental agent(s)-mediated cancers have been observed to share ten common traits that govern the transformation of normal cells to cancer cells (Hanahan and Weinberg 2011). Accumulating evidence has resulted in the acceptance of "chronic inflammation" to be one of the ten hallmarks of cancer. Cancers caused by environmental agents frequently occur in tissues with the greatest surface exposure to the agent(s), e.g., lungs, gastrointestinal tract, and skin (Loeb and Harris 2008). Skin cancer is the most common of all cancers. Therefore, this review focuses mainly on compiling available evidence and understanding the role of chronic inflammation in the development of skin cancer. Before presenting the available evidence on (a) the role of inflammatory molecules in the development of skin cancer in vitro and in vivo, and (b) observations on inhibitors of inflammation for the prevention and treatment of skin cancer, brief description of skin structure, function, types and prevalence of skin cancer, causative agents and risk factors, treatment modalities and survival, etc., has been included for enhancing the understanding and clarity of the presentation.

17.1.1 Skin Structure and Function

The skin is the largest and dynamic organ of the body, making up 16 % of body weight, with a surface area of 1.8 m^2 and situated at the interface between the body and environment. Skin serves as the armors for the body against mechanical, thermal, and physical injury and hazardous substances (Proksch et al. 2008). There are three structural layers of the skin: epidermis, dermis, and subcutaneous layer (Fig. 17.1).

Epidermis is an external and continually regenerative, stratified epithelium devoid of blood or nerve supplies of approximately 5–100 μm thickness. It is composed of several distinct cell populations, keratinocytes and melanocytes being the main constituents. Keratinocytes, which comprise 95 % of the epidermis, are arranged in four layers. The inner layer is the stratum germinativum (stratum basale, basal layer), from which columnar-shaped keratinocytes divide to migrate to the next layer. The stratum spinosum (spinous layer) is composed of polygonal keratinocytes that become eventually more condensed. Further differentiation of the cells leads to the stratum granulosum (granular layer), which contains basophilic granules. In thick skin areas, such as the soles of feet or the palms of hands, there is a clear layer of flattened cells called the stratum lucidum. The outermost layer is the stratum corneum (horny layer), which contains keratin and dead cells that confer to the skin its barrier function. Melanocytes are cells of neural crest embryogenic origin whose primary function is to produce melanin,

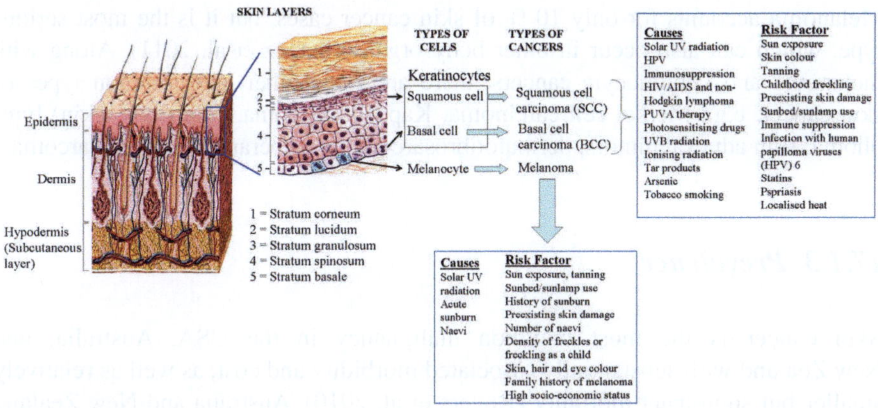

Fig. 17.1 Schematic presentation of skin structure, cell types, causes, and risk factors associated with skin cancer

the pigment that determines skin and hair color. They are located in the basal layer of the epidermis, which comprise from 5 to 10 % of the cells and in hair follicles, and are also found in other anatomical areas such as the inner ear, the eye, and the meninges (Costin and Hearing 2007).

Dermis, the middle layer of the skin found below the epidermis, is composed of a tough, supportive cell matrix. The dermis contains fibroblasts, which produce collagen, elastin, and structural proteoglycans, together with immune-competent mast cells and macrophages. Collagen fibers, which make up 70 % of the dermis, give skin its strength, elasticity, and toughness. Dermis contains hair follicles, sweat glands, blood vessels, and nerves that are held in place by collagen.

Subcutis or subcutaneous layer consists of loose connective tissue and fat. It helps the body conserve heat and has a shock-absorbing effect that helps protect the body's organs from injury.

Skin has several functions, the most important being to form a physical barrier to the environment, allowing and limiting the inward and outward passage of water, electrolytes, and various substances while providing protection against microorganisms, ultraviolet radiation (UVR), toxic agents, and mechanical insults. Its other functions are insulation, temperature regulation, sensation, and synthesis of vitamin D and the protection of vitamin B folates.

17.1.2 Types of Skin Cancer

There are four different types of skin cancer: basal cell carcinoma (BCC) and squamous cell carcinoma (SCC) collectively referred to as non-melanoma skin cancers (NMSC) or keratinocyte carcinoma; melanoma and other non-epithelial skin cancer. BCC and SCC account for approximately 80 and 16 % of all NMSC, respectively.

Melanoma accounts for only 10 % of skin cancer cases, but it is the most serious type, which can also occur in other body organs (Ibanez et al. 2011). Along with melanoma and keratinocyte cancers, there are some other less common types of skin cancer, e.g., Merkel cell carcinoma, Kaposi's sarcoma, cutaneous (skin) lymphoma, skin adnexal tumors, dermatofibrosarcoma protuberans, and angiosarcoma.

17.1.3 Prevalence

Skin cancer is the most common malignancy in the USA, Australia, and New Zealand with substantially associated morbidity and cost, as well as relatively smaller but significant mortality (Rogers et al. 2010). Australia and New Zealand have the highest rates of skin cancer incidence in the world, almost four times the rates registered in the USA, the UK, and Canada. Skin cancer is 10 times more common in whites than in African Americans. It is estimated that one American dies every hour from skin cancer, whereas the incidence of UV-induced NMSC has increased dramatically worldwide accounting for more than 40 % of all human cancers in the USA, with about 1.3 million new cases being diagnosed annually of which roughly 20–30 % is of SCC (Madan et al. 2010).

17.1.4 Causative Agents and Risk Factors

UVR from sun exposure is the main cause of skin cancer, accounting for at least 65 % of melanomas worldwide. The geographic variation and risk of development of NMSC are associated with ambient sun irradiance, genotypic, phenotypic, and environmental factors. Risk is greatest in residents of high ambient solar irradiance who have markers of UV susceptibility, such as light skin, eye and hair color, or an inability to tan, and those with benign sunlight-related skin disorders, e.g., actinic keratosis (AK) and solar lentigines. Incidence within countries is associated with increasing proximity to the equator. The thinner ozone layer and shorter distance traversed by UVB at lower latitudes than at high latitudes make residents of these regions most vulnerable to the effects of this radiation (Madan et al. 2010).

Individuals with familial genetic syndromes, viral infections such as human immunodeficiency virus (HIV), human herpesvirus 8 (HHV8), and human papilloma virus (HPV) or exposed to artificial UVR (tanning beds and lamps), aging, diet, and smoking are attributed risks. Some treatment modalities, including radiotherapy, phototherapy, psoralen, long-wave ultraviolet radiation (PUVA), and immunosuppressant drugs (cyclosporin A, methotrexate) besides work-related exposures such as arsenic, tar product, and chemical carcinogens (petroleum refining, pesticide manufacturing, etc.), also predispose individuals to skin cancers (Fig. 17.1) (IARC 1987; Boffetta et al. 2001). Skin cancers are also attributed to chronically injured or non-healing wounds and scars or ulcers that occur at sites of previous burns, sinuses, trauma, osteomyelitis, prolonged heat (Kangri cancer) and chronic friction (Saree/Dhoti cancer) (Aziz et al. 1998; Patil et al. 2005; Saladi and Persaud 2005). The incidence of malignancy in scar tissues is 0.1–2.5 %.

17.1.5 Treatment for Skin Cancer

A variety of modalities for the treatment of skin cancer is available, including surgery, radiation therapy, chemotherapy, photodynamic therapy (PDT), and biological therapy. Surgical options, including curettage with electrodessication, Mohs micrographic surgery, and surgical excision, are the most frequently used treatments, providing a high control rate and satisfactory cosmetic results. Radiation therapy, including brachytherapy techniques and external beam radiations such as superficial/orthovoltage X-rays, megavoltage photons, and electron beam radiation, has been used as primary and post-surgical adjuvant therapy for skin cancers. Chemotherapy includes the topical agents (in the form of ointment) such as fluorouracil, diclofenac sodium, and imiquimod. In PDT, a photosensitive drug and a certain type of laser light are used to kill cancer cells. However, in biological therapy (biotherapy or immunotherapy), substances such as interferon and imiquimod (made by the body or in a laboratory) are used to boost, direct, or restore the body's natural defenses against cancer.

17.1.6 Survival

Although the incidence of skin cancer is increasing, it is curable especially if it is detected or treated early and considered one of the most preventable types of cancer. The 5- and 10-year relative survival rates for persons with melanoma which is more likely than other skin tumors to spread to other parts of the body, are 91 and 89 %, respectively. For localized melanoma (84 % of cases), the 5-year survival rate is 98 %; survival declines to 62 and 15 % for regional- and distant-stage disease, respectively. BCC and SCC are highly treatable, and survival rates for NMSC are very high. The mortality rate of NMSC is around 0.3 %, causing 2,000 deaths per year in USA (American Cancer Society 2013).

17.1.7 Inflammation and Skin Cancer

Inflammation is a signal-mediated response to cellular insult by infectious agents, toxins, and physical stresses. Inflammation is caused by physical agents (e.g., UVR), mechanical injuries, chemical agents (tar products, arsenic, immunomodulatory drugs, toxins), biological agents (bacteria, viruses, fungi, parasites), immunologic

Table 17.1 Characteristics of inflammation

Characteristics	Acute inflammation	Chronic inflammation
Duration	Short	Relatively long
Pattern	Stereotyped	Varied
Predominant cell	Neutrophils, leukocytes	Lymphocytes, macrophages, plasma cells, giant cells, fibroblasts
Tissue destruction	Mild to moderate	Marked
Fibrosis	Absent	Present
Inflammatory reaction	Exudative	Productive

disorders (hypersensitivity reactions, autoimmunity, immunodeficiency states), etc. Inflammation can be acute or chronic with distinct characteristics (see Table 17.1) (Mueller 2006; Aggarwal et al. 2009). Acute inflammation is a rapid, self-limiting process, maybe prolonged and transformed to chronic inflammation. Chronic inflammation being more insidious lies at the basis of various diseases, including cardiovascular diseases, cancer, diabetes, arthritis, Alzheimer's disease, pulmonary diseases, and autoimmune diseases (Aggarwal et al. 2009).

As early as 1863, Virchow noted leukocytes in neoplastic tissues and made a connection between inflammation and cancer. He suggested that the "lymphoreticular infiltrate" reflected the origin of cancer at sites of chronic inflammation (Mantovani et al. 2008). The correlation between cancer and inflammation has been recognized for decades, but only in recent years, evidence begun to suggest that the inflammation is a prerequisite rather than a consequence of tumorigenesis (Balkwill and Coussens 2004). It is estimated that underlying infections and inflammatory responses are linked to 15–20 % of all deaths from cancer worldwide (Lu et al. 2006; Parkin 2006; Mantovani et al. 2008). Several clinical conditions such as discoid lupus erythematosus, dystrophic epidermolysis bullosa, and chronic wound sites are associated with cutaneous inflammation and appear to predispose the individual to increased susceptibility for skin cancer (Nickoloff et al. 2005).

Injury to the skin initiates a cascade of events including inflammation, new tissue formation, and tissue remodeling which leads to wound repair. In chronic inflammation, active inflammation, tissue destruction, and attempts at repair proceed simultaneously. The inflammatory response involves three major stages: dilation of capillaries to increase blood flow; microvascular structural changes and escape of plasma proteins from the bloodstream; and leukocyte transmigration through endothelium and accumulation at the site of injury (http://bme.virginia.edu/ley/). In addition to the defense functions [production of proteinase and reactive oxygen species (ROS)], inflammatory cells are also an important source of growth factors and cytokines such as interleukin-1 (IL-1) and tumor necrosis factor-alpha (TNF-α) that are necessary for cell recruitment, activation, and proliferation (Nickoloff et al. 2005; Mueller 2006). However, while normal inflammation, e.g., during wound healing, is a rapid self-limiting process, deregulation of the profile and level of any of cytokines/chemokines that persists at sites of inflammation result in the development of various pathologies including cancer. The mechanisms include induction of genomic instability, alterations in epigenetic events and subsequent inappropriate gene expression, enhanced proliferation of initiated cells, resistance to apoptosis, unlimited replicative potential, sustained angiogenesis (tumor neovascularization), tissue invasion, and metastasis (Colotta et al. 2009).

17.2 Inflammatory Signaling Pathways Associated with Skin Cancer

Inflammation is associated with different stages of tumor development, including initiation, promotion, malignant conversion, invasion, and metastasis (Fan et al. 2013). Cancer-related inflammation, which has been suggested to represent the seventh hallmark of cancer (Hanahan and Weinberg 2011), affects all the important aspects of cancer such as proliferation and survival of cancer cells, tumor response to chemotherapeutic drugs and hormones, metastasis and angiogenesis similar to that seen in chronic inflammatory responses, and tissue remodeling/repair (Kamp et al. 2011; Mantovani et al. 2008).

Two pathways connect cancer and inflammation: the intrinsic and extrinsic pathways (Fig. 17.2). The intrinsic pathway is activated by genetic events that cause neoplasia, including the activation of oncogenes (H-ras, N-ras, BRAF, c-MYC, human counterpart of MDM2 [HDM2], C-erbB) by mutation, chromosomal rearrangement or amplification, and inactivation of tumor suppressor genes (p16/INKA4 [cyclin-dependent kinase inhibitor 2A]; p14/ARF [ADP ribosylation factor]) (Soehnge et al. 1997; Hocker et al. 2008; Hanahan and Weinberg 2011). Cells, which are transformed in this manner, produce inflammatory mediators, thereby generating an inflammatory microenvironment in tumors. Moreover, there are other gene products frequently observed in skin cancer (mainly melanoma and NMSC) such as protein-patched homolog 1 (PTCH1), PTCH2, sonic hedgehog (Shh), cyclin-dependent kinase 4 (CDK4) and CDK6, melanocortin 1 receptor (MC1R), microphthalmia-associated transcription factor (MITF), cytochrome p450 (CYP), glutathione S-transferase theta 1 (GSTT1), Ras, xeroderma pigmentosum, complementation group C (XPC), and tumor protein 53 (TP53). Genes involved in UVR-induced skin cancer include the tumor suppressor gene p53, PTCH, and the ras oncogenes (Hocker et al. 2008; Madan et al. 2010).

In contrast, the extrinsic pathway represents inflammatory leukocytes and soluble mediators leading to conditions, which increase cancer risk (Fig. 17.2). The chronic inflammation related to malignancy is induced by infections with pathogens (HHV), mechanical, radiation, and chemical insults, which results in the production of oxidative stress (Del Prete et al. 2011). The two pathways unite, resulting in the activation of transcription factors, mainly nuclear factor kappa B (NF-κB), signal transducer and activator of transcription 3 (STAT3) and hypoxia-inducible factor-1 alpha (HIF-1α) in tumor cells. These transcription factors coordinate the production of pro-inflammatory mediators, including cytokines (TNF-α, IL-6, IL-1), chemokines (chemokine [C-C motif] ligand

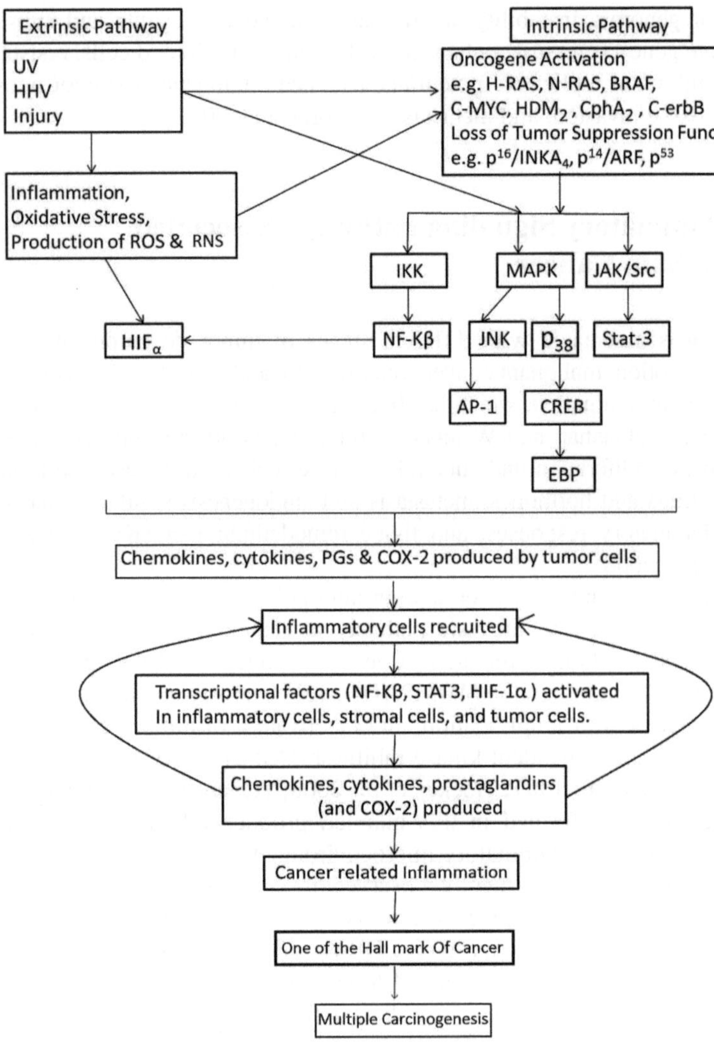

Fig. 17.2 Signaling pathways associated with inflammation and skin cancer

2 [CCL2], CXC chemokine ligand 8 [CXCL8]), as well as the production of cyclooxygenase-2 (COX-2) (which, in turn, results in the production of prostaglandins [PG]) (Mantovani et al. 2008; Del Prete et al. 2011). Pro-inflammatory cytokines, the important mediators of inflammation, have distinguished roles in skin cancer development and along with nitric oxide (NO) act as cell-to-cell messenger as well as help in the activation of NF-κB (Kundu and Surh 2008). The cytokines activate the same key transcription factors in inflammatory cells, stromal cells, and tumor cells, resulting in more mediators' production and cancer-related inflammatory microenvironment being generated.

In extrinsic pathway, exposure of skin to various physical, chemical, or biological agents induces infiltration of neutrophils at site of tissue injury which are key producers of ROS and reactive nitrogen species (RNS). ROS, an inherent part of the anabolism and catabolism of various body tissues, including skin, play important roles in the stimulation of molecules for metabolism, cell cycle, and intercellular transduction pathways (Ibanez et al. 2011) and are involved in all the three stages of carcinogenesis, viz. initiation, promotion, and progression. Furthermore, transient levels of ROS can activate cellular proliferation or survival signaling pathways, such as the NF-κB, activator protein-1 (AP-1), extracellular signal-regulated kinase-/mitogen-activated protein kinase (ERK/MAPK), and phosphoinositide 3-kinase/Akt8 virus oncogene cellular homolog (PI3K/Akt) pathways. In addition, ROS induce both the activation and synthesis of AP-1, a regulator of cell growth, proliferation, and apoptosis, and transcription factors such as STAT3, HIF-1α, and p53 (Reuter et al. 2010).

NF-κB and STAT3 are two most important transcription factors in inflammatory pathways that play major roles in tumorigenesis because they are constitutively active in most cancers, including skin (melanoma, SCC, Kaposi's sarcoma). Moreover, most gene products linked to inflammation, survival, proliferation, invasion, angiogenesis, and metastasis are regulated by NF-κB and STAT3, and most chemopreventive agents mediate their effects through inhibition of NF-κB and STAT3 activation pathways (Aggarwal et al. 2009; Zhu et al. 2011).

Many stimuli can induce NF-κB activity, such as TNF-α, IL-1β, bacterial lipopolysaccharides (LPS), UV, ionizing radiation, ROS, several skin-related microorganisms such as *Borrelia burgdorferi*, *Neisseria gonorrhoeae*, *Staphylococcus aureus*, herpes simplex virus (HSV), measles virus, and HIV-1 (Pahl 1999; Bell et al. 2003). NF-κB activation as core transcriptional mediator of inflammation is a central component of pro-carcinogenic innate immune responses. Functional nuclear NF-κB is necessary for the growth inhibition control during upward cellular migration and differentiation of epidermal cells, which have central role in skin carcinogenesis (Bell et al. 2003). Several NF-κB-dependent genes present in the skin are essential to the initiation of cutaneous inflammation, including genes for different chemokines (IL-1, IL-6, TNF) and cytokines, intercellular adhesion molecule-1 (ICAM-1), vascular cell adhesion molecule-1 (VCAM-1), urokinase plasminogen activator (uPA), and E-selectin (Pahl 1999; Bell et al. 2003). NF-κB also regulates pro-inflammatory enzymes, such as inducible nitric oxidase synthase (iNOS) and COX-2, which are involved in chronic inflammation of the skin and later in skin carcinogenesis. Additionally, NF-κB controls the expression of the genes linked with apoptosis (cellular inhibitor of apoptosis [c-IAP], XIAP, B cell lymphoma 2 [Bcl-2], Bcl-xL, cellular FLICE-like inhibitory protein [c-FLIP], survivin), proliferation (cyclins, c-Myc), invasion, angiogenesis, and metastasis (e.g., matrix metalloproteinase [MMP], vascular endothelial growth factor [VEGF], CXCL12, C-X-C chemokine receptor type 4 [CXCR4]) of cancer. Based on these evidences, NF-κB is believed to be closely associated with the whole process of tumorigenesis (Prasad et al. 2010; Zhu et al. 2011).

STATs are proteins that are activated by extracellular signaling proteins, growth factors such as epidermal growth factor receptor (EGFR), cytokines (IL-6, IL-17,

IL-22), and various peptides (Zhu et al. 2011). STAT3 regulates the expression of genes that mediate survival (survivin, Bcl-xl, myeloid cell leukemia sequence 1 [mcl-1], c-FLIP), proliferation (c-fos, c-myc, cyclin D1), invasion (MMP-2), and angiogenesis (VEGF) (Aggarwal et al. 2009). Along with NF-κB, STAT3 is a point of convergence for numerous oncogenic signaling pathways. Maintenance of NF-κB activation in tumors requires STAT3 which is constitutively activated both in tumors and in immune cells and plays a role in carcinogenesis (Colotta et al. 2009).

17.3 Role of Inflammatory Molecules in the Development of Skin Cancer: Evidence from In Vitro Studies

17.3.1 Role of Inflammatory Molecules in the Transformation of Skin Cells

Causal association between environmental (chemical/physical/biological) agent(s) in cancer development has been well established, while understanding and acceptance of the role of inflammation in cancer development are relatively recent. Due to this, evidence from available in vitro and/or in vivo experimental model systems pertaining to the role of inflammation in initiation of carcinogen-induced tumorigenicity is not clearly and conclusively addressed. One of the main reasons being non-inclusion of this aspect in the scope and planning of the experiments to address the question and/or complexity of experimental/real-life systems, wherein role of inflammation among multiple factors cannot easily be identified. Most of the environmental skin cancer-causing agents have been shown to induce spectrum of changes such as genotoxicity, cytotoxicity, and inflammation in cells exposed in vitro, and hence, biological significance and criticality of exact role of inflammation in the initiation of carcinogenesis are not established. Available evidence suggests the role of inflammatory molecules in the promotion of carcinogenesis in cells which have been initiated, wherein some products generated during inflammation do possess ability to damage/modify DNA, proteins, and lipids (Lu et al. 2006).

Several studies support the hypothesis that regulation of chemokines in certain cells in the presence of persistent autocrine and paracrine stimulation with specific CXC chemokine ligands can promote preneoplastic to neoplastic cellular transformation. Over-expression of CXCL1 (melanoma growth stimulatory activity/growth-regulated protein α) induced by IL-1, LPS, and TNF-α in immortalized melanocytes resulted in the transformation of these cells that had capability to form tumors in nude/SCID mice (Dhawan and Richmond 2002).

RAS-mediated tumor formation is commonly associated with up-regulation of cytokines and chemokines that mediate an inflammatory response relevant to oncogenesis (Cataisson et al. 2012). Over-expression of any of three normal Ras genes, N-Ras, H-Ras, or K-Ras, leads to in vitro transformation (Crespo and Leon 2000;

Dhawan and Richmond 2002). Studies using in vitro transformation assay have demonstrated that N-Ras could induce cellular transformation in a manner similar to CXCL1 in controlling melanocyte cells (Dhawan and Richmond 2002), indicating that CXCL1-mediated transformation requires Ras activation in melanocytes. Using both genetic and pharmacological approaches, it has been observed that the differentiation and pro-inflammatory effects of oncogenic RAS in keratinocytes require the establishment of an autocrine loop through IL-1α, IL-1R, and myeloid differentiation primary response gene (88) (MyD88), leading to the phosphorylation of IκBα (inhibitor of κBα) and NF-κB activation. Thus, MyD88 exerts a cell-intrinsic function in RAS-mediated transformation of keratinocytes (Cataisson et al. 2012).

The modulation of IL-1α production in the HaCaT keratinocyte cell line, wherein UVR induces keratinocytes to secrete other pro-inflammatory and immunomodulatory mediators, promotes inflammation and skin tumor development (Magcwebeba et al. 2012). Maximal production of these mediators appears to be due to overexpression of the slug (snail homolog 2 or zinc finger 2 [Snai2]) transcription factor in keratinocytes and normal human melanocytes, thereby stimulating growth and migration (Shirley et al. 2012). UVB exposure led to significant increase in the production of IL-1α in a dose-dependent manner with minimal necrotic and apoptotic effects. Moreover, induction of IL-6 production following short-wave UVR in normal human epidermal keratinocytes and epidermoid carcinoma cell line is mediated by DNA damage and that IL-6 release has been shown to be associated with enhanced levels of IL-6 mRNA transcripts (Petit-Frere et al. 1998).

In primary mouse keratinocyte cultures, prostaglandin E2 (PGE2) activated the EGFR and its downstream signaling pathways as well as increased cAMP production and activated the cAMP response element binding protein (CREB). Inhibitors of ERK1/2 and PI3K pathway attenuated the PGE2-induced proliferation, NF-κB, AP-1, and CREB binding to the promoter regions of the cyclin D1 and VEGF genes and expression of cyclin D1 and VEGF in primary mouse keratinocytes (Ansari et al. 2008).

Nuclear factor of activated T cells (NFAT), known to be expressed in both immune and non-immune cells, plays an essential role in inflammatory responses by regulating the expression of a wide range of pro-inflammatory cytokines. It has been demonstrated that NFAT transcriptional activity is preferentially induced by UVB wavelengths in HaCaT keratinocytes and retroviral Phoenix amphotropic (RPA) cells. Inhibiting UV-induced NFAT activation in keratinocytes led to reduced COX-2 protein induction and an increase in UV-induced apoptosis (Flockhart et al. 2008).

Pro-inflammatory cytokines have been shown to activate NF-κB by activating an NF-κB-inducing kinase (NIK)/MEKK–IκB kinase (IKK)–IκB signaling pathway in many cell types. Studies have reported that the suppression of phosphorylation of NF-κB/p65 on Ser536 reduced the activation and nuclear translocation of NF-κB and functionally led to the resistance of JB6 cells to TNF-α-induced transformation (Hu et al. 2005; Lu et al. 2006).

Different proteases also play important role in the transformation of skin cancer cells. Serpins constitute the most broadly distributed super family of protease inhibitors described in humans. Expression profiling of normal epidermal keratinocytes and transformed SCC cell lines revealed up-regulation of SerpinA1 in the latter and that the level of SerpinA1 mRNA has shown marked up-regulation as analyzed by quantitative RT-PCR. SerpinA1 production by SCC cells appears to be dependent on p38 MAPK activity and up-regulated by EGF, TNF-α, interferon-gamma (IFN-γ), and IL-1β (Farshchian et al. 2011). Other important protease is stromelysin-2 (MMP-10), which is known to be involved in the growth of skin tumors. The level of MMP-10 was up-regulated in a cutaneous SCC cell line (UT-SCC-7) by TNF-α and keratinocyte growth factor and by IFN-γ in combination with transforming growth factor (TGF)-β1 and TNF-α both in UT-SCC-7 and in HaCaT cells (Kerkela et al. 2001).

HPV are known to be additional cofactors in the development of cutaneous SCC. Several studies have evaluated the ability of the E6 and E7 proteins of HPV to transform cells in vitro. HPV 10 and HPV 20 E7 proteins do not display in vitro transforming activities. Moreover, E6 and E7 of HPV 38 have been shown to immortalize primary human keratinocytes, suggesting a role of HPV 38 infection in skin carcinogenesis. High-risk HPV E5 is considered tumorigenic because it transforms murine fibroblasts and keratinocytes in tissue culture, enhances the immortalization potential of E6 and E7, and, in cooperation with E7, stimulates the proliferation of human and mouse primary cells (IARC 2007).

17.3.2 Role of Inflammatory Molecules in the Survival and Proliferation of Skin Cancer Cells

Available experimental evidence suggests that the inflammatory response plays a role in providing survival and proliferative signals to initiated cells, thereby leading to tumor promotion (Balkwill and Coussens 2004). While NF-κB protein is a key player in inflammation, other molecular targets comprise cytokines, chemokines, ROS, oncogenes, inflammatory enzymes (COX-2, 5-lipoxygenase [5-LOX], MMP), anti-apoptotic proteins, transcription factors (STAT3, AP-1, CREB, nuclear factor erythroid 2-related factor 2 [Nrf2]) that regulate tumor cell proliferation, transformation, and survival (Shanmugam et al. 2012).

Expression of NF-κB has been shown to promote cell proliferation and contribute to cell survival mechanism. Cell lines from SCC are reported to constitutively express activated NF-κB (Balkwill and Coussens 2004). Definitive evidence that STAT3 (which is inducible by IL-6 signaling) contributes to oncogenesis has shown that interrupting STAT3 signaling blocks the transformation of fibroblasts by SRC oncoprotein (Yu et al. 2007; Hanahan and Weinberg 2011). Constitutively activated STAT3 is known to support tumor cell survival and proliferation by up-regulating expression of the anti-apoptotic protein, Bcl-2, in diverse human cancer cell lines, including melanoma cells. STAT3 also controls expression of cyclins D1, D2, and B, as well as the proto-oncogene c-Myc, and through them, it may stimulate cell proliferation (Yu et al. 2007).

The tumor- and progression-promoting effect of inflammatory cytokines is substantiated by the enhanced tumor growth of IL-6-transfected human BCC as well as by the malignant progression that is associated with the expression of G-colony-stimulating factor (G-CSF) and granulocyte/macrophage colony-stimulating factor (GM-CSF) in HaCaT keratinocyte cells (Mueller 2006). Studies on TNF-α signaling, the most extensively studied pro-inflammatory cytokines in skin carcinogenesis, revealed an involvement of both TNF-α receptor subtypes, as well as of protein kinase C-alpha (PKC-α) and transcription factors of the AP-1 family in tumor promotion-mediated inflammation and proliferation as well as angiogenesis and invasion (Balkwill and Coussens 2004; Mueller 2006; Mantovani et al. 2008). Cytokines also control the inflammatory milieu to either favor anti-tumor immunity (IL-12, TNF-related apoptosis-inducing ligand [TRAIL], IFN-γ) or enhance tumor progression (IL-6, IL-17, IL-23) and also have direct effects on cancer cell growth and survival (TRAIL, FasL, TNF-α, EGFR ligands, TGF-β, IL-6) as in the case of melanoma cells (Haghnegahdar et al. 2000).

Tumor progression locus 2 (Tpl2) is a MAP3 kinase at the crossroad of various pro-inflammatory and oncogenic signals with a major role in promoting cell proliferation and transformation through activation of the ERK MAPK. Studies have reported a link between naturally occurring high levels of Tpl2 expression and ERK phosphorylation in melanoma cell lines. The over-expression of Tpl2 in melanoma cells carrying mutated B-Raf is associated with resistance to the Raf kinase inhibitor PLX4720. Tpl2 can also stimulate the activation of JNK and to a lesser extent p38c and ERK5 by directly phosphorylating their upstream kinases MKK4, MKK6, and MEK5 (Vougioukalaki et al. 2011). Ras, which is mutated in approximately 25 % of all malignancies, promotes cell proliferation and tumor growth of malignant cells. During inflammatory stimuli, Ras induces the expression of various inflammatory gene products, including the pro-inflammatory cytokines IL-1, IL-6, and IL-11, and the chemokine IL-8. ROS have been reported to be tumorigenic by virtue of their ability to increase cell proliferation, survival, and cellular migration through the activation and synthesis of AP-1, a regulator of cell growth, proliferation, and apoptosis (Reuter et al. 2010).

PGE2, which plays a key role in normal skin homeostasis, has been shown to be a critical player mediating the contribution of the COX-2 pathway to cancer development and acts as a tumor promoter, controlling many of the behaviors typical of cancer cells. Studies have shown increased E prostanoid 1 (EP) receptor levels in murine skin tumor cells and that this receptor is critical for the mitogenic effects of PGE2 on these cells in vitro, a finding that has also been demonstrated in NIH-3T3 cells (Tober et al. 2006).

In vitro studies have implicated Bmx (bone marrow tyrosine kinase gene in chromosome X) gene signaling in cell migration and survival. Bmx over-expression accelerates keratinocyte proliferation and wound re-epithelialization and also induces chronic inflammation in the skin and that this occurs via cytokine-mediated recruitment of inflammatory cells (Paavonen et al. 2004).

Cylindromatosis (CYLD), which encodes a 956 amino acid enzyme that is ubiquitously expressed, contains a deubiquitinating domain at the C-terminus.

Mutations that inactivate the carboxyl-terminal-deubiquitinating domain of CYLD deregulate the NF-κB activity, underlying the development of skin appendage tumors in humans (Brummelkamp et al. 2003; Trompouki et al. 2003). It was demonstrated that the expression in tumorigenic epidermal cells of a catalytically inactive form of CYLD (CYLDC/S) that mimics the identified mutations of cyld in human tumors and competes with the endogenous CYLD results in enhanced cell proliferation and inhibition of apoptosis. These indicate an increased oncogenicity of the tumorigenic epidermal CYLDC/S mutant cells in vitro. The loss of CYLD in keratinocytes has been linked to hyperproliferation and elevation in cyclin D1 levels because of increased nuclear activity of Bcl-3-associated NF-κB p50 and p52 (Massoumi et al. 2006). A decrease in CYLD function results in an increase in the malignant behavior of the tumor epidermal cells and progression of skin carcinomas, as seen by an enhancement in proliferation and survival of the cells expressing the mutant CYLDC/S. Tumor epidermal cells expressing CYLDC/S also show an important increase in the nuclear localization of Bcl-3, p52, and β-catenin.

Tumor formation involves epigenetic modifications and microenvironmental changes as well as cumulative genetic alterations encompassing somatic mutations, loss of heterozygosity, and aneuploidy. The role of NF-κB in epidermal hyperproliferation arising from p120 loss appears rooted in its impact on epidermal microenvironment because p120-null keratinocytes display a growth-arrested phenotype in culture due to mitotic alterations and chronic inflammatory responses, resulting in unstable, binucleated cells in vitro (Perez-Moreno et al. 2008).

17.3.3 Role of Inflammatory Molecules in the Invasion, Metastasis, and Angiogenesis of Skin Cancer Cells

Several clinical observations and experimental findings indicate that the process of metastasis is non-random and involves a sequence of multistep events targeted for therapy. Metastatic cancer cells exploit the mechanisms of the inflammation process, which successfully migrate into distant organs. This implies a pivotal role for specific adhesive interactions between cancer cells and vascular endothelial cells and activation of migratory pathways in the cancer cells (Laferriere et al. 2002). The tumor cells follow the extravasation strategy of leukocytes in their migration toward inflammatory sites (Witz 2006). For instance, VCAM-1, an integrin receptor located on an endothelial cell, binds to the integrin α4 β1 (VLA-4—very late antigen-4), which are normally expressed on leukocyte plasma membranes, but they do not adhere to their appropriate ligands until the leukocytes are activated by chemotactic agents or other stimuli (Schadendorf et al. 1995).

Selectins have been involved in the progression of cancer. In fact, several types of tumor cells express functional ligands of selectins and contact selectins expressed on blood vessel walls (Laferriere et al. 2002; Witz 2006; Barthel et al. 2007). Keratinocyte cell lines—A431, HaCaT, SVK14—express selectin ligands including sialyl Lewis X and S-Le(a) expression, whereas normal human keratinocytes do not. These findings suggest a potential role for selectin-mediated events in the early and late metastasis (Groves et al. 1993). To this end, the study of the role of selectins in leukocyte and tumor cell extravasation merits particular attention in understanding the pathophysiology of inflammation and cancer and is substantiated by a number of recent studies (Witz 2006; Barthel et al. 2007). There is also growing awareness that platelets and leukocytes may potentiate and even enhance the hematogenous dissemination of cancer cells, suggesting a link between inflammation and cancer progression. Indeed, the tumor microenvironment often contains infiltrates of platelets, macrophages, dendritic cells, and lymphocytes (Mantovani et al. 2008). These cells may be critical sources of pro-inflammatory cytokines, including TGF-β, TNF-α, IL-1β, and IL-6, all of which may promote the up-regulation of selectin expression on the vascular wall and synergize with chemokines, such as IL-8, secreted by tumor cells.

Tumor invasion and metastasis represent a multistep process that depends on the activity of many proteins (Hua et al. 2011; Shanmugam et al. 2012; Ravi and Piva 2013). Several classes of proteases, including MMPs, serine proteases like furin, and cysteine proteases such as cathepsin have been implicated in the tumor cell-invasive process. Of these, MMPs appear to be primarily responsible for extracellular matrix (ECM) degradation observed during invasive processes (Hua et al. 2011; Pytliak et al. 2012; Ravi and Piva 2013). They contribute to tumor growth by degradation of the ECM as well as by the release of sequestered growth factors such as VEGF, b-fibroblast growth factor (b-FGF), or TGFβ, the suppression of tumor cell apoptosis and the destruction of immune-modulating chemokine gradients (Ravi and Piva 2013). In normal skin, MMPs are not constitutively expressed but can be induced temporarily in response to exogenous signals such as UVR. UVR is known to elevate the expression of MMP-1, MMP-3 (stromelysin-1), and MMP-9 in human skin. MMP-2 and MMP-9 have been frequently associated with the invasive and metastatic potential of tumor cells (Ramos et al. 2004; Dong et al. 2008; Ravi and Piva 2013).

Furin is a serine protease that is frequently over-expressed in several cancer cell lines and malignancies, including several murine cell lines derived from chemically induced skin tumors (Fu et al. 2012). Its activity results in proteolytic cleavage of substrates, leading to the activation of many cancer-related proteins including important growth factors and receptors such as insulin growth factor-1 (IGF-1) and its receptor IGF-1R, TGF-β, and VEGF. (Siegfried et al. 2003; Ravi and Piva 2013). Furin is also involved in the maturation of both TNF-alpha-converting enzyme (TACE) and MMP within skin cells and mainly activate MT1-MMP, which directly contributes to the motility and invasiveness of the tumor cell, thereby indicating that furin activity has an influence on the inflammation seen in the skin, following exposure to UVR (Ravi and Piva 2013). It has been shown that furin mRNA, protein, and enzyme activity increase immediately after UVA and UVB treatment in human epidermal keratinocytes (HaCaT cells). Furin/PC processing of substrates has been shown to contribute to tumor progression, aggressiveness, metastasis, and angiogenesis (Arsenault et al. 2012; Fu et al. 2012; Ravi and Piva 2013).

Cytokines play a crucial role in tumor progression. Pro-inflammatory cytokine, TNF-α, stimulates the secretion of active MMP-2, an enzyme that degrades type IV collagenase, in organ-cultured full-thickness human skin. TNF-α also induces MMP-2 activation in human skin and thus induces angiogenesis with the MMPs involved in wound healing or cancer cell invasion. As basement membrane components, type IV collagen and laminin are potential substrates for MMP-2, and activation of a type IV collagenase by this cytokine may provide a mechanistic explanation for the role of TNF-α during metastasis and angiogenesis (Han et al. 2001). TNF-α up-regulates malignant melanoma invasion and migration in vitro. In melanoma, TNF-α may exert its pro-invasive effect on human cutaneous melanoma cell line via an integrin-dependent mechanism as well as a modest up-regulation of degradative enzyme activity not readily detected in general protease assays (Katerinaki et al. 2003).

IL-6 is also one of the pro-inflammatory cytokines induced by UVR in keratinocytes (Schwarz and Luger 1989; Chung et al. 1996). IL-6 induced angiogenesis in human BCC cell line by up-regulation of bFGF via both Janus kinase (JAK)/STAT3 and PI3-kinase/Akt pathways. Blockage of COX-2 by siRNA reduced angiogenic activity in IL-6 over-expressing BCC cells, suggesting that COX-2 also plays a role in IL-6-induced angiogenesis (Jee et al. 2004). IL-6 also plays important role in tumor progression from benign to malignant, in invasive tumors in the HaCaT model of human skin carcinoma by activating STAT3, and directly stimulates proliferation and migration of the benign non-invasive HaCaT-ras A-5 cells in vitro. Furthermore, IL-6 induces inflammatory and angiogenic factors such as IL-8, GM-CSF, and CSF as well as VEGF and monocyte chemotactic protein-1 (MCP-1) in the tumor cells, leading to tumor cell invasion in organotypic cultures in vitro. Tumor invasion is supported by the IL-6 induced over-expression of MMP-1 in vitro and in vivo, thus demonstrating a key function of IL-6 in the progression of skin SCC by regulating a complex cytokine and protease network (Lederle et al. 2011).

A majority of cancers over-express COX-2, an enzyme responsible for the biosynthesis of PG metabolites. Enhanced production of PGs, and particularly PGE2, has been linked with tumor progression, invasion, and metastasis. Human epidermis actively synthesizes PGs, and previous studies have demonstrated that PGE2 generation can regulate epidermal cell proliferation in vitro. Elevated levels of PGE2 observed in SCC and BCC of the skin may correlate with an increased propensity for metastatic and invasive behavior (Singh and Katiyar 2011).

VEGF is known to be a key regulator of cutaneous angiogenesis and as such plays a role in several physiological and disease processes in the skin, including hair growth, cancer development, and psoriasis as well as wound healing. It has been shown that VEGF is essential for tumor development in multistage models of skin carcinogenesis, and the mechanism of action has been primarily attributed to the induction of angiogenesis (Johnson and Wilgus 2012). VEGFR-1, expressed in mouse and human skin tumor cells and in SCC cell lines, suggests that VEGF could affect tumor cells directly. UV up-regulates VEGF production in keratinocyte-derived cell lines both directly through transcription factor activation and indirectly through cytokine release. VEGF has also been shown to induce the migration of primary keratinocytes in vitro (Zhu et al. 2013).

17.4 Role of Inflammatory Molecules in the Development of Skin Cancer: Evidence from In Vivo Studies

Chemically induced mouse skin tumors using inflammatory agent, 12-O-tetradecanoylphorbol-13-acetate (TPA), for tumor promotion greatly contributed to our understanding of multistage carcinogenesis and have given important insights into the functional interaction between inflammatory microenvironment and epithelial tumor, especially when used in combination with transgenic animals. Data from these and additional new model systems clearly emphasize that the tumor-promoting microenvironment is indispensable for tumor formation and progression.

The two-stage mouse skin carcinogenesis and UV-induced photocarcinogenesis are well established in vivo models for the understanding of the multistage nature of tumor development to design novel therapeutic concepts for human epithelial neoplasia. In two-stage mouse skin model, tumor initiation is accomplished through a single topical application of a carcinogen, typically 7,12-dimethylbenz(a)anthracene (DMBA) that results in an initiated state of the epidermal keratinocytes, which frequently harbor one single genetic mutation (e.g., ras activation) and are more susceptible to subsequent genetic alterations (Mueller 2006). Tumor promotion achieved by repeated treatment with phorbol esters, such as TPA, resulted in benign papillomas, some of which spontaneously progress into malignant SCC. TPA activates a series of PKC isoenzymes and induces a pleiotropic tissue response, resulting in a strong inflammatory reaction (Rundhaug and Fischer 2010).

Tumor promoters, whether UV, chemicals, or endogenous factors, usually interact at the cell surfaces with specific receptors or other cell components that elicit several processes/responses, including enhanced DNA synthesis, increased production of eicosanoids, cytokines and growth factors, a pro-oxidant state, and alterations in cell surface properties, leading to changes in cell adhesion and cell-to-cell communication (Rundhaug and Fischer 2010).

Chronic exposure to UV leads to the up-regulation of COX-2 expression and chronic inflammation along with the accumulation of DNA damage and mutations, all of which combine to induce malignant changes in epidermal keratinocytes and skin cancers (Rundhaug and Fischer 2010). Topical application of a prototype tumor promoter, TPA, induces expression of COX-2 and its mRNA transcript in mouse skin in vivo by activating eukaryotic transcription factors such as NF-κB and AP-1. These in turn are regulated by a series of upstream kinases collectively known as MAP kinases such as ERK, p38 MAPK, and JUN amino-terminal kinase (JNK) (Chun et al. 2006; Kundu et al. 2006), thereby contributing to the inflammatory responses mediated by TPA and in arachidonic acid metabolite production (Kundu et al. 2006). Inappropriate up-regulation of COX-2 also prolongs the survival of malignant or transformed cells and leads to phenotypic changes associated with metastatic potential (Surh et al. 2001). COX-2 also has roles in keratinocyte differentiation, and the absence of COX-2 causes premature terminal differentiation of initiated keratinocytes and reduced tumor formation in DMBA/TPA-induced mouse skin carcinogenesis (Tiano et al. 2002). Increase in COX-2 results in a subsequent increase in the level of PGs, which inappropriately up-regulated in various premalignant and malignant tissues. Elevated levels of some PGs, especially PGE2 and PGF2-α, are functionally related to mouse skin tumor promotion (Furstenberger et al. 1989). Even topical application of a COX-2 product, 15-deoxy-D12,14-prostaglandin J2, has been shown to potentiate DMBA/TPA-induced mouse skin tumorigenesis (Millan et al. 2006), which indicated the important role of COX-2 in tumor promotion in vivo (Kundu et al. 2006). This was also evident by using transgenic mouse model, wherein COX-2 over-expressing transgenic mice (Muller-Decker et al. 2002) are highly susceptible to spontaneous skin tumor formation, while COX-2 knockout animals (Tiano et al. 2002) are less prone to experimentally induced tumorigenesis.

TGFβ1 and TNF-α, which play crucial role in the inflammatory process during wound healing, are the most comprehensively studied pro-inflammatory cytokines in skin carcinogenesis (Urban et al. 1986). TGFβ1 up-regulates PG generation and COX-1 and COX-2 expressions of mast cells and significantly affects skin tumor promotion by paradoxically enhancing epidermal proliferation, besides stimulating inflammation within a developing tumor (Perez-Lorenzo et al. 2010). This was evident by abrogation of TGF-β signaling by knocking out Smad3 (mothers against decapentaplegic homolog 3), which results in resistance to chemical carcinogenesis (Li et al. 2004; Mueller 2006).

TNF-α has been shown to activate neutrophils and mediate the cytotoxic effects of activated macrophages (Urban et al. 1986). The pro-inflammatory effect of TNF-α seems to be important for early stages of tumor promotion. This is evident from the observations, wherein TNF-α-deficient mouse is resistant to the development of benign and malignant skin tumors induced by repeated DMBA exposure or initiation with DMBA and promotion with TPA/okadaic acid. The resistance was associated with a clearly decreased inflammatory response in the dermis of the transgenic animals. Later stages of carcinogenesis were not affected by TNF-α as tumors in wild-type and TNF-α-deficient mice showed similar rates of malignant progression (Scott et al. 2004; Mueller 2006). TNF-α initiates the activation of NF-κB signaling through its receptor, TNFR1, by recruiting the IKK complex and through PKCζ and PI3K/Akt phosphorylation (Martin et al. 2001; Rundhaug and Fischer 2010). NF-κB signaling leads to the induction of a variety of anti-apoptotic factors. Another TNFR1-mediated signaling pathway is the activation of the JNK cascade. The activated JNK phosphorylates the AP-1 transcription factor, leading to transcriptional up-regulation of AP-1-responsive genes, such as GM-CSF, MMP-3, and MMP-9, which are involved in proliferation, differentiation, and apoptosis and promote inflammation and angiogenesis as well as invasion of tumor keratinocytes (Scott et al. 2004; Rundhaug and Fischer 2010).

IL-1 is another important cytokine secreted by monocytes and macrophages, which drive the acute phase of inflammation. Many cell types produce IL-1 after stimulation by microorganisms, cytokines, or other environmental insults. IL-1α activates adjacent cells (or IL-1β on distant cells) to induce the expression of additional pro-inflammatory genes, including IL-6, COX-2, and iNOS (Apte et al. 2006).

Various skin tumor promoters induce IL-1α mRNA and protein expression in the epidermis in vivo (Oberyszyn et al. 1993; Lee et al. 1994). Blocking the activity of IL-1α with intradermal injections of a neutralizing antibody inhibits TPA-induced vascular permeability, inflammatory cell infiltration, and epidermal hyperplasia, which demonstrates the central role of IL-1α in mediating these tumor promoter-related events (Lee et al. 1994). Transgenic mice over-expressing IL-1α in basal keratinocytes (K14 promoter) develop spontaneous inflammatory skin lesions, as well as dermal neutrophil infiltration even in non-lesional skin (Groves et al. 1995). Moreover, stable over-expression of antagonist of IL-1 (IL-1Ra) in mouse skin carcinoma cell line results in down-regulated COX-2 expression and slower in vitro and in vivo growth. These results indicate that IL-1 is contributing to malignant cell proliferation (Rundhaug and Fischer 2010). IL-12 and IL-23 also play role in skin tumorigenesis, wherein IL-12 acts as a tumor suppressor by inducing immune surveillance and IL-23 promotes skin tumorigenesis by driving inflammation and reducing immune surveillance. While IL-12p35-null mice develop papillomas earlier and more frequently than wild-type mice, IL-23p19-null mice, as well as p40-null mice, are resistant to DMBA/TPA induction of skin tumorigenesis (Langowski et al. 2006). In addition, IL-12p35- and IL-12p40-null mice are more sensitive to UV-induced skin carcinogenesis, with reduced repair of UV-induced DNA damage, increased number of tumors per mouse, more rapid growth, and greater malignant potential than wild-type mice. UV-induced tumors from IL-12p35-null mice also have increased angiogenesis and up-regulated expression of pro-inflammatory IL-6 and IL-23 (Meeran et al. 2007). Thus, IL-12 counteracts UV-induced immunosuppression, inflammation, and skin carcinogenesis.

Proteinases such as MMP-2 and MMP-9, provided by mast cells as well as granulocyte neutrophils in inflammatory microenvironment, play important roles as regulators of development, angiogenesis, and tumor progression. The essential role of stromal MMP-9 for tumor development in K14-HPV16 transgenic mice showed that mice deficient for MMP-9 resulted in decreased tumor incidence (Coussens et al. 1996). In addition, lack of MMP-9 was associated with delayed activation of angiogenesis in the stroma of the lesions (Mueller 2006). In another study, it has been shown that MMP-9 expressed by inflammatory cells is functionally involved in distinct processes of epithelial carcinogenesis such as regulation of oncogene-induced keratinocyte hyperproliferation, progression to invasive cancer, and end-stage malignancy (Coussens et al. 2000).

17.5 Evidence from Patients for the Role of Inflammation in Skin Cancer

The association between chronic inflammation and cancer including epithelial skin tumors was illustrated by epidemiologic and clinical studies for years (Lu et al. 2006). One of the earliest descriptions for the relationship between chronic inflammation and epithelial skin tumors is Marjolin's ulcer, which describes a relatively uncommon ulcerative condition associated with a thermal injury in which malignant transformation occurs within a chronic inflammatory focus. Various other similar associations have been observed for lupus erythematosus, leg ulcerations, osteomyelitis, perineal inflammatory disease, ulcerative lichen planus, and epidermolysis bullosa, where SCC development with inflammatory disorders had been seen in non-healing wounds. Inflammation also plays an important role in skin cancer progression. It is evident in a study, where progression of AK to SCC preceded by a short inflammatory phase in the AK. This is paralleled by an increase in the number of cells expressing detectable levels of p53 and Bcl-2 and a decrease in the number of cells expressing FasL, suggesting increasing resistance to cell cycle arrest and apoptosis (Mueller 2006).

It is established knowledge that there may be a mild-to-moderate chronic inflammatory cell infiltrate at the periphery of the tumors. In the cohort study of patients with head and neck cutaneous SCC, a dense infiltrate of lymphocytes was found in the dermis in 84/315 index tumors. Notably, the proportion of the presence of this infiltrate was significantly higher in those tumors that recurred (Kyrgidis et al. 2010). Moreover, peri-neoplastic inflammation in intraepithelial SCC is pronounced both in immune-competent patients and in organ transplant recipients (OTRs). Inflammation increases further in invasive SCC. OTRs show reduced proportions of regulatory T cells and CD123+ plasmacytoid dendritic cells. This distinct inflammatory infiltrate may result in the increased cutaneous carcinogenesis and more aggressive behavior of SCC in OTRs (Muhleisen et al. 2009).

In response to systemic inflammation, and in particular to elevated IL-6 levels, the liver produces C-reactive protein (CRP) used as a marker of systemic inflammation, which binds to dead or dying cells to activate the complement system. Elevated CRP concentration increases the risk for "all-cause" mortality compared to other subjects (Marsik et al. 2008). Cancer patients with highly elevated CRP showed increased mortality by a factor of 28, which confirms correlation between cancer progression and inflammation. Mikirova et al. (2012) observed that twenty-eight out of forty-five subjects had sharply elevated CRP levels in cancer patients, suggesting that inflammation is a prevalent problem for cancer patients. This is especially important since other reports indicate that inflammation, particularly elevated CRP, is a marker of a poor prognosis (St Sauver et al. 2009). They also observed higher level of pro-inflammatory cytokines IL-1α, IL-2, IL-8, TNF-α, chemokine eotaxin, which were reduced after treatment for vitamin C (Mikirova et al. 2012).

Prostaglandins generated by the arachidonic acid cascade particularly PGE2 have been involved in various models for tumorigenesis (Vanderveen et al. 1986). Squamous cell skin cancer appears to link with chronic activation of the PG biosynthetic pathway resulting from recurrent UVB exposure. In the series of tumor biopsies evaluated, COX-2 was highly expressed in SCC within the overlying sun-exposed epidermis as well as within the tumor nests. Positive staining was also observed within the endothelium and smooth muscle layers of the blood vessels and infiltrative macrophages of SCC biopsies (Buckman et al. 1998).

Taken together, the association of inflammation with enhanced tumor formation and tumor progression has been supported by a large number of clinical studies;

however, these studies do not allow any insight in the cellular and molecular mechanisms that lie at the basis of the tumor and progression-promoting effect of inflammation in epithelial skin cancers.

17.6 Inhibitors of Inflammation for the Prevention and Treatment of Skin Cancer

Evidence suggests that inflammation is causally linked to carcinogenesis (Balkwill and Coussens 2004). COX-2, the rate-limiting enzyme in arachidonic acid metabolism leading to PG synthesis, is up-regulated in murine and human NMSC. Inhibition of COX-2 by biochemical inhibitors or genetic deletion decreases chemical- or UV-induced skin tumor development (Wright et al. 2006). A number of animal models have shown that inhibition of COX-2 helps prevent skin cancer, including UVR-induced skin carcinogenesis and two-stage skin carcinogenesis model in mice.

17.6.1 Non-steroidal Anti-inflammatory Drugs (NSAIDs)

Drugs of this class include celecoxib, diclofenac, indomethacin, sulindac, aspirin, and ibuprofen. They act by repressing prostaglandin biosynthesis through inhibition of COX (Bode and Dong 2000). The expression of COX-2 is linked to excessive activation of intracellular signal transduction pathways comprising proline-directed serine/threonine kinases and their downstream transcription factors. There is an important relation between MAPK signaling and COX-2 expression, which further supports the idea that agents modulating MAPK signaling pathways can be effective in chemoprevention of skin cancer (Shrotriya et al. 2010).

Celecoxib, a COX-2 inhibitor, decreases macrophage and neutrophil infiltration into skin tumors, as well as inflammation induced by 50 Gy radiation (Liang et al. 2003). Celecoxib at the doses, determined to be equivalent to twice-daily doses in humans, was effective at increasing tumor latency and decreasing multiplicity in hairless mice exposed to UVR. This study showed a decrease in PG synthesis in the epidermis, as well as a statistically significant decrease in tumor yield (Fischer et al. 1999). Oral or topical administration of celecoxib has been reported to prevent new tumor formation after the onset of UV-induced photocarcinogenesis in hairless mice (Wilgus et al. 2003), while also suppressing PGE2 production induced by UVB. Such sensitization appears to be mediated through inhibition of AP-1, JNK, and p38 signaling pathways. In DMBA-initiated/TPA-promoted female ICR mouse skin, application of celecoxib also significantly reduced the multiplicity of papillomas, which was associated with decreased expression of COX-2 and VEGF, as well as inhibition of CCAAT (cytidine–cytidine–adenosine–adenosine–thymidine)/C/EBP (enhancer binding protein) activation (Chun et al. 2006). Oral administration of celecoxib is also effective in the prevention of SCC and BCC in individuals who have extensive actinic damage and are at high risk for the development of NMSC (Elmets et al. 2010).

Topical application of etodolac one week prior to and after the tumor initiation resulted in a significant delay of the tumor induction and inhibition of the tumor burden as well as multiplicity in the DMBA/TPA-induced skin tumorigenesis in ICR mouse. Treatment with oxyphenbutazone in drinking water increased the tumor latency period and decreased the tumor incidence as well as tumor burden in the peroxynitrite-induced/TPA-promoted skin tumors in the HOS-HR-1-specific pathogen-free mice (Kapadia et al. 2010).

The prototypical COX inhibitor, aspirin, blocks enzymatic activity covalently through the acetylation of Ser-530 in COX-1 and Ser-516 in COX-2 (Wennogle et al. 1995). Aspirin inhibits both UVC- and UVB-induced AP-1 activity in a dose-dependent manner, when the cells are treated with aspirin or before exposure to UVR. The inhibition of UVB-induced AP-1 activity appears to mediate through their ability to block the activation of ERKs, JNKs, and P38 kinases, whereas the inhibitory effect on UVC-induced AP-1 activity seems to be mediated only through the inhibition of JNKs. In the skin of AP-1/luciferase transgenic mice, topical pretreatment of mouse skin with aspirin blocked the UVB-induced AP-1 transactivation in vivo (Huang et al. 1997).

Topical application of indomethacin reduced skin tumor development by ~30 % in the DMBA/TPA-induced mouse skin tumorigenesis (Slaga et al. 1977). Indomethacin has also been shown to reduce photocarcinogenesis in mice and when administered through diet led to the decrease in tumor yield by 78 % in UV-induced skin tumor development in SKH:HR-1 hairless mice and also blocked PG synthesis in the epidermis (Fischer et al. 1999).

Diclofenac, a non-selective NSAID, is widely used in the treatment of AK. In a study of 32 organ transplant recipients with 3 or more AK, patients randomized to twice-daily treatment with 3 % diclofenac showed decrease in lesions and no patients in the diclofenac group had developed SCC in the treated areas. Thus, diclofenac may prevent the cancerous transformation of AK (Ulrich et al. 2010).

Sulindac is NO-releasing NSAIDs, which when synthesized reduces gastrointestinal and cardiovascular toxicities of NSAIDs and possess anti-proliferative, pro-apoptotic, and anti-cancer activities. In the skin, topical application of sulindac reduces UVB-induced cutaneous phototoxicity and significantly decreased the development of UVB-induced skin tumor in SKH-1 hairless mice, as indicated by a substantial reduction in tumor number and tumor volume. The inhibitory effect was corroborated by increase in Bax:Bcl-2 ratio and the expression of pro-apoptotic BCL-2-associated X protein (Bax), decrease in anti-apoptotic Bcl-2 expression indicating increased apoptosis, and reduced cell proliferation as evident by decreased expression of proliferating cell nuclear antigen (PCNA) and cyclin D1. Sulindac diminished UVB-induced inflammatory responses as observed by a remarkable reduction in the levels of phosphorylated MAPK such as ERK1/2, p38, and JNK1/2. It also inhibited NF-κB by enhancing IκBα as evidenced by the reduced expression of iNOS and COX-2, the direct NF-κB transcription target proteins. Moreover, sulindac also significantly reduced the progression of benign lesions to invasive carcinomas by suppressing the tumor aggressiveness and retarding epithelial–mesenchymal transition. Thus, sulindac is a potent inhibitor of UVB-induced and chemically induced skin carcinogenesis and acts by targeting proliferation regulatory pathways (Kim et al. 2006; Chaudhary et al. 2013).

17.6.2 Naturally Occurring Plant Products

Dietary polyphenols which are widely present in fruits, vegetables, dry legumes, and beverages (such as tea, coffee, juice, wine, beer) have gained considerable attention for the prevention of UV-induced skin photodamage including the risk of skin cancer. Experimental and epidemiologic studies have suggested that polyphenols protect the skin from the adverse effects of UV radiation. Polyphenols have been shown to (a) scavenge radical species such as ROS/RNS, e.g., O_2^-, H_2O_2, OH•, $ONOO^-$; (b) suppress ROS/RNS formation by inhibiting some enzymes or chelating trace metals involved in free radical production; and (c) up-regulate or protect antioxidant defense (Patel et al. 2007).

Oral administration of green tea polyphenols (GTPs) to SKH-1 hairless mice resulted in significant inhibition of UVR-induced cutaneous edema, erythema, and bifold skin thickness (a biomarker of inflammation). Administration of GTPs in drinking water decreased COX-2, PGE2, PCNA, and cyclin D1 and also significantly reduced the levels of various pro-inflammatory cytokines in chronically UVB-exposed skin/skin tumors of mice (Meeran et al. 2009). Topical treatment with GTPs prior to UV exposure reduced the UV-induced hyperplastic response, myeloperoxidase (MPO) activity, and the numbers of infiltrating inflammatory leukocytes in the skin (Afaq et al. 2003). Moreover, similar administration of both agents in the untanned backs of humans resulted in significantly less development of erythema as compared to the UV-irradiated skin that was not treated with GTPs (Katiyar et al. 2001). Topical application of EGCG, an active constituent of green tea, in mice and humans, resulted in the inhibition of UVB-induced production of PG metabolites (PGE2, PGF2-α, and PGD2), which play a critical role in inflammatory disorders, free radical generation, proliferative skin diseases, and skin tumor promotion (Katiyar et al. 2001; Katiyar and Mukhtar 2001). The inhibitory effects of GTPs on these biomarkers of inflammation in UV-exposed skin provide mechanistic evidence of the anti-carcinogenic effects of GTPs. Studies have also shown that topical pretreatment with polymeric black tea polyphenols in Swiss bare mouse skin decreased TPA-induced inflammatory protein (COX-2) and cellular proliferation through decreasing activation of cellular kinases (JNK, ERK, p38, and Akt) and transcription factors (AP-1 and NF-κB) as well as apoptosis (Patel et al. 2008). The above in vivo observations generated using both animal and human systems provide insights into the possible protective mechanisms involved in the anti-initiating and/or anti-inflammatory effects of tea polyphenols.

Dietary intake or topical treatment of silymarin as well as resveratrol in UVR-exposed mice also resulted in similar inhibitory effects in terms of inflammation-related biomarkers as observed with GTPs (Gu et al. 2007). These products also inhibited the expression of ornithine decarboxylase (ODC), an enzyme required for polyamine biosynthesis, which has a role in tumor promotion in UVB-exposed skin. Moreover, topical pretreatment with resveratrol in mouse skin is reported to inhibit the TPA-induced (a) AP-1 (c-jun and c-fos) via modulation of p38 and JNK; (b) nuclear translocation of p65 and subsequent DNA binding of NF-κB by blocking the degradation of IκBα; (c) phosphorylation of p65 and its interaction with CREB-binding protein (CBP)/p300, rendering NF-κB transcriptionally inactive; and (d) mRNA levels of COX-1, COX-2, c-myc, c-fos, c-Jun, TGF-β1, and TNF-α and protein levels of COX-2 (Jang and Pezzuto 1999; Kundu et al. 2006). Topical application of rosemary was observed to decrease TPA-induced tumor promotion through inhibition of hyperplasia, ODC activity, and inflammatory responses (Osakabe et al. 2004).

Bromelain derived from pineapple, when applied topically, resulted in delay in onset and thereby inhibition of tumor development in DMBA-initiated/TPA-promoted skin tumors in female Swiss albino mice. The mechanism involved in anti-carcinogenic activity is underlined by induction of p53, shift in Bax/Bcl-2 ratio, induction of caspases, decrease in COX-2 expression, and inhibition of NF-κB pathway by regulating MAPK and Akt/PKB pathways (Bhui et al. 2009). Pretreatment with oligonol has been shown to significantly inhibit the expression of COX-2 in skin papillomas and carcinomas in DMBA/TPA-induced skin carcinogenesis (Kundu et al. 2009).

Administration of polyphenol fraction from dried fruits of *Crataegus pinnatifida* (CF-TP), diallyl trisulfide (DATS), organosulfur compounds from garlic, and D-limonene exhibited an inhibitory effect on DMBA/TPA-mediated mouse skin tumorigenesis. These effects are evidenced by reduction in TPA-mediated inflammatory responses (edema, hyperplasia, COX-2, iNOS expression), activation of ODC, and oxidative stress, which were attributed to the inhibition of Ras/Raf/ERK1/2 signaling pathway, blockade of AP-1 activation via downregulation of upstream Akt and JNK signaling pathways, and promotion to pro-apoptotic state (Chaudhary et al. 2012; Shrotriya et al. 2010). Moreover, CF-TP inhibited the activation of NF-κB and AP-1 induced by TPA in JB6 P+ cells as well as benzo[a]pyrene (B[a]P)/TPA-induced skin tumor formation and decreased the incidence of tumor. CF-TP also suppressed TPA-induced MPO activation, which is used as a marker to quantitate the extent to which leukocytes that have infiltrated into the dermis produce reactive oxygen intermediates in response to topical stimuli (Kao et al. 2007). Apigenin exerts chemopreventive effects on UVB-induced COX-2 and skin inflammation in JB6 P+ mouse epidermal cells and SKH-1 hairless mice by directly suppressing Src kinase activity (Byun et al. 2013).

Topical application of euphol isolated from the roots of *Euphorbia kansui* markedly inhibited TPA-induced ear edema and skin inflammation in DMBA/TPA-treated male CD 1 mice (Yasukawa et al. 2000). Euphol also inhibited activation of downstream signaling proteins, namely PKC and MAPKs, which in turn decreased the levels of CXC chemokines and COX-2, following topical application of TPA. Thus, euphol exhibits strong topical anti-inflammatory actions on mouse ear through a mechanism that involves its ability to regulate PKC and ERK activation, resulting in reduced COX-2, MIP-2, and CXCL1/KC up-regulation and leukocyte infiltration (Passos et al. 2013).

Female Swiss albino mice pretreated topically with geraniol (GOH) prior to TPA administration significantly inhibited TPA-induced lipid peroxidation (LPO), inflammatory responses, pro-inflammatory cytokine release, reduced glutathione (GSH) content, and the activity of different antioxidant enzymes. GOH attenuated early tumor promotional changes through TPA-induced altered expression of NF-κB (p65) and COX-2 and inhibited TPA-induced altered activity of p38 MAPK. GOH also effectively suppresses the production of the TNF-α, IL-1β, and IL-6 cytokines (Khan et al. 2013).

Topical treatment of UVB-induced mice with honokiol, magnolol, or silibinin decreased tumor multiplicity and volume. These effects are corroborated by decrease in the UVB-induced expression of markers of inflammation and proliferation, e.g., COX-2, PGE2, PCNA, cyclins, Cdc25B, and associated Cdks (2, 4, 6) besides phosphorylation and nuclear translocation of STAT3 (Tyr 705, Ser536) and NF-κB/its DNA-binding activity, which are potential upstream regulators of iNOS and COX-2 in the skin/skin tumors of mice. Moreover, these products increased the levels of CDK-interacting protein 1 (Cip)/p21, Kip/p27, cleavage of caspase-8, and poly-ADP-ribose polymerase (PARP) by inhibiting the levels of PI3K and the phosphorylation of Akt (Mallikarjuna et al. 2004; Vaid et al. 2010; Chilampalli et al. 2011). Treatment with honokiol also significantly inhibited UVB-induced expression of pro-inflammatory cytokines, such as TNF-α, IL-1β, and IL-6, in the mouse skin/skin tumors and that may have contributed in the inhibition of tumor development (Vaid et al. 2010). Topical pretreatment with delphinidin inhibits the UVB-induced MAPKK and PI3K activity directly to suppress COX-2 over-expression in mouse skin (Kwon et al. 2009).

Caffeine is effective in inhibiting the UVB-induced AKT/COX-2 pathway independent of ATR in human HaCaT keratinocyte, which results in the induction of UVB-induced apoptosis. Blocking the AKT/COX-2 signaling by caffeine specifically eliminates UVB-damaged keratinocytes without complete DNA repair through apoptosis (Han et al. 2011).

Benzene fraction of *Selaginella bryopteris* inhibited the expression of the inflammatory cytokines IL-8, IL-1β, and TNF-α in methyl isocyanate-stimulated HEK-293 cells. In a parallel study involving a two-stage protocol of DMBA/croton oil-induced skin carcinogenesis, oral administration of the flavonoid-rich benzene fraction of *S. bryopteris* prior to croton oil application caused significant reduction in tumor incidence and multiplicity with significant delay in the latency period, providing evidence to the effect of polyphenolic flavonoids as anti-carcinogenic and/or anti-tumor-promoting agents (Mishra et al. 2011).

Collectively, the results concerning the inhibitory effects of these naturally occurring plant products on UV- and phorbol ester-induced inflammatory responses revealed that anti-carcinogenic activity of naturally occurring plant products is mediated in part through their anti-inflammatory effects.

17.7 Conclusions and Future Directions

Melanoma and non-melanoma skin cancers are among the most prevalent cancers in human. Epidemiological and experimental evidence suggests "chronic inflammation" to be one of the hallmarks in solar UVR and several other environmental agent-mediated skin cancers. The identification of transcription factors, i.e., NF-κB, STAT3, and HIF-1α, and their gene products, i.e., COX-2, cytokines, chemokines, and chemokine receptors, suggests critical role of inflammation in skin carcinogenesis. Considering the potential role of inflammation in initiation and its major as well as convincing role in promotion, progression as well as tumor angiogenesis and metastasis, inflammatory pathways may become attractive targets for skin cancer prevention. Efforts to prevent or minimize the exposure to known skin carcinogens and ongoing studies on evaluating the role of various pro-inflammatory mediators in carcinogenesis and assessing them as potential targets for chemoprevention of skin cancers need to be enhanced/encouraged.

Acknowledgments We thank Dr. Vikram Gota for useful discussion and Council of Scientific and Industrial Research (CSIR) and ACTREC, Government of India, for awarding fellowship to Mr. Gaurav Kumar.

References

Afaq F, Ahmad N, Mukhtar H (2003) Suppression of UVB-induced phosphorylation of mitogen-activated protein kinases and nuclear factor kappa B by green tea polyphenol in SKH-1 hairless mice. Oncogene 22(58):9254–9264. doi:10.1038/sj.onc.1207035

Aggarwal BB, Vijayalekshmi RV, Sung B (2009) Targeting inflammatory pathways for prevention and therapy of cancer: short-term friend, long-term foe. Clin Cancer Res: Official J Am Assoc Cancer Res 15(2):425–430. doi:10.1158/1078-0432.CCR-08-0149

American Cancer Society (2013) Cancer facts and figures 2013. American Cancer Society, Atlanta

Ansari KM, Rundhaug JE, Fischer SM (2008) Multiple signaling pathways are responsible for prostaglandin E2-induced murine keratinocyte proliferation. Mol Cancer Res 6(6):1003–1016. doi:10.1158/1541-7786.MCR-07-2144

Apte RN, Krelin Y, Song X, Dotan S, Recih E, Elkabets M, Carmi Y, Dvorkin T, White RM, Gayvoronsky L, Segal S, Voronov E (2006) Effects of micro-environment- and malignant cell-derived interleukin-1 in carcinogenesis, tumour invasiveness and tumour-host interactions. Eur J Cancer 42(6):751–759. doi:10.1016/j.ejca.2006.01.010

Arsenault D, Lucien F, Dubois CM (2012) Hypoxia enhances cancer cell invasion through relocalization of the proprotein convertase furin from the trans-Golgi network to the cell surface. J Cell Physiol 227(2):789–800. doi:10.1002/jcp.22792

Aziz SA, Hussain KS, Ahmad KN, Ahmed M, Kharadi MY, Bhat JR (1998) Profile of Kangari cancer: a prospective study. Burns: J Int Soc Burn Injuries 24(8):763–766

Balkwill F, Coussens LM (2004) Cancer: an inflammatory link. Nature 431(7007):405–406. doi:10.1038/431405a

Barthel SR, Gavino JD, Descheny L, Dimitroff CJ (2007) Targeting selectins and selectin ligands in inflammation and cancer. Expert Opin Ther Targets 11(11):1473–1491. doi:10.1517/14728222.11.11.1473

Bell S, Degitz K, Quirling M, Jilg N, Page S, Brand K (2003) Involvement of NF-kappaB signalling in skin physiology and disease. Cell Signal 15(1):1–7

Bhui K, Prasad S, George J, Shukla Y (2009) Bromelain inhibits COX-2 expression by blocking the activation of MAPK regulated NF-kappa B against skin tumor-initiation triggering mitochondrial death pathway. Cancer Lett 282(2):167–176. doi:10.1016/j.canlet.2009.03.003

Bode AM, Dong Z (2000) Signal transduction pathways: targets for chemoprevention of skin cancer. Lancet Oncol 1:181–188

Boffetta P, Gridley G, Lindelof B (2001) Cancer risk in a population-based cohort of patients hospitalized for psoriasis in Sweden. J Invest Dermatol 117(6):1531–1537. doi:10.1046/j.0022-202x.2001.01520.x

Brummelkamp TR, Nijman SM, Dirac AM, Bernards R (2003) Loss of the cylindromatosis tumour suppressor inhibits apoptosis by activating NF-kappaB. Nature 424(6950):797–801. doi:10.1038/nature01811

Buckman SY, Gresham A, Hale P, Hruza G, Anast J, Masferrer J, Pentland AP (1998) COX-2 expression is induced by UVB exposure in human skin: implications for the development of skin cancer. Carcinogenesis 19(5):723–729

Byun S, Park J, Lee E, Lim S, Yu JG, Lee SJ, Chen H, Dong Z, Lee KW, Lee HJ (2013) Src kinase is a direct target of apigenin against UVB-induced skin inflammation. Carcinogenesis 34(2):397–405. doi:10.1093/carcin/bgs358

Cataisson C, Salcedo R, Hakim S, Moffitt BA, Wright L, Yi M, Stephens R, Dai RM, Lyakh L, Schenten D, Yuspa HS, Trinchieri G (2012) IL-1R-MyD88 signaling in keratinocyte transformation and carcinogenesis. J Exp Med 209(9):1689–1702. doi:10.1084/jem.20101355

Chaudhary SC, Siddiqui MS, Athar M, Alam MS (2012) D-Limonene modulates inflammation, oxidative stress and Ras-ERK pathway to inhibit murine skin tumorigenesis. Hum Exp Toxicol 31(8):798–811. doi:10.1177/0960327111434948

Chaudhary SC, Singh T, Kapur P, Weng Z, Arumugam A, Elmets CA, Kopelovich L, Athar M (2013) Nitric oxide-releasing sulindac is a novel skin cancer chemopreventive agent for UVB-induced photocarcinogenesis. Toxicol Appl Pharmacol 268(3):249–255. doi:10.1016/j.taap.2012.12.009

Chilampalli C, Guillermo R, Zhang X, Kaushik RS, Young A, Zeman D, Hildreth MB, Fahmy H, Dwivedi C (2011) Effects of magnolol on UVB-induced skin cancer development in mice and its possible mechanism of action. BMC Cancer 11:456. doi:10.1186/1471-2407-11-456

Chun KS, Kundu JK, Park KK, Chung WY, Surh YJ (2006) Inhibition of phorbol ester-induced mouse skin tumor promotion and COX-2 expression by celecoxib: C/EBP as a potential molecular target. Cancer Res Treat: Official J Korean Cancer Assoc 38(3):152–158. doi:10.4143/crt.2006.38.1.152

Chung JH, Youn SH, Koh WS, Eun HC, Cho KH, Park KC, Youn JI (1996) Ultraviolet B irradiation-enhanced interleukin (IL)-6 production and mRNA expression are mediated by IL-1 alpha in cultured human keratinocytes. J Invest Dermatol 106(4):715–720

Colotta F, Allavena P, Sica A, Garlanda C, Mantovani A (2009) Cancer-related inflammation, the seventh hallmark of cancer: links to genetic instability. Carcinogenesis 30(7):1073–1081. doi:10.1093/carcin/bgp127

Costin GE, Hearing VJ (2007) Human skin pigmentation: melanocytes modulate skin color in response to stress. FASEB J: Official Publ Fed Am Soc Exp Biol 21(4):976–994. doi:10.1096/fj.06-6649rev

Coussens LM, Hanahan D, Arbeit JM (1996) Genetic predisposition and parameters of malignant progression in K14-HPV16 transgenic mice. Am J Pathol 149(6):1899–1917

Coussens LM, Tinkle CL, Hanahan D, Werb Z (2000) MMP-9 supplied by bone marrow-derived cells contributes to skin carcinogenesis. Cell 103(3):481–490

Crespo P, Leon J (2000) Ras proteins in the control of the cell cycle and cell differentiation. Cell Mol Life Sci: CMLS 57(11):1613–1636

Del Prete A, Allavena P, Santoro G, Fumarulo R, Corsi MM, Mantovani A (2011) Molecular pathways in cancer-related inflammation. Biochemia Med: Casopis Hrvatskoga Drus Medicinskih Biokemicara/HDMB 21(3):264–275

Dhawan P, Richmond A (2002) Role of CXCL1 in tumorigenesis of melanoma. J Leukoc Biol 72(1):9–18

Dong KK, Damaghi N, Picart SD, Markova NG, Obayashi K, Okano Y, Masaki H, Grether-Beck S, Krutmann J, Smiles KA, Yarosh DB (2008) UV-induced DNA damage initiates release of MMP-1 in human skin. Exp Dermatol 17(12):1037–1044. doi:10.1111/j.1600-0625.2008.00747.x

Elmets CA, Viner JL, Pentland AP, Cantrell W, Lin HY, Bailey H, Kang S, Linden KG, Heffernan M, Duvic M, Richmond E, Elewski BE, Umar A, Bell W, Gordon GB (2010) Chemoprevention of nonmelanoma skin cancer with celecoxib: a randomized, double-blind, placebo-controlled trial. J Natl Cancer Inst 102(24):1835–1844. doi:10.1093/jnci/djq442

Fan Y, Mao R, Yang J (2013) NF-κB and STAT3 signaling pathways collaboratively link inflammation to cancer. Protein Cell 4(3):176–185. doi:10.1007/s13238-013-2084-3

Farshchian M, Kivisaari A, Ala-Aho R, Riihila P, Kallajoki M, Grenman R, Peltonen J, Pihlajaniemi T, Heljasvaara R, Kahari VM (2011) Serpin peptidase inhibitor clade A member 1 (SerpinA1) is a novel biomarker for progression of cutaneous squamous cell carcinoma. Am J Pathol 179(3):1110–1119. doi:10.1016/j.ajpath.2011.05.012

Fischer SM, Lo HH, Gordon GB, Seibert K, Kelloff G, Lubet RA, Conti CJ (1999) Chemopreventive activity of celecoxib, a specific cyclooxygenase-2 inhibitor, and indomethacin against ultraviolet light-induced skin carcinogenesis. Mol Carcinog 25(4):231–240

Flockhart RJ, Diffey BL, Farr PM, Lloyd J, Reynolds NJ (2008) NFAT regulates induction of COX-2 and apoptosis of keratinocytes in response to ultraviolet radiation exposure. FASEB J: Official Publ Fed Am Soc Exp Biol 22(12):4218–4227. doi:10.1096/fj.08-113076

Fu J, Bassi DE, Zhang J, Li T, Nicolas E, Klein-Szanto AJ (2012) Transgenic overexpression of the proprotein convertase furin enhances skin tumor growth. Neoplasia 14(4):271–282

Furstenberger G, Gross M, Marks F (1989) Eicosanoids and multistage carcinogenesis in NMRI mouse skin: role of prostaglandins E and F in conversion (first stage of tumor promotion) and promotion (second stage of tumor promotion). Carcinogenesis 10(1):91–96

Groves RW, Allen MH, Ross EL, Ahsan G, Barker JN, MacDonald DM (1993) Expression of selectin ligands by cutaneous squamous cell carcinoma. Am J Pathol 143(4):1220–1225

Groves RW, Mizutani H, Kieffer JD, Kupper TS (1995) Inflammatory skin disease in transgenic mice that express high levels of interleukin 1 alpha in basal epidermis. Proc Natl Acad Sci USA 92(25):11874–11878

Gu M, Singh RP, Dhanalakshmi S, Agarwal C, Agarwal R (2007) Silibinin inhibits inflammatory and angiogenic attributes in photocarcinogenesis in SKH-1 hairless mice. Cancer Res 67(7):3483–3491. doi:10.1158/0008-5472.CAN-06-3955

Haghnegahdar H, Du J, Wang D, Strieter RM, Burdick MD, Nanney LB, Cardwell N, Luan J, Shattuck-Brandt R, Richmond A (2000) The tumorigenic and angiogenic effects of MGSA/GRO proteins in melanoma. J Leukoc Biol 67(1):53–62

Han W, Ming M, He YY (2011) Caffeine promotes ultraviolet B-induced apoptosis in human keratinocytes without complete DNA repair. J Biol Chem 286(26):22825–22832. doi:10.1074/jbc.M111.222349

Han YP, Tuan TL, Wu H, Hughes M, Garner WL (2001) TNF-alpha stimulates activation of pro-MMP2 in human skin through NF-(kappa) B mediated induction of MT1-MMP. J Cell Sci 114(Pt 1):131–139

Hanahan D, Weinberg RA (2011) Hallmarks of cancer: the next generation. Cell 144(5):646–674. doi:10.1016/j.cell.2011.02.013

Hocker TL, Singh MK, Tsao H (2008) Melanoma genetics and therapeutic approaches in the 21st century: moving from the benchside to the bedside. J Invest Dermatol 128(11):2575–2595. doi:10.1038/jid.2008.226

Hu J, Haseebuddin M, Young M, Colburn NH (2005) Suppression of p65 phosphorylation coincides with inhibition of IκBα polyubiquitination and degradation. Mol Carcinog 44(4): 274–284. doi:10.1002/mc.20142

Hua H, Li M, Luo T, Yin Y, Jiang Y (2011) Matrix metalloproteinases in tumorigenesis: an evolving paradigm. Cell Mol Life Sci: CMLS 68(23):3853–3868. doi:10.1007/s00018-011-0763-x

Huang C, Ma WY, Hanenberger D, Cleary MP, Bowden GT, Dong Z (1997) Inhibition of ultraviolet B-induced activator protein-1 (AP-1) activity by aspirin in AP-1-luciferase transgenic mice. J Biol Chem 272(42):26325–26331

IARC (1987) Overall evaluations of carcinogenicity. An updating IARC monographs, vols 1–42. IARC monographs evaluation carcinogenic risk chemicals humans, Suppl 7, Lyon

IARC (2007) Molecular mechanisms of HPV-induced carcinogenesis. Monograoh on human papilloma virus, vol 90. IARC monographs evaluation carcinogenic risk chemicals humans, Lyon, pp 432–465

Ibanez IL, Notcovich C, Policastro LL, Duran H (2011) Reactive oxygen species in the biology of melanoma. Breakthroughs in Melanoma Research. InTech

Jang M, Pezzuto JM (1999) Cancer chemopreventive activity of resveratrol. Drugs Exp Clin Res 25(2–3):65–77

Jee SH, Chu CY, Chiu HC, Huang YL, Tsai WL, Liao YH, Kuo ML (2004) Interleukin-6 induced basic fibroblast growth factor-dependent angiogenesis in basal cell carcinoma cell line via JAK/STAT3 and PI3-kinase/Akt pathways. J Invest Dermatol 123(6):1169–1175. doi:10.1111/j.0022-202X.2004.23497.x

Johnson KE, Wilgus TA (2012) Multiple roles for VEGF in non-melanoma skin cancer: angiogenesis and beyond. J Skin Cancer 2012:483. doi:10.1155/2012/483439

Kamp DW, Shacter E, Weitzman SA (2011) Chronic inflammation and cancer: the role of the mitochondria. Oncology (Williston Park) 25(5):400–410, 413

Kao ES, Wang CJ, Lin WL, Chu CY, Tseng TH (2007) Effects of polyphenols derived from fruit of Crataegus pinnatifida on cell transformation, dermal edema and skin tumor formation by phorbol ester application. Food Chem Toxicol: Int J Publ Br Ind Biol Res Assoc 45(10):1795–1804. doi:10.1016/j.fct.2007.03.016

Kapadia GJ, Azuine MA, Shigeta Y, Suzuki N, Tokuda H (2010) Chemopreventive activities of etodolac and oxyphenbutazone against mouse skin carcinogenesis. Bioorg Med Chem Lett 20(8):2546–2548. doi:10.1016/j.bmcl.2010.02.093

Katerinaki E, Evans GS, Lorigan PC, MacNeil S (2003) TNF-α increases human melanoma cell invasion and migration in vitro: the role of proteolytic enzymes. Br J Cancer 89(6):1123–1129. doi:10.1038/sj.bjc.6601257

Katiyar SK, Afaq F, Perez A, Mukhtar H (2001) Green tea polyphenol (−)-epigallocatechin-3-gallate treatment of human skin inhibits ultraviolet radiation-induced oxidative stress. Carcinogenesis 22(2):287–294

Katiyar SK, Mukhtar H (2001) Green tea polyphenol (−)-epigallocatechin-3-gallate treatment to mouse skin prevents UVB-induced infiltration of leukocytes, depletion of antigen-presenting cells, and oxidative stress. J Leukoc Biol 69(5):719–726

Kerkelä E, Ala-Aho R, Lohi J, Grénman R, Saarialho-Kere U (2001) Differential patterns of stromelysin-2 (MMP-10) and MT1-MMP (MMP-14) expression in epithelial skin cancers. Br J Cancer 84(5):659–669. doi:10.1054/bjoc.2000.1634

Khan AQ, Khan R, Qamar W, Lateef A, Rehman MU, Tahir M, Ali F, Hamiza OO, Hasan SK, Sultana S (2013) Geraniol attenuates 12-O-tetradecanoylphorbol-13-acetate (TPA)-induced oxidative stress and inflammation in mouse skin: Possible role of p38 MAP Kinase and NF-kappaB. Exp Mol Pathol 94(3):419–429. doi:10.1016/j.yexmp.2013.01.006

Kim DJ, Prabhu KS, Gonzalez FJ, Peters JM (2006) Inhibition of chemically induced skin carcinogenesis by sulindac is independent of peroxisome proliferator-activated receptor-beta/delta (PPARbeta/delta). Carcinogenesis 27(5):1105–1112. doi:10.1093/carcin/bgi346

Kundu JK, Hwang DM, Lee JC, Chang EJ, Shin YK, Fujii H, Sun B, Surh YJ (2009) Inhibitory effects of oligonol on phorbol ester-induced tumor promotion and COX-2 expression in mouse skin: NF-kappaB and C/EBP as potential targets. Cancer Lett 273(1):86–97. doi:10.1016/j.canlet.2008.07.039

Kundu JK, Shin YK, Surh YJ (2006) Resveratrol modulates phorbol ester-induced pro-inflammatory signal transduction pathways in mouse skin in vivo: NF-kappaB and AP-1 as prime targets. Biochem Pharmacol 72(11):1506–1515. doi:10.1016/j.bcp.2006.08.005

Kundu JK, Surh YJ (2008) Inflammation: gearing the journey to cancer. Mutat Res 659(1–2): 15–30. doi:10.1016/j.mrrev.2008.03.002

Kwon JY, Lee KW, Kim JE, Jung SK, Kang NJ, Hwang MK, Heo YS, Bode AM, Dong Z, Lee HJ (2009) Delphinidin suppresses ultraviolet B-induced cyclooxygenases-2 expression through inhibition of MAPKK4 and PI-3 kinase. Carcinogenesis 30(11):1932–1940. doi:10.1093/carcin/bgp216

Kyrgidis A, Vahtsevanos K, Tzellos TG, Xirou P, Kitikidou K, Antoniades K, Zouboulis CC, Triaridis S (2010) Clinical, histological and demographic predictors for recurrence and second primary tumours of head and neck basal cell carcinoma. A 1062 patient-cohort study from a tertiary cancer referral hospital. Eur J Dermatol: EJD 20(3):276–282. doi:10.1684/ejd.2010.0903

Laferriere J, Houle F, Huot J (2002) Regulation of the metastatic process by E-selectin and stress-activated protein kinase-2/p38. Ann NY Acad Sci 973:562–572

Langowski JL, Zhang X, Wu L, Mattson JD, Chen T, Smith K, Basham B, McClanahan T, Kastelein RA, Oft M (2006) IL-23 promotes tumour incidence and growth. Nature 442(7101):461–465. doi:10.1038/nature04808

Lederle W, Depner S, Schnur S, Obermueller E, Catone N, Just A, Fusenig NE, Mueller MM (2011) IL-6 promotes malignant growth of skin SCCs by regulating a network of autocrine and paracrine cytokines. Int J Cancer J Int du Cancer 128(12):2803–2814. doi:10.1002/ijc.25621

Lee WY, Lockniskar MF, Fischer SM (1994) Interleukin-1 alpha mediates phorbol ester-induced inflammation and epidermal hyperplasia. FASEB Journal: Official Publ Fed Am Soc Exp Biol 8(13):1081–1087

Li AG, Lu SL, Zhang MX, Deng C, Wang XJ (2004) Smad3 knockout mice exhibit a resistance to skin chemical carcinogenesis. Cancer Res 64(21):7836–7845. doi:10.1158/0008-5472.CAN-04-1331

Liang L, Hu D, Liu W, Williams JP, Okunieff P, Ding I (2003) Celecoxib reduces skin damage after radiation: selective reduction of chemokine and receptor mRNA expression in irradiated skin but not in irradiated mammary tumor. Am J Clin Oncol 26(4):S114–S121. doi:10.1097/01.COC.0000074149.95710.40

Loeb LA, Harris CC (2008) Advances in chemical carcinogenesis: a historical review and prospective. Cancer Res 68(17):6863–6872. doi:10.1158/0008-5472.CAN-08-2852

Lu H, Ouyang W, Huang C (2006) Inflammation, a key event in cancer development. Molecular Cancer Res: MCR 4(4):221–233. doi:10.1158/1541-7786.MCR-05-0261

Madan V, Lear JT, Szeimies RM (2010) Non-melanoma skin cancer. Lancet 375(9715):673–685. doi:10.1016/S0140-6736(09)61196-X

Magcwebeba T, Riedel S, Swanevelder S, Bouic P, Swart P, Gelderblom W (2012) Interleukin-1alpha induction in human keratinocytes (HaCaT): an in vitro model for chemoprevention in skin. J Skin Cancer 2012:393681. doi:10.1155/2012/393681

Mallikarjuna G, Dhanalakshmi S, Singh RP, Agarwal C, Agarwal R (2004) Silibinin protects against photocarcinogenesis via modulation of cell cycle regulators, mitogen-activated protein kinases, and Akt signaling. Cancer Res 64(17):6349–6356. doi:10.1158/0008-5472.CAN-04-1632

Mantovani A, Allavena P, Sica A, Balkwill F (2008) Cancer-related inflammation. Nature 454(7203):436–444. doi:10.1038/nature07205

Marsik C, Kazemi-Shirazi L, Schickbauer T, Winkler S, Joukhadar C, Wagner OF, Endler G (2008) C-reactive protein and all-cause mortality in a large hospital-based cohort. Clin Chem 54(2):343–349. doi:10.1373/clinchem.2007.091959

Martin AG, San-Antonio B, Fresno M (2001) Regulation of nuclear factor kappa B transactivation. Implication of phosphatidylinositol 3-kinase and protein kinase C zeta in c-Rel activation by tumor necrosis factor alpha. J Biol Chem 276(19):15840–15849. doi:10.1074/jbc.M011313200

Massoumi R, Chmielarska K, Hennecke K, Pfeifer A, Fassler R (2006) Cyld inhibits tumor cell proliferation by blocking Bcl-3-dependent NF-kappaB signaling. Cell 125(4):665–677. doi:10.1016/j.cell.2006.03.041

Meeran SM, Akhtar S, Katiyar SK (2009) Inhibition of UVB-induced skin tumor development by drinking green tea polyphenols is mediated through DNA repair and subsequent inhibition of inflammation. J Invest Dermatol 129(5):1258–1270. doi:10.1038/jid.2008.354

Meeran SM, Katiyar S, Elmets CA, Katiyar SK (2007) Interleukin-12 deficiency is permissive for angiogenesis in UV radiation-induced skin tumors. Cancer Res 67(8):3785–3793. doi:10.1158/0008-5472.CAN-06-3134

Mikirova N, Casciari J, Rogers A, Taylor P (2012) Effect of high-dose intravenous vitamin C on inflammation in cancer patients. J Transl Med 10:189. doi:10.1186/1479-5876-10-189

Millan O, Rico D, Peinado H, Zarich N, Stamatakis K, Perez-Sala D, Rojas JM, Cano A, Bosca L (2006) Potentiation of tumor formation by topical administration of 15-deoxy-delta12,14-prostaglandin J2 in a model of skin carcinogenesis. Carcinogenesis 27(2):328–336. doi:10.1093/carcin/bgi213

Mishra PK, Raghuram GV, Bhargava A, Ahirwar A, Samarth R, Upadhyaya R, Jain SK, Pathak N (2011) In vitro and in vivo evaluation of the anticarcinogenic and cancer chemopreventive potential of a flavonoid-rich fraction from a traditional Indian herb Selaginella bryopteris. Br J Nutr 106(8):1154–1168. doi:10.1017/S0007114511001498

Mueller MM (2006) Inflammation in epithelial skin tumours: old stories and new ideas. Eur J Cancer 42(6):735–744. doi:10.1016/j.ejca.2006.01.014

Muhleisen B, Petrov I, Gachter T, Kurrer M, Scharer L, Dummer R, French LE, Hofbauer GF (2009) Progression of cutaneous squamous cell carcinoma in immunosuppressed patients is associated with reduced CD123+ and FOXP3+ cells in the perineoplastic inflammatory infiltrate. Histopathology 55(1):67–76. doi:10.1111/j.1365-2559.2009.03324.x

Muller-Decker K, Neufang G, Berger I, Neumann M, Marks F, Furstenberger G (2002) Transgenic cyclooxygenase-2 overexpression sensitizes mouse skin for carcinogenesis. Proc Natl Acad Sci USA 99(19):12483–12488. doi:10.1073/pnas.192323799

Nickoloff BJ, Ben-Neriah Y, Pikarsky E (2005) Inflammation and cancer: is the link as simple as we think? J Invest Dermatol 124(6):x–xiv. doi:10.1111/j.0022-202X.2005.23724.x

Oberyszyn TM, Sabourin CL, Bijur GN, Oberyszyn AS, Boros LG, Robertson FM (1993) Interleukin-1 alpha gene expression and localization of interleukin-1 alpha protein during tumor promotion. Mol Carcinog 7(4):238–248

Osakabe N, Yasuda A, Natsume M, Yoshikawa T (2004) Rosmarinic acid inhibits epidermal inflammatory responses: anticarcinogenic effect of Perilla frutescens extract in the murine two-stage skin model. Carcinogenesis 25(4):549–557. doi:10.1093/carcin/bgh034

Paavonen K, Ekman N, Wirzenius M, Rajantie I, Poutanen M, Alitalo K (2004) Bmx tyrosine kinase transgene induces skin hyperplasia, inflammatory angiogenesis, and accelerated wound healing. Mol Biol Cell 15(9):4226–4233. doi:10.1091/mbc.E04-03-0241

Pahl HL (1999) Activators and target genes of Rel/NF-kappaB transcription factors. Oncogene 18(49):6853–6866. doi:10.1038/sj.onc.1203239

Parkin DM (2006) The global health burden of infection-associated cancers in the year 2002. Int J Cancer J Int du Cancer 118(12):3030–3044. doi:10.1002/ijc.21731

Passos GF, Medeiros R, Marcon R, Nascimento AF, Calixto JB, Pianowski LF (2013) The role of PKC/ERK1/2 signaling in the anti-inflammatory effect of tetracyclic triterpene euphol on TPA-induced skin inflammation in mice. Eur J Pharmacol 698(1–3):413–420. doi:10.1016/j.ejphar.2012.10.019

Patel R, Garg R, Erande S, BM G (2007) Chemopreventive herbal anti-oxidants: current status and future perspectives. J Clin Biochem Nutr 40(2):82–91. doi:10.3164/jcbn.40.82

Patel R, Krishnan R, Ramchandani A, Maru G (2008) Polymeric black tea polyphenols inhibit mouse skin chemical carcinogenesis by decreasing cell proliferation. Cell Prolif 41(3): 532–553. doi:10.1111/j.1365-2184.2008.00528.x

Patil AS, Puri YS, Gedham MC, Naik AV, Joshi RK (2005) Saree cancer. Bombay Hosp J 47(3):302–303

Perez-Lorenzo R, Markell LM, Hogan KA, Yuspa SH, Glick AB (2010) Transforming growth factor beta1 enhances tumor promotion in mouse skin carcinogenesis. Carcinogenesis 31(6):1116–1123. doi:10.1093/carcin/bgq041

Perez-Moreno M, Song W, Pasolli HA, Williams SE, Fuchs E (2008) Loss of p120 catenin and links to mitotic alterations, inflammation, and skin cancer. Proc Natl Acad Sci USA 105(40):15399–15404. doi:10.1073/pnas.0807301105

Petit-Frere C, Clingen PH, Grewe M, Krutmann J, Roza L, Arlett CF, Green MH (1998) Induction of interleukin-6 production by ultraviolet radiation in normal human epidermal keratinocytes and in a human keratinocyte cell line is mediated by DNA damage. J Invest Dermatol 111(3):354–359. doi:10.1038/sj.jid.5602962

Prasad S, Ravindran J, Aggarwal BB (2010) NF-κB and cancer: how intimate is this relationship. Mol Cell Biochem 336(1–2):25–37. doi:10.1007/s11010-009-0267-2

Proksch E, Brandner JM, Jensen JM (2008) The skin: an indispensable barrier. Exp Dermatol 17(12):1063–1072

Pytliak M, Vargova V, Mechirova V (2012) Matrix metalloproteinases and their role in oncogenesis: a review. Onkologie 35(1–2):49–53. doi:10.1159/000336304

Ramos MC, Steinbrenner H, Stuhlmann D, Sies H, Brenneisen P (2004) Induction of MMP-10 and MMP-1 in a squamous cell carcinoma cell line by ultraviolet radiation. Biol Chem 385(1):75–86. doi:10.1515/BC.2004.010

Ravi R, Piva TJ (2013) The role of furin in the development of skin cancer. In: Vereecken DP (ed.) Highlights in skin cancer. InTech, UK. doi:10.5772/55569

Reuter S, Gupta SC, Chaturvedi MM, Aggarwal BB (2010) Oxidative stress, inflammation, and cancer: how are they linked? Free Radical Biol Med 49(11):1603–1616. doi:10.1016/j.freeradbiomed.2010.09.006

Rogers HW, Weinstock MA, Harris AR, Hinckley MR, Feldman SR, Fleischer AB, Coldiron BM (2010) Incidence estimate of nonmelanoma skin cancer in the United States, 2006. Arch Dermatol 146(3):283–287. doi:10.1001/archdermatol.2010.19

Rundhaug JE, Fischer SM (2010) Molecular mechanisms of mouse skin tumor promotion. Cancers 2(2):436–482. doi:10.3390/cancers2020436

Saladi RN, Persaud AN (2005) The causes of skin cancer: a comprehensive review. Drugs Today (Barc) 41(1):37–53. doi:10.1358/dot.2005.41.1.875777

Schadendorf D, Heidel J, Gawlik C, Suter L, Czarnetzki BM (1995) Association with clinical outcome of expression of VLA-4 in primary cutaneous malignant melanoma as well as P-selectin and E-selectin on intratumoral vessels. J Natl Cancer Inst 87(5):366–371

Schwarz T, Luger TA (1989) Effect of UV irradiation on epidermal cell cytokine production. J Photochem Photobiol B 4(1):1–13

Scott KA, Arnott CH, Robinson SC, Moore RJ, Thompson RG, Marshall JF, Balkwill FR (2004) TNF-α regulates epithelial expression of MMP-9 and integrin αvβ6 during tumour promotion. A role for TNF-α in keratinocyte migration? Oncogene 23(41):6954–6966. doi:10.1038/sj.onc.1207915

Shanmugam MK, Nguyen AH, Kumar AP, Tan BK, Sethi G (2012) Targeted inhibition of tumor proliferation, survival, and metastasis by pentacyclic triterpenoids: potential role in prevention and therapy of cancer. Cancer Lett 320(2):158–170. doi:10.1016/j.canlet.2012.02.037

Shirley SH, Grimm EA, Kusewitt DF (2012) Ultraviolet radiation and the slug transcription factor induce proinflammatory and immunomodulatory mediator expression in melanocytes. J Skin Cancer 2012:410925. doi:10.1155/2012/410925

Shrotriya S, Kundu JK, Na HK, Surh YJ (2010) Diallyl trisulfide inhibits phorbol ester-induced tumor promotion, activation of AP-1, and expression of COX-2 in mouse skin by blocking JNK and Akt signaling. Cancer Res 70(5):1932–1940. doi:10.1158/0008-5472.CAN-09-3501

Siegfried G, Basak A, Cromlish JA, Benjannet S, Marcinkiewicz J, Chretien M, Seidah NG, Khatib AM (2003) The secretory proprotein convertases furin, PC5, and PC7 activate VEGF-C to induce tumorigenesis. J Clin Investig 111(11):1723–1732. doi:10.1172/JCI17220

Singh T, Katiyar SK (2011) Green tea catechins reduce invasive potential of human melanoma cells by targeting COX-2, PGE2 receptors and epithelial-to-mesenchymal transition. PLoS One 6(10):e25224. doi:10.1371/journal.pone.0025224

Slaga TJ, Viaje A, Bracken W (1977) The effects of anti-inflammatory agents on skin tumor initiation and aryl hydrocarbon hydroxylase. Res Commun Chem Pathol Pharmacol 16(2):337–350

Soehnge H, Ouhtit A, Ananthaswamy ON (1997) Mechanisms of induction of skin cancer by UV radiation. Frontiers Biosci: J Virtual Libr 2:d538–d551

St Sauver JL, Sarma AV, Jacobson DJ, McGree ME, Lieber MM, Girman CJ, Nehra A, Jacobsen SJ (2009) Associations between C-reactive protein and benign prostatic hyperplasia/lower urinary tract symptom outcomes in a population-based cohort. Am J Epidemiol 169(11):1281–1290. doi:10.1093/aje/kwp085

Surh YJ, Chun KS, Cha HH, Han SS, Keum YS, Park KK, Lee SS (2001) Molecular mechanisms underlying chemopreventive activities of anti-inflammatory phytochemicals: down-regulation of COX-2 and iNOS through suppression of NF-κB activation. Mutat Res 480–481:243–268

Tiano HF, Loftin CD, Akunda J, Lee CA, Spalding J, Sessoms A, Dunson DB, Rogan EG, Morham SG, Smart RC, Langenbach R (2002) Deficiency of either cyclooxygenase (COX)-1 or COX-2 alters epidermal differentiation and reduces mouse skin tumorigenesis. Cancer Res 62(12):3395–3401

Tober KL, Wilgus TA, Kusewitt DF, Thomas-Ahner JM, Maruyama T, Oberyszyn TM (2006) Importance of the EP(1) receptor in cutaneous UVB-induced inflammation and tumor development. J Invest Dermatol 126(1):205–211. doi:10.1038/sj.jid.5700014

Trompouki E, Hatzivassiliou E, Tsichritzis T, Farmer H, Ashworth A, Mosialos G (2003) CYLD is a deubiquitinating enzyme that negatively regulates NF-kappaB activation by TNFR family members. Nature 424(6950):793–796. doi:10.1038/nature01803

Ulrich C, Johannsen A, Rowert-Huber J, Ulrich M, Sterry W, Stockfleth E (2010) Results of a randomized, placebo-controlled safety and efficacy study of topical diclofenac 3 % gel in organ transplant patients with multiple actinic keratoses. Eur J Dermatol 20(4):482–488. doi:10.1684/ejd.2010.1010

Urban JL, Shepard HM, Rothstein JL, Sugarman BJ, Schreiber H (1986) Tumor necrosis factor: a potent effector molecule for tumor cell killing by activated macrophages. Proc Natl Acad Sci USA 83(14):5233–5237

Vaid M, Sharma SD, Katiyar SK (2010) Honokiol, a phytochemical from the Magnolia plant, inhibits photocarcinogenesis by targeting UVB-induced inflammatory mediators and cell cycle regulators: development of topical formulation. Carcinogenesis 31(11):2004–2011. doi:10.1093/carcin/bgq186

Vanderveen EE, Grekin RC, Swanson NA, Kragballe K (1986) Arachidonic acid metabolites in cutaneous carcinomas. Evidence suggesting that elevated levels of prostaglandins in basal cell carcinomas are associated with an aggressive growth pattern. Arch Dermatol 122(4):407–412

Vougioukalaki M, Kanellis DC, Gkouskou K, Eliopoulos AG (2011) Tpl2 kinase signal transduction in inflammation and cancer. Cancer Lett 304(2):80–89. doi:10.1016/j.canlet.2011.02.004

Wennogle LP, Liang H, Quintavalla JC, Bowen BR, Wasvary J, Miller DB, Allentoff A, Boyer W, Kelly M, Marshall P (1995) Comparison of recombinant cyclooxygenase-2 to native isoforms: aspirin labeling of the active site. FEBS Lett 371(3):315–320

Wilgus TA, Koki AT, Zweifel BS, Kusewitt DF, Rubal PA, Oberyszyn TM (2003) Inhibition of cutaneous ultraviolet light B-mediated inflammation and tumor formation with topical celecoxib treatment. Mol Carcinog 38(2):49–58. doi:10.1002/mc.10141

Witz IP (2006) Tumor-microenvironment interactions: the selectin-selectin ligand axis in tumor-endothelium cross talk. Cancer Treat Res 130:125–140

Wright TI, Spencer JM, Flowers FP (2006) Chemoprevention of nonmelanoma skin cancer. J Am Acad Dermatol 54(6):933–946; quiz 947–950. doi:10.1016/j.jaad.2005.08.062

Yasukawa K, Akihisa T, Yoshida ZY, Takido M (2000) Inhibitory effect of euphol, a triterpene alcohol from the roots of Euphorbia kansui, on tumour promotion by 12-O-tetradecanoylphorbol-13-acetate in two-stage carcinogenesis in mouse skin. J Pharm Pharmacol 52(1):119–124

Yu H, Kortylewski M, Pardoll D (2007) Crosstalk between cancer and immune cells: role of STAT3 in the tumour microenvironment. Nat Rev Immunol 7(1):41–51. doi:10.1038/nri1995

Zhu JW, Wu XJ, Lu ZF, Luo D, Cai SQ, Zheng M (2013) Role of VEGF receptors in normal and psoriatic human keratinocytes: evidence from irradiation with different UV sources. PLoS One 8(1):e55463. doi:10.1371/journal.pone.0055463

Zhu Z, Zhong S, Shen Z (2011) Targeting the inflammatory pathways to enhance chemotherapy of cancer. Cancer Biol Ther 12(2):95–105

Erratum to:
The Role of Inflammation in Leukaemia

**Janusz Krawczyk, Michael O'Dwyer, Ronan Swords,
Ciara Freeman and Francis J Giles**

Erratum to:
Chapter 13 in: B. B. Aggarwal et al. (eds.), *Inflammation and Cancer*, DOI 10.1007/978-3-0348-0837-8_13

Please note that the sequence of authors' names was incorrect in the original version. The correct sequence should read as:

Janusz Krawczyk, Michael O'Dwyer, Ronan Swords, Ciara Freeman, and Francis J Giles

---

The online version of the original chapter can be found under DOI 10.1007/978-3-0348-0837-8_13

J. Krawczyk
Department of Haematology, Galway University Hospital, Galway, Ireland

M. O'Dwyer
Biosciences, National University of Ireland Galway, Upper Newcastle, Galway, Ireland

R. Swords
Sylvester Comprehensive Cancer Center, University of Miami, Miami, USA

C. Freeman
Department of Haematology, Barts and the Royal London NHS Trust, London, UK

F. J. Giles (✉)
Northwestern Medicine Developmental Therapeutics Institute, Robert H. Lurie Comprehensive Cancer Center of Northwestern University, Chicago, USA
e-mail: frankgiles@aol.com

Editors

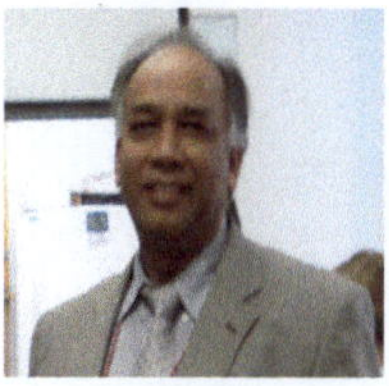

Bharat B. Aggarwal, Ph.D.
Department of Experimental Therapeutics
Division of Cancer Medicine
The University of Texas, MD Anderson Cancer Center
1515 Holcombe Boulevard, 1401 East Road, Unit 1950
Houston, TX 77054
USA
E-Mail: aggarwal@mdanderson.org

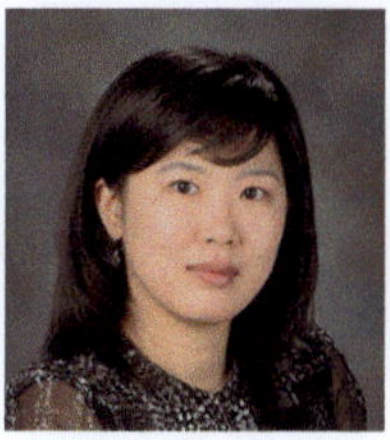

Bokyung Sung, Ph.D.
Department of Experimental Therapeutics
Division of Cancer Medicine
The University of Texas, MD Anderson Cancer Center
1515 Holcombe Boulevard, 1401 East Road, Unit 1950
Houston, TX 77054
USA
E-Mail: auvers1516@gmail.com

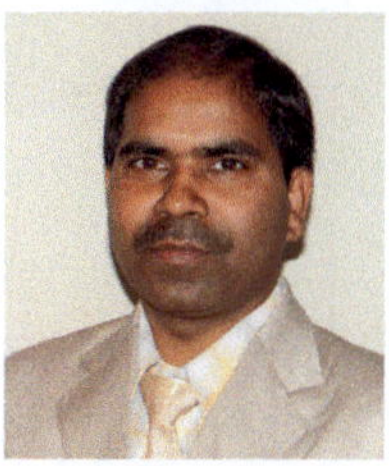

Subash Chandra Gupta, Ph.D.
Department of Experimental Therapeutics
The University of Texas, MD Anderson Cancer Center
1901 East Road, 4SCR3.1320.03, Unit 1950
Houston, Texas, 77054-3005
USA
E-Mail: subhashg167@gmail.com

B. B. Aggarwal et al. (eds.), *Inflammation and Cancer*, Advances in Experimental Medicine and Biology 816, DOI: 10.1007/978-3-0348-0837-8, © Springer Basel 2014

Index

Page numbers followed by "*f*" and "*t*" indicate figures and tables respectively

B. B. Aggarwal et al. (eds.), *Inflammation and Cancer*, Advances in Experimental Medicine and Biology 816, DOI: 10.1007/978-3-0348-0837-8, © Springer Basel 2014

I

Microvessel density (MVD), 327
Mitogen-activated protein extracellular kinase (MEK), 278, 281, 282, 283, 403
  MEK inhibitors, 279, 282, 283
ML-IAP, 411
MnSOD, 291
Monocytes chemoattractant protein (MCP), 37
  MCP-1, 7, 29, 363
  MCP-3, 365
  MCP-4, 365
Morin, 416*t*, 420
Mouse double minute 2 homolog (MDM2), 79
Mouse double minute 4 protein (MDM4), 79
Mouse mammary tumor virus (MMTV), 61, 62
Mucin-depleted foci (MDFs), 39
Mucosa-associated lymphoid tissue (MALT) lymphomas, 240, 317
Multiple myeloma (MM), 367
  cytokines, 370
  immunomodulatory drugs (IMiDs), 369–370
  monoclonal gammopathy of undetermined significance (MGUS), 367
  neovascularization
    macrophages in, 367–368
    mast cells in, 368–369
  non-active MM, 367
  pentraxin 3 (PTX3), 370
Mutator phenotype, 275
Myelodysplastic syndrome (MDS), 339
  NF-κB activation, 342
Myeloid differentiation primary response gene (88) (MyD88), 346, 405, 447
Myeloid-derived suppressor cells (MDSCs), 116, 118, 119, 120, 142, 156, 166, 214, 215–216
  suppressive MDSCs, 220–221
Myeloperoxidase (MPO), 86, 87, 459, 460

N

MIX
Papier aus verantwortungsvollen Quellen
Paper from responsible sources
FSC® C105338

If you have any concerns about our products,
you can contact us on
ProductSafety@springernature.com

In case Publisher is established outside the EU,
the EU authorized representative is:
Springer Nature Customer Service Center GmbH
Europaplatz 3, 69115 Heidelberg, Germany

Printed by Libri Plureos GmbH
in Hamburg, Germany